Learning Veterinary Terminology

Learning Veterinary Terminology

DOUGLAS F. MCBRIDE, DVM
Former Director
Veterinary Technology Program
LaGuardia Community College
Long Island City, New York

SECOND EDITION

with 121 *illustrations*

Mosby
An Affiliate of Elsevier

Mosby
An Affiliate of Elsevier

Publisher: John A. Schrefer
Editorial Manager: Linda L. Duncan
Developmental Editor: Teri Merchant
Project Manager: Linda McKinley
Senior Production Editor: Julie Eddy
Design: Julia Ramirez
Cover Design: Julia Ramirez

SECOND EDITION

Mosby, Inc.
An Affiliate of Elsevier
11830 Westline Industrial Drive
St. Louis, Missouri 63146

Printed in the United States of America

ISBN-13: 978-0-323-01329-1
ISBN-10: 0-323-01329-5

Library of Congress Cataloging in Publication Data

McBride, Douglas F.
Learning veterinary terminology / Douglas F. McBride.—2nd ed.
p. cm.
Includes bibliographical references (p.).
ISBN-13: 978-0-323-01329-1 ISBN-10: 0-323-01329-5
1. Veterinary medicine—Terminology. I. Title.

SF610 .M38 2001
636.089'01'4—dc21 2001034562

05 GW/QWF 9 8 7 6

Contributors

ALLEN R. BALAY, DVM

Director of Veterinary Technology
Ridgewater College
Willmar, Minnesota

DIANE CAMILLERI, VMD

Former Director
Veterinary Technology Program
LaGuardia Community College
Long Island City, New York

GARY P. CAMPBELL, PhD

Professor
Veterinary Science Technology
Suffolk Community College
Brentwood, New York

THOMAS M. DONNELLY, DVM

The Kenneth S. Warren Institute
712 Kitchawan Rd.
Ossining, New York

BETH HARRIES, MEd, LVT

Educational Designer
William Beaumont Hospital
Royal Oak, Michigan

KAREN L. HRAPKIEWICZ, DVM, Dipl ACLAM

Director
Veterinary Technology Program
Wayne County Community College
Wayne State University
Detroit, Michigan

BERNADINE KLICKNER LEAHY, LVT, LATG

Senior Veterinary Technician
Central Park Wildlife Center
Wildlife Conservation Society
New York, New York

DOUGLAS F. MCBRIDE, DVM

Former Director
Veterinary Technology Program
LaGuardia Community College
Long Island City, New York

KATHLEEN RIDER, BA, AAS

Licensed Veterinary Technician
Veterinary Technology Program
LaGuardia Community College
Long Island City, New York

Dedication

To the memory of Dennis E. J. Baker, friend, teacher,
raconteur and connoisseur of language

Preface

Several goals have guided this second edition of *Learning Veterinary Terminology.* Of course, we planned to include new developments and items we had overlooked before. We wanted to respond to changes in veterinary practice and areas of increasing interest. There was also the harder task of cutting out seldom-used words and obscure meanings. We have tried to do all these things. But the primary goal has been to make the book more valuable for teachers and helpful to students.

We have added a new chapter on exotic animals. They are increasingly important not just because of their popularity as pets but because of environmental concerns. The format of this chapter differs somewhat from that of the other species because exotic animals as a group present such a wide variety and include so many unique features. With the help of two new contributors we have provided material that will give students a sound basis in the terminology of this subject.

Other changes have been made to improve the book's usefulness. A set of study tips has been added. We have dropped word roots that have only one or two usages. New illustrations have been added and others have been improved. The reviews and exercises have been extensively rewritten to make them more interesting and challenging while minimizing the use of arcane words. In the Section I exercises, whole words are used instead of isolated prefixes, suffixes, and roots. In Section IV the order in which species are introduced has been changed to reflect the fact that students are more likely to have had personal experience with dogs and cats than any other species. Finally, the index has been greatly expanded to enable finding all occurrences of any word or word part in the text.

With these improvements we have retained the same general organization and features. The book is divided into four sections. Section I presents the basic foundation of veterinary language, beginning with extensive lists of prefixes, suffixes, roots, and combining forms. It then introduces the systems approach using internal and external anatomic terms. The section concludes with additional word roots along with lists of body fluids, substances, chemicals, and colors. Review questions are provided at frequent intervals to enable students to test their knowledge while studying the text. At the end of each chapter, exercises cover the chapter's content and provide a good resource for subsequent study. Crossword puzzles afford an additional opportunity for the student to use newly learned words.

Section II introduces the student to the language of body structure and the skeletal, muscular, and integumentary systems. The remaining body systems are covered in the seven chapters of Section III. The use of exercises, review questions, and crossword puzzles is continued, giving students immediate feedback on their progress. We emphasize the similarities shared by species but describe major comparative aspects where necessary. Each chapter concludes with a glossary of the terms introduced in the text and additional words germane to the subject. The multiple small glossaries are meant to be read through and not used just as references. An extensive index at the end of the book obviates a single glossary.

Section IV gives the student an overview of the terminology used with specific animals. Just as medical terminology must be related to the systems of the body, animal terminology makes sense most readily in the many different contexts in which people use the various species. The section is arranged by species or species group. The terminology of each group is explained as an outgrowth of management practices. We have attempted to distill the most important aspects so that the student can see how terminology has been determined by the different ways in which humans interact with various animals. Exercises, puzzles, and glossaries are provided, as in earlier sections.

The appendices contain information that relates to terminology, including abbreviations, Latin and Greek combining forms for numbers, and the metric system with common equivalents. There is a list of terms relating to disease, a chart of species names, and a list of specialty boards in veterinary medicine.

The book is suitable for introductory courses in veterinary technology, veterinary science, and related fields. Students in preveterinary courses may also find the book useful. The large number of exercises and reviews should make the book worthwhile for self-study by nontraditional students or others outside the conventional educational system. The book should also be a valuable reference for practicing technicians and office personnel.

Learning Veterinary Terminology would not have been possible without the continuing guidance and encouragement of Linda Duncan of Mosby. I am grateful also to Miriam G. Austrin and Harvey R. Austrin for permission to use *Learning Medical Terminology* as the basis for the first edition. Pauline Thomas deserves special praise for providing several new drawings. Once again, she has worked tirelessly to achieve artistic simplification without loss of accuracy. Ultimate credit is due to students, past and future, whose needs provided the impetus for the book's creation.

Douglas F. McBride

Contents

SECTION IV
TERMINOLOGY OF THE ANIMAL INDUSTRY

APPENDIX

I

THE BASIC FOUNDATION OF VETERINARY TERMINOLOGY

Section I of LEARNING VETERINARY TERMINOLOGY consists of four chapters that introduce the student to the basic foundation of veterinary language.

Chapter 1 is a brief introduction to the separate parts of words, with examples to help the student understand the construction of veterinary terms.

Chapter 2 presents the initial step in building and learning the vocabulary. The most essential components of the language, prefixes and suffixes, are conveniently arranged in chart form with meanings and examples.

Chapter 3, which introduces the second step in building the vocabulary, adds the roots and combining forms that relate to the structures of the body. The chapter is divided into two sections, external and internal body parts, arranged in chart form with pronunciations and identification of the parts.

Chapter 4, illustrating the third step in vocabulary development, presents descriptive words and roots. They are divided into separate charts, defining actions, conditions, characteristics, substances, and colors.

1 An Introduction to Veterinary Terminology

CHAPTER OVERVIEW

This chapter introduces word elements (prefixes, suffixes, roots, and combining forms), their meanings, and ways of combining them to build veterinary terms. Basic pronunciation rules are presented, with pertinent examples.

OBJECTIVE

The primary objective of this book is to enable you, the student, to learn veterinary terminology. When you are first confronted with veterinary terms, you may be bewildered by their strange spelling and pronunciation. This is understandable when you consider that approximately 75% of these terms are based on either Greek or Latin. New terms are constantly being coined, but most are derivatives of Greek or Latin words. The Greeks were the founders of modern medicine, although Latin has become the universal source of medical language. Veterinary terminology is a subset of medical terminology.

When you complete this worktext, you will have a basic, workable vocabulary, applicable to any branch of veterinary medicine. You do not need prior knowledge of Greek, Latin, anatomy, or physiology to build a veterinary vocabulary, but you will need to know some fundamentals. These fundamentals are presented in this worktext and will help you to learn and be comfortable with veterinary language.

This is accomplished by:

1. breaking down a word and identifying its parts (prefix, suffix, root, and combining form).
2. the presentation of simplified anatomy and physiology of each of the body systems, with some reference to species differences.
3. relating the words and their parts to each of the body systems.
4. providing basic terminology used in various segments of the animal industry.
5. using illustrations, diagrams, and charts to assist in the learning process.
6. including review questions (and answers) throughout, and exercises at the end of each chapter.

Most veterinary terms are a combination of two or more word parts or elements. The identification of a word involves a search for the meaning of each of its parts. When they are translated separately and combined into a word, the parts give the essential meaning of the entire word.

The fundamental method of building a veterinary vocabulary, as it is outlined in this book, consists of breaking down a word and identifying its elements: prefix, suffix, root or roots, and combining form. A prefix is the beginning part of a word, and a suffix is the end part. A root is the foundation or basic meaning of a word and may appear with a prefix or a suffix or between a prefix and a suffix. Prefixes and suffixes can never stand alone; they must always be attached to a root. A combining form is a root with an added vowel, known as a combining vowel, which combines the root with a suffix or with another root.

For example:

antisepsis—The prefix *anti-* means against; the root *-sepsis* means infection; antisepsis means against infection.

rhinitis—The root *rhin-* means nose; the suffix *-itis* means inflammation; rhinitis means inflammation of the nose.

arteriosclerosis—The root *arteri-* means artery; with the combining vowel "o" arteri- becomes the combining form *arterio-*; the root *scler-* means hardening; the suffix *-osis* means state or condition; arteriosclerosis means hardening of the arteries.

Some words contain more than one root, each of which retains its basic meaning. Such words, called *compounds,* are very common in medicine. *Arteriosclerosis,* previously shown as an example of a combining form, is a compound word. Another example of a compound word is *osteoarthritis.* The combining form *osteo-* comes from the root *oste,* meaning bone; the root *arthr-* means joint or joints; and the suffix *-itis* means inflammation. Therefore the compound word *osteoarthritis* means inflammation of the bone joints.

Specific Suggestions for Learning Veterinary Terminology

The identification of prefixes, suffixes, and anatomic roots of words is the first step in building a veterinary vocabulary. The next step is to learn to recognize the most common roots referring to conditions, actions, characteristics, fluids, substances, and colors. This will help you to understand the anatomic structures, diseases, procedures, and other descriptive terms by simply breaking each word into its components, defining the components separately, and then combining them to discover the meaning of the word as a whole. If you practice analyzing veterinary words that you see or hear, you will find, in time, that you are able to define words at a glance, much the same as you would learn a foreign language.

It is possible to memorize some veterinary words without regard to a breakdown of the components, but you cannot memorize the entire veterinary dictionary. Although most veterinary terms can be learned easily from their components, there is no way to use components to analyze those terms that are derived from proper names. Use your veterinary dictionary when you do not recognize a term that bears a proper name, when you cannot arrive at a definition by analysis, or when the meaning is not clear. This book does not pretend to break down all veterinary terms into components, but it does give you the key to analysis by listing over 400 specific roots and combining forms you will find in the majority of veterinary words. Treat each veterinary word as if it were a puzzle you were attempting to solve, and you will see how enjoyable and rewarding it will be to define the word without reference to a veterinary dictionary.

Pronunciation of Veterinary Terms

Some veterinary terms are hard to pronounce, especially if you have never heard them spoken. Here are some shortcuts you will find helpful:

ch is sometimes pronounced like *k.*
Examples—chromatin, chronic.

ps is pronounced like *s.*
Examples—psychiatry, psychology.

pn is pronounced with only the *n* sound.
Examples—pneumonia, pneusis.

c and *g* are given the soft sound of *s* and *j*, respectively, before *e*, *i*, and *y* words.
Examples—generic, giant, cycle, cytoplasm.

c and *g* have a hard sound before other letters.
Examples—cast, cardiac, gastric, gonad.

ae and *oe* are pronounced *ee*.
Examples—fasciae, coelom.

i at the end of a word is pronounced *eye* (to form a plural).
Examples—alveoli, glomeruli, fasciculi.

es when forming the final letters of a word, is often pronounced as a separate syllable.
Examples—stases (stay' seez), nares (nah' reez).

The phonetic spelling of words is given throughout the text, where necessary, for purposes of pronunciation only.

Plurals

The plural of most English words is formed by adding *s* or *es*, but in veterinary terms the plural may be formed by changing the ending:

ae, in fasciae (singular form, *fascia*).

ia, as in crania (singular form, *cranium*).

i, as in glomeruli (singular form, *glomerulus*). When the singular form ends in *us*, the plural form is made by dropping the *us* and adding *i*.

ata, as in adenomata (singular form, *adenoma*).

Spelling

Rules for pronunciation and the formation of plurals are essential for spelling, but it is very important that you consult a veterinary dictionary if you are not sure. Phonetic spelling has no place in veterinary medicine.

Some terms sound alike but are spelled differently. For example, *ileum* is a part of the intestinal tract, but *ilium* is a pelvic bone. A misspelled word may lead to the wrong meaning, creating confusion and possibly an incorrect diagnosis.

STUDY TIPS

The beginning student may feel overwhelmed by the mass of words to be learned. Veterinary terminology is indeed complicated, as it must be if it is to describe the increasingly complex world of veterinary medicine. You need to develop strategies for learning that work for you. Here are some pointers that have helped others. Try them; they may work for you too.

1. Organize the material so it makes sense to you. Divide large masses of detail into smaller segments that you can handle. Don't tackle too much in one gulp. Be sure you understand how each part of each chapter fits into the overall organization. This book represents only one way of organizing veterinary terminology.
2. Make connections with what you already know. Words like *anemia, bronchitis, antibiotic, prenatal, heterosexual* and *orthopedic* are in everyday usage. Take them apart and see the word forms that you already know.
3. Do the review questions as soon as you've read a section. Write your answers on a separate piece of paper before you check the answers in the book. That way you can test yourself again when you re-read the chapter. Do the same with the exercises at the end of each chapter.
4. Write the words down on paper. Just the act of writing the words helps you to learn them. Make lists of the words you find difficult. Make lists of syn-

onyms, like the prefixes *anti-* and *contra-*. Do the same with antonyms, like *pre-* and *post-*, and homonyms like *dis-* and *dys-*. Write down similar forms like *inter-*, *intra-*, and *intro-* so they don't trip you up.

5. Speak the words out loud. It's easier to remember something you've spoken. Don't worry too much about pronunciation—it will come with practice. It's better to say it wrong than not at all.
6. Study in groups of two or more. Test each other verbally and in writing. After all, the main purpose of learning terminology is to communicate with others. You can't do that when you're alone.
7. Work the puzzles.

Chapter 1 EXERCISES

AN INTRODUCTION TO VETERINARY TERMINOLOGY

Exercise 1: Name the part of the word that is underlined.

1. arteritis suffix
2. epicarditis root
3. nephrosis suffix
4. antibiotic prefix
5. polyarthritis root
6. dermatitis root
7. macrocytosis root
8. asepsis prefix
9. hyperkeratosis root

Exercise 2: Match the definition in the right column with the word part in the left column by placing its letter in the blank provided.

Study

h	1. -osis	A. inflammation -itis
f	2. anti-	B. nose rhin-
a	3. -itis	C. hardening scler-
g	4. -sepsis	D. joint arthr-
b	5. rhin-	E. bone oste-
i	6. arteri-	F. against anti-
E	7. oste-	G. infection -sepsis
C	8. scler-	H. state or condition -osis
d	9. arthr-	I. artery arteri-

Exercise 3: Identify the principal parts of each word. The first one is done for you.

1. dermat/o/myc/osis root/combining vowel/root/suffix
2. scler/o/derma root/cv/root
3. arthr/osis root/suf artery condition
4. oste/o/arthr/osis root/cv/root/suf bone condition
5. oste/o/chondr/itis root/cv/root/suf bone Condition
6. anti/dote pre/root
7. enter/itis root/suf
8. gloss/itis root/suf
9. bio/logy root suf
10. arteri/o/ven/ous root/cv/root/suf

CHAPTER 1 PUZZLE

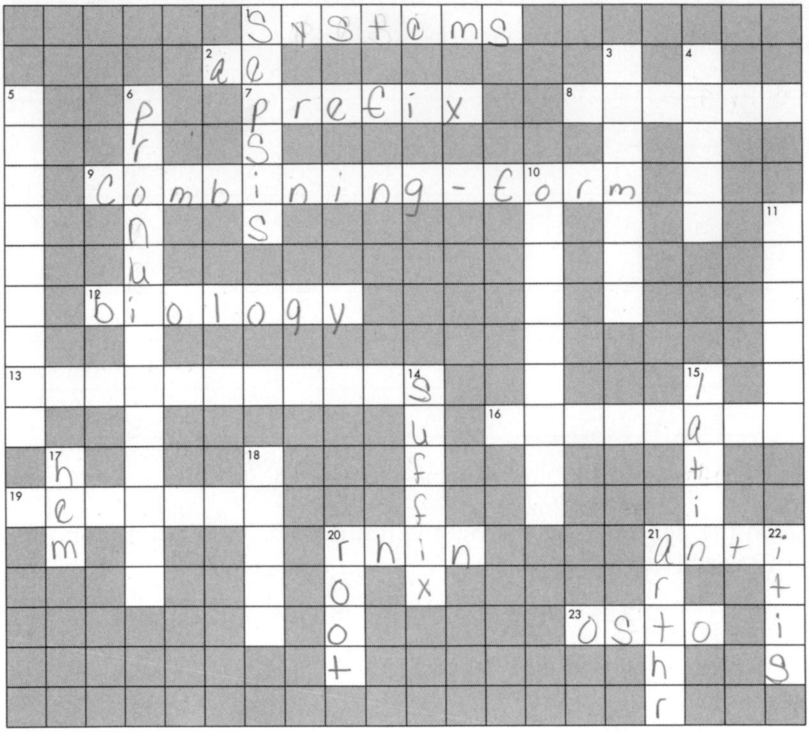
systems
prefix
combining-form
biology
rhin
anti
osto
hem
root
suffix
latin
arthr
itis

ACROSS CLUES

1. Many roots relate to the ____ of the body.
2. The plural suffix of fascia.
7. Beginning word part.
8. Founders of modern medicine.
9. A word part.
12. Science related to the study of the parts of the body.
13. Words that come from proper name or other words.
16. A type of visual aid to assist in learning.
19. Type of dictionary.
20. A root meaning nose.
21. A prefix meaning against.
23. Means bone.

DOWN CLUES

1. Infection.
3. First.
4. Opposite of teach.
5. Words with more than one root.
6. Phonetic sounding out of a word.
10. Learning veterinary terminology is the ____ of this text.
11. Additional visual aids to assist in learning.
14. Ending word part.
15. Source of veterinary language.
17. Means blood.
18. Part of intestinal tract that sounds like a pelvic bone.
20. A foundation word part.
21. A root meaning joint.
22. Inflammation.

Chapter 1 Answers

Exercise 1

1. suffix	6. root
2. root	7. root
3. suffix	8. prefix
4. prefix	9. root
5. root	

Exercise 2

1. H	6. I
2. F	7. E
3. A	8. C
4. G	9. D
5. B	

Exercise 3

1. dermat/o/myc/osis root/combining vowel/root/suffix
2. scler/o/derma root/combining vowel/root
3. arthr/osis root/suffix
4. oste/o/arthr/osis root/combining vowel/root/suffix
5. oste/o/chondr/itis root/combining vowel/root/suffix
6. anti/dote prefix/root
7. enter/itis root/suffix
8. gloss/itis root/suffix
9. bio/logy root/suffix
10. arteri/o/ven/ous root/combining vowel/root/suffix

Note: The combination of root and combining vowel in numbers 1, 2, 4, 5 and 10 becomes a combining form.

ANSWERS: CHAPTER 1 PUZZLE

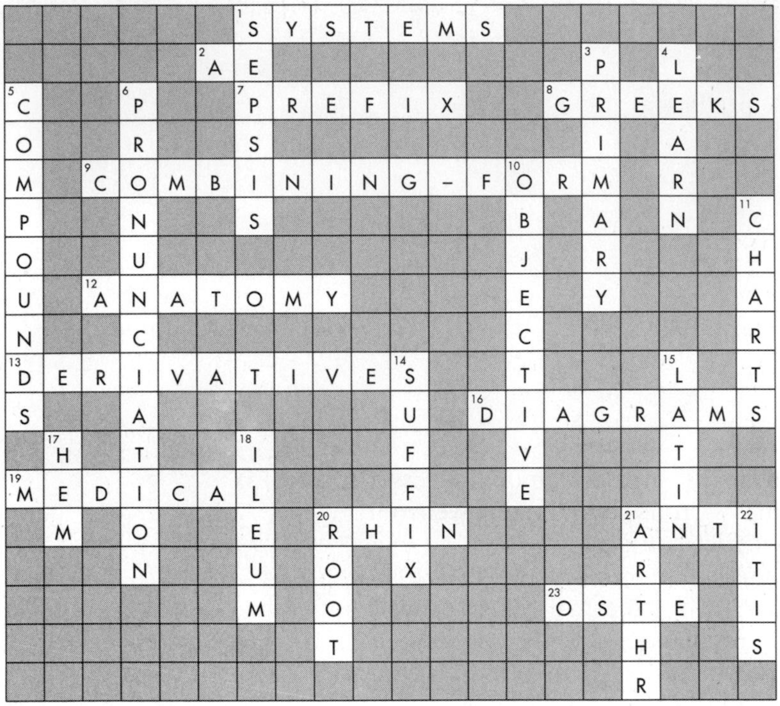
1 SYSTEMS
2 AE
3 PRIMARY
4 LEARN
5 COMPOUNDS
6 PRONUNCIATION
7 PREFIX
8 GREEKS
9 COMBINING-FORM
10 OBJECTIVE
11 CHARTS
12 ANATOMY
13 DERIVATIVES
14 SUFFIX
15 LATTI
16 DIAGRAMS
17 HEM
18 ILEUM
19 MEDICAL
20 RHIN
ROOT
21 ANTI
ARTHR
22 ITIS
23 OSTE

2 Building a Veterinary Vocabulary

CHAPTER OVERVIEW

In this chapter you become familiar with prefixes (the beginnings of words) and suffixes (the endings of words) through definitions and word examples. These word parts are listed alphabetically in chart form to enhance learning.

STEP 1: PREFIXES AND SUFFIXES

The next three chapters present the basic building blocks of a veterinary vocabulary. To know the meaning of a complete word, you want to be able to break down the terms into their separate parts. To do this you need to learn the roots and combining forms as well as the prefixes and suffixes that modify their meaning.

By learning the meanings of the word parts as given in these chapters, you will find that you can define most veterinary words appearing in the chapters that follow. The meanings of the word parts presented in these chapters will generally *not* be repeated in following chapters; however, these chapters can be used for reference whenever you do not recognize the meaning of a word part. To quickly find the page reference for a word part, look in the index.

Prefixes

Prefixes consist of one or more syllables placed at the beginning of a word. A prefix never stands alone. It is placed in front of a verb, adjective, or noun to modify its meaning. Most prefixes are parts of words in ordinary language and do not specifically refer to veterinary terminology. However, many prefixes do occur frequently in veterinary language, and studying them is an important first step in learning veterinary terms. The principal prefixes used in veterinary terminology are given in Table 2-1.

Table 2-1 PREFIXES

Prefix	Meaning	Examples
a-, an-	without, lack of, not	Afebrile (without fever) Anemia (lack of blood)
ab-	away from	Abductor (leading away from) Aboral (away from mouth)
ad-	toward, to, near	Adductor (leading toward) Adrenal (near the kidney)
ambi-, amphi-, ampho-	both	Ambidextrous (ability to use both hands equally) Amphoteric (both acid and base) Amphibious (living both on land and in water)
ana-	up, toward, apart	Anatomy (to cut apart) Anabolism (building up)
ante-	before, in front of, forward	Antenatal (before birth) Antemortem (before death)
anti-	against, opposing	Antisepsis (against infection) Antibiotic (against microbial life)
apo-	separation from, derived from	Apocrine (secretion containing cell parts) Apomorphine (drug derived from morphine)
auto-	self	Autogenous (self-generating) Autolysis (self-dissolving)
bi-	two, double, twice	Biceps (muscle with two heads) Bifurcate (divide into two branches)
cata-	down, under, lower, against	Catabolism (breaking down) Catalepsy (reduced movement)
circum-	around	Circumflex (winding around) Circumanal (surrounding the anus)
co-,* com-,† con-	with, together	Commissure (coming together) Conductor (leading together)
contra-	opposed, against	Contralateral (opposite side) Contraception (prevention of conception)
de-	reverse, remove	Dehydrate (remove water from) Defibrillate (stop fibrillation)
di-	two, twice	Diphasic (having two stages) Dichromic (having two colors)
dia-	between, through, apart, across, completely	Diapedesis (ooze through) Diaphragm (wall across) Diagnosis (complete knowledge)
dis-	apart from, free from	Disinfection (to free from infection) Dissect (cut apart) Disarticulation (separation at a joint)
dys-	difficult, painful, abnormal	Dyspnea (difficult breathing) Dyscrasia (abnormal condition) Dysuria (difficult or painful urination)

*co- before a vowel.
†com- before b, m, and p.

Table 2-1 PREFIXES—cont'd

Prefix	Meaning	Examples
e-, ec- ex-	out of, from, away from	Enucleate (remove whole from) Ectopic (out of place) Exostosis (outgrowth of bone)
ecto-, exo-	outer, outside, situated on	Ectoderm (outer skin) Ectoparasite (organism living on the outside) Exogenous (originating outside)
em,* en-	in	Empyema (pus in) Enzootic (in a population of animals)
endo-	within, inner	Endogenous (originating inside) Endoplasm (inner portion of cytoplasm) Endoderm (inner cell layer)
ep-, epi-	upon, on, over, above	Epicostal (upon a rib) Epidermis (outer skin layer)
eu-	normal, good, well, healthy	Eupnea (normal breathing) Euthanasia (inducing death painlessly)
extra-	outside of, beyond	Extracellular (outside the cells) Extraocular (outside the eye)
hemi-	half	Hemiplegia (paralysis of one side of body) Hemisphere (half of a sphere or globe)
hyper-	excessive, above, beyond	Hyperactive (overactive) Hyperesthesia (excessive sensitivity)
hyp-, hypo-	under, deficient, beneath	Hypoxia (reduced oxygen) Hypothyroidism (deficiency of thyroid activity)
im-,† in-	in, into, within, not	Implant (insert into) Injection (forcing fluid into) Immature (not mature) Involuntary (not voluntary)
infra-	below, beneath	Infraorbital (beneath eye) Infrastructure (underlying support system)
inter-	between	Intercostal (between ribs) Internodal (between nodes)
intra-	within	Intracardiac (within heart) Intraocular (within the eye)
intro-	into, within	Introversion (turning inward) Introduce (lead into)
mes-, meso-	middle	Mesencephalon (midbrain) Mesoderm (middle cell layer)
meta-	change, beyond, after	Metacarpus (bone beyond the carpus) Metamorphosis (change shape or structure)
micr-, micro-	small	Microphthalmos (abnormally small eye) Microbe (minute organism)
mult-, multi-	many	Multiangular (many angles) Multiform (many shapes)
neo-	new, recent	Neoplastic (new tissue growth) Neonatal (newborn)

*em- before b, m, and p.
†im- before b, m, and p.

Continued

Table 2-1 PREFIXES—cont'd

Prefix	Meaning	Examples
pan-	all, entire	Panacea (cure-all) Panzootic (throughout an animal population)
para-	beside, beyond	Paravertebral (beside the vertebrae) Paranormal (beyond scientific explanation)
per-	through, excessive	Permeable (may pass through) Peracute (excessively sharp)
peri-	around	Periosteum (around bone) Peribulbar (around eye bulb)
poly-	many, much, excessive	Polycystic (many cysts) Polydipsia (excessive thirst)
post-	after, behind	Postoperative (after surgery) Postorbital (behind the eye)
pre-, pro-	before, in front of	Prenatal (before birth) Project (throw forward)
pseudo-	false	Pseudoparasite (false parasite) Pseudocyesis (false pregnancy)
re-	again, backward	Reflex (bend back) Regurgitation (vomiting)
retro-	backward, behind	Retrograde (going backward) Retroperitoneal (behind peritoneum)
semi-	half, partial	Semilunar (half-moon shaped) Semipermeable (partly permeable)
sub-	under, beneath	Subcutaneous (under the skin) Sublingual (beneath the tongue)
super-, supra-	above, superior, excess	Supernumerary (excessive number) Suprarenal (above kidneys)
sym-,* syn	together, with	Symbiosis (two organisms living in close association) Syndactyly (fusion of digits)
trans-	across, through	Transection (cut across) Transfix (to pierce across)
ultra-	beyond, excess	Ultravirus (very small virus) Ultrasonic (beyond upper limit of hearing)

*sym- before b, m, p, and ph.

REVIEW QUESTIONS: PREFIXES

Fill in the blanks:

1. A prefix (sometimes) (always) (never) stands alone.
2. The prefix ante- means in front of ________________.
3. A prefix meaning two or twice is bi, di ________________.

4. The prefix meaning around is peri or circum.
5. The prefix for half is hemi or semi.
6. Super- has a similar meaning to the prefix supra.
7. The prefix sym- is used before the letters b, m, p, and ph.
8. The prefix for false is pseudo.
9. The prefix pan- means all, entire.
10. The prefixes mes- and meso- mean middle.

Matching:

Study

____	1. a-, an-	A. self auto
____	2. ambi,	B. difficult, painful dys-
____	3. contra-	C. apart, free from dis-
____	4. dys-	D. without, lack of, not a-, an-
____	5. ep-, epi-	E. below, beneath infra-
____	6. auto	F. upon, on, over ep-, epi-
____	7. multi-	G. oppose, against contra-
____	8. dis-	H. both ambi
____	9. infra-	I. normal, good eu-
____	10. eu-	J. many multi-

REVIEW QUESTIONS: PREFIXES
Answers

Fill in the blanks:

1. never
2. before, in front of
3. bi-, di-
4. circum-, peri-
5. hemi-, semi-
6. supra-
7. b, m, p, and ph
8. pseudo-
9. all, entire
10. middle

Matching:

1. D
2. H
3. G
4. B
5. F
6. A
7. J
8. C
9. E
10. I

Suffixes

Suffixes consist of one or more syllables placed at the ends of words. Like a prefix, a suffix never stands alone. Suffixes are added to the roots of words to modify their meanings. To make pronunciation easier, the last letter or letters of the root may be changed before adding the suffix. For this purpose, there are two general rules:

1. The last vowel of the root may be changed to another vowel. Usually, but not always, an "o," or another vowel, may be inserted between the root and a suffix that begins with a consonant. This vowel is known as a *combining vowel.*
   For example:
   Cardiology means study of the heart.
   To the root *cardi-*, meaning heart, the combining vowel "o" is added, producing the combining form *cardio-*, to which is added the suffix *-logy,* which means study of.
2. When a suffix begins with a vowel, the last vowel of the root may be dropped before adding the suffix.
   For example:
   Carditis means inflammation of the heart.
   The ending vowel "i" of the root *cardi-* is dropped before adding the suffix *-itis,* which means inflammation.

Most suffixes are in common use, but there are some that are specific to veterinary language. The most common suffixes encountered are listed in Table 2-2.

Table 2-2 SUFFIXES

Suffix	Meaning	Examples
-ac, -al, -ic, -ous, -tic	pertaining to, relating to	Cardiac (pertaining to the heart) Neural (pertaining to nerve) Hemorrhagic (relating to bleeding) Delirious (relating to mental disturbance) Acoustic (pertaining to sound)
-algia	pain	Neuralgia (pain in nerves) Myalgia (muscular pain)
-ate	having, resembling, acting upon	Impregnate (to make pregnant) Caudate (having a tail) Pinnate (resembling a feather)
-cele	protrusion (hernia)	Cystocele (bladder hernia) Rectocele (rectal protrusion into vagina)
-centesis	surgical puncture to remove fluid	Paracentesis (from a body cavity) Thoracentesis (from chest cavity)
-cle, -cule, -ole, -ola, -ule, -ulum, -ulus	small (diminutive)	Follicle (little bag) Molecule (small mass) Arteriole, arteriola (small artery) Nodule (small node) Ovulum (small egglike structure) Homunculus (small man)
-cyte	cell	Leukocyte (white blood cell) Erythrocyte (red blood cell)
-ectomy	cutting out	Hysterectomy (surgical removal of uterus) Appendectomy (cutting out of the appendix)
-emesis	vomit	Hematemesis (vomiting blood) Hyperemesis (excessive vomiting)
-emia	blood condition	Leukemia (malignant blood disease) Hyperemia (increased blood flow)
-ent, -er, -ist, -or	person or agent	Recipient (one who receives) Examiner (one who examines) Anesthetist (one who anesthetizes) Donor (one who donates)
-esis, -ia, -iasis, -ism, -ity, -osis, -sis, -tion, -y	state or condition	Paresis (partial paralysis) Anesthesia (loss of sensation) Trichiasis (hair growing against the eye) Priapism (persistent erection) Acidity (excess acid) Dermatosis (skin condition) Inhalation (inhaling) Therapy (treatment condition)
-form, -oid	resembling, shaped like	Fusiform (spindle-shaped) Ovoid (egg-shaped)
-genesis	development, origin	Pathogenesis (origin of disease) Carcinogenesis (development of cancer)
-gram, -graphy	recording, written record	Hemogram (record of blood examination) Cardiography (heart action record)

Continued

Table 2-2 SUFFIXES—cont'd

Suffix	Meaning	Examples
-graph	instrument that records	Cardiograph (heart action) Encephalograph (brain function)
-ible, -ile	capable, able	Flexible (capable of bending) Contractile (able to contract)
-itis	inflammation	Otitis (inflammation of ear) Adenitis (inflammation of gland)
-ize	use, subject to (makes a noun or adjective into a verb)	Anesthetize (subject to anesthesia) Euthanatize (subject to euthanasia) Cauterize (burn with a cautery)
-logy	science, study of	Biology (science of life) Histology (study of tissues)
-oma	tumor	Carcinoma (cancerous growth) Adenoma (tumor arising from gland)
-penia	deficiency of, lack of	Eosinopenia (deficiency of eosinophils) Leukopenia (deficiency of white blood cells)
-pexy, -pexis	fixation	Gastropexy (fixation of stomach) Abomasopexy (fixation of abomasum)
-phage, -phagy	eating	Coprophagy (eating feces) Macrophage (large engulfing cell)
-phobia	abnormal fear or intolerance	Ailurophobia (fear or hatred of cats) Photophobia (intolerance to light)
-plasia, -plastic, -plasty	forming, growing, changing	Anaplasia (changing structure of cells) Aplastic (lack of cell growth) Otoplasty (surgical change to ear)
-pnea	breathing	Apnea (absence of breathing) Dyspnea (difficult breathing)
-rrhaphy	suturing in place	Herniorrhaphy (repair of hernia) Osteorrhaphy (wiring of bone)
-rrhea	flow or discharge	Seborrhea (excessive sebum secretion) Diarrhea (watery feces)
-rrhexis	rupture	Enterorrhexis (intestinal rupture) Karyorrhexis (break up of cell nucleus)
-scope	instrument for examining	Microscope (instrument for examining minute objects) Endoscope (instrument for examining body interior)
-scopy	act of examining	Microscopy (act of examining minute objects) Endoscopy (using an endoscope)
-stomy	surgical opening	Colostomy (surgical opening of colon to body surface) Gastrostomy (surgical opening into stomach)
-tome	instrument for cutting	Fetotome (instrument for cutting up dead fetus) Microtome (for cutting thin sections for microscopy)
-tomy	cutting, incision	Cystotomy (cutting of urinary bladder) Rumenotomy (incision into rumen)

REVIEW QUESTIONS: SUFFIXES

Fill in the blanks:

1. The suffix for cutting or incision is toma.
2. A suffix meaning eating is phage, phagy.
3. A suffix meaning cell is cyte.
4. A suffix for breath is pnea.
5. State or condition is indicated by several suffixes. Two of these suffixes are iasis and osis.
6. A suffix meaning instrument that records is graph.
7. The suffix -emia means blood condition.
8. The suffix oma means tumor.
9. The suffix for origin or development is genesis.
10. The suffix -phobia means intolerance.

Matching:

g	1. -al, -ic	A. surgical puncture
j	2. -ectomy	B. vomit
f	3. -penia	C. resembling, shaped like
e	4. -scopy	D. use, subject to
b	5. -emesis	E. act of examining
a	6. -centesis	F. deficiency of, lack of
h	7. -stomy	G. pertaining to
i	8. -logy	H. surgical opening
d	9. -ize	I. science of, study of
c	10. -form, -oid	J. cutting out

study

REVIEW QUESTIONS: SUFFIXES

Answers

Fill in the blanks:

1. -tomy
2. -phage, -phagy
3. -cyte
4. -pnea
5. -esis, -ia, -iasis, -ity, -osis, -sis, -tion, -y
6. -graph
7. blood condition
8. -oma
9. -genesis
10. abnormal fear or intolerance

Matching:

1. G
2. J
3. F
4. E
5. B
6. A
7. H
8. I
9. D
10. C

Chapter 2 — EXERCISES

BUILDING A VETERINARY VOCABULARY

STEP 1: PREFIXES AND SUFFIXES

Use the following exercises as an additional opportunity to review and employ the preceding prefixes and suffixes. As in the review questions, the answers are provided after the last page of questions. To make the best use of these exercises, if you find that you cannot answer a given question, we strongly suggest that you look it up in the preceding text material. You should use the answers provided only to check your accuracy and not as a short route to completion of these exercises.

Exercise 1: In the blank following each pair of words, indicate whether the underlined prefixes or suffixes have the same or opposite meanings.

1. dystrophy ______________________
   eucaryote
2. exotoxin ______________________
   endocrine
3. semilunar ______________________
   hemiarthrosis
4. hyperparathyroid ______________________
   hypocalcemia
5. submandibular ______________________
   infraspinous
6. achlorhydria ______________________
   analgesia
7. circumarticular ______________________
   pericardium
8. psoriasis ______________________
   narcosis
9. bicornuate ______________________
   dicephalous
10. lobectomy ______________________
    cysticorrhaphy
11. hepatic ______________________
    renal
12. antipyretic ______________________
    contraindication
13. reducible ______________________
    refractile
14. myelogram ______________________
    pyelography
15. anteflex ______________________
    anticholinergic

Exercise 2: Define the prefix in each word.

1. postmortem ______________________
2. dysplasia ______________________
3. aseptic ______________________
4. infrared ______________________
5. retrospective ______________________
6. endothelium ______________________
7. interface ______________________
8. paralumbar ______________________
9. ambivalent ______________________
10. catatonic ______________________

Exercise 3: Define the suffix in each word.

1. enucleate ate
2. osteogenesis esis
3. hepatitis itis
4. lymphoma oma
5. zoophobia ia
6. rectocele
7. physiology logy
8. osteotome ome
9. rhinorrhea hea
10. microphage age

Exercise 4: Match the underlined prefixes and suffixes with their meanings:

k	1. reticulocyte	A. blood condition emia
l	2. otic	B. away from ab
m	3. hemizygote	C. instrument scope
i	4. percutaneous	D. rupture rrhexis
j	5. congenital	E. between, through dia
a	6. polycythemia	F. breathing pnea
B	7. abaxial	G. upon, on, over epi
O	8. symphysis	H. resembling, shaped like oid
N	9. autoclave	I. through per
D	10. metrorrhexis	J. with, together con
E	11. diaphoresis	K. cell cyte
C	12. theloscope	L. pertaining to ic
H	13. odontoid	M. half hemi
G	14. epicondyle	N. self auto
f	15. hypercapnea	O. together sym

CHAPTER 2 PUZZLE

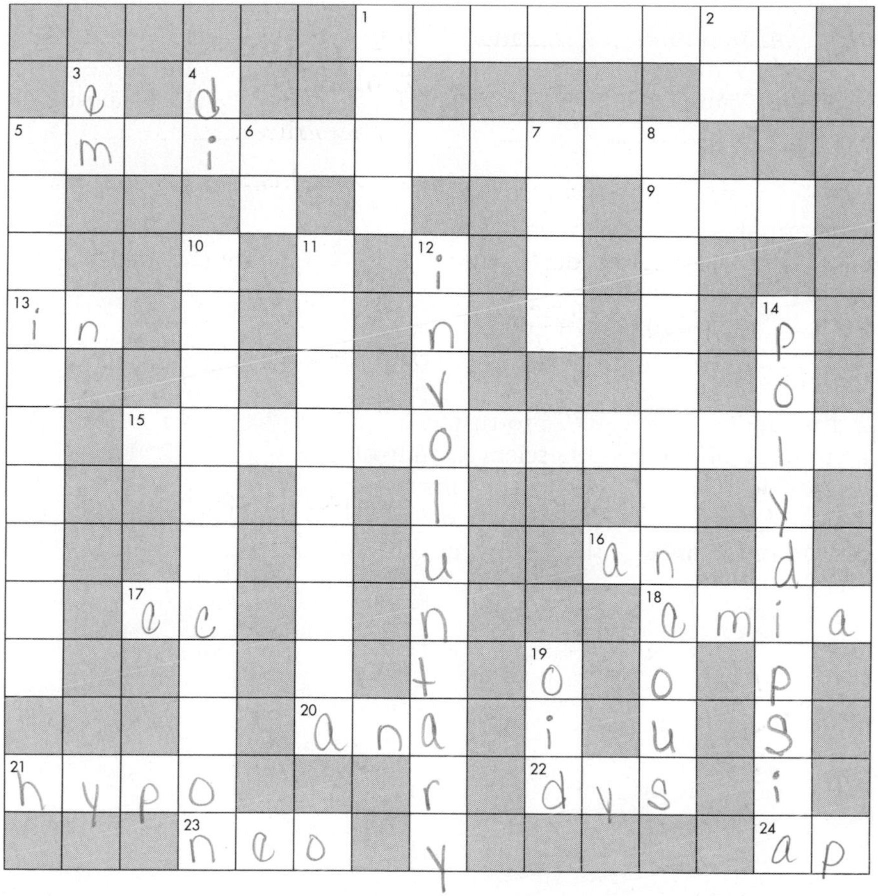

ACROSS CLUES

1. before birth
5. ability to use both hands equally
9. suffix meaning small
13. prefix meaning not in
15. beneath the eye
16. prefix meaning without an
17. prefix meaning out of ec
18. suffix meaning blood condition emia
20. prefix meaning up or apart ana
21. prefix meaning under or beneath hypo
22. prefix meaning difficult dys
23. prefix meaning new neo
24. prefix meaning separation from ap

DOWN CLUES

1. suffix meaning fixation
2. prefix meaning away from
3. prefix meaning in em
4. prefix meaning two or twice di
5. against infection
6. prefix meaning down or from
7. suffix meaning state or condition
8. under the skin
10. cut across
11. pain in nerves
12. not voluntary
14. excessive thirst polydipsia
19. suffix for resembling oid

Chapter 2 Answers

Exercise 1

1. opposite
2. opposite
3. same
4. opposite
5. same
6. same
7. same
8. same
9. same
10. opposite
11. same
12. same
13. same
14. same
15. opposite

Exercise 2

1. behind, after
2. difficult, abnormal
3. without
4. below
5. behind
6. within
7. between
8. beside, beyond
9. both
10. down, under

Exercise 3

1. having, acting upon
2. beginning process, origin
3. inflammation
4. tumor
5. abnormal fear, intolerance
6. protrusion
7. science, study of
8. cutting instrument
9. flow or discharge
10. eating, devouring

Exercise 4

1. K
2. L
3. M
4. I
5. J
6. A
7. B
8. O
9. N
10. D
11. E
12. C
13. H
14. G
15. F

ANSWERS: CHAPTER 2 PUZZLE

						1 P	R	E	N	A	T	2 A	L	
	3 E		4 D			E						B		
5 A	M	B	I	6 D	E	X	T	R	7 O	U	8 S			
N				E		Y			S		9 U	L	E	
T			10 T		11 N		12 I		I		B			
13 I	N		R		E		N		S		C		14 P	
S			A		U		V				U		O	
E		15 I	N	F	R	A	O	R	B	I	T	A	L	
P			S		A		L				A		Y	
S			E		L		U			16 A	N		D	
I		17 E	C		G		N				18 E	M	I	A
S			T		I		T		19 O		O		P	
			I		20 A	N	A		I		U		S	
21 H	Y	P	O				R		22 D	Y	S		I	
			23 N	E	O		Y						24 A	P

3 Adding to the Foundation

CHAPTER OVERVIEW

This chapter presents word roots that name the parts of the animal body. Word lists are divided into two groups. External anatomy refers to visible parts of the body. Internal anatomy refers to organs, bones and other tissues within the body.

STEP 2: ROOTS AND COMBINING FORMS

You will remember that a root is the foundation or basic meaning of a word. A combining form is a root with a combining vowel added, attaching the root to a suffix or another root. The first list, Table 3-1, relates to external anatomy—that which can be seen with the naked eye. This list is arranged alphabetically, with the pronunciation and body part relating to each root. The combining form is divided with a slash mark (/) separating the root and the combining vowel, which is usually, but not always, an "o."

Table 3-1 EXTERNAL ANATOMY

Root/combining form	Pronunciation	Body part
blephar/o-	blef'ahr-o	Eyelid or eyelash
brachi/o-	bra'ke-o	Arm (foreleg in quadrupeds)
bucc/o-	buk'o	Cheek
canth/o-	kan'tho	Angle at either end of the slit between the eyelids
capit/o-	kap'it-o	Head
carp/o-	karp'o	Area corresponding to the human wrist
cephal/o-	sef'al-o	Head
cervic/o-	ser'vik-o	Neck (also refers to necklike projection of the cervix uteri, which is internal anatomy)
cheil/o-, chil/o-	kile'o	Lip
cili/o-	sil'ee-o	Eyelid, eyelash, or small hairlike processes
cor/e-, cor/o-	kor'ee, kor'o	Pupil of eye

Table 3-1 EXTERNAL ANATOMY—cont'd

Root/combining form	Pronunciation	Body part
dactyl/o-	dak'til-o	Digit, toe
dent/i-, dent/o-	dent'ee, dent'o	Tooth or teeth
derm/a-, derm/o-, dermat/o-	derm'a, derm'o, derm'at-o	Skin
dors/i-, dors/o-	dor'see, dor'so	Back
faci/o-	fa'she-o	Face
gingiv/o-	jin'jiv-o	Gums
gloss/o-	glos'o	Tongue
gnath/o-	nath'o	Jaw
irid/o-	ir'id-o	Iris of eye
labi/o-	lay'be-o	Lip, especially lips of mouth
lapar/o-	lap'ahr-o	Flank; abdomen
later/o-	lat'er-o	Side
lingu/o-	ling'wo	Tongue
mamm/a-, mamm/o-	mam'ah, mam'o	Mammary gland
mast/o-	mast'o	Mammary gland
nas/o-	naze'o	Nose
occipit/o-	ock-si'pit-o	Back of head
ocul/o-	ock'ule-o	Eye
odont/o-	oh-dont'o	Tooth or teeth
omphal/o-	om'fah-lo	Navel or umbilicus
onych/o-	on'ik-o	Nail or claw
ophthalm/o-	of-thal'mo	Eye or eyes
or/o-	or'o	Mouth
ot/o-	oh'toe	Ear
papill/o-	pah-pill'o	Nipple or nipple-shaped projection
phall/o-	fal'o	Penis
pil/o-	pile'o	Hair
pod/o-	pod'o	Foot or foot-shaped part
rhin/o-	rine'o	Nose
somat/o-, somatic/o-	sew-mat'o, sew-mat'ik-o	Body
steth/o-	steth'o	Chest
stom-, stomat/o-	sto'mah-toe	Mouth
tars/o-	tahr'so	Area corresponding to the human ankle or the edge of the eyelid
thorac/o-	tho'rah-ko	Chest or thorax
trich/o-	trik'o	Hair or hairlike structure
ventr/i-, ventr/o-	ven'tree, ven'tro	Belly, underside of quadruped

REVIEW QUESTIONS: EXTERNAL ANATOMY ROOTS AND COMBINING FORMS

Fill in the blanks:

1. Blepharo and cilio mean ______________________ and ______________________.
2. The combining forms for head are ______________________ and ______________________.
3. A combining form for hair is ______________________.
4. A combining form for lip is ______________________.
5. Rhino and naso both refer to ______________________.
6. Two combining forms for mammary gland are ______________ and ______________.
7. Cervico means ______________________.
8. A combining form for mouth is ______________________.
9. Ophthalmo and ______________________ are combining forms for eye.
10. Stetho and ______________________ are combining forms for chest.

Matching:

G	1. carpo-	A.	tongue
I	2. derma-, dermo-, dermato-	B.	pupil of eye
H ~~B~~	3. brachio-	C.	ear
a	4. glosso-	D.	back of head
J	5. ventri-, ventro-	E.	foot
C	6. oto-	F.	cheek
_____	7. core-, coro-	G.	wrist
_____	8. occipito-	H.	arm
_____	9. podo-	I.	skin
_____	10. bucco-	J.	belly

REVIEW QUESTIONS: EXTERNAL ANATOMY ROOTS AND COMBINING FORMS

Answers

Fill in the blanks:

_____ 1. eyelid, eyelash

_____ 2. capito-, cephalo-

_____ 3. tricho- or pilo-

_____ 4. cheilo-, chilo-, labio-

_____ 5. nose

_____ 6. mamma- or mammo-, masto-

_____ 7. neck (or necklike structure)

_____ 8. oro- or stomato-

_____ 9. oculo-

_____ 10. thoraco-

Matching:

1. G
2. I
3. H
4. A
5. J
6. C
7. B
8. D
9. E
10. F

Table 3-2 relates to internal anatomy—that which is inside the body. This list is arranged alphabetically, with the pronunciation and body part relating to each root. The combining form is divided with a slash (/) separating the root and the combining vowel, which is usually, but not always, an "o."

Table 3-2 INTERNAL ANATOMY

Root/combining form	Pronunciation	Body part
aden/o-	ad'e-no	Gland
adren/o-	ad-re'no	Adrenal gland
angi/o-	an'je-o	Vessel, usually a blood vessel
arteri/o-	ar-te're-o	Artery
arteriol/o-	ar-te're-o"lo	Arteriole
arthr/o-	ar'throe	Joint
atri/o-	a'tree-o	Atrium or upper heart chamber
balan/o-	bal'ah-no	Glans penis or glans clitoridis
bronch/i-, bronch/o-	brong'ke, brong'ko	Bronchus
bronchiol/o-	brong'ke-olo	Bronchiolus
cardi/o-	kar'de-o	Heart
cerebell/o-	ser"e-bel'o	Cerebellum part of brain
cerebr/i-, cerebr/o-	ser'e-bri, ser'e-bro	Cerebrum part of brain
choledoch/o-	ko-lee'dok-o	Common bile duct
chondr/i-, chondr/io-, chondr/o-	kon'dree, kon'dree-o, kon'dro	Cartilage

Continued

Table 3-2 INTERNAL ANATOMY—cont'd

Root/combining form	Pronunciation	Body part
chord/o-	kor'do	Cord, string
cleid/o-	kli'do	Clavicle (collarbone)
colp/o-	kol'po	Vagina
cost/o-	kos'to	Rib
cyst/i-, cyst/o-	sis'ti, sis'to	Bladder, cyst, sac
cyt/o-	si'to	Cell
duoden/o-	du"o-de'no	Duodenum section of intestine
encephal/o-	en-sef'ah-lo	Brain
enter/o-	en'ter-o	Intestine
episi/o-	e-peez'e-o	Vulva
fibr/o-	fie'bro	Fibers
gastr/o-	gas'tro	Stomach
gli/o-	glee'o	Gluey substance
hepat/ico-, hepat/o-	he-pat'i-ko, he-pat'o	Liver
hist/o-	his'to	Tissue
hyster/o-	his'ter-o	Uterus
ile/o-	ill'e-o	Ileum section of intestine
ili/o-	ill'e-o	Ilium (upper part of hipbone)
jejun/o-	je-joo'no	Jejunum section of intestine
kerat/o-	ker'ah-to	Horny tissue (and cornea of eye)
laryng/o-	lah-ring'go	Larynx (voice box)
lymph/o-	lim'fo	Lymphatic vessels, lymphocytes
mening/o-	me-ning'go	Membranes covering brain and spinal cord
metr/a-, metr/o-	me'trah, me'tro	Uterus
myel/o-	my'el-o	Bone marrow or spinal cord
my/o-	my'o	Muscle
myring/o-	mi-ring'o	Eardrum
nephr/o-	nef'ro	Kidney
neur/o-	nu'ro	Nerve, nerves, nervous system
oophor/o-	o-of'or-o	Ovary
orchi/o-, orchi/do-	or'ke-o, or'ki-do	Testis, testes
oss/eo-, oss/i-, ost/e-, ost/eo-	os'se-o, os'see, os'tee, os'tee-o	Bone or bones
ovari/o-	o-var'e-o	Ovary
palat/o-	pal'ah-to	Palate (roof of mouth)
pharyng/o-	fah-ring'go	Pharynx (throat)
phleb/o-	fleb'o	Vein or veins
phren/i-, phren/ico-, phren/o-	fren'ee, fren'i-ko, fren'o	Diaphragm, mind
pleur/o-	ploor'o	Pleura, rib (or side)
pneum/a-, pneum/o-, pneum/ato-, pneum/ono-	nu'mah, nu'mo, nu-mat'o, nu-mon'o	Lungs, respiration (air, breath)

Table 3-2 INTERNAL ANATOMY—cont'd

Root/combining form	Pronunciation	Body part
proct/o-	prok'to	Rectum or anus
pulm/o-	pull'mo	Lungs
pyel/o-	pi'el-o	Pelvis or kidney
rect/o-	rek'to	Rectum
ren/i-, ren/o-	ren'i, ren'o	Kidney
sacr/o-	sa'kro	Sacrum
salping/o-	sal-ping'go	Fallopian or eustachian tube
sarc/o-	sar'ko	Flesh, muscular substance
splen/o-	splen'o	Spleen
spondyl/o-	spon'di-lo	Vertebra, spinal column
stern/o-	stern'no	Sternum (breastbone)
tend/o-, ten/o-	ten'doe, ten'o	Tendon
thym/o-	thi'mo	Thymus gland
thyr/o-	thi'ro	Thyroid gland
trache/o-	tra'ke-o	Trachea
ureter/o-	u-re'ter-o	Ureter (kidney to bladder tube)
urethr/o-	u-re'thro	Urethra (bladder to outside)
vas/o-	vaz'o	Vessel or duct
ven/e-, ven/i-, ven/o-	vene'eh, vene'ee, vene'o	Vein or veins
viscer/o-	vis'er-o	Viscera

REVIEW QUESTIONS: INTERNAL ANATOMY ROOTS AND COMBINING FORMS

Fill in the blanks:

1. The combining form for gland is ____________________.
2. A combining form for uterus is ____________________.
3. Ileo- is the combining form meaning ____________________.
4. Gastro- is the combining form meaning ____________________.
5. The combining form for testis is ____________________.
6. Pneuma- or pulmo- refers to ____________________.
7. The combining form for spleen is ____________________.
8. Osteo- refers to ____________________.
9. A combining form for vein is ____________________.
10. Chordo- is a combining form meaning ____________________.

Matching:

_____	1. urethro-	A. viscera
_____	2. recto-	B. tendon
_____	3. tracheo-	C. kidney
_____	4. viscero-	D. bone marrow, spinal cord
_____	5. sarco-	E. muscle
_____	6. myelo-	F. urethra
_____	7. teno-	G. trachea
_____	8. kerato-	H. flesh
_____	9. myo-	I. rectum
_____	10. reni-	J. horny tissue, cornea

REVIEW QUESTIONS: INTERNAL ANATOMY ROOTS AND COMBINING FORMS

Answers

Fill in the blanks:

1. adeno-
2. hystero-, metra-, or metro-
3. ileum
4. stomach
5. orchio-, orchido-
6. lungs
7. spleno-
8. bone
9. phlebo-, vene-, veni-, or veno-
10. cord

Matching:

1. F
2. I
3. G
4. A
5. H
6. D
7. B
8. J
9. E
10. C

Chapter 3 — EXERCISES

ADDING TO THE FOUNDATION:
STEP 2: ROOTS AND COMBINING FORMS

The following exercises provide further review opportunity for learning the roots and combining forms presented in this chapter. Once again, we urge you to consult the answers only after you have completed the exercises.

Exercise 1: In the blank following each pair of words indicate whether the underlined roots and combining forms are similar or different.

1. blepharitis
   facial ________________
2. angiogenesis
   vascular ________________
3. capitulum
   encephalitis ________________
4. iliocecal
   ileostomy ________________
5. oculomotor
   ophthalmoscope ________________
6. oropharynx
   otolaryngology ________________
7. tenotomy
   tibiotarsal ________________
8. rhinencephalon
   nasolacrimal ________________
9. vasodilator
   visceral ________________
10. pilomotor
    trichobezoar ________________
11. myofibril
    metamyelocyte ________________
12. sublingual
    hypoglossal ________________
13. odontoid
    dental ________________
14. renal
    glomerulonephritis ________________
15. anisocoria
    iridocyclitis ________________
16. phlebotomy
    venipuncture ________________
17. splenomegaly
    spondylitis ________________
18. colpotomy
    hysterotomy ________________
19. omphalitis
    orchitis ________________
20. stethoscope
    thoracotomy ________________

Exercise 2: In the blank after each word write a word from the list on the right that contains a combining form for that body part. Underline the combining form.

1. Bladder or sac cystocentesis
2. Cartilage Chohdroma
3. Fibers fibroblast
4. Horny tissue hyerkeratosis
5. Kidney pelvis pyelonephritis
6. Larynx larynogospasm
7. Membranes covering brain and spinal cord meningitis
8. Muscle myo globin
9. Nose rhinovirus
10. Tendon tenosynovitis
11. Thymus Thymic
12. Thyroid gland thyrotropic

athymic
chondroma
cystocentesis
fibroblast
hyperkeratosis
laryngospasm
meningitis
myoglobin
pyelonephritis
rhinovirus
tenosynovitis
thyrotropic

Exercise 3: Match the following roots and combining forms with their meanings:

D	1. brachio-	A. back of head occipito
K	2. cantho-	B. gum gingivo
J	3. ovario-	C. head cephalo
B	4. gingivo-	D. foreleg, arm brachio
G	5. derma-	E. body stomato
H	6. glosso-	F. intestine entero
A	7. occipito-	G. skin derma
L	8. oto-	H. tongue glosso
F	9. entero-	I. belly, underside ventro
I	10. ventro-	J. ovary ovario
E	11. somato-	K. angle at either end of eyelid slit cantho
C	12. cephalo-	L. ear oto

Exercise 4: Define the underlined root in each word:

1. buccal Cheek
2. cheilitis lip
3. polydactyly toe/digit
4. lateral Side
5. onychectomy Claw, nail
6. laparotomy flank abdomn
7. somatoplasm Body
8. mastitis mammary gland
9. stomatitis ~~Body~~ mouth
10. pododermatitis foot

ilium hip
ileum intestine

ilium
ileum

ilium hip
ileum intestine

phreno diphragm
poikilo irragular

Conjunctivitis
inflammation of
Conary & Conjunctive

dry eye

CHAPTER 3 PUZZLE

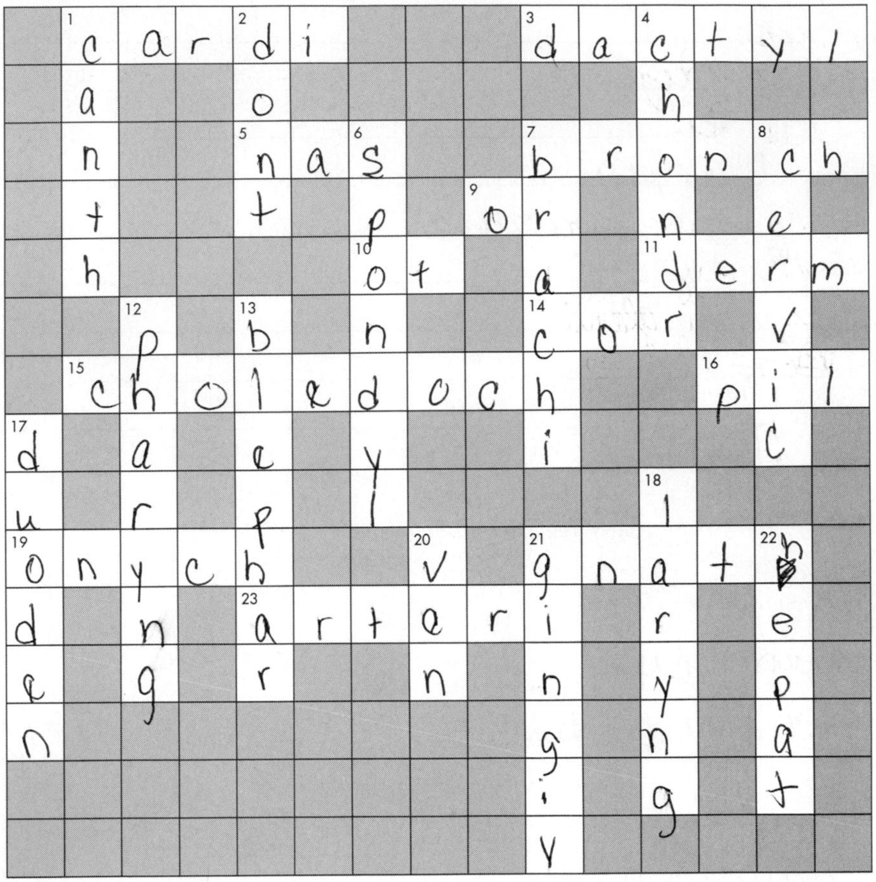

ACROSS CLUES

1. heart
3. digit
5. nose
7. bronchus
9. mouth
10. ear
11. skin
14. ~~heart~~ pupil of eye
15. common bile duct
16. hair
19. nail or claw
21. jaw
23. artery

DOWN CLUES

1. angle at ends of eyelid slits
2. tooth or teeth
4. cartilage
6. vertebra or spinal column
7. arm
8. neck
12. pharynx
13. eyelid or eyelash
17. duodenum
18. larynx
20. vein
21. gums
22. liver

Chapter 3 Answers

Exercise 1

1. different
2. similar
3. similar
4. different
5. similar
6. different
7. different
8. similar
9. different
10. similar
11. different
12. similar
13. similar
14. similar
15. different
16. similar
17. different
18. different
19. different
20. similar

Exercise 2

1. cystocentesis
2. chondroma
3. fibroblast
4. hyperkeratosis
5. pyelonephritis
6. laryngospasm
7. meningitis
8. myoglobin
9. rhinovirus
10. tenosynovitis
11. athymic
12. thyrotropic

Exercise 3

1. D
2. K
3. J
4. B
5. G
6. H
7. A
8. L
9. F
10. I
11. E
12. C

Exercise 4

1. cheek
2. lip
3. digit
4. side
5. nail or claw
6. abdomen, flank
7. body
8. mammary gland
9. mouth
10. foot

ANSWERS: CHAPTER 3 PUZZLE

	1 C	A	R	2 D	I				3 D	A	4 C	T	Y	L
	A			E							H			
	N			5 N	A	6 S			7 B	R	O	N	8 C	H
	T			T		P		9 O	R		N		E	
	H					10 O	T		A		11 D	E	R	M
		12 P		13 B		N			14 C	O	R		V	
	15 C	H	O	L	E	D	O	C	H			16 P	I	L
17 D		A		E		Y			I				C	
U		R		P		L					18 L			
19 O	N	Y	C	H			20 V		21 G	N	A	T	22 H	
D		N		23 A	R	T	E	R	I		R		E	
E		G		R			N		N		Y		P	
N									G		N		A	
									I		G		T	
									V					

4 Completing the Foundation

CHAPTER OVERVIEW

This chapter presents important verbal and adjectival roots. The names of various chemicals, body fluids, and other substances are also presented, along with a list of colors.

STEP 3: ADDITIONAL ROOTS AND COMBINING FORMS

The following lists of roots and combining forms relate to action or description. Table 4-1 lists verbal roots and combining forms that show an activity, a condition, or an action. The roots and combining forms are marked with slash marks showing the root and its combining vowel.

Table 4-1 VERBAL ROOTS AND COMBINING FORMS

Root/combining form	Meaning	Examples
audi/o-	hearing	Auditory (sense or organs of hearing) Audiology (study of hearing)
bio-	life	Biology (study of living things) Biogenesis (origin of life)
caus-, caut-	burn	Caustic (burning material) Cautery (device to scar or burn)
-clas-, -clast	break	Osteoclasis (surgical fracture) Clastothrix (splitting of hair)
duct-	lead	Abduct (lead away from) Duct (tube leading to or from)
-ectas-	dilate	Phlebectasia (dilation of veins) Venectasia (dilation of veins)
-edem-	swelling	Cephaledema (swelling of head) Edematous (swollen)
-esthes-	sensation	Anesthesia (without sensation) Paresthesia (abnormal sensation)
gen/o-	producing	Pathogen (disease producing) Antigenic (producing a reaction)

Continued

Table 4-1 VERBAL ROOTS AND COMBINING FORMS—cont'd

Root/combining form	Meaning	Examples
-iatr/o-	treatment	Geriatrics (treatment of aging) Iatrogenic (caused by treatment)
kin/e-, kin/o-	movement, motion	Kinetogenic (producing movement) Kinetics (study of motion)
-lysis, -lys/o-, -lytic	breaking down	Lysis (destruction of a cell) Lysozyme (bacteria-destroying enzyme)
-morph/o-	form, structure, shape	Amorphous (no definite form) Polymorphic (many forms)
-op/ia, -ops/ia, -opsy	vision	Myopia (nearsightedness) Chromatopsia (color vision)
-path-, -pathy	disease	Pathogenic (disease causing) Enteropathy (intestinal disease)
-phage, phag/o-	eating	Phagocyte (engulfing cell) Macrophage (large phagocyte)
-phas-	speech	Aphasia (loss of speech functions) Dysphasia (difficulty in speaking)
-phil	affinity, love for	Philanthropy (love of mankind) Acidophilic (acid-loving)
-plegia	paralysis	Hemiplegia (one-sided paralysis) Paraplegia (paralysis of hind legs)
-poiesis	formation, production	Hemopoiesis (blood cell formation) Leukopoiesis (white blood cell production)
schist/o-, schiz/o-	split, cleft, division	Schistocyte (broken red cell) Schizogony (type of asexual reproduction)
spasm/o-	spasm	Spasmogenic (causing spasm) Spasmolysis (relieving spasm)
-stasis	standing still, stoppage	Homeostasis (constant internal environment) Hemostasis (stoppage of blood flow)
troph/o-	nourishment, food	Trophism (nutrition) Dystrophy (defective nutrition)

REVIEW QUESTIONS: VERBAL ROOTS AND COMBINING FORMS

Fill in the blanks: Give the meaning of the underlined combining forms.

1. pathogen producing
2. inaudible hearing
3. atelectasis dilate
4. osteoclast break
5. cardiopathy disease

Give the verbal root or combining form for each word.

6. standing still, stoppage ____________
7. eating ____________
8. vision ____________
9. affinity, love for ____________
10. spasm ____________

Matching: Match each underlined word part with its meaning:

____ 1. conduct	A. burn
____ 2. morphogenesis	B. sensation
____ 3. psychiatric	C. movement
____ 4. lymphedema	D. lead
____ 5. biosynthesis	E. breaking down
____ 6. hyperesthesia	F. formation
____ 7. karyolysis	G. shape
____ 8. cauterization	H. swelling
____ 9. lymphopoiesis	I. life
____ 10. kinesthetic	J. treatment

REVIEW QUESTIONS: VERBAL ROOTS AND COMBINING FORMS

Answers

Fill in the blanks:

1. producing
2. hearing
3. dilate
4. break
5. disease
6. -stasis
7. -phage, -phago-
8. -opia, -opsia, -opsy
9. -phil-
10. spasmo-

Matching:

1. D
2. G
3. J
4. H
5. I
6. B
7. E
8. A
9. F
10. C

Table 4-2 lists adjectival roots and combining forms that describe a quality or characteristic. Each root and its combining form is marked with slash marks showing the root and its combining vowel.

Table 4-2 ADJECTIVAL ROOTS AND COMBINING FORMS

Root/combining form	Meaning	Examples
brachy-	short	Brachycephalic (short head) Brachygnathous (receding underjaw)
brady-	slow	Bradycardia (slow heartbeat) Bradypnea (slow breathing)
brev/i-	short	Brevicollis (short neck) Brevicaudate (short tail)
cry/o-	cold	Cryotherapy (treatment using cold) Cryoanesthesia (freezing body part)
crypt/o-	hidden	Cryptorchidism (undescended testis) Cryptic (hidden)
dextr/o-	right, right side	Dextrocardia (heart on right side) Dextromanual (right-handed)
dipl/o-	double, twice	Diplocoria (double pupil in eye) Diplococcus (bacteria in pairs)
dolich/o-	long	Dolichocephalic (long head) Dolichoderus (long neck)
glyc/o-, gluc/o-	sugar, sweet	Glycemia (glucose in the blood) Glucosuria, Glycosuria (sugar in the urine)
heter/o-	other, different	Heterocellular (of different cells) Heterochromatic (of different colors)
hom/eo-, hom/o-	same, alike	Homeostasis (staying the same) Homozygous (having identical genes)
hydr/o-	wet, water, fluid	Hydrothorax (fluid in pleural cavity) Hydrocephalus (excess fluid in brain)
is/o-	equal, alike	Isotonic (of equal tension) Isocoria (equal-sized pupils)
lept/o-	slender, small, thin	Leptocyte (thin-walled red blood cell) Leptomeninges (two thinner meninges)
lev/o-	left, to the left	Levoduction (eyes turn left) Levorotation (turning to the left)
macr/o-	large	Macrocyte (large cell) Macroscopic (visible to naked eye)
mal-	ill, bad	Malady (illness) Malnutrition (any nutritional disorder)
malac/o-	soft, softening	Malacia (softening) Osteomalacia (softening of bones)
meg/a-, meg/alo-, meg/aly-	large, oversized	Megacolon (enlarged colon) Megaloblast (large immature blood cell) Hepatomegaly (enlarged liver)

Table 4-2 ADJECTIVAL ROOTS AND COMBINING FORMS—cont'd

Root/combining form	Meaning	Examples
necr/o-	death	Necrosis (localized tissue death) Necropsy (examination of dead animal)
olig/o-	few, little	Oliguria (scanty urine formation) Oligospermia (few sperm)
orth/o-	straight, normal, correct	Orthodontics (straightening teeth) Orthodox (commonly accepted)
pachy-	thick	Pachyderm (thick-skinned animal) Pachymeninges (thick meninges)
pale/o-	old, primitive	Paleogenetic (originated in past) Paleontology (study of primitive life)
platy-	flat, wide	Platyhelminth (flatworm) Platyrrhine (wide nose)
ple/o-	more, many	Pleomorphic (many forms) Pleochromatic (many colors)
poikil/o-	irregular, varied	Poikilocytosis (irregular red cell shapes) Poikilothermic (cold-blooded)
-scler/o-	hardness	Sclerosis (hardening) Arteriosclerosis (artery hardening)
sinistr/o-	left, to the left	Sinistrad (toward the left) Sinistromanual (left-handed)
sten/o-	narrow, contracted	Stenosed (narrowed, contracted) Stenosis (abnormal constriction)
stere/o-	solid, three-dimensional	Stereoscopic (solid appearance) Stereopsis (three-dimensional vision)
tachy-	rapid, fast	Tachypnea (fast breathing) Tachycardia (rapid heart rate)
tel/e-, tel/o-	distant, end	Telophase (final stage) Telencephalon (end brain)
therm/o-	heat	Thermogenic (producing heat) Thermolabile (destruction by heat)
xer/o-	dry	Xerophthalmia (dry eyes) Xeroderma (dry skin)

REVIEW QUESTIONS: ADJECTIVAL ROOTS AND COMBINING FORMS

Fill in the blanks: Give the meaning of the underlined combining forms:

1. anhydrous wet
2. glycogen sugar
3. isograft equal
4. homeopathy same
5. necrotizing death

Give the verbal root or combining form for each word:

6. different hetero
7. short brachy
8. double diplo
9. large megaly
10. rapid, fast tachy

Matching: Match each underlined word part with its meaning:

heat	F	1. thermophilic	A. thick patchy
narrow	J	2. stenotic	B. left levo
ill	I	3. malocclusion	C. hidden crypt
hardening	H	4. sclerotic	D. cold cryo
thick	A	5. pachymeter	E. slow brachy
normal	G	6. orthopedic	F. heat thermo
hidden	C	7. cryptogenic	G. straight, normal ortho
left	B	8. levotorsion	H. hardness scelur
slow	E	9. bradykinin	I. ill, bad mal
cold	D	10. cryosurgery	J. narrow stamight

REVIEW QUESTIONS: ADJECTIVAL ROOTS AND COMBINING FORMS

Answers

Fill in the blanks:

1. water, wet, fluid
2. sweet, sugar
3. equal, alike
4. same, alike
5. death
6. hetero-
7. brachy-
8. diplo-
9. macro- or mega-, megalo-, megaly-
10. tachy-

Matching:

1. F
2. J
3. I
4. H
5. A
6. G
7. C
8. B
9. E
10. D

The following tables list a number of additional terms used in veterinary language. Collectively, these terms complete the basic foundation for learning veterinary terminology. They are presented as words, roots, and combining forms, in separate tables relating to body fluids, substances, chemicals, and colors (Tables 4-3 to 4-5). In the tables, the roots and combining forms are marked with slash marks to show the root and the combining vowel, whereas the words are unmarked.

Table 4-3 BODY FLUIDS

Word, root/combining form	Meaning
aqua, hydr/o-	water
chol/e-, chol/o-	bile
chyle, chyl/o-	milky fluid—product of digestion
dacry/o-, lacrima	tears
galact/o-, lact/o-	milk
hem/a-, hemat/o-, hem/o-	blood
hidr/o-, sudor	sweat
lymph/o-	lymph
mucus, muco-	secretion of mucous membranes
myx/o-	mucus
plasma	fluid portion of blood
ptyal/o-	saliva

Continued

Table 4-3 BODY FLUIDS—cont'd

Word, root/combining form	Meaning
pus	liquid product of inflammation
py/o-	pus
sangui-, sanguin/o-	blood, bloody
serum, ser/o-	clear portion of blood fluid
sial/o-	saliva, salivary glands
ur/e-, ur/ea-, ur/eo-, ur/in-, ur/ino-, ur/o-	urine or urea

Table 4-4 BODY SUBSTANCES AND CHEMICALS

Word, root/combining form	Meaning
adip/o-	fat
amyl/o-	starch
cerumen, cerumin/o-	earwax
collagen	fibrous protein of connective tissue, cartilage, bone, and skin
ele/o-, ole/o-	oil
ferrum, ferr/o-	iron
gluco-, glyc/o-, sacchar/o-, sacchar/i-	sugar
hal/o-	salt
heme	iron-based, pigment part of hemoglobin
hormone	body-produced chemical substance
hyal/o-, hyalin	glassy, translucent substance
lip/o-, lipid	fat, fatty acids
lith/o-	stone or calculus
mel/i-	honey or sugar
natrium	sodium
petrous	stony hardness
sal	salt
sebum	sebaceous gland secretion

Table 4-5 COLORS

Word, root/combining form	Meaning
albus, alba, alb-	white
chlor/o-, chloros	green
chrom/o-, chromat/o-	color (as compared with no color)
cirrhos	orange-yellow
cyan/o-	blue
erythr/o-	red
leuc/o-, leuk/o-	white
lutein	saffron yellow
melan/o-	black
photo-	light
poli/o-	gray (relating to gray matter of the nervous system)
rhod/o-	red
ruber, rubor	red, redness
xanth/o-	yellow, yellowish

REVIEW QUESTIONS: BODY FLUIDS, SUBSTANCES, CHEMICALS, AND COLORS

Fill in the blanks: Give the meaning of the underlined combining forms:

1. ceruminolytic ______________________.
2. hyperhidrosis ______________________.
3. adipocyte ______________________.
4. cyanmethemoglobin ______________________.
5. melanocyte ______________________.

Give the word, root, and/or combining form for each word:

6. water ______________________.
7. mucus ______________________.
8. pus ______________________.
9. clear blood fluid ______________________
10. milk ______________________

Matching: Match the underlined word or word part with its meaning:

G.	1. rubor red	A. stony hardness petrous
E	2. leukorrhea white	B. saliva ptyal
J	3. poliomyelitis ~~stony hardness~~ gray	C. sugar saracc
I	4. urogenital urine	D. salt sal
H	5. cholecyst bile	E. white leuk
a	6. petrous stony hard	F. iron ferr
C	7. polysaccharide sugar	G. red rubar
B	8. ptyalism saliva	H. bile chole
D	9. saline ~~bile~~ salt	I. urine uro
F	10. ferritin iron	J. gray polio

REVIEW QUESTIONS: BODY FLUIDS, SUBSTANCES, CHEMICALS AND COLORS

Answers

Fill in the blanks:

1. earwax
2. sweat
3. fat
4. blue
5. black
6. aqua, hydro-
7. muco-, myxo-
8. pyo-
9. plasma, serum, sero-
10. galacto-, lacto-

Matching:

1. G
2. E
3. J
4. I
5. H
6. A
7. C
8. B
9. D
10. F

Chapters 2, 3, and 4 — EXERCISES

THE COMPLETE FOUNDATION

The following exercises provide a review of the basic foundation material presented. The word parts are not necessarily clustered according to use, as was done in the preceding exercises. Approach the exercises as a challenge. You may find it necessary to look back through Chapter 2 and Chapter 3, as well as this one, to locate answers you may not remember. Once more, try to avoid using the answer page except as a final check.

Exercise 1: For each pair of words, indicate whether the underlined parts have the same or opposite meanings.

1. oligodendrocyte
   polymorphonuclear ______
2. macronutrient
   splenomegaly ______
3. leptomeninges
   pachyderm ______
4. levorotary
   dextrorotary ______
5. erythrocyte
   rhodopsin ______
6. poikilocytosis
   homeothermic ______
7. sinistrad
   dextrose ______
8. hydrolysis
   xerophthalmia ______
9. leukocyte
   linea alba ______
10. hematoma
    sanguine ______
11. hydrophobic
    basophil ______
12. diphasic
    biconcave ______
13. osteomalacia
    atherosclerosis ______
14. bronchiectasis
    aortostenosis ______

Exercise 2: This exercise is to help you learn to break veterinary medical words into their component parts to define them. Write the meaning of each component in the space provided, and then define the word. Do not define those suffixes following a slash (/) mark.

1. postocular:
   post after behind
   ocul/ar eye
   behind the eye.

2. gluconeogenesis:
   gluco sugar
   neo new
   genesis formation
   new sugar formation

3. hypoglycemia:
   hypo ~~[illegible]~~ deficicent
   glyc Sugar
   emia blood condition
   dificient sugar in blood
4. microscope:
   micro to small for naked eye
   scope examing insterment
   ~~[illegible]~~ examing insterment for small objects
5. oophorectomy:
   oophor ovary
   ectomy SX remove
   removing ovary SX
6. hematopoiesis:
   hemato blood
   poiesis formation
   formation of blood
7. endocardium:
   endo inner
   cardi/um heart
   inner heart lining
8. intercostal:
   inter between
   cost/al ribs
   between the ribs
9. thoracotomy:
   thoraco Chest
   tomy to remove SX
   SX opening chest
10. osteomalacia:
    osteo bone
    malac/ia Softening
    Softening of the bone
11. xerography:
    xero dry
    graphy record
    dry imaging process
12. onychectomy:
    onych nail
    ectomy SX remove
    declawing
13. anisocoria:
    an not
    iso equal
    cor/ia pupil of eye
    unequal size pupil
14. pleomorphism:
    pleo many
    morph/ism form
    many forms
15. hydronephrosis:
    hydro water
    nephr kidney
    osis codition
    collecting fluid in kidney
16. retrocervical:
    retro behind
    cervic/al refering to cervix
    behind the cervix

17. leukocytopenia:
    leuko white
    cyto Cell
    penia lack of
    lack of WBC

18. urethrostomy:
    urethro urethra
    stomy Sx opening
    Sx opening up urethra

19. polychromatophilia:
    poly many
    chromato colors
    philia affinaty
    Attracting many colors

20. achromatopsia:
    a Not
    chromat color
    opsia vision
    lack of color vision

21. mucolytic:
    muco mucous
    lytic breaking down
    ~~...~~ breaking down mucous

22. panophthalmitis:
    pan All
    ophthalm eye
    itis inflammation
    inflammation of entire eye

23. cardiomyopathy:
    cardio heart
    myo muscle
    pathy disease
    disease of the heart muscle

24. pyometra:
    pyo pus
    metra uritus
    pus in~~fected~~ uritus

25. sialodacryoadenitis:
    sialo saliva
    dacryo tears
    aden glands
    itis inflammation
    inflammation of the saliva & tear glands

Exercise 3: In the blank space provided opposite each word, fill in the appropriate word, root, or combining form.

1. Bile Chole cholo
2. Sweat hidro, sudor
3. Saliva ptyalo, sialo
4. Iron ferrum ~~ferro~~
5. Fluid portion of blood plasma serum
6. Salt sal
7. Sugar gluco, glyco, sacchero sacchari
8. Oil eleo oleo
9. Starch amylo
10. Sebaceous gland secretions sebum

Exercise 4: In the blank write the meaning of the underlined part of each word:

1. abrade away from
2. adsorb toward
3. costochondral rib
4. exophthalmia out of
5. extravasation beyond
6. genotype producing
7. hemagglutination blood
8. hepatectomy liver
9. homozygote same, alike
10. intraventricular within
11. liposome fat
12. proteolysis breaking down
13. metazoa change
14. neurotoxin nerve
15. chromatophobe abnormal fear
16. photoreceptor light
17. neoplasia new
18. presynaptic before
19. tarsometatarsal human ankle
20. transudate across
21. urolithiasis urine

CHAPTER 4 PUZZLE

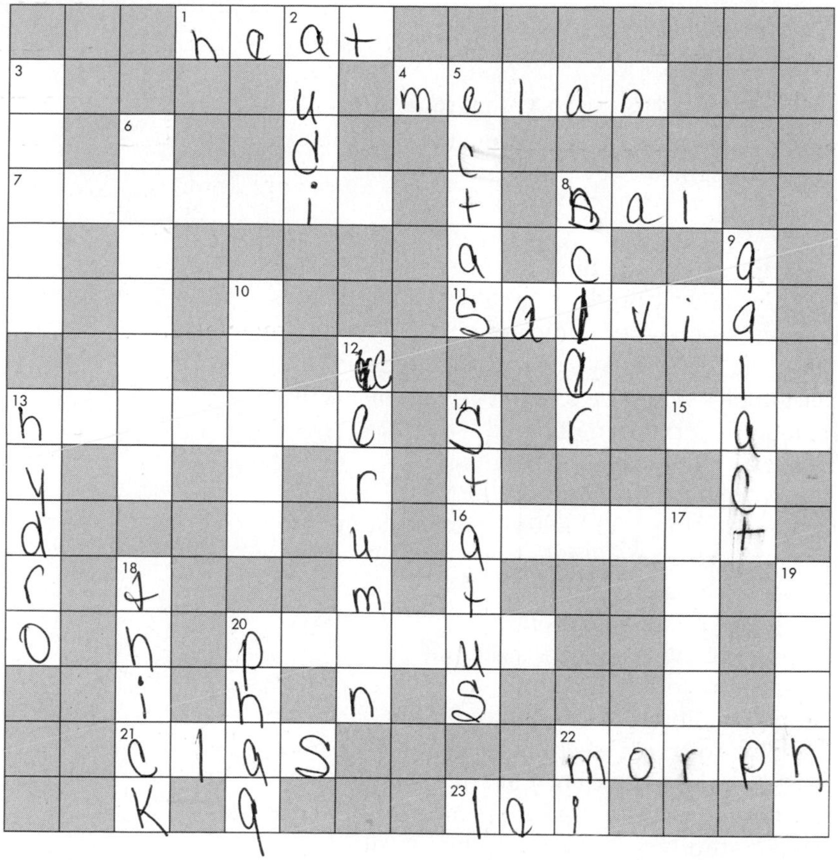

ACROSS CLUES

1. meaning of therm
4. root for black
7. root for formation
8. root for salt
11. meaning of the root ptyal
13. chemical substance produced by the body
15. meaning of the root mal
16. word meaning lead away from
20. root meaning paralysis
21. root meaning break
22. root meaning form, shape, structure
23. root meaning smooth

DOWN CLUES

2. root meaning hearing
3. root meaning stone
5. root meaning dilate
6. a cleft or groove
8. root meaning hardness
9. root meaning milk
10. root meaning twisted or crooked
12. word for earwax
13. root for wet or water
14. root for standing still
17. meaning of the root chrom
18. meaning of the root pachy
19. root meaning fast
20. root for eating

Chapters 2, 3, and 4 Answers

Exercise 1

1. opposite
2. same
3. opposite
4. opposite
5. same
6. opposite
7. opposite
8. opposite
9. same
10. same
11. opposite
12. same
13. opposite
14. opposite

Exercise 2

1. behind; referring to eye—behind the eye
2. sugar; new; formation—production of new sugar
3. deficient; sugar; blood—deficient sugar in the blood
4. small; examining instrument—instrument to examine small objects
5. ovary; excision of—surgical excision of ovary or ovaries
6. blood; formation—formation of blood
7. within or inner; heart—inner heart lining
8. between; referring to ribs—between the ribs
9. chest or thorax; cutting, incision—surgical opening into the chest
10. bone; softening—softening of bone
11. dry; record—a dry imaging process
12. nail; cut out—declawing operation
13. not; equal; pupil of eye—unequal sized pupils
14. many; form—many forms
15. water; kidney; condition—collection of fluid in kidney(s)
16. behind; referring to cervix—behind the (uterine) cervix
17. white; cell; deficiency—deficiency of white blood cells
18. urethra; surgical opening—surgical opening into the urethra
19. many; color(s); affinity for—attracting many colors
20. not; color; vision—lack of color vision
21. mucus; breaking down—breaking down mucus
22. all; eye; inflammation—inflammation of entire eye
23. heart; muscle; disease—disease of heart muscle
24. pus; uterus—pus in the uterus
25. saliva; tears; gland; inflammation—inflammation of the salivary and tear glands

Exercise 3

1. chole- cholo-
2. hidro- sudor
3. sialo-, ptyalo-
4. ferrum
5. plasma, serum
6. sal
7. glyco-, saccharo-, sacchari-
8. eleo-, oleo-
9. amylo-
10. sebum

Exercise 4

1. away from
2. toward, to
3. rib
4. out of, from
5. outside of, beyond
6. producing
7. blood
8. liver
9. same, alike
10. within
11. fat, fatty acids
12. breaking down
13. change, beyond, after
14. nerve
15. fear or intolerance
16. light
17. new
18. before, in front of
19. area corresponding to human ankle
20. across, through
21. urine or urea

ANSWERS: CHAPTER 4 PUZZLE

			1 H	E	2 A	T								
3 L					U		4 M	5 E	L	A	N			
A		6 F			D			C						
7 P	O	I	E	S	I	S		T		8 S	A	L		
I		S						A		C			9 G	
S		S		10 S				11 S	A	L	I	V	A	
		U		C		12 C				E			L	
13 H	O	R	M	O	N	E		14 S		R		15 B	A	D
Y		E		L		R		T					C	
D				I		U		16 A	B	D	U	17 C	T	
R		18 T				M		S				O		19 T
A		H		20 P	L	E	G	I	A			L		A
		I		H		N		S				O		C
		21 C	L	A	S					22 M	O	R	P	H
		K		G				23 L	E	I				Y

II

THE BODY SHELL AND ITS SUPPORTS

Section II of LEARNING VETERINARY TERMINOLOGY consists of four chapters introducing the student to the language of body structure and the systems that support, move, and protect it.

Chapter 5 acquaints the student with the branches of science that deal with the study of the animal body, body structure development, and the terms used to describe directions, planes, positions, and regions of the body. Beginning with this chapter, a glossary relating to the material in the text will be found at the end of each chapter.

Chapter 6 discusses the skeletal system and its function as a supporting framework for the body.

Chapter 7 presents the muscular system, which, in conjunction with the skeletal system, produces body movement.

Chapter 8 describes the integumentary system (the skin and its accessory structures) and its various functions.

Drawings illustrate the principal parts of the anatomy in each chapter.

5 Understanding the Animal Body and Its Structure

CHAPTER OVERVIEW

This chapter describes the basic structures of the animal body, their characteristics, and their composition. Descriptive anatomic terms are introduced in chart form.

STUDY OF THE ANIMAL BODY

Six major disciplines (branches of science) deal with the study of the body: anatomy, physiology, pathology, embryology, histology, and biology.

Anatomy, which literally means cutting apart, is the study of the structure of the body and the relationship of its parts. Examination of the structures of various animal species is called *comparative anatomy.* Knowledge of these characteristics helps to classify animals.

Physiology is the study of the normal functions and activities of organisms.

Pathology is the study of the changes caused by disease in the structure and functions of living things.

Embryology is the study of the origin and development of an individual organism. It begins after conception, or fertilization of the egg, through *parturition,* or birth.

Histology is the microscopic study of the minute structure, composition, and function of normal cells and tissues.

Biology is the study of all forms of life.

Veterinarians also combine these words to specify particular areas of concern. *Histopathology,* for example, is the microscopic study of diseased tissues. *Pathophysiology* is the study of abnormal function of cells and tissues. Many other combinations are used.

BASIC STRUCTURE

The body may be compared with a machine, its many parts working together to promote good health, growth, and life itself. It is a combination of organs and systems supported by a framework of muscles and bones, with an external covering of skin for protection.

The *cell* is the smallest unit of life from which tissues, organs, and systems are constructed (*cyt-* is the root for *cell*). Cells similar in structure and function form a mass called a *tissue.* Groups of different tissues combine to form an *organ* (for example, liver, heart, or lungs), each of which performs a special function. The organs are grouped into *systems* that perform specific and more complicated functions. A complete set of systems (cardiovascular, respiratory, gastrointestinal, etc.) makes up each *organism,* or individual animal.

CHARACTERISTICS OF LIVING MATTER

Animals are maintained by a process called *metabolism* (*meta-* means change, *bolus* refers to mass, and *-ism* means condition). Metabolism is the sum of the processes of *anabolism*

Cell
↓
A group of cells
↓
Forms a tissue
↓
A group of tissues
↓
Forms an organ
↓
A group of organs
↓
Forms a system
↓
All systems together
↓
Form an organism

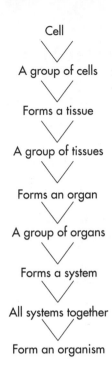

(*ana*- means building up) and *catabolism* (*cata*- means breaking down). When metabolism ceases, the organism dies.

All living matter is irritable and excitable: It reacts to stimulation. With appropriate stimulation, nerve cells conduct impulses, muscle cells contract, and gland cells secrete substances.

CELLS

Understanding the structure and function of animals begins with the smallest unit of life, the cell. Specialized cells carry out the functions of growth, secretion, excretion, irritability, nutrition, and reproduction. They are activated by mechanical, chemical, or nervous stimulation.

Each cell of the body is enclosed by a membrane called the *plasma membrane*. This membrane protects the internal structure of the cell and regulates the passage of materials in and out of the cell. Inside the membrane is a jellylike substance, *cytoplasm*, surrounding a centrally located body, the *nucleus* (Fig. 5-1).

The cytoplasm contains *fibers* that provide a support lattice for the cell framework and huge numbers of *organelles* (little organs) outside the nucleus, including the following:

The *endoplasmic reticulum* is a network of canals consisting of smooth and rough portions. The smooth portion manufactures carbohydrates and some fats. Attached to the rough portion are thousands of granules called *ribosomes,* made up of ribonucleic acid (RNA). The ribosomes make proteins before passing them on to the Golgi apparatus.

The *Golgi apparatus* consists of vesicles, or small sacs, believed to manufacture carbohydrates and combine them with protein in a closed globule secreted by the cell.

The *mitochondria* (singular is *mitochondrion*) are microscopic sacs with enzyme molecules attached to their membranous walls. These organelles are the "power plants" of the cell, supplying its energy.

The *lysosomes* are membranous closed sacs containing enzymes that digest large molecules and particles for use by the cell. They also protect the cell by digesting invading bacteria by *phagocytosis* (*phago*- means eating).

The *nucleus,* enclosed in a membrane called the *nuclear membrane,* is a *spheroid* (round), centrally located body. The nucleus is a highly specialized part of the cell, regulating growth and reproduction. It contains deoxyribonucleic acid (DNA) molecules, which determine heredity. During cell divi-

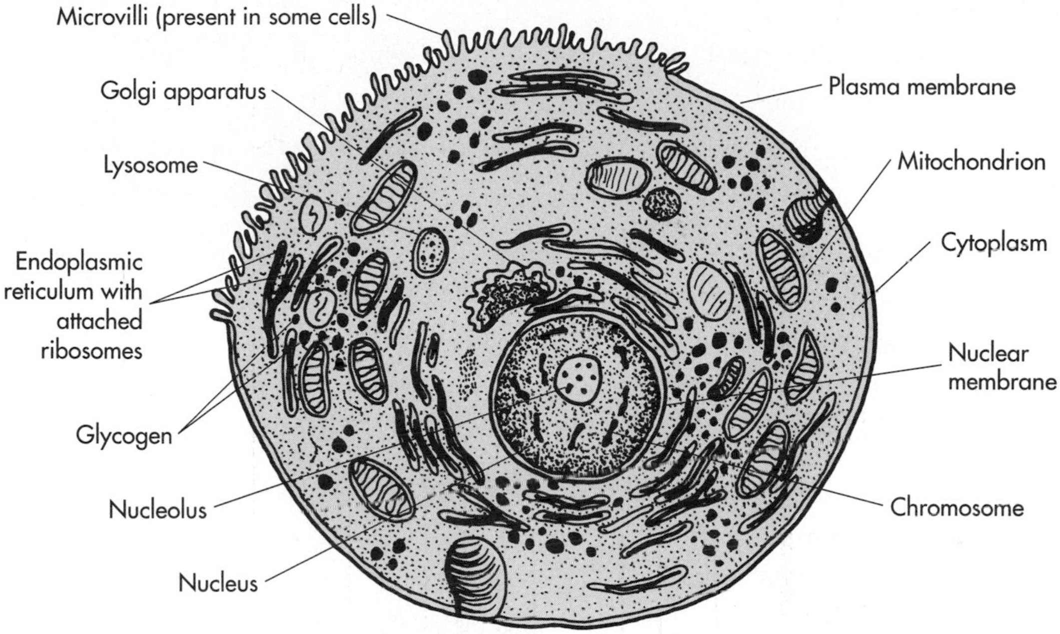
Microvilli (present in some cells)
Golgi apparatus
Lysosome
Endoplasmic reticulum with attached ribosomes
Glycogen
Nucleolus
Nucleus
Plasma membrane
Mitochondrion
Cytoplasm
Nuclear membrane
Chromosome

FIG. 5-1 Diagram of a cell showing cellular structures, as seen with the electron microscope.

sion, the DNA molecules become short and rodlike and are then called *chromosomes.*

There are 60 chromosomes (30 pairs) in all bovine cells. The exception is mature sex cells, which have only half this number (30 total). At conception the mature male and female sex (reproductive) cells unite. They each contribute a chance combination of 30 chromosomes out of innumerable possible combinations.

All individuals within a species have the same number of chromosomes, but there is variation between animal species in the number of chromosomes. Some common animals and their total chromosome number are as follows:

Species	Chromosome number
Dog	78
Horse	64
Cattle	60
Goat	60
Sheep	54
Swine	38
Cat	38

The *nucleolus* is a round body within the nucleus, consisting mainly of RNA. It combines RNA with protein to form the ribosomes.

REVIEW A

1. The disciplines that deal with structure and function of animal bodies are __________________ and __________________, respectively.
2. __________________ is the study of the origin and development of an individual organism.
3. The microscopic study of diseased tissues is called __________________ .
4. The metabolic processes involved with building up are called __________________, whereas the processes involved with breaking down are called __________________ .
5. Name the organelles described in each of the following:
   a. Consists of smooth and rough portions __________________
   b. Is made up of vesicles, or small sacs __________________
   c. Are the "power plants" of the cell __________________
   d. Are sacs of enzymes __________________
   e. Are extranuclear RNA granules __________________
6. DNA molecules become short and rodlike during cell division, when they are called __________________ .
7. The nucleolus consists mainly of __________________ .

TISSUES

Tissues are groups of specialized cells that are similar in structure and function but have different characteristics in accordance with their function. The basic types of tissue are *epithelial, connective, muscle,* and *nerve.*

Epithelial Tissue

Epithelial tissue (*epi-* means upon, on, or over) is found throughout the animal. It makes up the outer covering of external and internal body surfaces such as the skin, mucous membranes, serous membranes, and the lining of the digestive, respiratory, and urinary tracts.

The main functions of epithelial tissue are to protect, absorb, and secrete. For example, the skin protects underlying structures; other types allow substances to pass through them and serve as absorbing tissue (lungs and intestines) or secreting tissue (mucous membranes and glands).

A special type of epithelial tissue called *endothelium* (*endo-* means within or inner) lines the heart, blood and lymph vessels, and other serous body cavities. *Mesothelium* (*meso-* means middle), another type of epithelial tissue, covers the surface of serous membranes (pleura, pericardium, and peritoneum).

There are various types of epithelial tissue (Fig. 5-2), classified according to the number of layers of cells:

Simple epithelial tissue has one layer of cells.

Stratified epithelial tissue has three or more layers of cells.

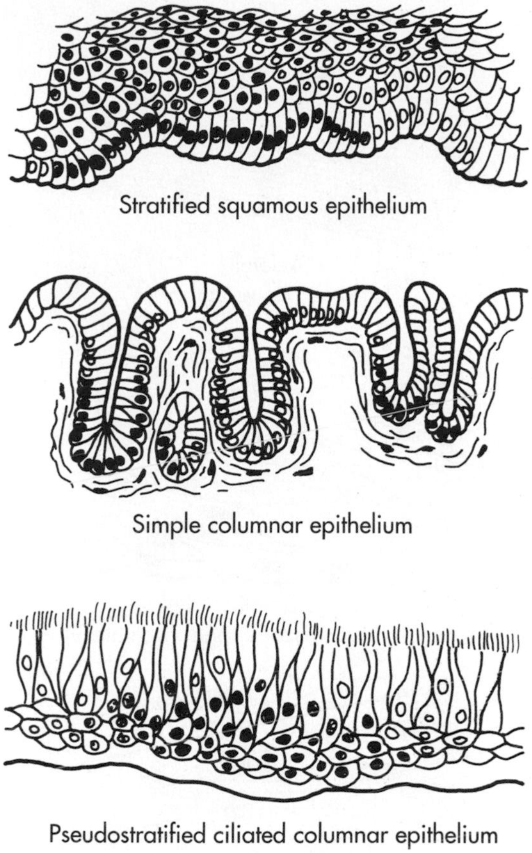
Stratified squamous epithelium
Simple columnar epithelium
Pseudostratified ciliated columnar epithelium

FIG. 5-2 Types of epithelial tissue.

Pseudostratified epithelial tissue has one layer of cells but appears to have more.

Epithelial tissue is further subdivided according to the shape of the surface layer of the cells:

Squamous cells have a flat appearance.

Cuboidal cells have a cubelike appearance.

Columnar cells resemble columns.

Transitional cells vary from squamous to cuboidal because they are found only in the urinary tract and change appearance according to the amount of pressure to which they are subjected.

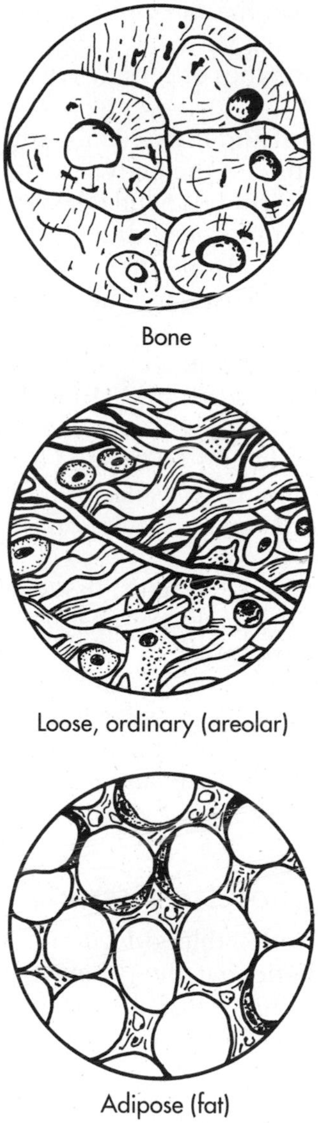
Bone
Loose, ordinary (areolar)
Adipose (fat)

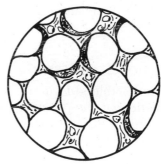

FIG. 5-3 Three types of connective tissue.

All types are composed largely or entirely of cells that undergo *mitosis* (cell division) to replace old or damaged cells.

Connective Tissue

Connective tissue, the most widespread tissue, forms the framework of animals, holds organs in place, and connects body parts to each other (Fig. 5-3).

The main types of connective tissue are as follows:

Bone, hard and unbendable, supports and protects the body.

Cartilage, firm but bendable, is found throughout the body.

Dense fibrous tissue, strong and bendable, is found mostly in tendons and ligaments.

Reticular tissue, in weblike networks, supports nerves and capillaries; provides the framework for the spleen, lymph nodes, and bone marrow; and destroys harmful matter. *Reticular* is from a Latin word meaning network.

Loose, ordinary (areolar) tissue, elastic and stretchable, connects adjacent body structures.

Adipose, fatty tissue, pads and protects organs, stores excess fat, and insulates against body heat loss.

Hematopoietic tissue and *blood* are included by some histologists.

Hematopoietic Tissue

Hematopoietic (blood-forming) tissue is found in bone marrow (Chapter 6) and the lymphatic system (Chapter 9).

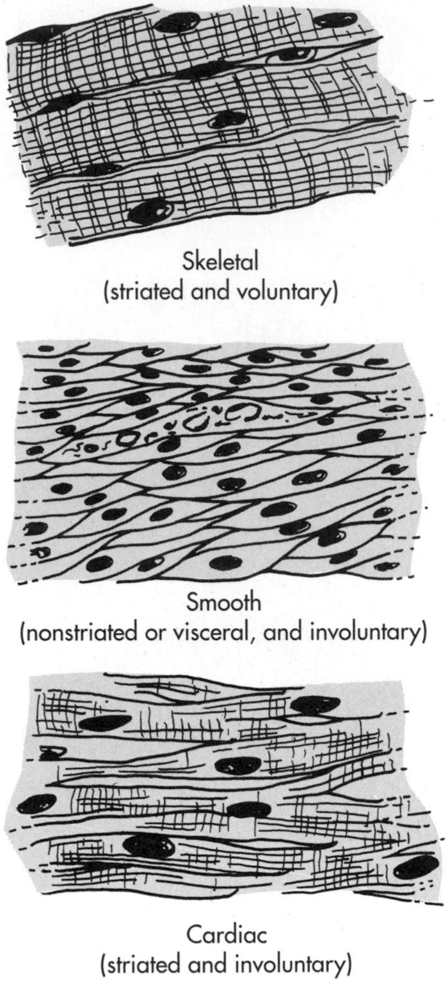
Skeletal
(striated and voluntary)
Smooth
(nonstriated or visceral, and involuntary)
Cardiac
(striated and involuntary)

FIG. 5-4 Types of muscle tissue.

Blood Tissue

Blood tissue is found in the blood vessels (Chapter 9).

Muscle Tissue

There are three types of muscle tissue: *skeletal,* which is *striated* (striped) and *voluntary* (movable at will); *smooth,* which is *nonstriated* (visceral) and involuntary; and *cardiac,* which is striated but involuntary. Skeletal muscles move bones. Visceral muscles are in the walls of hollow internal structures (blood vessels, intestines, and the uterus). Cardiac muscle makes up the heart (Fig. 5-4).

The main function of muscle tissue is to contract. Muscle cells are long and slender and are called *fibers.* The fibers decrease in length and increase in thickness during muscle contraction.

Nervous Tissue

Nervous tissue is composed of nerve cells called *neurons,* nerve fibers, and supporting tissue between the cells and fibers to keep them in position (see Fig. 14-1). The supporting structure of nervous tissue is *neuroglia* (*neuro-* means nerve; *-glia* means glue). Nervous tissue is the most highly specialized tissue in the body, needing more oxygen and more nutrition than any other body tissue. Nerve structure is described more completely in Chapter 14.

REVIEW B

1. The inside of the heart and blood vessels is lined with a special type of epithelium called ________________ .
2. When an epithelial tissue is described as *simple,* it means that ________________ .
3. What shape are *squamous* epithelial cells? ________________
4. Weblike networks of connective tissue are called ________________ connective tissue.
5. Loose, ordinary connective tissue is also called ________________ connective tissue.
6. Circle the correct word in each pair of parentheses.
   a. Skeletal muscle is (striated, nonstriated) and (voluntary, involuntary).
   b. Smooth muscle is (striated, nonstriated) and (voluntary, involuntary).
   c. Cardiac muscle is (striated, nonstriated) and (voluntary, involuntary).
7. The stem *-glia* in *neuroglia* means ________________ .

ORGANS

In the body, groups of cells form tissues, and similar tissues form organs (e.g., the heart, lungs, liver, and kidneys). Although they act as units, organs do not function independently; several combine to form a system, with each system having a special function.

SYSTEMS

A *system* is a combination of organs that performs a particular function. The systems of the body and their functions are as follows:

Skeletal—framework of the body; supports organs, furnishes a place of attachment for muscles.

Muscular—permits motion and movement of the body.

Integumentary—includes skin, hair, nails, sweat, and sebaceous glands. Covers and protects the body, aids in temperature regulation, and has functions in sensation and excretion.

Cardiovascular—transports the blood and includes the *lymphatic* system, which retrieves plasma and tissue fluids and protects against disease organisms.

Respiratory—absorbs oxygen and discharges carbon dioxide.

Gastrointestinal—digests and absorbs food and excretes waste.

Urogenital—provides for reproduction and urine excretion.

Endocrine—manufactures hormones.

Nervous—with the *special senses,* processes stimuli and enables the body to act and respond.

DIRECTIONS AND ANATOMIC PLANES

A number of anatomic terms are used in describing the animal body and determining direction. The terms listed refer to the quadrupedal vertebrate, standing on four limbs. Directions generally refer to relative locations, not absolute points (Fig. 5-5).

CLARIFICATION OF DIRECTIONS

Anterior—situated at the front. In bipeds, *anterior* is synonymous with *ventral.* In quadrupeds, *anterior* should correctly be limited to use within the head. However, *anterior* is commonly used to mean *cranial.*

Posterior—situated toward the back. In bipeds, *posterior* is synonymous with *dorsal.* In quadrupeds, *posterior* should correctly be limited to use within the head. However, *posterior* is commonly used to mean *caudal.*

Superior—above.

Inferior—below. These words, like *anterior* and *posterior,* make less sense when referring to quadrupeds than to bipeds. They are seldom used in veterinary terminology.

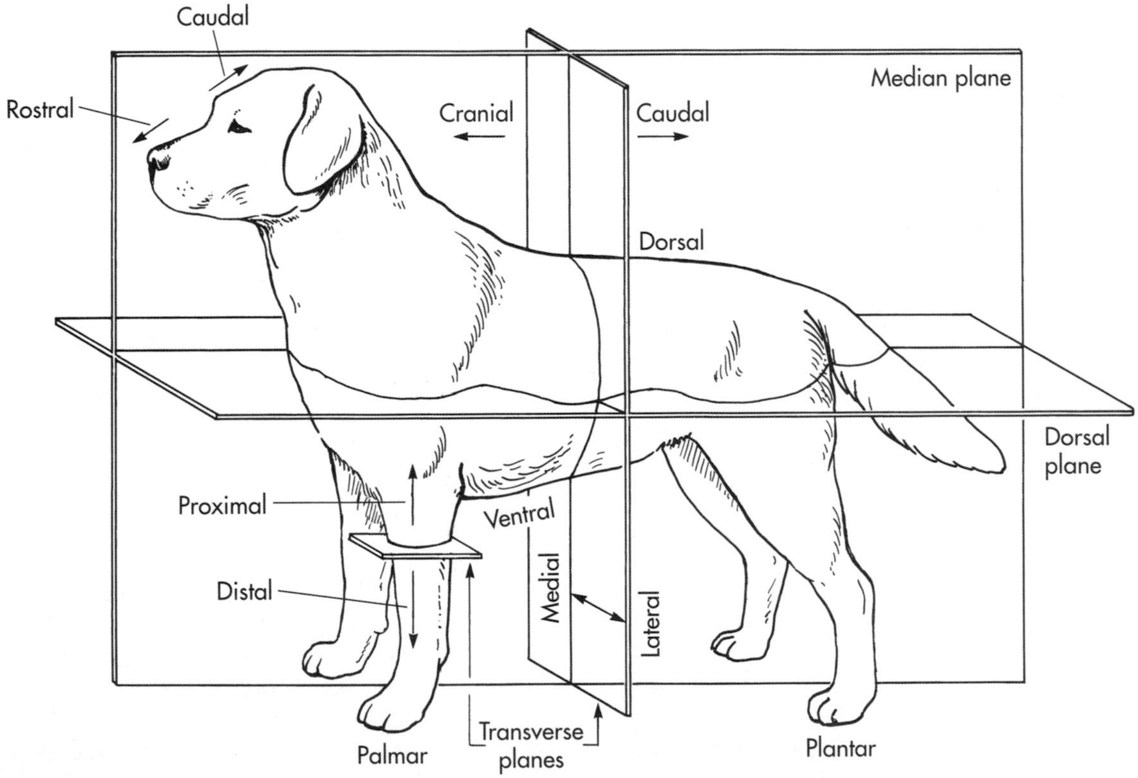
Caudal
Rostral
Cranial
Caudal
Median plane
Dorsal
Dorsal plane
Proximal
Ventral
Distal
Medial
Lateral
Palmar
Transverse planes
Plantar

FIG. 5-5 Anatomic directions and planes.

DIRECTIONS

Cranial—toward the head (cranium).

Caudal—toward the tail (cauda). *Caudal* also describes the direction specifically within the head and toward the tail.

Rostral—within the head and toward the muzzle (rostrum, beak).

Medial—nearer to or toward the midline (*medianus,* in the middle).

Lateral—farther from the midline or toward the side (*latus,* flank) of the body.

Dorsal—toward the back *(dorsum).*

Ventral—toward the belly *(venter).*

Proximal—nearer to the point of origin or closer (*proximus,* near) to the body.

Distal—farther from the point of origin or away (*distantia,* distance) from the body.

Palmar (volar)—caudal surface of the forelimb below the *carpus* (knee).

Plantar—caudal surface of the hind limb below the tarsus *(hock).*

Internal (deep)—inside.

External (superficial)—outside.

ANATOMIC PLANES

Dorsal (frontal) plane—a section through the side of the body, passing at right angles to the median plane and dividing the body into dorsal and ventral portions

Median (midsagittal, midline) plane—an imaginary plane that passes from the front to the back through the center of the body and divides the body into right and left equal portions

Sagittal plane—a section parallel to the long axis of the body or parallel to the median plane, dividing the body into right and left unequal parts

Transverse plane (cross-sectional)—a perpendicular transection to the long axis of the trunk, head, limb, or other appendage

ANATOMIC POSITIONS

Numerous terms describe anatomic positions. Some of the more common terms are listed here:

Recumbent—lying down

Ventrally recumbent—lying down on the belly

Sternally recumbent (prone)—lying down on the breastbone (sternum)

Dorsally recumbent (supine)—lying down on the backbone (vertebrae)

Laterally recumbent—lying down on the side

Left laterally recumbent—lying down on the left side

Right laterally recumbent—lying down on the right side

EXTERNAL PARTS OF THE GOAT (Fig. 5-6)

Poll—dorsal surface of the cranium
Horn butt—site of previous horn growth on the poll region of the head between the eyes and ears
Forehead—region of the head between the eyes and ears
Bridge of nose—the nasal bone
Muzzle—part of the face including the nasal bone and upper and lower lips
Jaw—either of the two bones of the mouth (maxilla or mandible)
Neck—the area connecting the head to the trunk of the body
Shoulder—the region around the joint connecting the scapula and the humerus
Brisket—the cranial portion of the chest
Chest floor—the ventral region of the sternum
Elbow—the joint connecting the humerus with the radius and ulna
Forearm—the portion of the forelimb between the elbow and carpus, containing the radius, ulna, and carpal bones
Knee—carpal bones
Shank (cannon)—the metacarpal (metatarsal) bone
Fetlock—the joint connecting the metacarpal (metatarsal) and the proximal phalanx
Dewclaw—an accessory claw that projects caudally from the fetlock
Pastern—joint connecting the proximal and middle phalanges
Hoof (foot)—the horny covering of the distal phalanx
Toe—the cranial end of the hoof
Heel (bulb)—the rear or caudal region of the hoof
Sole—the underside or ventral aspect of the hoof
Topline—the area of the vertebral column that extends from the withers to the tail head
Withers—the junction of the dorsal margins of the scapulae
Heartgirth—the circumference of the chest, measured just behind the withers and elbows, in inches
Back—the part of the vertebral column consisting of the chine and the loin
Chine—the thoracic region of the back
Loin—the lumbar region of the back
Rump—the region of the topline extending from the sacrum to the tail head
Tail head—the base of the tail where it lies between the pinbones
Ribs—the paired curved bones extending from the thoracic vertebrae to the ventral portion of the trunk
Barrel—the abdominal cavity of the animal body
Hipbone (hook)—the point of the hip or tuber coxae
Pinbone (pin)—the caudal prominence of the ischium, called tuber ischii
Flank—the side of the body extending from the last rib to the hind limb
Stifle (corresponds to the human knee)—the joint connecting the femur with the tibia and fibula
Hock—the tarsal bones
Udder—the mammary gland of farm animals
Teat—the nipple of the mammary gland
Milk vein—the large subcutaneous abdominal blood vessel that transports blood away from the udder

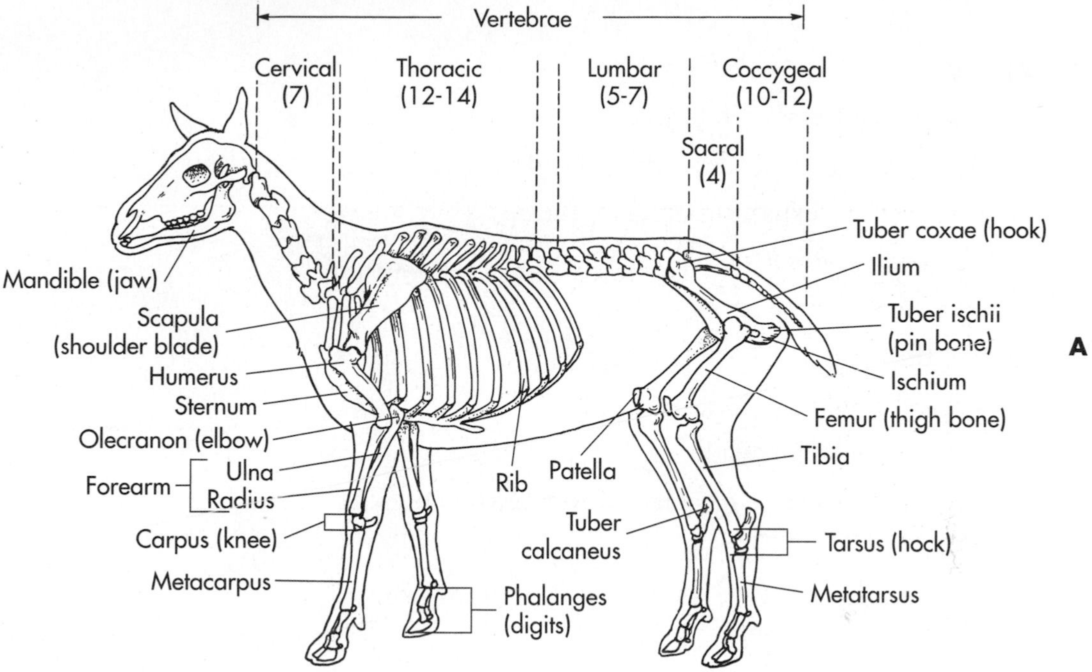
Vertebrae
Cervical
(7)
Thoracic
(12-14)
Lumbar
(5-7)
Coccygeal
(10-12)
Sacral
(4)
Tuber coxae (hook)
Ilium
Tuber ischii
(pin bone)
Ischium
Femur (thigh bone)
Tibia
Tarsus (hock)
Metatarsus
Mandible (jaw)
Scapula
(shoulder blade)
Humerus
Sternum
Olecranon (elbow)
Forearm
Ulna
Radius
Carpus (knee)
Metacarpus
Rib
Patella
Tuber
calcaneus
Phalanges
(digits)
A

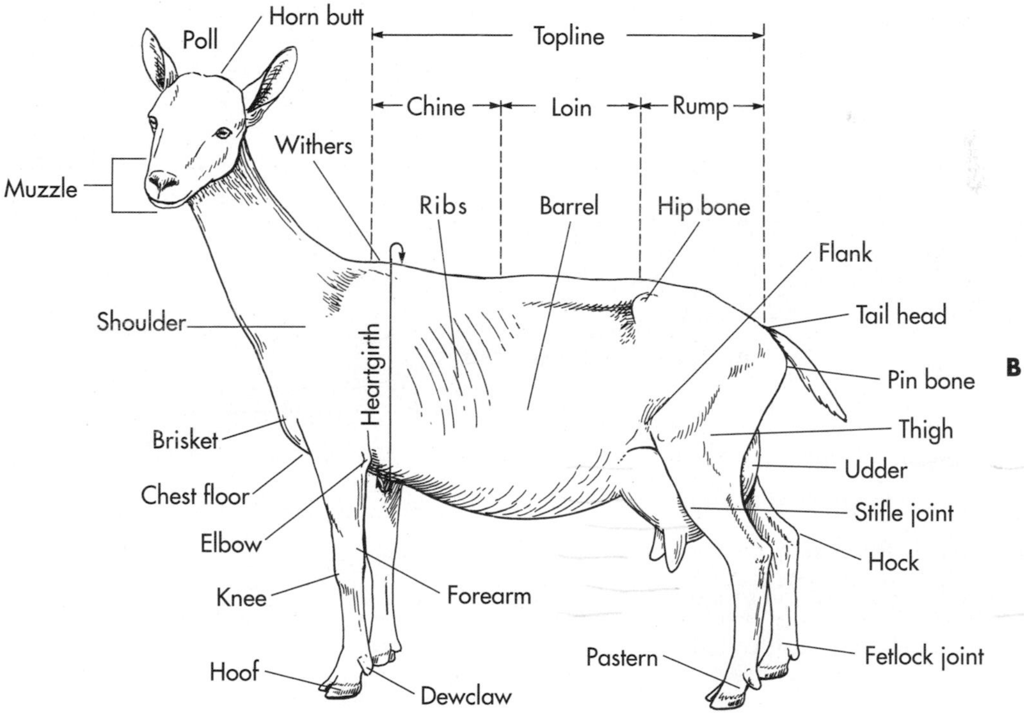
Poll
Horn butt
Topline
Chine
Loin
Rump
Withers
Muzzle
Ribs
Barrel
Hip bone
Flank
Tail head
Shoulder
Heartgirth
Pin bone
Thigh
Brisket
Udder
Chest floor
Stifle joint
Elbow
Hock
Knee
Forearm
Fetlock joint
Pastern
Hoof
Dewclaw
B

FIG. 5-6 Anatomy of the goat. **A,** Skeleton. **B,** External parts.

REVIEW C

1. Which system performs each function?
   a. Absorbs oxygen, discharges carbon dioxide ____________________
   b. Covers the body exterior ____________________
   c. Digests and absorbs food ____________________
   d. Manufactures hormones ____________________
   e. Moves the body ____________________
   f. Processes stimuli ____________________
   g. Provides a solid framework ____________________
   h. Provides for both reproduction and urine excretion ____________________
   i. Transports blood ____________________
2. Give the directional term that means the opposite of each:
   a. Cranial ____________________
   b. Distal ____________________
   c. Lateral ____________________
   d. Plantar ____________________
   e. Posterior ____________________
   f. Rostral ____________________
   g. Superficial ____________________
   h. Ventral ____________________
   i. Volar ____________________
3. Name the anatomic plane described in each case:
   a. Divides the body into right and left unequal parts ____________________
   b. Is perpendicular to the long axis of a leg ____________________
   c. Divides the body into right and left equal parts ____________________
   d. Divides the body into dorsal and ventral parts ____________________
4. The anatomic position of a dog lying down on its right side is __________________________. The supine position is also called ____________________ .

Chapter 5 Answers

Review A

1. anatomy, physiology
2. embryology
3. histopathology
4. anabolism, catabolism
5. a. endoplasmic reticulum
   b. Golgi apparatus
   c. mitochondria
   d. lysosomes
   e. ribosomes
6. chromosomes
7. RNA

Review B

1. endothelium
2. there is only a single layer
3. flat
4. reticular
5. areolar
6. a. striated, voluntary
   b. nonstriated, involuntary
   c. striated, involuntary
7. glue

Review C

1. a. respiratory
   b. integumentary
   c. gastrointestinal
   d. endocrine
   e. muscular
   f. nervous
   g. skeletal
   h. urogenital
   i. cardiovascular
2. a. caudal
   b. proximal
   c. medial
   d. dorsal
   e. anterior
   f. caudal
   g. deep
   h. dorsal
   i. dorsal
3. a. sagittal
   b. transverse
   c. median, midsagittal, midline
   d. dorsal, frontal
4. right lateral recumbency, dorsal recumbency

Chapter 5 EXERCISES

THE BODY SHELL AND ITS SUPPORTS

Exercise 1: Complete the following:

1. Epithelial tissue with three or more layers of cells is called ________________ .
2. *Hematopoietic* means ________________ . Where is tissue of this type found? ________________
3. Two types of involuntary muscle are ________________ and ________________ . Two types of striated muscle are ________________ and ________________ .
4. Name the direction of movement indicated in each:
   a. From the brisket to the shoulder ________________
   b. From the elbow to the heart ________________
   c. From the elbow to the hoof on the same leg ________________
   d. From the first lumbar vertebra to the last thoracic vertebra ________________
   e. From the hock to the stifle on the same leg ________________
   f. From the midline to the ear ________________
   g. From the poll to the muzzle ________________
   h. From the thoracic vertebrae to the sternum ________________
   i. From the withers to the hip bone ________________
5. The ________________ surface of the hind foot touches the ground when the goat is standing. In the front foot the same surface is called the ________________ or ________________ surface.
6. The anatomic position of a dog lying down on its belly is ________________ .
7. The hock is composed of the ________________ bones.
8. An animal that walks on four feet is called a(n) ________________ .
9. The junction of the dorsal margins of the scapulae is called the ________________ .
10. An accessory and non–weight-bearing claw that projects caudally from the fetlock is called a ________________ .
11. The stifle joint corresponds to the human ________________ joint.

Exercise 2:

Match the definitions in the right column with the terms in the left column by placing the appropriate letter in the blank space provided.

_____ 1. Ventral	A. Lying on the backbone
_____ 2. Distal	B. Toward the head
_____ 3. Cranial	C. Lying down on the side
_____ 4. Caudal	D. Away from the body
_____ 5. Prone	E. Lying down on the breastbone
_____ 6. Supine	F. Cross section view of the body
_____ 7. Laterally recumbent	G. Toward the abdomen
_____ 8. Transverse plane	H. Caudal surface of the metatarsus
_____ 9. Rostral	I. Toward the muzzle
_____ 10. Plantar	J. Toward the tail

CHAPTER 5 PUZZLE

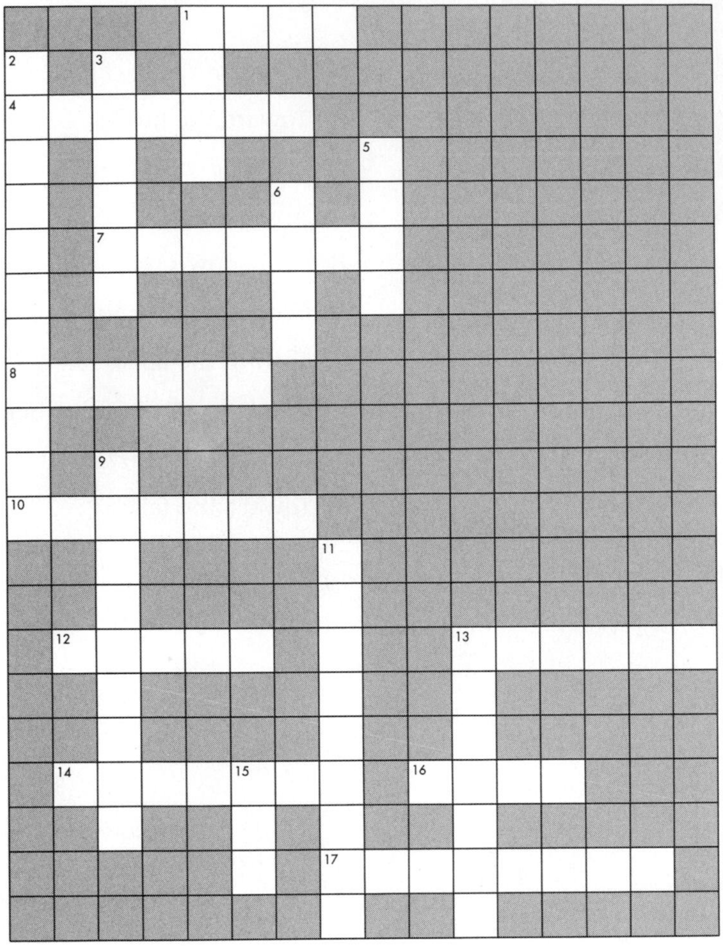
1
2
3
4
5
6
7
8
9
10
11
12
13
14
15
16
17

ACROSS CLUES

1. Hipbone.
4. Study of body structures.
7. Fatty tissue.
8. What a group of cells form.
10. Nerve cells.
12. Sternally recumbent.
13. Toward the midline.
14. Toward the belly.
16. Tarsus.
17. Striped.

DOWN CLUES

1. Horny covering of distal phalanx.
2. Birth.
3. Toward the tail.
5. Carpus.
6. Type of hard connective tissue.
9. Animal with four feet.
11. Jellylike substance of cells.
13. Type of cell division.
15. Ribonucleic acid.

Chapter 5 Answers

Exercise 1

1. stratified
2. blood-forming, bone marrow
3. smooth, cardiac; skeletal, cardiac
4. a. dorsally
   b. medially
   c. distally
   d. cranially
   e. proximally
   f. laterally
   g. rostrally
   h. ventrally
   i. caudally
5. plantar; palmar, volar
6. ventrally recumbent, sternally recumbent, prone
7. tarsal
8. quadruped
9. withers
10. dewclaw
11. knee

Exercise 2

1. G	6. A
2. D	7. C
3. B	8. F
4. J	9. I
5. E	10. H

ANSWERS: CHAPTER 5 PUZZLE

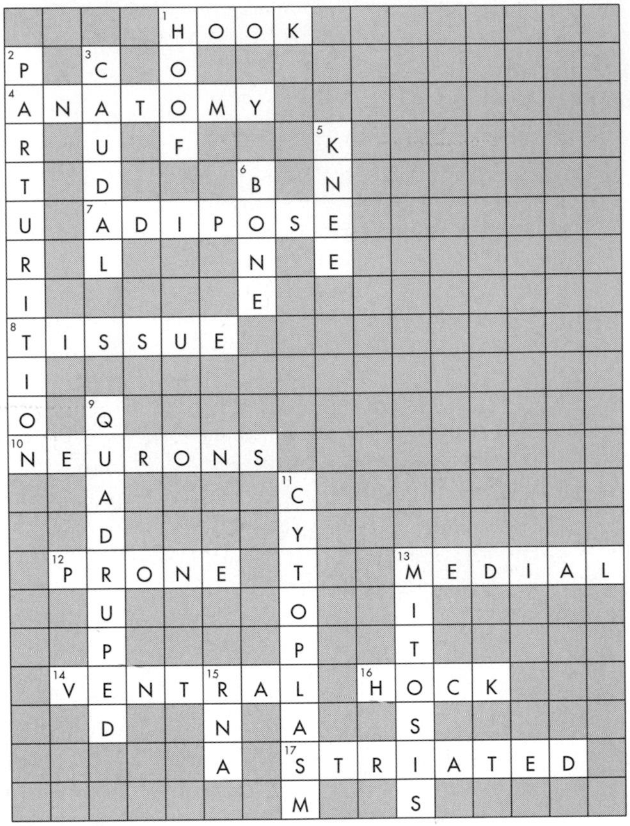
1 HOOK
4 ANATOMY
7 ADIPOSE
8 TISSUE
10 NEURONS
12 PRONE
13 MEDIAL
14 VENTRAL
16 HOCK
17 STRIATED
1 HOOF
2 PARTURITION
3 CAUDAL
5 KNEE
6 BONE
9 QUADRUPED
11 CYTOPLASM
13 MITOSIS
15 RNA

Beginning with this chapter, a *glossary* (word list with definitions) with phonetic pronunciation guides will be found at the end of each chapter to help you understand the terminology that relates to the material. Each glossary is organized according to its text, with some review material and some additions, including anatomic terms, diseases, conditions, procedures, and other descriptive terms.

GLOSSARY

adipose tissue (ad'ĭ-pōs): fatty connective tissue.

areolar tissue (ah-re'o-lar): elastic connective tissue connecting adjacent structures of the body.

biped (bi'ped): animal with two feet.

bony tissue: dense connective tissue that forms the skeletal framework of the body.

cardiac muscle tissue: heart muscle.

cartilage (kar'ti-lĭj): firm, elastic, somewhat dense connective tissue that forms many parts of the skeleton.

centrosome (sen'tro-som): area of cell cytoplasm near nucleus, containing *centrioles* (minute cells), which play an important part in *mitosis* (cell division).

chromosomes (kro'mo-sōmz): rodlike bodies in the nucleus composed mainly of DNA and containing the *genes,* which transmit the hereditary codes.

columnar epithelium (ko-lum'nar ep"ĭ-the'le-um): cells arranged in one layer, resembling columns.

connective tissue: forms framework of body, holds organs in place, and connects body parts to each other.

cuboidal epithelium: surface layer of cells having a cube-shaped appearance.

cytoplasm (si'to-plazm"): jelly-like substance of a cell within the plasma membrane, surrounding the nucleus.

dense fibrous tissue: strong, pliant connective tissue of the body, found where organs are subjected to stress or strain.

deoxyribonucleic (de-ok'se-ri"bo-nu-kle'ic) *acid* (DNA): large molecule that is the main constituent of chromosomes.

endothelium (en"do-the'le-um): layer of simple squamous cells lining the inner surfaces of the circulatory organs and serous body cavities.

enzyme (en'zīm): protein able to *catalyze* (speed up or change) chemical reactions in living cells.

epithelium (ep"i-the'le-um): tissue covering the external and internal body surfaces.

Golgi (gol'je) *apparatus:* cellular component of the cytoplasm, believed to condense substances before they leave the cell as secretions.

inorganic matter: mineral.

invertebrata (in-ver"tĕ-bra'tah): division of the animal kingdom including all forms with no backbone.

involuntary muscle tissue: muscle tissue that cannot be controlled at will; types are *visceral* (smooth, nonstriated) and *cardiac* (striated, striped).

lysosomes (li'so-sōmz): microscopic membranous sacs in the cytoplasm that contain enzymes capable of *phagocytosis* (digesting for nutrition and protection of the cell).

mesothelium (mes"o-the'le-um): epithelial tissue forming the surface cover of serous membranes that line the abdominal and chest cavities.

metabolism (mĕ-tab'o-lizm): sum of all physical and chemical processes by which living organisms are maintained.

mitochondria (mi"to-kon'dre-ah): organelles containing enzymes that are considered to be the source of energy for the cell (singular is *mitochondrion*).

mitosis (mi-to'sis): process of cell division.

molecule (mol'ĕ-kūl): chemical combination of two or more atoms that form a specific chemical substance (DNA and RNA are molecules).

nervous tissue: substance of which nerves and nerve centers are composed.

neuron (nur'-on): nerve cell.

nucleolus (nu-kle'o-lus): spherical body within the nucleus composed mainly of RNA and some protein (plural is *nucleoli*).

nucleus (nu'kle-us): spheroid body in a cell containing the chromosomes and nucleoli (plural is *nuclei*).

organelle: a differentiated structure within a cell, such as a ribosome or mitochondrion.

organic matter: animal and vegetable (living) matter.

organism: an individual form of life.

parturition (par-tur-ish'-un): act of giving birth.
phagocytosis (fag"o-si-to'sis): ingestion and digestion of particulate matter by cells.
phalanges (fa-lan'jez): plural form of *phalanx.*
phalanx (fa'-lanks): any principal bone segment of the digits of vertebrates.
quadruped (kwah'-dri-ped): animal having four feet.
ribonucleic (ri"bo-nu-kle'ik) *acid:* three types of molecules similar to DNA that relate to the function of the ribosomes.
ribosomes (ri'bo-sōmz): organelles in the cytoplasm attached to the endoplasmic reticulum that build and transmit proteins.
squamous (skwa'mus) *epithelium:* flat epithelial cells arranged in one or more layers.
stratified epithelium: cells arranged in three or more layers; may be columnar or squamous.
striated (stri'at-ed): striped.
transitional epithelium: tissue made up of cells varying from squamous to cuboidal according to the amount of pressure to which they are subjected.
vertebrata (ver"tĕ-bra'tah): division of the animal kingdom comprising all animals that have a vertebral column or backbone, including mammals, reptiles, fish, and birds.
voluntary muscle tissue: striated muscle tissue that can be controlled at will (also called skeletal muscle).

6 Skeletal System

The framework of the body

CHAPTER OVERVIEW

In this chapter we describe the bones of the body and the ways in which they connect and are moved. Evolutionary change has produced significant species differences in skeletal anatomy. Bones may be more developed, less developed, or even absent in some species.

The inorganic matter that gives bone its hardness contains higher proportions of calcium and phosphorus as the body ages, causing the bones to become brittle and fracture more easily in old age. The bones of young animals are thus more flexible and less subject to fracture than those of mature animals.

BONE

Bones support and give shape to the body in a jointed framework called the *skeleton*. This framework helps protect vital and delicate organs from external injury and furnishes attachment points for muscles, ligaments, and tendons, making body movement possible. Bones store mineral salts, and particular bones contain the hematopoietic (blood cell–forming) red bone marrow. The study of bone is called *osteology* (*os*- and *ost*- are roots meaning bone).

Bone Composition

Bone (osseous tissue), a specialized form of connective tissue, is about 50% water and 50% solid matter. Part of the solid matter consists of inorganic (mineral) salts, which give bone its hardness. When the embryonic skeleton is first formed, it is made of cartilage and fibrous membrane in the shape of bones, which harden and become bone before birth. Ossification continues until maturity; the length of time depends on the species.

Bone Structure

Bone consists of a hard outer shell called *compact bone tissue* and an inner, spongy, latticelike structure called *cancellated* or *cancellous* bone. The dense, compact bone is thick in the midshaft to avoid bending under stress and tapers to paper thinness at the ends. When a long bone in an adult animal is sectioned longitudinally, the *medullary cavity* (innermost part) of the *diaphysis* (shaft) is seen to be filled with yellow marrow, which stores fat. The yellow marrow has replaced red marrow, which is hematopoietic (red blood cell–forming) tissue containing red blood cells in various stages of growth (Fig. 6-1). In the adult animal, most red marrow has disappeared except for that found in spaces in cancellated bone, such as the flat bones of the skull, pelvis, vertebrae, ribs, and sternum and the upper ends of the shafts of the humerus and femur.

The bone surfaces, with the exception of the cartilage-covered articular surfaces, are covered by a tough, fibrous, vascular membrane called the *periosteum*, which is very thick, except where muscles are attached to the bone. The outer layer is vascular, and the inner layer in the growing bone is lined with *osteoblasts* (immature bone cells). The deposition of bone from this layer of osteoblasts on the surface of the shaft provides for bone growth and repair when a bone is fractured. The periosteum also provides a confining membrane for the bone. It contains blood vessels that enter the canals of the bone to supply it with nutrients. Nerves in the periosteum account for the pain experienced after an injury to a bone.

Arteries that nourish bone tunnel into the *medullary* (bone marrow) cavity and make *anastomoses* (connections) with the blood vessels of the periosteum. The bones have a poor capillary network but have many minute arterioles. Venous blood of the marrow and bone is returned to the circulation by large veins that leave the bone by *foramina* (openings) at the extremities.

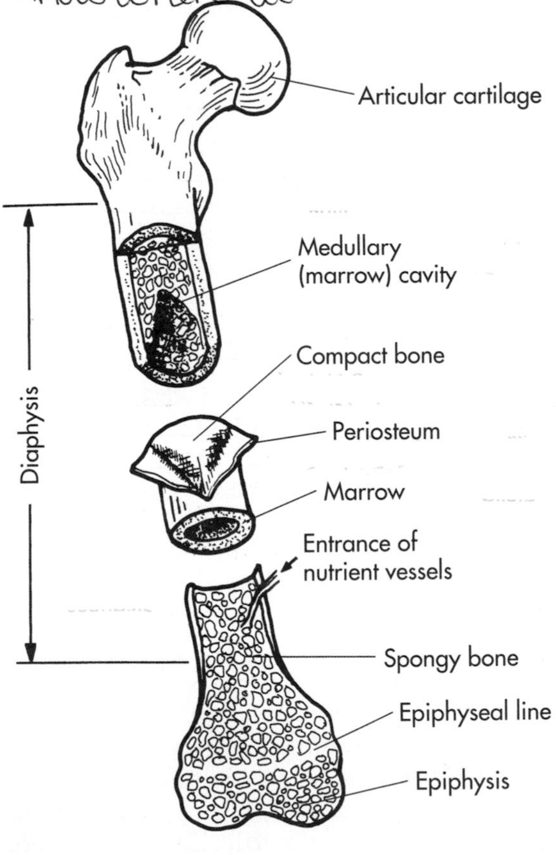
Articular cartilage
Medullary (marrow) cavity
Compact bone
Periosteum
Marrow
Entrance of nutrient vessels
Spongy bone
Epiphyseal line
Epiphysis
Diaphysis

FIG. 6-1 Structure of bone.

Bone Growth

The long bones grow in length at the junctions of the *epiphyses* (ends of the developing bones) with the *diaphyses* (shafts) and in thickness (through the activity of the osteoblasts) in the deep layers of the periosteum. Growth of the long bones is produced by the initial cartilage growth, followed by bone deposition to the diaphyses along the epiphyseal line. Bone growth is controlled by a hormone secreted by the anterior lobe of the pituitary gland.

Bone growth is precisely balanced between the teamwork of the osteoblasts and *osteoclasts* (large phagocytic cells). The osteoblasts produce bony tissue, and the osteoclasts eat away bony tissue in the medullary cavity, preventing the bone from becoming too thick. Healthy bone is constantly being broken down, reabsorbed, and repaired, but the process slows with increasing age.

Bone Classification

Bones are classified according to their shape: long, flat, short, and irregular. The *femur* (bone between the hip joint and the stifle) and the *humerus* (bone between the shoulder and the elbow) are examples of long bones. The short bones are those of the carpus and tarsus. The flat bones are those of the *sternum* (breastbone), *scapula* (shoulder blade), and pelvis. Sesamoid bones, which are found in some joint capsules of certain species, are also considered short bones. Examples of irregular bones include the vertebrae, bones of the inner ear, and os penis of the dog.

SKELETON

The skeleton is divided into two main parts: axial and appendicular (Fig. 6-2). The *axial skeleton* includes the bones of the skull, *hyoid bones* (U-shaped bones located in the neck), vertebral column, ribs, and sternum. The *appendicular skeleton* is made up of the bones of the limb: clavicle (when present), scapula, humerus, radius, ulna, carpus, metacarpals, phalanges, pelvis, femur, patella, tibia, fibula, tarsus, and metatarsals.

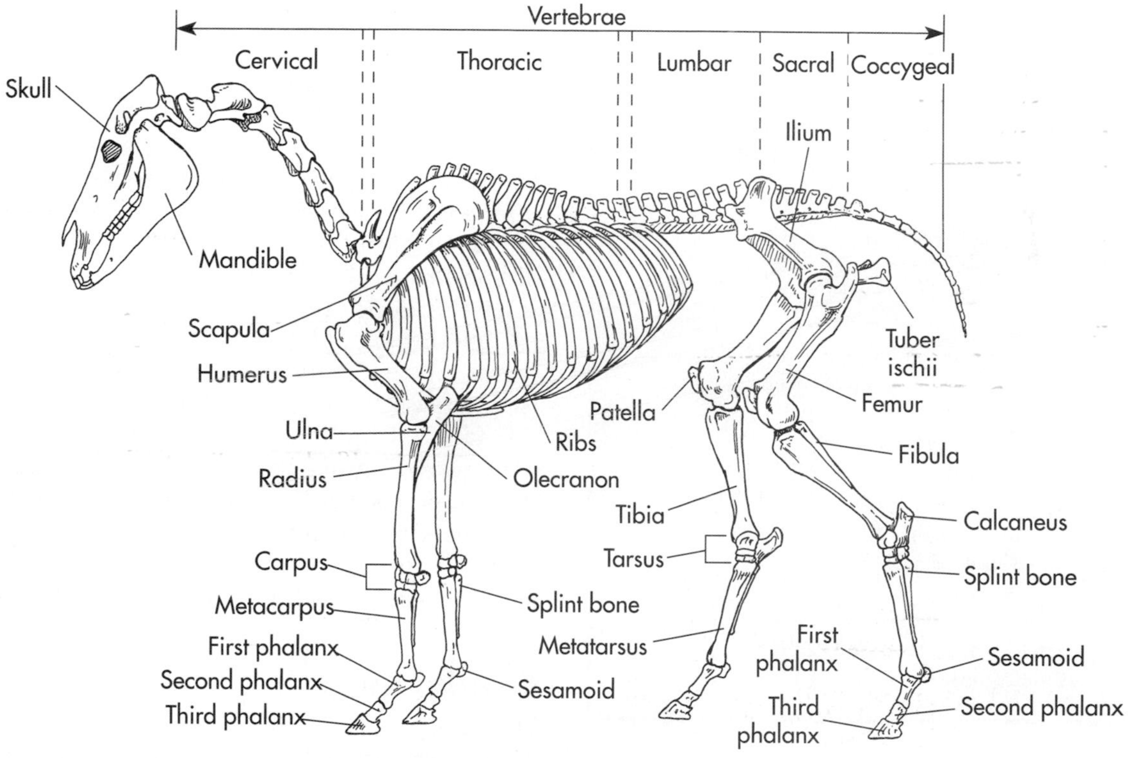

Vertebrae
Cervical
Thoracic
Lumbar
Sacral
Coccygeal
Skull
Ilium
Mandible
Scapula
Humerus
Tuber ischii
Femur
Patella
Ulna
Ribs
Fibula
Radius
Olecranon
Tibia
Calcaneus
Carpus
Tarsus
Splint bone
Metacarpus
Splint bone
Metatarsus
First phalanx
First phalanx
Sesamoid
Second phalanx
Sesamoid
Third phalanx
Third phalanx
Second phalanx

FIG. 6-2 Equine skeleton.

REVIEW A

Complete the following statements.

1. The two main parts of the skeleton are the ________________ and the ________________.
2. The shaft of long bones is called the ________________.
3. Bone marrow is contained in the ________________ cavity of long bones.
4. The outer membrane covering bones is called ________________.
5. Immature bone cells are called ________________.
6. Bones are classified according to shapes, which are ________________, ________________, ________________, and ________________.
7. The humerus is an example of a ________________ bone.
8. The bones of the carpus and tarsus are classified as ________________ bones.
9. An example of an irregular bone is ________________.
10. The U-shaped bones in the neck are called the ________________ bones.

STRUCTURAL DESCRIPTIVE TERMS OF BONES

Canal—tunnel
Condyle—rounded projection
Crest, crista—high ridge
Facet—small, smooth area
Foramen (plural: *foramina*)—opening or hole
Fossa, fovea—basinlike depression
Head—rounded eminence or projection
Line—low ridge
Meatus—passage or opening
Process—any projection
Sinus—cavity or channel
Spine—sharp projection
Sulcus—open, ditchlike groove
Suture—seam
Trochanter—broad, flat process
Tubercle—small, rounded eminence
Tuberosity—protuberance

AXIAL SKELETON

Skull

The skull includes two major segments: the *cranium* (brain case) and the facial bones. The skull protects the brain and the organs of special sense: hearing, sight, taste, and smell (Fig. 6-3). All skull bones are immobile except the *mandible* (lower jawbone). The bones of the skull are united by *sutures* (seams). Within the bones of the skull and the face are hollows called *sinuses,* which have varied functions including lessening the bone weight, providing resonating chambers for vocalization, and moistening and warming air. Sinuses usually are named for the skull bone that contains the sinus.

Cranial Bones

The *frontal* bone forms the forehead and helps form the *orbits* (eye sockets) and the front part of the cranial floor. Horns, when present in some species, are an extension of

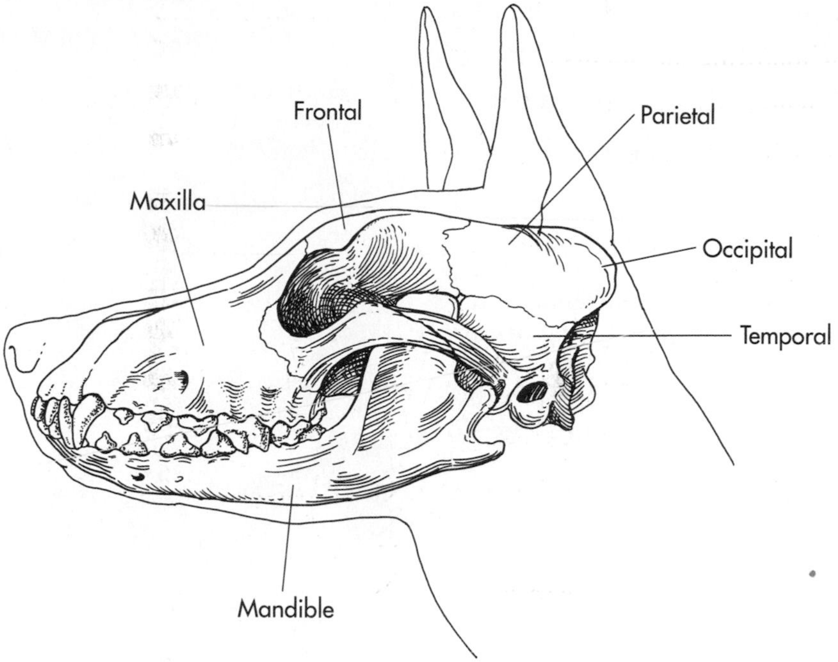
Frontal
Parietal
Maxilla
Occipital
Temporal
Mandible

FIG. 6-3 Principal bones of the canine skull.

the frontal bone that is covered with a modified epithelium. Two *parietal* bones form the roof and the upper part of each side of the skull. The *occipital* bone forms the back of the skull and can be prominent in species such as dogs. At the base of the occipital bone is a large opening, the *foramen magnum* (meaning large hole or opening) for the passage of the spinal cord from the skull into the spine. Two *temporal* bones form part of the cranial floor and the lower part of the sides. These bones contain the middle and inner ear structures. The *sphenoid* is a bone at the base of the skull that extends laterally to support parts of the orbit and forms the lateral walls of the skull. The *ethmoid* bone lies in front of the sphenoid but behind the nasal bones of the face, forming the front of the base of the skull, the medial walls of the orbits, and part of the roof and lateral walls of the nose.

Facial Bones

There are several facial bones. The most significant are the *maxilla* and *mandible.* Two maxillary bones form the upper jaw, nose, orbits, and roof of the mouth. The mandible, which forms the lower jaw, is the only movable bone in the skull. Within the maxillary bones are the *turbinate* bones of the upper respiratory tract. The turbinates are covered with a highly vascular mucous membrane that warms and moistens the air as animals inspire.

Hyoid Bone

The *hyoid* bone (or apparatus) is composed of numerous parts that may be cartilage or bone. This U-shaped apparatus does not form a joint with any other bone. It is located above the larynx and below the mandible and is suspended from the temporal bones by ligaments. The muscles of the tongue and the floor of the mouth are inserted into it.

VERTEBRAL COLUMN

The *vertebral* or *spinal column* (backbone) is made up of numerous *vertebrae* (plural of *vertebra*). The vertebral column shelters the spinal cord, supports the skull and thorax, lends stiffening to the trunk, anchors the pelvis, and provides attachment points for many of the muscles. It is made up of five different types of vertebrae, and there are species variations in the number of each different type. The types of vertebrae are as follows:

- *Cervical* (neck) vertebrae, the first of which is the *atlas.* It supports the skull and rotates on the *axis,* which is the second cervical vertebra. There are seven cervical vertebrae in all common species.
- *Thoracic* (chest) vertebrae, to which the ribs are attached. The number of thoracic vertebrae ranges from 13 in most species to 14 or 15 in the porcine and 18 in equines.
- *Lumbar* (lower back) vertebrae, which support the abdomen and vary from six to seven, depending on the species.
- *Sacrum,* which is one bone resulting from the fusion of three to five vertebrae, to which the pelvis is attached.
- *Coccygeal* (caudal or tail) which is composed of 2 to 23 vertebrae, depending on the species and whether the tail has been docked (surgically removed).

Each vertebra has a body and an arch. The body bears the weight, and the arch forms the canal that houses the spinal cord. Between the vertebral bodies are intervertebral disks, which are made up of cartilage and serve as shock absorbers or cushions.

VERTEBRAL FORMULAS

Vertebral formulas are written in a specific fashion with abbreviations. These formulas are based on the number of each type of vertebra in different species. The abbreviations for the different types of vertebra are as follows:

C, cervical
T, thoracic
L, lumbar
S, sacral
Cy, coccygeal (caudal)

Canine and feline	C-7, T-13, L-7, S-3, Cy-6 to 23
Equine	C-7, T-18, L-7, S-5, Cy-15 to 21
Bovine	C-7, T-13, L-6, S-5, Cy-18 to 20
Porcine	C-7, T-14 or 15, L-6 or 7, S-4, Cy-20 to 23
Ovine	C-7, T-13, L-6 or 7, S-4, Cy-16 to 18

Tail docking reduces the number of coccygeal vertebrae listed for each species. Docking usually is done for management or cosmetic purposes unless an animal has had a traumatic injury necessitating surgical amputation.

RIBS

There are 13 to 18 pairs of ribs, depending on the species. *Ribs* are flat, curved bones attached dorsally to the thoracic vertebrae. The first pairs that are attached to the sternum by cartilage are the *true ribs.* The cartilage at the end of the rib where it attaches to the sternum is the *costal cartilage.* The remaining pairs are called *false ribs,* some of which are attached to the distal sternal cartilage and some of which are not. Ribs not attached to cartilage are known as *floating ribs.* The ribs form the thoracic wall and protect the heart and lungs.

STERNUM

The *sternum* (breastbone) is composed of an unpaired series of flat bones called *sternebrae* and cartilages located on the ventral midline of the chest. The ventral ends of the first pairs of ribs (true ribs) attach to the sternum. The caudalmost sternebra is called the *xiphoid process.*

Most domestic mammals do not have a *clavicle,* which is present in humans and birds. The thoracic vertebrae, the ribs and costal cartilages, and the sternum make up the *thoracic cage,* the bony structure that protects vital organs of the chest and allows them to expand and contract during respiration (breathing).

human feline Birds only have

REVIEW B

Complete the following statements:

1. An opening or passage in bone is called a foramen.
2. A sharp projection is called a Spine.
3. All skull bones are immobile except for the mandible.
4. Sutures unite the bones of the skull.
5. The prominent bone at the back of the skull is the occipital bone.
6. The bones that support the membranous framework that warms and moistens the air are called turbinate bones.
7. The first vertebra of the neck that is modified to support the skull is called atlas.
8. The equine has 18 pairs of ribs.
9. The cushions of cartilage between the vertebrae are known as intervertbal disks.
10. The series of flat bones called Sternebrea make up the sternum.

APPENDICULAR SKELETON

Forelimbs

The different species vary in the number and development of the bones in the legs. The canine foot has *digits* similar to those of a human hand. However, *ungulates* (animals having hooves) have developed a digit (or digits) that is encased distally in a hoof. Significant species differences will be mentioned as the bones are listed.

The bones of the forelimb are as follows (Fig 6-4):

Clavicle (collarbone), a small, flat bone in the feline species attached to the scapula. The dog's clavicle is a vestigial bone that is not *articulated* (joined) with any other bone and may be absent in some dogs. Large animal species have only a small cartilaginous rudiment of the clavicle.

Scapula (shoulder blade), a large triangular bone on the side of the thorax.

Humerus, a long bone extending from the shoulder to the elbow. The humerus articulates with the scapula at the shoulder and with the ulna and radius at the elbow.

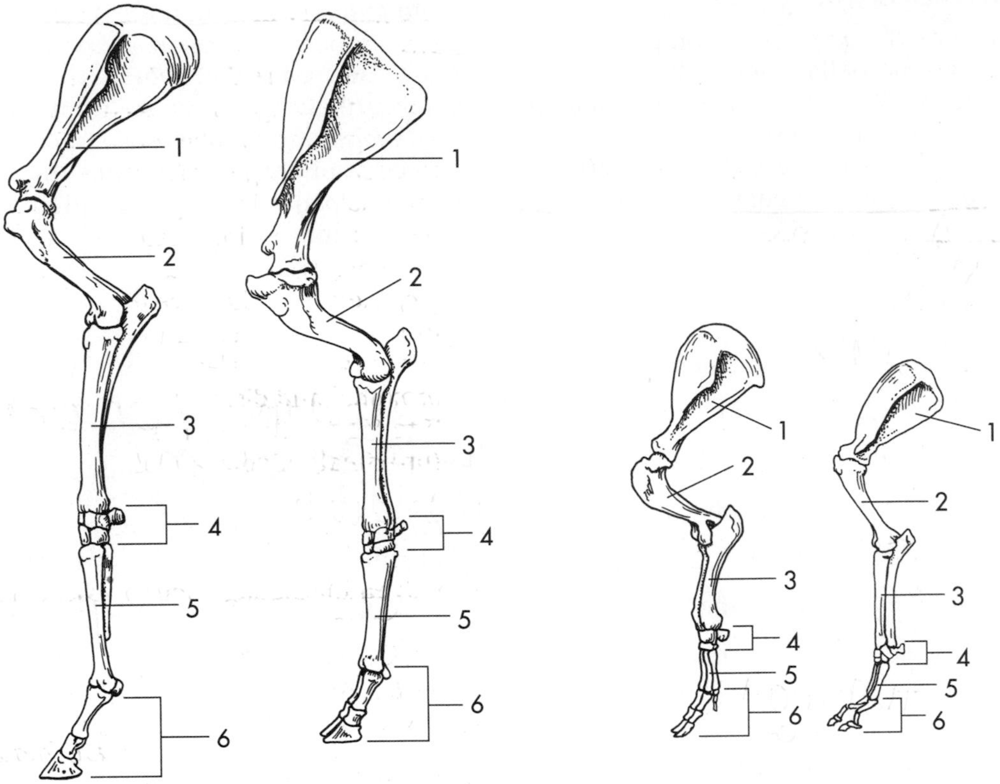
1
2
3
4
5
6
1
2
3
4
5
6
1
2
3
4
5
6
1
2
3
4
5
6

Know **FIG. 6-4** Bones of the forelimb of four species: from left, horse, cow, pig, and dog. *1,* Scapula; *2,* humerus; *3,* radius, ulna; *4,* carpus; *5,* metacarpals; *6,* phalanges.

Ulna, the caudal long bone of the forelimb, which forms the elbow joint by articulation with the humerus at the *olecranon.* In some species such as the horse, the ulna is fused to the radius to form one large bone (Fig. 6-5).

Radius, the cranial long bone of the forelimb, which articulates with the ulna, the humerus at the elbow, and the carpus, forming the carpal joint.

Carpus, composed of numerous (usually seven to eight) irregularly shaped carpal bones in two rows. The term *carpus* refers not only to the bones but to the entire joint. This joint is commonly called the wrist in humans, but this term is rarely used in animals. In large animal species, especially the equine, the carpus is commonly called the *knee.* The term knee is not commonly used to describe any joint in the hind limb of animals.

The *metacarpal* bones vary widely in the number and development of the bones between the different species. In the dog, five metacarpals articulate proximally with the carpus and distally with five digits to form a paw. The horse is at the other extreme, with three metacarpals (two are quite small) that articulate with only one

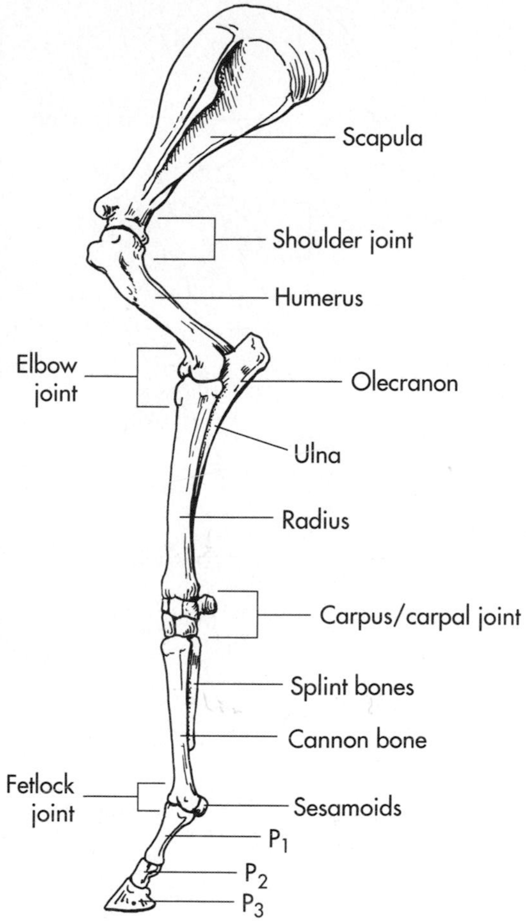
Scapula
Shoulder joint
Humerus
Elbow joint
Olecranon
Ulna
Radius
Carpus/carpal joint
Splint bones
Cannon bone
Fetlock joint
Sesamoids
P1
P2
P3

FIG. 6-5 Bones of the equine forelimb.

digit. The metacarpals are numbered from medial to lateral for identification purposes (usually using roman numerals). In species in which some of the metacarpals are small and do not articulate distally with the digits (the horse, for example), the metacarpals are commonly called *splint* bones. Splint bones are attached to a large third metacarpal bone called the *cannon* bone by a ligament called the *interosseous* ligament.

The digits vary in number and size between species. Commonly, but not always, there are three *phalanges* (*phalanx* is the singular) in each digit. The digits are numbered from medial to lateral (using roman numerals), and the phalanges in a digit are numbered 1 to 3 (using Arabic numerals) from proximal to distal. For example, the canine has five digits on the forelimb. The medialmost digit (digit I) has only two phalanges (named proximal and distal or 1 and 3). Digits II to V have three phalanges each (proximal, middle, and distal or 1, 2, and 3). In some dog breeds, the medial digit or digit I (commonly called the *dewclaw*) is surgically removed for management or cosmetic purposes.

Animals that are considered to have a *cloven* (split) hoof, such as cattle, goats, and sheep, have two digits (III and IV), each having three phalanx bones. Digits II and V are vestiges and are found on the palmar surface. These vestiges do not articulate and are also known as dewclaws. The distalmost phalanx (III or third) is encased in a hoof, which is a modified epithelial structure.

The equine has only one digit (III), which has three phalanx bones. Because of the large size and relative structural importance of these bones in the horse, each bone and joint distal to the metacarpus has its own common name. The joint between metacarpal III and the digit is called the *fetlock or fetlock joint* (commonly called ankle). The first phalanx (phalanx 1) is commonly called the long *pastern* bone. The second phalanx is commonly called the short pastern bone, and the first and second phalanges collectively are called the pastern. The distal phalanx (third or phalanx 3) is referred to by several terms: *coffin* bone, *pedal* bone, or P3.

In some large animal species there is significant development and importance of the *sesamoid bones.* Sesamoids are found within the joint capsule of some joints. Particularly in the horse, sesamoids have clinical significance and therefore have been named. On the caudal or palmar aspect of the fetlock joint, there are two large sesamoids correctly called proximal sesamoids. These two bones commonly are just called sesamoids. Inside the hoof on the palmar or plantar aspect and behind the third phalanx is a distal sesamoid called the *navicular* bone.

Hind Limbs

Different species vary in the number and development of the bones of the hind limbs. The bones of the hind limb are as follows (Fig. 6-6):

Pelvis, which consists of three pairs of bones that fuse early in life into one solid, irregular bone. The pelvis connects to the sacrum and coccygeal vertebrae and forms a basinlike structure that supports the caudal half of the body, affords an attachment for the hind limbs at the hip joint, and protects the caudal abdominal organs. The three pairs of bones that fuse are the *ilium,* the largest pair, flaring to the side; the *ischium,* the strongest and most caudal pair; and the *pubis,* the most ventral pair, which meets at the *pubic symphysis,* a cartilaginous joint.

Femur, the longest bone in the body, which articulates with the *acetabulum* (hip socket) at the proximal end and with the *tibia* at the distal end.

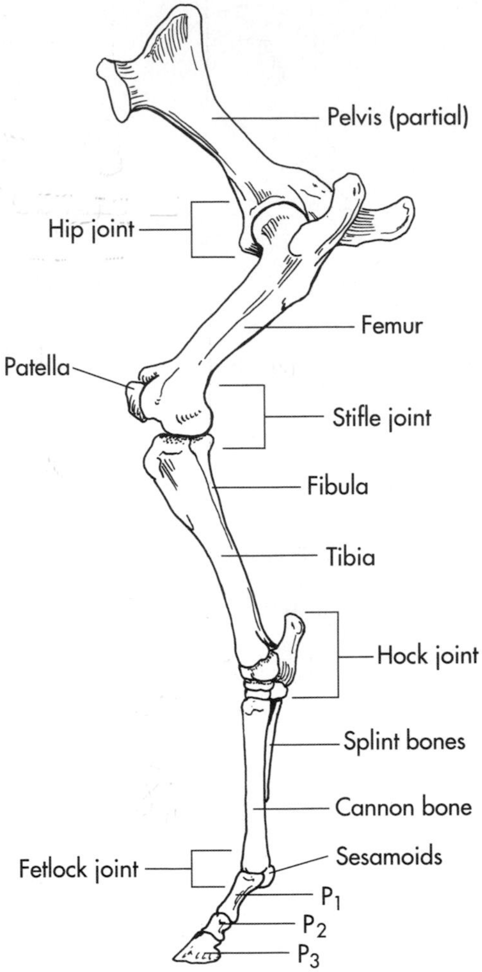
Pelvis (partial)
Hip joint
Femur
Patella
Stifle joint
Fibula
Tibia
Hock joint
Splint bones
Cannon bone
Sesamoids
Fetlock joint
P1
P2
P3

FIG. 6-6 Bones of the equine hind limb.

The *greater* and *lesser trochanters* are two processes on the femur for attachment of muscles. The *lateral* and *medial condyles,* two bony prominences at the lower end of the femur, articulate with the tibia and *patella.* The joint between the femur and the tibia is called the *stifle* joint.

Patella, a flat bone inserted in a ligament that glides over the stifle joint. In humans the stifle joint is called the knee. The term *knee* is not used in the

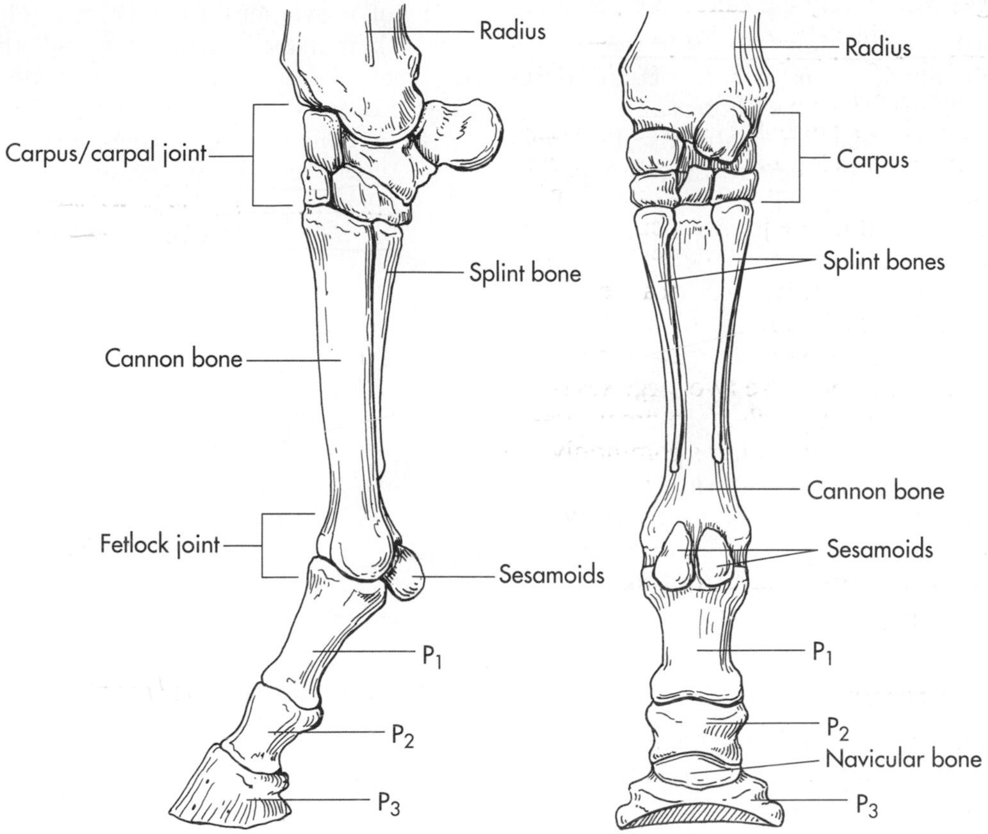
Radius
Carpus/carpal joint
Splint bone
Cannon bone
Fetlock joint
Sesamoids
P1
P2
P3
Radius
Carpus
Splint bones
Cannon bone
Sesamoids
P1
P2
Navicular bone
P3

FIG. 6-7 Bones of the equine lower limb.

hind limb of quadrupeds. The term *knee* is used for the carpus (forelimb) in species such as the horse.

Tibia, the larger, more weight-bearing, medially placed bone of the two leg bones, articulating at its proximal end with the femur and at its distal end in some species with the *fibula* and the tarsus.

Fibula, a long, slender, lateral bone, articulating at the proximal end with the tibia and at the distal end with the tibia and tarsus in some species. The horse has a small fibula that does not extend or articulate at the distal end.

Tarsus, composed of numerous (usually seven) irregularly shaped tarsal bones arranged in several rows. The term *tarsus* is used collectively for this entire joint. The term *ankle* is used for this joint in humans; however, the tarsus is usually called the *hock* in animals.

Metatarsals vary in number between species, like the forelimb. The number of digits also varies, but the terminology used for the hind limb is similar to that of the forelimb. The numbering system used for metatarsals and phalanges in the hind limb is the same as that of the forelimb (Fig. 6-7).

JOINTS

The study of the joints is *arthrology* (*arthr-* means joints). A *joint* is an articulation between bones or between bones and cartilage and is held in place by ligaments of connective tissue, which may or may not permit motion between them.

Joints are classified according to the degree of movement they permit (Fig. 6-8) and their tissue structure, and there is a direct relationship between these two classifications.

Degree of movement (Figs. 6-8 and 6-9)

Synarthroses allow no movement.

Amphiarthroses allow slight movement.

Diarthroses freely permit movement.

A

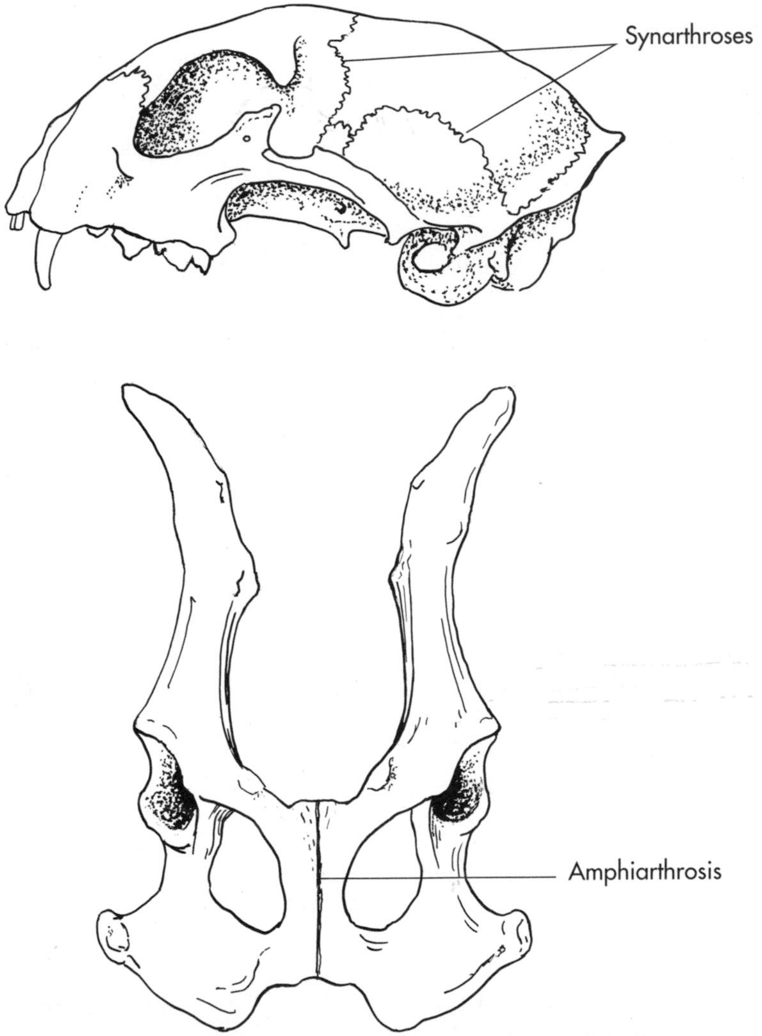
Synarthroses
Amphiarthrosis

B

FIG. 6-8 Types of joints. **A,** Cat skull, lateral view, showing synarthroses (fibrous joints). **B,** Dog pelvis, ventral view, showing an amphiarthrosis (cartilaginous joint).

Tissue structure

Fibrous (synarthroses) joints contain fibrous tissue that unites bones and permits no movement. An example of this type is found in the sutures of the skull.

Cartilaginous (amphiarthroses) joints contain cartilage that connects the bones and permits slight movement. Examples of this type are found in the vertebrae and the symphysis pubis.

Synovial (diarthroses) joints are freely movable, the most numerous, and the most complex in the body. They have six characteristic structures, as noted in the accompanying box.

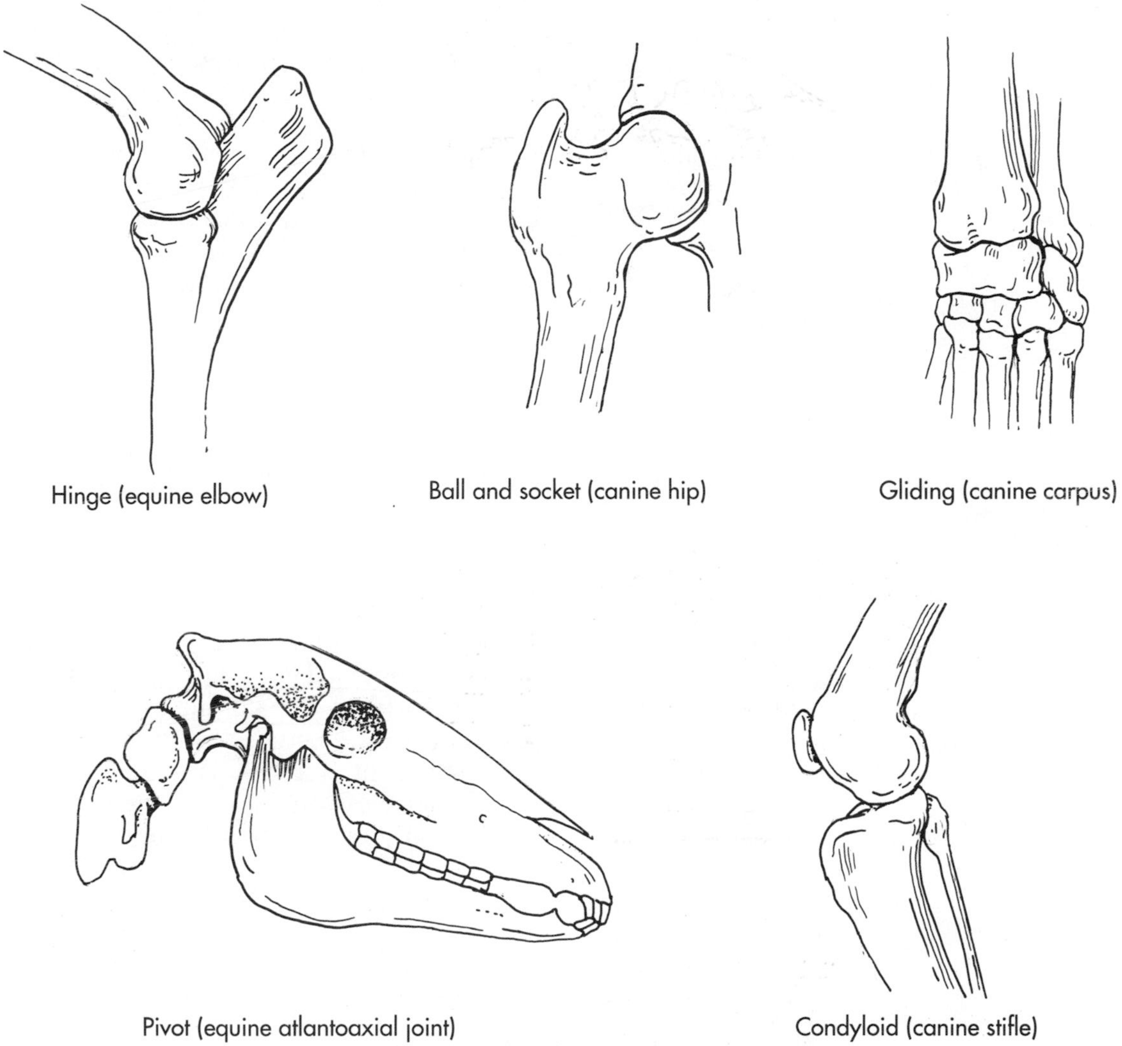
Hinge (equine elbow)
Ball and socket (canine hip)
Gliding (canine carpus)
Pivot (equine atlantoaxial joint)
Condyloid (canine stifle)

FIG. 6-9 Types of diarthroses (synovial joints).

CHARACTERISTICS OF SYNOVIAL JOINTS

Joint capsule—forms a covering around the articulating ends of the bones, holding them to each other

Synovial membrane—lines the joint capsule and secretes synovial fluid, lubricating opposing surfaces of the bones

Joint cavity—space between the opposing surfaces of bones of the joint

Articular cartilage—Thin covering of cartilage that cushions the articulating bone surfaces

Ligaments—Cords of white, dense, fibrous tissue that help to bind the bones together

Articular disks—Pads of cartilage between articulating surfaces in some synovial joints

The movable joints are further divided into subtypes (Fig. 6-9):

Hinge joints—those that permit movement in only one direction, as in the elbow.

Ball-and-socket joints—the round head of one bone fits into a cuplike cavity of another, permitting movement in different directions, as in the hip joint.

Gliding joints—the least movable of this group, in which the adjacent bone surfaces glide against each other to permit movement, such as that of the carpus and tarsus.

Pivot (rotary) joints—one bone pivots around a stationary bone, such as the axis and atlas (first two cervical vertebrae).

Condyloid joints—the oval head of one bone fits into a shallow depression in another, such as the stifle joint.

TYPES OF MOVEMENT

The following are descriptive terms for defining the different types of motion:

Flexion—bending at a joint, as the elbow.

Extension—straightening or unbending of a joint; this movement is the opposite of flexion.

Abduction—movement that draws a body part away from the midline of the body.

Adduction—movement that draws a body part toward the midline of the body.

Rotation—movement that turns a body part on its own axis, such as the turning of the head.

Circumduction—a movement describing a circle.

Not all joints can perform all the movements listed in the box above. The immovable joints cannot perform any of them. Of the freely movable joints, only the ball-and-socket can perform all the movements listed. The hinge joints can perform only flexion and extension. The slightly movable joints can perform rotation.

BURSAE

The *bursae* (singular: *bursa*) are sacs of connective tissue lined with synovial membrane and filled with synovial fluid. Synovial fluid relieves pressure between moving parts. Inflammation of a bursa is called bursitis. Some bursae of animals can have particular clinical significance when inflamed.

REVIEW C

Complete the following statements.

1. Which species has a well-developed clavicle? feline
2. The shoulder blades are called scapulae.
3. The long bones of the forelimb are humoras, ulna, and radius.
4. The carpal bones are located in the capus.
5. The pelvis is formed by these three bones: ilium, ischium, and pubis.
6. The joint including the patella is called the stifle.
7. The tarsal joint is commonly called the hock.
8. The first and second phalanges in the equine are commonly called the pastern.
9. The joint type allowing the greatest range of movement is ball n socket.
10. The bending of a joint is called flexion.

Chapter 6 Answers

Review A

1. axial and appendicular
2. diaphysis
3. medullary
4. periosteum
5. osteoblasts
6. long, flat, short, irregular
7. long
8. short
9. vertebrae, os penis, or bones of inner ear
10. hyoid

Review B

1. meatus or foramen
2. spine
3. mandible (lower jawbone)
4. Sutures
5. occipital
6. turbinate
7. atlas
8. 18
9. intervertebral disks
10. sternebrae

Review C

1. feline
2. scapulae
3. humerus, ulna, radius
4. carpus
5. ilium, ischium, pubis
6. stifle
7. hock
8. pastern
9. ball-and-socket
10. flexion

Chapter 6 EXERCISES

SKELETAL SYSTEM: THE FRAMEWORK OF THE BODY

Exercise 1: Complete the following.

1. The hard outer shell of bone is called compact bone tissue.
2. The inner, latticelike, spongy structure of bone is called ~~osteoblast~~ cancellated bone.
3. The shaft of a long bone is called diaphysis.
4. The developing ends of long bones are called epiphyses.
5. The anatomic classifications of the skeleton are axial and appendicular

Exercise 2: Match the definition in the right column with the terms in the left column by placing the appropriate letter in the blank space provided.

B	1. periosteum	A. seam
H	2. red bone marrow	B. tough, fibrous membrane covering
D	3. osteoblast	C. phagocytic cell
~~B~~C	4. osteoclast	D. immature bone cell
F	5. fossa	E. small, smooth area
J	6. sulcus	F. basinlike depression
E	7. facet	G. high ridge
G	8. crest	H. hematopoietic tissue
A	9. suture	I. opening or hole
I	10. foramen	J. open, ditchlike groove

Exercise 3: Multiple choice.

1. Which of the following bones is the only movable bone of the skull?
   a. Frontal
   (b.) Mandible
   c. Maxilla
   d. Temporal
2. Horns are an extension of which bone?
   (a.) Frontal
   b. Mandible

c. Maxilla

d. Temporal

3. Which bones are covered with a vascular membrane that warms and moistens the air during inspiration?

a. Frontal

b. Sphenoid

c. Turbinates

d. Temporal

4. Which bone is composed of numerous parts, supports the floor of the mouth, and supports the insertion of the tongue?

a. Maxilla

b. Mandible

c. Occipital

d. Hyoid

5. At the base of the skull is an opening called the foramen magnum. At the base of which bone is this opening?

a. Occipital

b. Temporal

c. Ethmoid

d. Frontal

Exercise 4: Multiple choice.

1. The second cervical vertebra is called

a. Axis

b. Atlas

c. Pubis

d. Occipital

2. To which type of vertebrae are the ribs attached?

a. Cervical

b. Thoracic

c. Lumbar

d. Sacral

3. What type of vertebrae forms the tail?
   a. Thoracic
   b. Lumbar
   c. Sacral
   d. Coccygeal
4. Which species has 18 pairs of ribs?
   a. Bovine
   b. Equine
   c. Canine
   d. Porcine
5. What type of ribs are attached directly to the sternum by cartilage?
   a. False ribs
   b. Floating ribs
   c. True ribs
   d. Costal ribs

Exercise 5: Multiple choice.

1. What is the lateral long bone of the forelimb that articulates with the ulna and the humerus at the elbow and with the carpus distally?
   a. Humerus
   b. Radius
   c. Tibia
   d. Scapula
2. In the horse, metacarpals II and IV are small and do not articulate distally with the phalanges. What is the common name for these metacarpal bones?
   a. Sesamoids
   b. Navicular
   c. Pastern
   d. Splint
3. What are the first and second phalanges in the horse commonly called?
   a. Sesamoids
   b. Navicular

c. Pastern

d. Splint

4. What is the distal sesamoid found on the palmar or plantar aspect inside the hoof of the horse called?

   a. Sesamoids

   b. Navicular

   c. Pastern

   d. Splint

5. How do we describe the distal extremity in animals such as the cow that have two split digits, each having three phalanx bones?

   a. Cloven hoof

   b. Paw

   c. Hoof

   d. Dewclaw

Exercise 6: Multiple choice.

1. What three bones compose the pelvis?

   a. Fibula, ilium, pubis

   b. Ischium, pelvis, ilium

   c. Ilium, ischium, pubis

   d. Pubis, femur, ilium

2. What is the name of the joint at the distal end of the femur and proximal end of the tibia that the patella overlaps?

   a. Stifle

   b. Hip

   c. Hock

   d. Acetabulum

3. Where is the fibula in relation to the tibia?

   a. Medial

   b. Lateral

   c. Proximal

   d. Distal

4. What is the common name for the tarsus?

   a. Hock

   b. Ankle

   c. Knee

   d. Wrist

5. What is the name of bones that are found within the joint capsules of some joints?

   a. Navicular

   b. Synovial

   c. Condyle

   d. Sesamoid

Exercise 7: Multiple choice.

1. What are sacs of connective tissue lined with synovial membrane that are filled with synovial fluid called?

   a. Sesamoids

   b. Synovial

   c. Bursae

   d. Diarthroses

2. Which type of joint permits the greatest amount of movement?

   a. Synarthroses

   b. Amphiarthroses

   c. Diarthroses

   d. Fibrous

3. Which of the following movable joint subtypes permits movement in different directions?

   a. Ball-and-socket

   b. Gliding

   c. Hinge

   d. Condyloid

4. What type of movement involves a movable body part that is drawn toward the midline of the body?

   a. Flexion

   b. Adduction

c. Extension

d. Abduction

5. What type of joint is the most numerous and most complex in the body?

a. Condyloid

b. Synarthroses

c. Amphiarthroses

d. Diarthroses

CHAPTER 6 PUZZLE

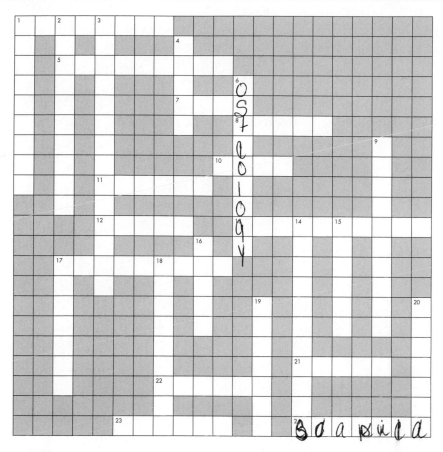

ACROSS CLUES

1. Inflammation of bone
5. Acute or chronic inflammation of joint
7. Second cervical vertebra
8. Large bone next to fibula
10. Tarsal joint
11. Composed of tarsal bones
12. Sac of fluid near joint
13. Fracture on only one side of bone
17. Bones of digits
21. Cranial bone of pelvis
22. Vertebrae of the back
23. Joint composed of carpal bones
24. Shoulder blade

DOWN CLUES

1. Bone forming back of skull
2. Fracture of bone at right angles to its axis
3. Between vertebrae
4. First cervical vertebra
6. The study of bone
9. Bones in nasal cavity
14. Inflammation of epiphysis
15. Fused vertebrae to which pelvis is attached
16. Upper bone in hind limb
17. First phalanx in horse
18. Distal sesamoid of horse
19. Most proximal bone of forearm
20. Bone of upper jaw

Chapter 6 Answers

Exercise 1

1. compact bone tissue
2. cancellated or cancellous bone
3. diaphysis
4. epiphyses
5. appendicular, axial

Exercise 2

1. B
2. H
3. D
4. C
5. F
6. J
7. E
8. G
9. A
10. I

Exercise 3

1. B
2. A
3. C
4. D
5. A

Exercise 4

1. A
2. B
3. D
4. B
5. C

Exercise 5

1. B
2. D
3. C
4. B
5. A

Exercise 6

1. C
2. A
3. B
4. A
5. D

Exercise 7

1. C
2. C
3. A
4. B
5. D

ANSWERS: CHAPTER 6 PUZZLE

1 O	S	2 T	E	3 I	T	I	S													
C		R		N				4 A												
C		5 A	R	T	H	R	I	T	I	S										
I		N		E				L			6 O									
P		S		R				7 A	X	I	S									
I		V		V				S			8 T	I	B	I	A					
T		E		E							E							9 T		
A		R		R						10 H	O	C	K					U		
L		S		11 T	A	R	S	U	S		L							R		
		E		E							O							B		
				12 B	U	R	S	A			13 G	R	E	14 E	N	15 S	T	I	C	K
				R					16 F		Y			P		A		N		
		17 P	H	A	L	A	18 N	G	E	S				I		C		A		
		A		L			A		M					P		R		T		
		S					V		U			19 H		H		U		E		20 M
		T					I		R			U		Y		M		S		A
		E					C					M		S						X
		R					U					E		21 I	L	I	U	M		I
		N					22 L	U	M	B	A	R		T						L
							A					U		I						L
					23 C	A	R	P	U	S		S		24 S	C	A	P	U	L	A

GLOSSARY

BONES AND RELATED ANATOMIC TERMS

Acetabulum: cup-shaped socket in the pelvis.
Appendicular skeleton: bones of the limbs.
Atlas: first cervical vertebra.
Axial skeleton: bones of the skull, vertebral column, ribs, and sternum.
Axis: second cervical vertebra.
Cancellous bone: inner spongy surface of long bones.
Cannon bone: common name for metacarpal and metatarsal III in horses.
Cervical: vertebrae of the neck.
Clavicle: bone found in some species that serves as portion of the chest; collarbone.
Coccygeal: vertebrae of the tail.
Coffin, pedal bone: distal phalanx of the horse.
Compact bone: outer hard shell of bone.
Costal cartilages: cartilage of ribs.
Cranium: portion of the skull encasing the brain.
Dewclaw: digit I or the medial digit in some species such as dogs, also vestigial digits II and V in sheep, goats, and cattle.
Diaphysis: central part of the bone shaft.
Digit: distal extremity made up of phalanges (e.g., toes, claws, hoofs).
Epiphysis: end part of developing bone.
Epiphysitis: inflammation of the epiphysis of a bone.
Femur: upper bone in hind limb.
Fibula: more lateral and smaller of the two bones distal to the stifle joint (next to the tibia).
Foramen (*foramina* is plural): opening in bone.
Foramen magnum: large opening in the occipital bone connecting the cranial cavity to the vertebral canal.
Frontal bone: bone forming the forepart of the cranium.
Humerus: large bone of the forelimb, between the shoulder and the elbow.
Hyoid: U-shaped bone at the base of the tongue.
Ilium: cranial bones of the pelvis.
Interosseous ligament: ligament between splint and cannon bone in the horse.
Intervertebral disks: cushions found between the bodies of vertebrae.
Ischium: caudal bones of the pelvis; most caudal projections are called pin bones.
Lumbar: vertebrae of the back.
Mandible: movable portion of the skull; lower jaw.
Maxilla: portion of the skull; upper jaw.
Medullary cavity: innermost portion of bones.
Metacarpals: bones distal to the carpus and proximal to the phalanges, variable in number between species.
Metatarsals: bones distal to the tarsus and proximal to the phalanges, variable in number between species.
Navicular: boat-shaped, distal sesamoid in the hoof of the horse.
Occipital: bone forming the back of the skull.
Olecranon: proximal process of the ulna at the elbow joint.
Os penis: bone found within the penis of the dog.
Osteoblasts: bone-forming cells.
Osteoclasts: bone-remodeling cells.
Osteology: the study of bone.
Parietal: lateral bones of the cranium.
Patella: bone over the stifle joint.
Pelvis: girdle of bone encircling the caudal abdomen and providing attachment for the hind limb.
Periosteum: membrane covering bone.
Phalanges (singular, *phalanx*): bones of the digits.
Pubis: ventral bones of the pelvis.
Quadruped: a four-footed animal.
Radius: more medial bone of two bones distal to the elbow (next to the ulna).
Ribs: flat, curved bones forming the thoracic wall and protecting the lungs and heart.
Sacrum: fused sacral vertebrae resulting in one bone to which the pelvis is attached.
Scapula: shoulder blade.
Sesamoid: any small flat bone embedded in tendon or joint capsule.
Sinuses: air spaces within the skull.
Sphenoid: wedge-shaped bone at the base of the skull.
Splint bones: common name for metacarpals or metatarsals II and IV in the horse.
Sternebrae: series of unpaired bones on ventral chest that make up the sternum.
Sternum: breastbone, bone on ventral chest.
Sutures: seams of the bones of the skull.
Temporal: bones forming the sides and base of the skull.

Thoracic: vertebrae of the chest or thorax.
Tibia: more medial and larger of the two bones distal to the stifle joint (next to the fibula).
Turbinates: scroll-like bones in the nasal cavity.
Ulna: more lateral of the two bones distal to the elbow (next to the radius).
Ungulates: animals with hooves.
Vertebra: spinal column bone.
Xiphoid process: caudalmost sternebra.

JOINTS AND RELATED ANATOMIC TERMS

Amphiarthroses: a joint type that only allows slight movement; also called cartilaginous joints.
Arthrology: the study of joints.
Articulation: the joining or connecting together as in a joint (verb: to articulate).
Bursa: sacs of synovial fluid found near joint surfaces.
Carpus: joint made up of carpal bones, between the radius/ulna and the metacarpals.
Cartilaginous: joints containing cartilage that connect bone and permit slight movement, such as joints between vertebrae.
Diarthroses: a joint type that allows free movement; also known as synovial joints.
Fetlock: joint between the metacarpals (or metatarsals) and digits in some species such as the horse or cow.
Fibrous: joints that contain fibrous tissue that unites bone and permits no movement, such as skull sutures.
Hock: common term for the tarsus or tarsal joint.
Pastern: joint between the first and second phalanges, also a collective term for the first and second phalanges in the horse.
Pubic symphysis: cartilaginous joint on the ventral aspect of the pelvis.
Stifle: large joint between the femur and the tibia.
Synarthroses: a joint type that allows no movement; also called fibrous joints.
Synovial: freely movable joints that are the most numerous joints in the body and are complex, with six characteristics of structure.
Tarsus: joint made up of tarsal bones, between the tibia/fibula and the metatarsals.

PATHOLOGIC CONDITIONS

Arthritis: acute or chronic inflammation of one or more joints.
Bursitis: inflammation of bursa.
Chondroma: tumor of cartilage cell origin.
Comminuted: fracture in which there are multiple pieces or splinters.
Compound: type of fracture in which there is an open wound.
Desmitis: inflammation of a ligament.
Greenstick: fracture in which one side of the bone is broken and the other side may be bent.
Osteitis: inflammation of bone.
Osteoarthritis: degenerative joint disease affecting articular cartilage and the synovial membranes.
Osteochondritis: inflammation of cartilage of bone.
Osteoma: bone tissue tumor.
Osteomalacia: softening of bone.
Osteomyelitis: inflammation of bone involving periosteum and cancellous and marrow tissues.
Osteoporosis: abnormal loss of bone density.
Osteosarcoma: malignant bone tumor.
Spondylitis: inflammation of the spinal column vertebrae.
Synovitis: inflammation of the synovial membrane of a joint.
Transverse: fracture in which the bone is fractured at right angles to its axis.
Tendinitis: inflammation of a tendon (also spelled tendonitis).
Tendosynovitis: inflammation of tendon and its surrounding sheath (sometimes also called tenosynovitis).

7 The Muscular System

The moving force

CHAPTER OVERVIEW

This chapter presents the different muscles of the body, their composition, their classification, and their relationship to other structures that aid in movement.

THE WHOLE SYSTEM

The study of muscles is called *myology.* All physical activity is carried on by muscles in conjunction with the skeleton to achieve movement. Although the skeleton provides attachment points and support for the muscles, it is the muscle tissue and its ability to extend and contract that affect movement.

There are more than 600 muscles in the body (Fig. 7-1). Muscles constitute the major part of the fleshy portions of the body and one half of its weight, varying in proportion to the size of the animal. The form of the body is determined largely by the muscles covering the bones.

In addition to movement, the muscles have other roles, such as supporting and maintaining posture and producing body heat. They help form many of the internal organs (such as the heart, uterus, lungs, and intestines). There is never a time when all the muscles are in a quiescent state because the muscles of the heart, intestines, arteries, and stomach are at work, even though we are not aware of it.

ALLIED MUSCULAR STRUCTURES

Tendon

Tendons are the strong, fibrous white bands that attach muscles to bones, enabling the movement of a part located some distance from the contracting muscle (Fig. 7-2). An example is seen in the muscles of the leg, which, through their tendons, control the movement of the distal extremities. If the movement of the lower leg depended on its own muscles, that part would have to be many times its present size. Therefore the phalanges are controlled by the muscles of the upper limb through their tendons. One particular type of tendon that is flat and ribbonlike is called an *aponeurosis.* Where there is a long distance from the tendons to their distal attachments or where the tendon pulls over a joint, the tendons are surrounded by a *tendon sheath.*

Fascia

Fascia is a sheet of fibrous membrane that encloses muscles and separates them into groups.

Ligament

Ligaments are strong bands of fibrous tissue connecting bones or cartilage (Fig. 7-2). They aid or restrict movement and support organs.

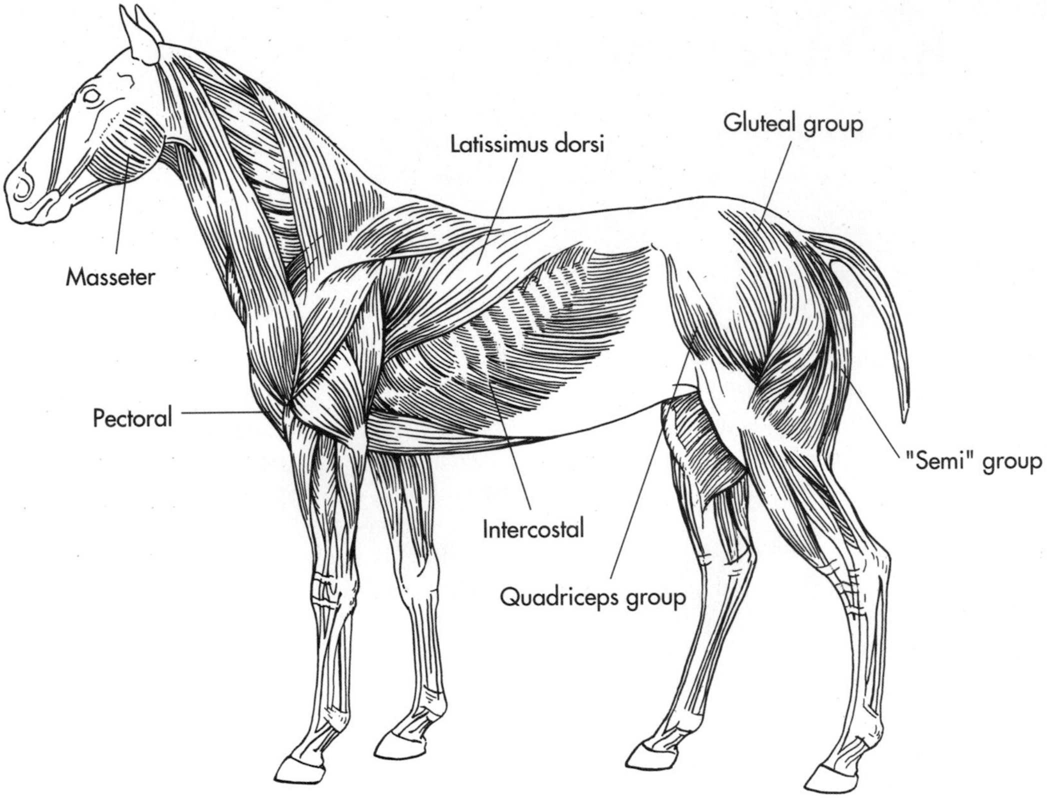
Latissimus dorsi
Gluteal group
Masseter
Pectoral
"Semi" group
Intercostal
Quadriceps group

FIG. 7-1 Major superficial muscles of the horse.

Aponeurosis

An *aponeurosis* is a broad sheet of fibrous connective tissue that serves as a tendon to attach muscles to bone or as fascia to bind muscles together.

Origin

The *origin* is the less movable of the two points of attachment of a muscle (Fig. 7-2). It is also the end of the muscle that is attached to the more fixed part of the skeleton.

Insertion

The *insertion* is the point of attachment by a muscle (Fig. 7-2). The insertion moves when that particular muscle is contracted.

Motor Nerve

A *motor nerve* causes muscle to move by stimulating a group of muscle fibers. The combination of the nerve cell and its group of muscle cells is called a *motor* or *neuromotor unit.*

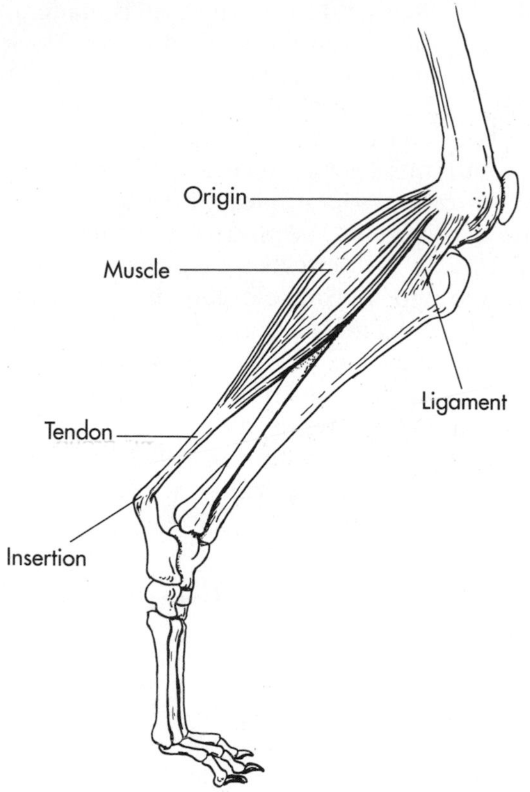
Origin
Muscle
Tendon
Insertion
Ligament

FIG. 7-2 Hind limb of dog showing attachments of soft tissue to bone.

REVIEW A

1. The study of muscles is called ______________________________.
2. Movement is produced by the ability of muscle to ______________ and ______________.
3. The immovable bone to which a muscle is attached is known as its ______________.
4. The movable bone to which a muscle is attached is known as its ______________.
5. The sheet of fibrous membrane that encloses muscles is called ______________.

COMPOSITION OF MUSCLE

Like other tissues of the body, muscle tissue is composed of cells. Muscle cells are long and slender and because of their shape are called *fibers*. These fibers vary greatly in size, depending on their function, but they are large compared with other body cells.

The plasma membrane of a muscle cell is called a *sarcolemma,* and its cytoplasm is called *sarcoplasm*. The muscle fibers are held together by connective tissue and enclosed in *fascia* (fibrous membrane sheath). The fibers contract, producing movement of the body or its organs.

The speed of muscle contraction varies with individual muscles and the size of the structure to be moved. The smaller the structure to be moved, the more rapid is the muscle action. For example, the muscles that move the eye contract much more rapidly than those that move a large muscle, such as the muscles of the hip.

Many movements of the body are carried out by several muscles or muscle groups acting together. The muscles have a rich vascular (blood) supply. Exercise increases muscle fiber thickness but does not produce new fibers.

CLASSIFICATION OF MUSCLES

Muscles are divided into three types according to their function, shape, and structure: skeletal, smooth, and cardiac (Fig. 5-4).

Skeletal (Voluntary, Striated) Muscle

Skeletal muscles, which are attached to the skeleton, are called voluntary because they are controlled at will. They are called striated because, under a microscope, they have a cross-striated (striped) appearance. Other voluntary muscles not attached to the skeleton are those that move the eyes, tongue, pharynx, and some portions of the skin. A typical voluntary muscle is made up of a fleshy mass of elongated muscle fibers held together in a casing of white, fibrous tissue and supplied with a nerve that makes it contract and extend. When muscles contract, the fibers become shorter and thicker. Skeletal muscle is supplied by both the central and peripheral nervous systems (see Chapter 14).

Smooth (Visceral or Nonstriated, Involuntary) Muscle

Smooth muscle, which is found in parts of the body such as the stomach, intestines, uterus, blood vessels, and iris of the eye, is made up of nonstriated, spindle-shaped fibers. These muscles are involuntary (not controllable at will) and are controlled by the autonomic nervous system (see Chapter 14). Some smooth muscles may be under the influence of hormones. Examples of these are the muscle fibers in the uterus and the udder, which are influenced by hormones, especially oxytocin. Some organs may be composed of combinations of skeletal and smooth muscle fibers. An example of this is the esophagus of ruminants, which allows the animal to regurgitate its food when chewing cud. Combining skeletal fibers with smooth gives voluntary control to these organs.

Cardiac (Striated, Involuntary) Muscle

The *cardiac* (heart) *muscle,* although involuntary, shows fine, transverse striations under the microscope. Its appearance is unlike that of other involuntary muscle tissue. The cardiac muscle is controlled by the autonomic nervous system (see Chapters 9 and 14).

ATTACHMENT OF MUSCLES

The attachment of muscles to tendons, which extend to the phalanges, results in movement and reduction of bulk that would be necessary if muscles extended to the digits. Voluntary muscles usually attach to bone, but in the larynx and thorax, muscle is attached to cartilage. Usually muscle is attached to the capsule of joints over which its tendon passes. Other muscles may be attached to the skin, as in the cheeks, or to mucous membrane, as in the tongue. Muscles may also be attached to fascia of other muscles, such as the flat muscles of the abdomen, or to body structures, such as the eye.

MOVEMENT OF MUSCLES

A muscle does not act alone but depends on other muscles to assist in executing a desired movement. For this reason, muscles are called prime movers, antagonists, and synergists (*syn-* means together; *erg* refers to work). The *prime movers* are those that actively produce a movement. The *antagonists* are those in opposition to the prime movers, relaxing as the prime movers contract. The *synergists* contract simultaneously with the prime movers to help execute a movement or steady a part. The muscles, in conjunction with the skeleton, move the body. The different types of movements are described in Chapter 6, p. 92.

REVIEW B

1. In shape, muscle cells are ______________ and ______________.
2. ______________ is the plasma membrane of a muscle cell.
3. Three types of muscle tissue are ______________, ______________, and ______________.
4. Muscles are classified according to how they produce movement and are called ______________, ______________, and ______________.
5. Voluntary, striated muscles are also known as the ______________ muscle type.

HOW MUSCLES ARE NAMED

The names of muscles are based on six points of identification.

- Muscles may be named for their action. Example: extensor carpi radialis (extends the carpus)
- Muscles may be named for their origin and insertion. Example: occipitofrontal (between occipital and frontal skull bones)
- Muscles may be named for their location. Example: external oblique muscle of abdomen
- Muscles may be named for their shape or use. Example: pyramidal (shaped like a pyramid)
- Muscles may be named for the direction of their fibers. Example: orbicular muscle of eye (around eye)
- Muscles may be named according to the number of their sections. Example: biceps (*bi-* means two, *-cep* means head)

ADDITIONAL ADJECTIVES USED IN MUSCLE NAMES

The following are some important adjectives that are not given in the list in Chapter 4 but aid in the description of muscles:

Azygous—not paired
Bi-, *tri-*, and *quadri-*—two, three, and four
Externus—external or outer
Gracilis—slender
Latissimus—wide
Longissimus—long
Longus—long
Medius—intermediate
Orbicularis—surrounding
Quadratus—square
Rectus—straight
Rhomboideus—diamond-shaped or shaped like a kite
Scalenus—irregularly triangular or unequally three-sided
Serratus—sawtoothed
Teres—round or cylindrical
Transversus—crosswise
Vastus—great

REVIEW C

1. *Externus,* in relation to muscle, means ______________________________.
2. *Orbicularis,* in relation to muscle, means ______________________________.
3. *Quadratus,* in relation to muscle, means ______________________________.
4. *Rhomboideus,* in relation to muscle, means ______________________________.
5. *Teres,* in relation to muscle, means ______________________________.

MUSCLE GROUPS

The following paragraphs name and describe various muscles and their actions according to location in the body. Only a few muscles are covered to provide you with a basic understanding of this system. The significance and development of muscle groups vary between species. Muscle groups that are routinely used for intramuscular injections are included. A more complete list of the muscles and their related anatomic terms is found in the glossary.

Facial Muscles

There are many facial muscles that produce a variety of movements. Some of these are

Orbicularis oculi (*ocul-* means eye): muscle that moves the eyelids

Masseters: muscles of *mastication* (chewing), which raise the mandible (and close the jaw)

Muscles of the Neck, Back, and Thorax

Muscles in the neck and thorax assist in rotation of the head, flexion and extension of the head on the neck, breathing, and attachment of the thoracic limb or forelimb to the body. Important muscles are

Serratus muscle group: important for respiration and for supporting the trunk of the body in all quadruped species

Pectoral muscle group: forms chest and adducts forelimb

Latissimus dorsi: broadest muscle in the back; supports forelimb and aids in flexion of shoulder

The important muscles of the dorsum include the *epaxial* group. This group is composed of three muscles:

Iliocostalis
Longissimus
Transversospinalis

These muscles act as extensors of the vertebral column and produce lateral movements of the trunk.

Three important muscles of the thorax are

External intercostals
Internal intercostals
Diaphragm

During respiration, the external intercostals lift the ribs, the internal intercostals lower the ribs, and the diaphragm contracts and flattens out, causing the thorax to enlarge and the lungs to expand.

Muscles of the Forelimbs

In addition to the action of the muscles of the shoulder, back, and upper thorax, the muscles of the upper forelimb also contribute to movement of the distal extremity. Included are

Triceps brachii: extends forelimb

Biceps brachii: flexes forelimb

The groups of flexor and extensor muscles control the movement of the toes and hooves.

Abdominal Muscles

The abdominal muscles are

External oblique
Internal oblique
Rectus abdominis
Transversus abdominis

These muscles keep the viscera in place, support and compress the abdomen, and contract during parturition, defecation, urination, and coughing. Additionally, they assist in rotating the vertebral column. The *linea alba* is a fibrous band of connective tissue running the entire length of the center of the ventral abdominal floor. The linea alba is the center attachment of the abdominal muscles and is an important landmark for many surgical incisions into the abdomen.

Muscles of the Hind Limb

The muscles of the hind limb have several functions in movement. The most important muscles are

Gluteal group: major muscles over pelvis, extends and abducts limb.

Quadriceps femoris group: includes the following muscles:
- *Rectus femoris:* flexes and extends leg
- *Vastus lateralis:* extends leg
- *Vastus medialis:* extends leg
- *Vastus intermedius:* extends leg

"Semi" group: descends on the posterior of hind limb, its tendons forming the "hamstrings" (Fig. 7-3). This group includes
- *Semimembranosus*
- *Semitendinosus*
- *Biceps femoris*

These three muscles work together to flex the distal extremity.

Gastrocnemius: flexes leg and foot. The tendon of insertion of the gastrocnemius at the hock is commonly called the *Achilles tendon.*

Miscellaneous Muscles

Some species may have muscles that are of particular significance. A specific example is the *arrector pili* muscles of the dog and cat. These are smooth muscles that attach to hairs on the dorsum. When stimulated,

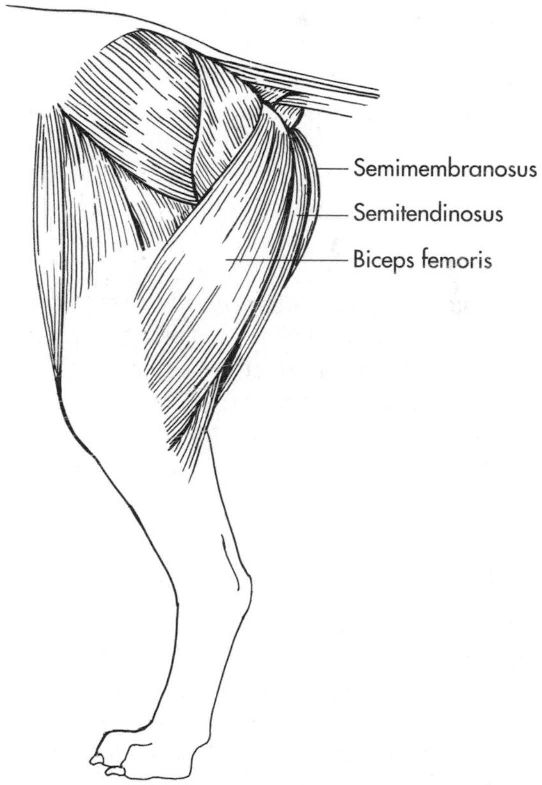
Semimembranosus
Semitendinosus
Biceps femoris

FIG. 7-3 Hind limb of dog showing "semi" group of muscles.

these muscles contract to raise the hair on the back.

The *cutaneous trunci* is an important muscle that attaches to the dermis and is responsible for the insect-repelling skin twitch in some large animals, such as the horse.

Another muscle of significance in large animal species is the *cremaster*. This muscle is part of the spermatic cord of male animals and attaches to the scrotum. The cremaster contracts and relaxes in response to ambient temperatures, raising and lowering the testicles. This movement of the testes away from or closer to the body is important for sperm viability.

REVIEW D

1. The diaphragm is a muscle of respiration located in the ______________________.
2. The muscles used for mastication are ______________________.
3. The muscle group that is important for supporting the trunk of the body by the forelimbs and aiding in respiration is the ______________________ group.
4. The fibrous band of connective tissue at the center of the ventral abdominal floor is called the ______________________.
5. The smooth muscles that attach to the hair on the dorsum and raise the hairs when stimulated in dogs and cats are the ______________________.
6. An important muscle attaching to the dermis that is responsible for the skin twitch response to insects is called the ______________________.
7. The muscle that raises and lowers the scrotum is the ______________________.
8. The major flexors of the hind limbs that form the "hamstrings" belong to a group called the ______________________.

Chapter 7 Answers

Review A

1. myology
2. extend, contract
3. origin
4. insertion
5. fascia

Review B

1. long, slender
2. sarcolemma
3. skeletal, smooth, cardiac
4. prime movers, antagonists, synergists
5. skeletal

Review C

1. external or outer
2. surrounding
3. square
4. diamond-shaped or kite-shaped
5. round

Review D

1. thorax
2. masseters
3. serratus
4. linea alba
5. arrector pili
6. cutaneous trunci
7. cremaster
8. "semis"

Chapter 7 — EXERCISES

THE MUSCULAR SYSTEM

Exercise 1: Complete the following statements.

1. The strong, fibrous, white bands that attach muscles to bones are called ______________________.
2. The strong bands of tissue that hold bones together and support organs are called ______________________.
3. A particular type of tendon that is flat and ribbonlike is called ______________________.
4. The immovable attachment of a muscle or the point at which it is anchored by a tendon to a bone is called its ______________________.
5. The nerve that causes a muscle to move is called a/an ______________________.

Exercise 2: Matching.

_____	1. Skeletal muscle	A. Muscles that work together
_____	2. Smooth muscle	B. Muscle that actively produces movement
_____	3. Cardiac muscle	C. Striped
_____	4. Prime mover	D. Muscle that moves voluntarily
_____	5. Antagonist	E. Smooth
_____	6. Sarcolemma	F. Muscle that cannot move at will
_____	7. Synergists	G. Muscle acting in opposition to another
_____	8. Insertion	H. Heart muscle
_____	9. Striated	I. Movable bone attached
_____	10. Nonstriated	J. Plasma membrane of a muscle cell

Exercise 3: Multiple choice.

1. The muscle adjective for unpaired muscles is
   a. Azygous
   b. Gracilis
   c. Serratus
2. The muscle adjective meaning long is
   a. Latissimus

b. Longissimus

c. Medius

3. The muscle adjective for surrounding a part is

a. Externus

b. Orbicularis

c. Transversus

4. Muscles that have four insertions may be called

a. Bi-

b. Tri-

c. Quadri-

5. A round or cylindrical muscle may be described as

a. Azygous

b. Orbicularis

c. Teres

Exercise 4: Multiple choice.

1. The masseter muscles are used for

a. Flexing the forelimb

b. Supporting the back

c. Chewing

d. Skin twitch reflex

2. The muscle that raises and lowers the scrotum is

a. Rectus abdominis

b. Longissimus

c. Serratus

d. Cremaster

3. The linea alba is found on the ____________ surface of the abdomen.

a. Ventral

b. Dorsal

c. Lateral

d. Caudal

4. An important muscle group needed for respiration that supports the trunk of the body from the forelimbs is
   a. Epaxials
   b. Serratus
   c. Semimembranosus
   d. Pectorals
5. The muscles that are used for intramuscular injections in the back or loin and are important extensors of the back are called the
   a. Triceps
   b. Semis
   c. Epaxials
   d. Gluteals
6. The muscle that contracts to cause the thorax to enlarge and the lungs to expand during inspiration is
   a. Transversus abdominis
   b. Diaphragm
   c. Iliocostalis
   d. External oblique

Exercise 5: Matching.

_____	1. Orbicularis oculi	A. Flexes the hind limb
_____	2. Masseters	B. Surrounding the eye
_____	3. Cremaster	C. Forms the chest and adducts the forelimbs
_____	4. Pectorals	D. Portion of the spermatic cord
_____	5. Triceps brachii	E. Abdominal wall muscle
_____	6. Cutaneous trunci	F. Skin twitch muscle
_____	7. Serratus	G. Extends distal forelimb
_____	8. Gluteals	H. Hip muscle
_____	9. Latissimus dorsi	I. Sawtooth muscle that supports trunk
_____	10. Rectus abdominis	J. Broadest muscle of the back
_____	11. Semimembranosus	K. Facial muscle for chewing

CHAPTER 7 PUZZLE

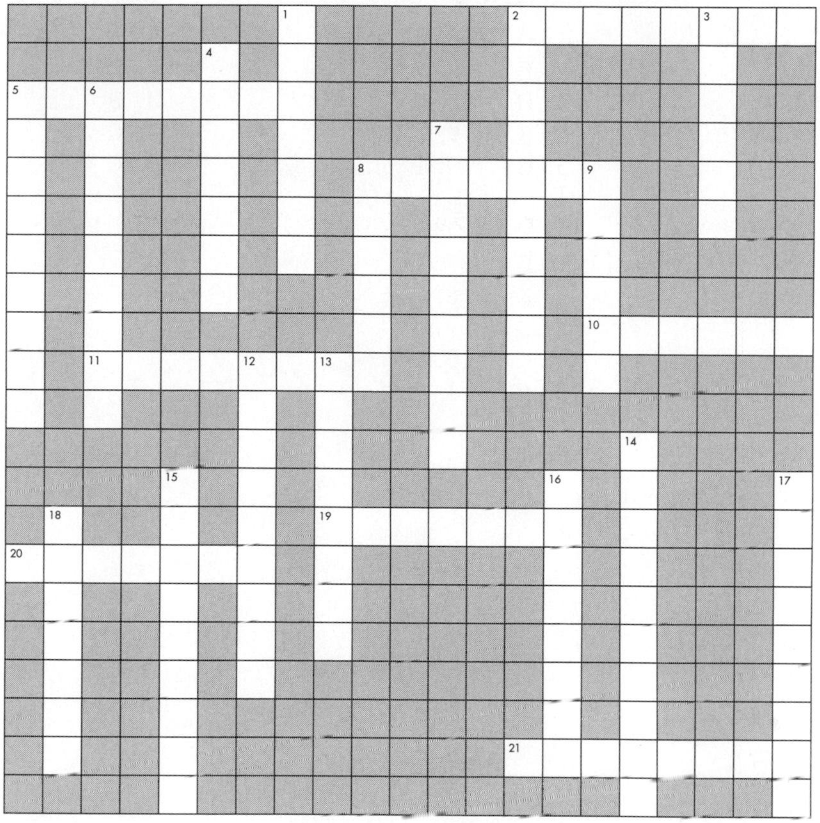

ACROSS CLUES

2. Voluntary striated muscle fiber
5. Muscles that move body part away from midline
8. Muscles that flex body part
10. Spasms
11. Muscles of dorsal pelvis
19. Study of muscles
20. ____________ brachii extends distal foreleg
21. Inflammation of voluntary muscles

DOWN CLUES

1. Muscle type found in heart
2. Plasma membrane of muscle cells
3. Connects muscle to bone
4. Wasting away of muscle
5. Movement toward midline
6. Wall between chest and abdominal cavities
7. Chest muscles
8. Muscle threads or filaments
9. Involuntary, nonstriated muscle fiber
12. Muscles that extend body parts
13. Connects bone to bone
14. Cytoplasm of muscle cells
15. Muscle in spermatic cord
16. Disease of muscles
17. Muscle that works with others
18. Triceps ____________, extensor of distal foreleg

Chapter 7 Answers

Exercise 1

1. tendons
2. ligaments
3. aponeurosis
4. origin
5. motor nerve

Exercise 2

1. D
2. F
3. H
4. B
5. G
6. J
7. A
8. I
9. C
10. E

Exercise 3

1. A
2. B
3. B
4. C
5. C

Exercise 4

1. C
2. D
3. A
4. B
5. C
6. B

Exercise 5

1. B
2. K
3. D
4. C
5. G
6. F
7. I
8. H
9. J
10. E
11. A

ANSWERS: CHAPTER 7 PUZZLE

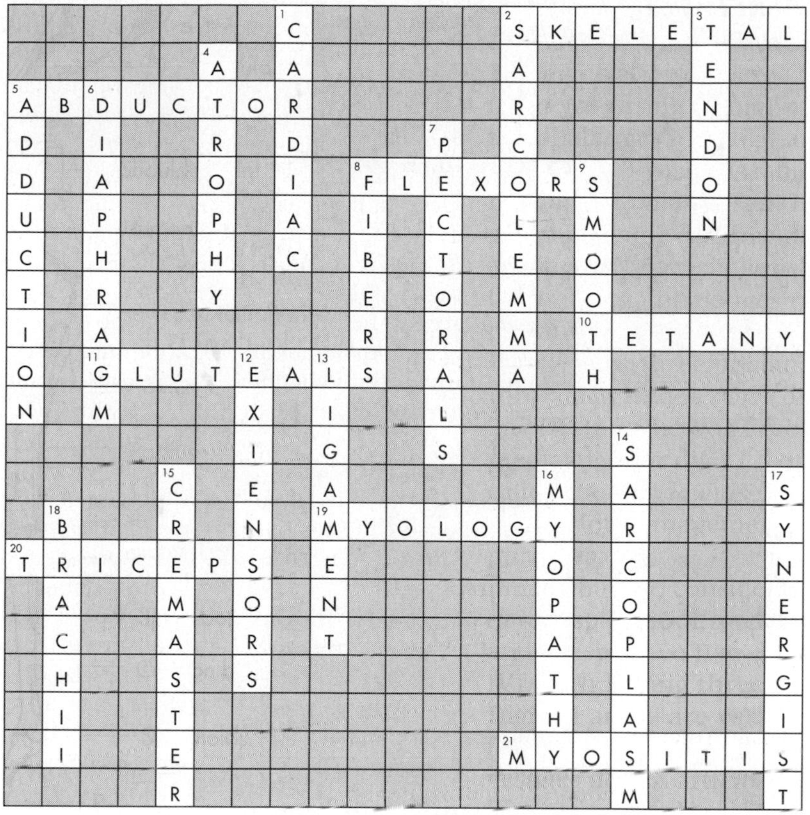
1 CARDIAC
2 SKELETAL
2 SARCOLEMMA
3 TENDON
4 ATROPHY
5 ABDUCTOR
5 ADDUCTION
6 DIAPHRAGM
7 PECTORALS
8 FLEXORS
8 FIBERS
9 SMOOTH
10 TETANY
11 GLUTEALS
12 EXTENSORS
13 LIGAMENT
14 SARCOPLASM
15 CREMASTER
16 MYOPATHY
17 SYNERGIST
18 BRACHII
19 MYOLOGY
20 TRICEPS
21 MYOSITIS

GLOSSARY

MUSCLES AND RELATED ANATOMIC TERMS

abduction: movement that draws a body part away from the midline of the body.

Achilles tendon: tendon of the gastrocnemius that inserts at the tarsus or hock.

adduction: movement that draws a body part toward the midline of the body.

antagonist: a muscle acting in opposition to another.

aponeurosis: broad sheet of fibrous connective tissue that serves as a tendon to attach muscles to bone or to bind muscles together.

arrector pili: smooth muscles in dorsum that act to raise the hairs on the back.

biceps brachii: flexor of distal foreleg.

biceps femoris: portion of "semi" group of muscles, flexor of the distal hind limb.

cardiac: type of striated muscle fiber found in the heart.

cremaster: muscle found in spermatic cord that raises and lowers the testicles.

cutaneous trunci: muscle of the dermis that is responsible for insect-repelling skin twitch.

diaphragm: musculomembranous wall between abdominal and thoracic cavities.

epaxial group: muscles of the dorsal back sometimes used for intramuscular injections.

extensors: muscles that extend a part of the body.

external intercostals: respiratory muscles situated between the ribs.

external oblique: muscle that compresses and supports the abdomen.

fascia: sheet of fibrous membrane that encloses muscles and separates them into groups.

fibers: muscle threads or filaments, usually in bundles.

flexors: muscles that flex a part of the body.

gastrocnemius: muscle of the distal hind limb that flexes the leg and extends the foot.

gluteal group: a group of muscles on the dorsal pelvis sometimes used for intramuscular injections.

iliocostalis: portion of epaxial group of muscles in dorsum.

insertion: the more movable of the two points of attachment of a muscle.

internal intercostals: respiratory muscles situated between the ribs.

internal oblique: muscle that compresses and supports the abdomen.

latissimus dorsi: the broadest muscle of the back; supports the forelimb and aids in flexing the shoulder.

ligament: strong bands of fibrous tissue connecting bones or cartilage that aid or restrict movement and support organs.

linea alba: fibrous band of connective tissue that is the center attachment of the abdominal muscles on the ventral abdominal wall.

longissimus: portion of epaxial group of muscles in dorsum.

masseter: muscle of mastication.

mastication: the process of grinding or chewing food.

motor nerve: the nerve that connects to a muscle.

myology: the study of muscles.

neuromotor unit: combination of the nerve cell and its group of muscles that are stimulated to cause muscle contraction.

orbicularis oculi: muscle that moves the eyelids.

origin: the less movable of the two points of attachment of a muscle.

pectoral group: group of muscles on the chest sometimes used for intramuscular injections.

prime movers: muscles that actively produce a movement.

quadriceps femoris group: group of muscles important for extension of the hind limb.

rectus abdominis: muscle that compresses and supports the abdomen.

rectus femoris: portion of the quadriceps femoris group of muscles of the hind limb.

sarcolemma: plasma membrane of muscle cells.

sarcoplasm: cytoplasm of muscle cells.

"semi" group: sometimes called the hamstring group, flexors of distal hind limb.

semimembranosus: portion of "semi" group of muscles, flexor of distal hind limb.

semitendinosus: portion of "semi" group of muscles, flexor of distal hind limb.

serratus group: group of muscles important for supporting the trunk of the body and for respiration.

skeletal: type of striated muscle fiber that is voluntary (controlled at will).

smooth: type of nonstriated muscle fiber that is involuntary (not controlled at will).

synergists: muscles that work together.

tendon: strong, white bands of connective tissue that attach muscle to bone.

tendon sheath: connective tissue surrounding tendons where there is a long distance to the distal attachment or where the tendon pulls over a joint.

transversospinalis: portion of epaxial group of muscles in dorsum.

transversus abdominis: muscle that compresses and supports the abdomen.

triceps brachii: extensor of distal foreleg.

vastus intermedius: portion of the quadriceps femoris group of muscles of the hind limb.

vastus lateralis: portion of the quadriceps femoris group of muscles of the hind limb.

vastus medialis: portion of the quadriceps femoris group of muscles of the hind limb.

PATHOLOGY

atrophy: wasting away of muscle tissue.

fasciitis: inflammation of the fascia.

leiomyoma: benign tumor of smooth muscle.

leiomyosarcoma: malignant tumor of smooth muscle.

myalgia: muscle pain or pain in a muscle.

myoma: a tumor of muscular tissue.

myopathy: any abnormal condition or disease of the muscular tissues.

myosarcoma: a malignant tumor composed of muscular tissue.

myositis: inflammation of voluntary muscles.

myotonia: increased muscular irritability and contractility.

rhabdomyoma: benign tumor arising from striated muscle.

rhabdomyosarcoma: malignant tumor of striated muscle.

tenosynovitis: inflammation of a tendon sheath.

tetany: spasms or abnormal contracture of muscle.

8 The Integumentary System

The skin and its accessory structures

CHAPTER OVERVIEW

This chapter describes the integumentary system, which includes the skin, the largest organ of the body. Also included are the accessory organs: hair, sweat glands, sebaceous glands, nails, and the variations of these special parts.

SKIN

The study of skin is called *dermatology.* The skin, which covers the body, has a variety of functions necessary for survival. It acts as a barrier against the invasion of microorganisms, protects underlying structures from injury, prevents the body from drying out (and, conversely, inhibits excess water intake in aquatic species), helps maintain and regulate body temperature, and acts as a receptor for the sensations of touch, heat, cold, pressure, and pain. Along with the kidneys, intestines, and lungs, the skin plays a crucial role in disposing of waste products.

Under normal conditions body temperature is maintained through a heat-regulating mechanisms that keeps a balance between heat production and heat loss. The body produces heat by metabolizing the food ingested, and the amount of heat produced is directly connected to the amount of work done by the muscles.

Most body heat loss occurs through the skin in the following ways:

Radiation: Heat energy is transmitted as rays to the surrounding area. Neither direct contact nor a medium is necessary for this form of energy transfer.

Conduction: Heat energy passes by direct contact through a nonmoving medium. When an animal lies on a cold surface, for example, it loses heat directly to that surface by conduction.

Convection: Heat transfer occurs in a gas or liquid by the circulation of currents from one region to another. This is the heat loss mechanism responsible for the windchill factor.

Evaporation: As perspiration or other fluids on the skin and hair change to vapor, they absorb heat. Air currents can increase evaporative heat loss through convection.

Most of the remainder of heat loss occurs through the mucous membranes of the respiratory tract, with lesser amounts lost through the digestive and urinary tracts.

REVIEW A

1. The accessory organs of the skin are the ____________, ____________, ____________, and ____________.
2. The study of skin is called ____________.
3. The body produces heat by ____________ of food taken in.
4. Heat loss resulting from perspiration is called ____________.
5. The largest organ of the body is the ____________.

Composition of the Skin

The skin is composed of two principal layers: the *epidermis,* the outer, thinner layer visible to the naked eye; and the *dermis* (or *corium*), the inner, thicker layer (Fig. 8-1).

EPIDERMIS

The epidermis is made up of stratified squamous epithelial tissue. The layers of the epidermis, from the dermis outward, are as follows:

Stratum germinativum (basal layer): The cells in this innermost layer multiply continuously to compensate for the constant loss of cells from the surface of the epidermis. These new cells push upward into each succeeding layer, eventually die, and are sloughed off. The process is continuous.

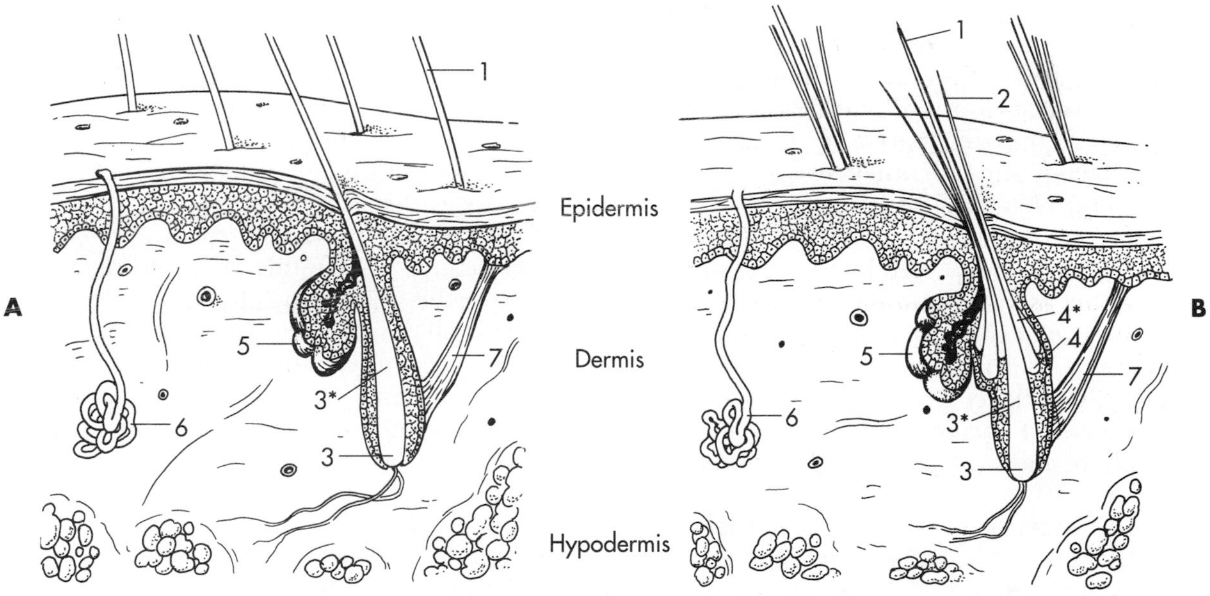
A
B
Epidermis
Dermis
Hypodermis
1
2
3
3*
4
4*
5
6
7

FIG. 8-1 Composition of skin and hair. **A,** Simple hair follicle. **B,** Compound hair follicle. *1,* Primary hair shaft; *2,* secondary hair shaft; *3,* primary hair papilla; *3**, primary hair follicle; *4,* secondary hair papilla; *4**, secondary hair follicle; *5,* sebaceous gland; *6,* sweat gland; *7,* arrector pili muscle.

Stratum spinosum (spinous layer): Cells begin to shrink and draw apart. The layer is one or two cells thick. It is thicker in body regions of rugged wear, such as footpads on dogs.

Stratum granulosum (granular layer): This layer is so called because it contains granules visible in the cytoplasm of the cells, which begin to die in this layer. The stratum granulosum may not be present in some areas of thin skin. *Keratinization* (*kerat* means horny tissue) or *cornification* packs the cells with a fibrous protein, called *keratin*. Keratinization begins in the granular layer.

Stratum lucidum (clear layer): This layer is so called because of its closely packed, clear cells. When present, this layer is found in areas of rugged wear.

Stratum corneum (horny layer): This layer is composed of flat, lifeless, cornified cells, which appear as overlapping, dry scales making up the outer skin layer. If these scales are unbroken, they can prevent the entrance of microorganisms. Keratinization gives the special epidermal parts (horns, hooves, beaks, and hair) their strength and is completed in this layer. Dead cells are continuously sloughed off this layer and replaced by new ones from the stratum germinativum.

Skin color is determined by the amount of *melanin* (skin pigment) in the stratum germinativum layer of the epidermis. Heredity is the chief factor influencing skin color. Sunlight and some hormones also affect skin color.

The absence of normal pigmentation in skin results in *albinism*. True albinism prevents pigmentation of the hair, skin, and eyes. Albinos may suffer from associated lethal traits. They also lack protection from some of the damaging effects of sunlight.

Skin color can be affected by the blood supply in nonpigmented skin. For instance, skin color may take on a blue hue *(cyanosis)* when oxygen supply is reduced. Lower forms of life, such as the chameleon, change skin color quickly to mimic their environment as a means of defense.

DERMIS

The dermis (corium) is made up of dense, fibrous, connective tissue containing blood vessels and nerves. Small bundles of involuntary muscle, called the *arrector pili,* are attached to hair follicles. When arrector pili muscles contract, hairs stiffen. This action increases the insulating ability of an animal's coat during cold weather. Another function of this smooth muscle contraction is noticed in the fight-or-flight reaction initiated by the sympathetic nervous system. When an animal raises its *hackles* (the hairs along the neck and back), it is enlarging its apparent size to bluff an opponent during battle. *Sebaceous* (oil-producing, to lubricate the hair) glands, sweat glands, and receptors for the sensations of touch, heat, cold, and pain are also found in the dermis.

A subcutaneous layer under the dermis is called the *hypodermis* or *subcutis.* It consists of loose, areolar connective tissue and *adipose* (fatty) tissue. Skin tends to conform and adhere to the underlying elements. The hypodermis allows the skin to move over the deeper structures without tearing.

Skin structure differs throughout the body. It is tough and stretchable and varies in thickness. It is thickest in areas where the skin is most exposed to hard usage, such as the footpads of dogs. Thick skin can also be found on the forehead, dorsal neck, dorsal thorax, rump, and base of the tail. Skin is usually thicker in larger animals. Skin of some animals, particularly cattle, is cleaned and preserved in a process called *tanning* to produce leather. Thin skin generally is located on the pinna of the ear and on the axillary, inguinal, and perianal regions.

The looseness of skin varies with the species. Rodents have abundant loose skin about the neck and shoulders, thus permitting picking up such animals by the scruff. Swine, on the other hand, have little excess loose skin.

REVIEW B

1. Skin is composed of two principal layers: ______________________________ and ______________________________.
2. Skin contains receptors for the sensations of ______________, ______________, ______________, and ______________.
3. The outermost layer of the epidermis is called ______________.
4. Skin color is determined by the pigment called ______________.
5. The hypodermis layer is also known as the ______________.
6. Horns and hooves get their strength from the fibrous protein ______________.

HAIR

Hair covers most animals as a thick coat, except the areas of the muzzle and foot surfaces. Some species, such as the pig, are almost hairless. Many animals have fur coats rather than hair coats. *Fur* is short, fine, soft hair. Pelts of fur are commonly worn in cold climates and used for fashion garments.

Mammals have three types of hair: primary, secondary, and tactile. *Primary hairs* are also called guard hairs and make up the *topcoat.* These hairs are stiff, with a smooth appearance. This arrangement allows rain to run off the coat, thereby preventing chilling of the animal. There are variations of primary hair, which include coarse manes and tails of horses, long tail hairs on cattle, sparse bristles of pigs, and feathering of tails and limbs on dogs.

Secondary hairs are known as wool hairs and make up the *undercoat.* Secondary hairs are soft, thin, and wavy. Sheep have abundant wool hairs in their fleeces, and guard hairs are present on their faces and limbs.

Tactile hairs are usually thicker and longer than primary hairs and are most often found about the face. Tactile hairs grow deep from the hypodermis or superficial muscle layer. Each hair is accompanied by a venous sinus that is generously innervated, aiding the function of the tactile hair as a touch receptor. Cat whiskers or vibrissae are a prime example of tactile hairs. A *vibrissa* is any large tactile hair.

Hair develops from a structure in the dermis called the *hair papilla.* The hair papilla is located at the base of a tube, the *hair follicle.* Cells at the base of the follicle increase, push upward, and keratinize, forming the visible *hair shaft* at the surface. Hair follicles are positioned at a 30- to 60-degree angle to the skin. There are two basic arrangements for hair growth: simple and compound. Cows and horses demonstrate the simple pattern. Primary hairs grow from separate follicular openings. Dogs and cats exhibit a compound style. Two to five long guard hairs erupt from a single follicle. They are surrounded by clusters of wool hairs emerging from a common pore (Fig. 8-1).

Hair color, governed by genetics, is important for thermal regulation. In general, light-colored coats are cooler in hot, sunny climates. Many animals, such as dogs, cats, gerbils, and rabbits demonstrate a unique color pattern called *agouti.* In this coloration, individual hairs have several bands of light and dark pigment with black tips. The name *agouti* originates from the South American rodent that also bears this color pattern.

On animals, hair grows during cycles. The process of losing hair is called *shedding* and occurs seasonally as a factor of photoperiod, temperature, nutrition, hormones, genetics, general state of health, and other intrinsic factors. Shedding peaks every spring and fall.

SWEAT GLANDS

The *sweat* (sudoriferous) *glands* are excretory organs of the skin that cool the body. *Apocrine sweat glands* are found throughout the animal body. They secrete a strong-smelling albuminous substance into the hair follicles.

An *eccrine sweat gland* is a coiled tubular structure embedded in the dermis, with its duct emerging on the skin surface. Eccrine glands produce a watery sweat. Eccrine glands are not distributed over the entire body but are found in limited areas, usually the footpads and between the nostrils. (See Fig. 8-1.)

The amount of sweating is masked by the generous hair coat of most mammals. Dogs and cats sweat very little. Instead they pant, slobber, and smear saliva on their coats to dissipate heat. Horses sweat generously, as evidenced by the lathering up of sweat.

The *sebaceous glands* are *holocrine glands,* secreting a substance called *sebum,* which lubricates the skin and hair. Sebum also waterproofs the coat, gives the coat a glossy sheen, increases the spread of sweat, slows bacterial growth, and serves as a territorial marker recognized by other members of the species.

A few examples of sebaceous glands include the following:

Circumoral glands: These glands are found in the lips of cats. During grooming or when a cat rubs its head against an object, the secretion is deposited to mark territory.

Horn glands: These scent glands produce a strong musk odor that attracts females to male goats during breeding season. The glands are located caudomedially to the horn base of bucks and does.

Anal sacs: The anal sacs are cutaneous pouches located in the four o'clock and eight o'clock positions about the anus of carnivores. The secretion is foul smelling and is expressed during defecation as a territorial marker. Skunks empty these sacs to ward off aggressors.

CERUMINOUS GLANDS

Ceruminous glands are classified as modified sweat glands, located in the external ear canal, secreting a yellowish, waxy substance called *cerumen* (earwax).

NAILS, CLAWS, AND HOOVES

The distal phalanges of animals are covered by modified epidermal structures known as nails, claws, or hooves. Nails, claws, or hooves have the following parts in common: wall, sole, and pad. However, there are variations in each. In primates the nail is the wall. It grows from the epidermis, adhering to the slightly curved form of the dermis below. The sparse sole is located beneath the nail at the open end. The pad corresponds with the finger (toe) tips.

The claw in carnivores is the wall, which has been compressed laterally to form a sharp dorsal border. The sole is the underside of the claw and is somewhat flaky in texture. There is also diversity in footpads.

Humans and bears are examples of plantigrade animals. *Plantigrades* have well-developed footpads. Individual digital pads, as well as metacarpal (metatarsal) and carpal (tarsal) pads, are present. Dogs and cats belong to the *digitigrade* category. In these animals, only the digital and metacarpal (metatarsal) pads make ground contact. The carpal pad is obvious on the forelimb, but the tarsal pad is absent from the hind limb (Fig. 8-2).

Hoffed animals are called *ungulates*. The hoof, which is visible as the animal stands, is the wall of the foot. Hooves differ in appearance. The horse hoof is a solid structure with curved sides. Ruminants and pigs have two cloven toes that make up the hoof. The sole is essentially the underside of the hoof. The sole is abundant in the horse and much less abundant in ruminants and pigs. The footpad of ruminants and pigs is the bulb or heel. Ruminant bulbs are harder than pig heels. Pig bulbs are also set apart from the wall and sole. The horse hoof has a complex structure known as the *frog*, which is the pad of the hoof. The frog and bulbs offer shock absorption to the hoof as it strikes the ground. (See Fig. 8-2.)

The nail, claw, or hoof protects the deeper structures and can also be used for scratching, digging, or defense in battle. The underlying dermis is richly innervated and vascularized. Trimming the nail, claw, or hoof too far is known as *cutting the quick* and results in bleeding and pain.

DEWCLAWS, CHESTNUTS, AND ERGOTS

Dewclaws, chestnuts, and ergots are modified epidermal structures. The dewclaw has a rudimentary bone in the dog and pig. In ruminants dewclaws are like miniature hooves, consisting mainly of wall and bulb. They serve no practical purpose. However, they can bear weight on soft ground or when the animal has weak pasterns.

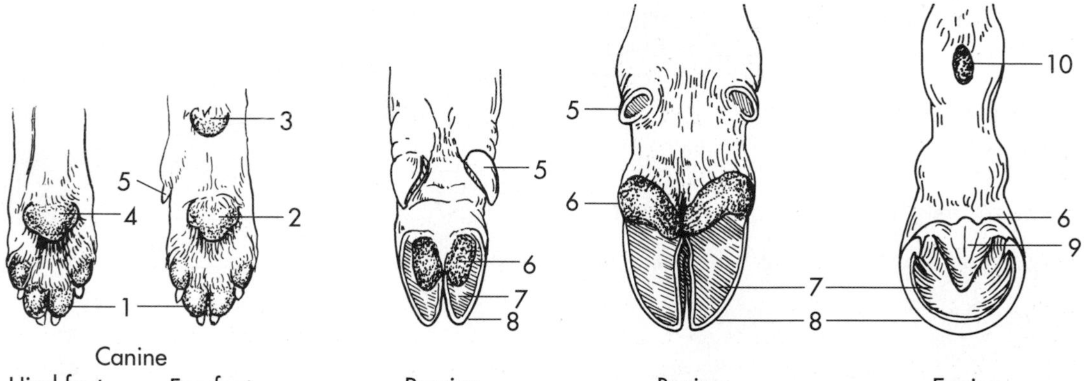
3
5
4
2
1
5
6
7
8
10
6
9
Canine
Hind foot
Forefoot
Porcine
Bovine
Equine

FIG. 8-2 Comparative anatomy of animal feet. From left, canine, hind foot and forefoot; porcine foot; bovine foot; equine foot. *1,* Digital pad; *2,* metacarpal pad; *3,* carpal pad; *4,* metatarsal pad; *5,* dewclaw; *6,* bulb/heel (digital pad); *7,* sole; *8,* wall; *9,* frog; *10,* ergot.

Horses have unique growths called chestnuts and ergots. *Chestnuts* are hornlike protrusions on the medial surface of the legs. In the forelimb, they are located above the carpus. In the hind limb, chestnuts are medial to the hock. Draft horses have larger chestnuts, and they may be absent from some lighter-weight horses. *Ergots* are keratinized epithelium found in the center of the caudal aspect of the fetlock. Fetlock hair usually covers ergots. (See Fig. 8-2.)

HORNS AND ANTLERS

Some species have protrusions from the skull called horns or antlers, which are used for defense. Some breeds are naturally hornless, or *polled.* Breed characteristics, sex, and age determine the size and shape of horns. Generally horns of males are larger than horns of females.

A *horn* is a permanent structure that grows continuously soon after birth. Horns grow over a horn process that stems from the frontal bones of the skull. The horn wall originates from keratinized epithelium. The sensitive dermis of the horn is supplied by nerves and blood. Horns of cows tend to be located in a temporal position, whereas sheep and goat horns are in a parietal position. Goat horns grow caudally. Sheep horns have a more complex appearance. They first protrude caudally and then ventrally and dorsally. The horns may grow very close to the skin of sheep, causing necrosis if the horns are not trimmed periodically. For safety reasons horns often are removed from domestic animals.

Antlers are shed and regrown each year. Antlers, like horns, also grow from the skull but are composed of bone rather than keratin. Initially antlers are covered with skin called *velvet.* As the skin dies, the velvet is rubbed off, exposing the underlying bony process. When the bony process is exposed, the antlers lose blood supply and are shed.

REVIEW C

1. The three types of animal hair are ____________________, ____________________, and ____________________.
2. "Cutting the quick" means ____________________.
3. Another word for sweat gland is ____________________ gland.
4. Sebaceous glands secrete ____________________.
5. New antlers are covered with skin called ____________________.
6. What animals have chestnuts and ergots on their legs? ____________________
7. Large hairs that function as touch receptors are called ____________________.

Chapter 8 Answers

Review A

1. hair, sweat glands, sebaceous glands, nails
2. dermatology
3. metabolism
4. evaporation
5. skin

Review B

1. epidermis, dermis
2. touch, heat, cold, pain
3. stratum corneum
4. melanin
5. subcutis
6. keratin

Review C

1. primary, secondary, tactile
2. cutting the hoof, nail, or claw too deeply
3. sudoriferous
4. sebum
5. velvet
6. horses
7. vibrissae

Chapter 8 EXERCISES

THE INTEGUMENTARY SYSTEM

Exercise 1: Complete the following statements.

1. The epidermis is composed of five layers of cells. They are ____________________, ____________________, ____________________, ____________________, and ____________________.
2. Primary hairs are also called ____________________ hairs.
3. An animal that sweats profusely after rigorous exercise is the ____________________.
4. The footpad of a horse's hoof is known as the ____________________.
5. Absence of normal skin pigmentation is called ____________________.
6. Primary hairs make up the ____________________ coat; secondary hairs make up the ____________________ coat.
7. Cats use secretions from the ____________________ glands to mark territory when rubbing their lips and head against an object.
8. A hornlike growth on the medial surface of an equine limb is called a ____________________.
9. A naturally hornless animal is called ____________________.
10. The word ____________________ describes skin color with a bluish hue.

Exercise 2: Match the definitions in the right column with the terms in the left column by placing the appropriate letter in the blank spaces provided.

_____ 1. Sebaceous glands
_____ 2. Eccrine glands
_____ 3. Ceruminous glands
_____ 4. Dermis
_____ 5. Ungulate
_____ 6. Arrector pili
_____ 7. Antlers
_____ 8. Melanin
_____ 9. Sebum
_____ 10. Skin

A. Barrier, receptor, waste disposal
B. Glands that produce watery sweat
C. Large sweat glands with strong-smelling secretions that waterproof the coat and mark territory
D. Pigment of skin or hair
E. Secretion of sebaceous glands
F. Dense, fibrous connective tissue
G. Bony protrusions that are shed and regrown annually
H. Animal with hooves
I. Modified sweat glands located in the external ear canal
J. Small muscles of the skin that produce "raising of the hackles"

Exercise 3: Using the following list of terms, identify the parts in Fig. 8-3 by placing their names in the corresponding blanks.

Primary hair papilla	1. ____________
Epidermis	2. ____________
Dermis	3. ____________
Hypodermis	4. ____________
Secondary hair papilla	5. ____________
Duct of sweat gland	6. ____________
Sebaceous gland	7. ____________
Arrector pili muscle	8. ____________
Primary hair shaft	9. ____________
Secondary hair shaft	10. ____________

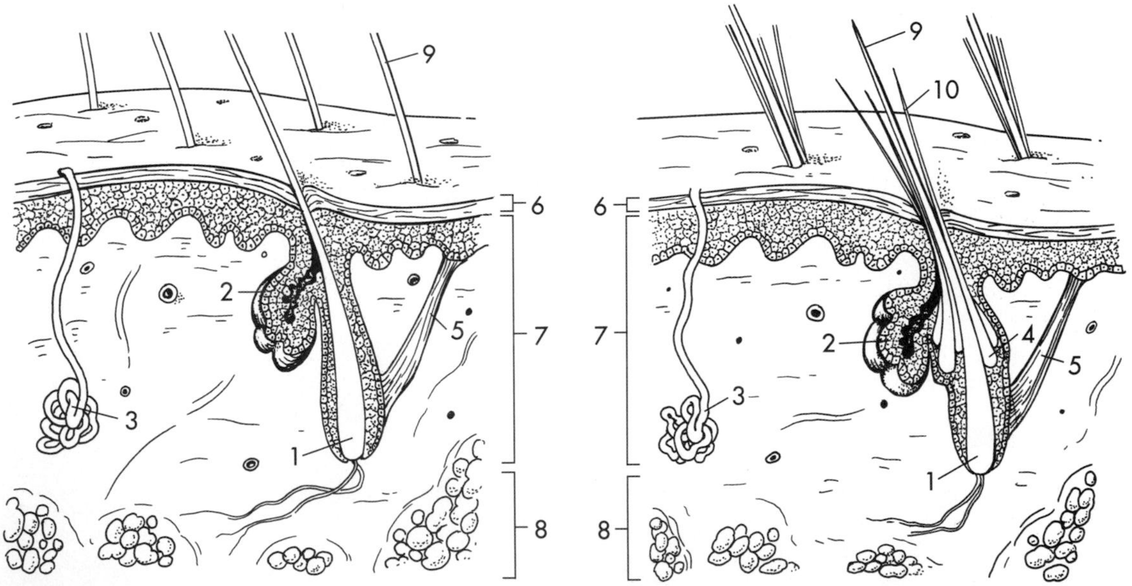
9
6
2
5
7
3
1
8
9
10
6
7
2
4
5
3
1
8

FIG. 8-3 Composition of skin and hair.

Exercise 4: Give the meaning of the components in the following words, and then define the word as a whole. Suffixes meaning "pertaining to" or "state or condition" are not to be defined separately and are preceded by a slash (/) mark. Before reaching for your medical dictionary, check the glossary at the end of the chapter.

1. Dermatofibroma

   dermato ______________________

   fibr ______________________

   oma ______________________

   ____

2. Hyperkeratosis

   hyper ______________________

   kerat/osis ______________________

   ____

3. Pyoderma

   pyo ______________________

   derma ______________________

   ____

4. Onychectomy

   onych ______________________

   ectomy ______________________

   ____

5. Autograft

   auto ______________________

   graft ______________________

   ____

6. Anhidrosis

   an ______________________

   hidr/osis ______________________

   ____

7. Dyskeratosis

   dys ______________________

   kerat/osis ______________________

   ____

8. Intradermal

   intra ______________________

   dermal ______________________

   ____

9. Seborrheic dermatitis

   sebo ______________________

   rrheic ______________________

   dermat ______________________

   itis ______________________

   ____

CHAPTER 8 PUZZLE

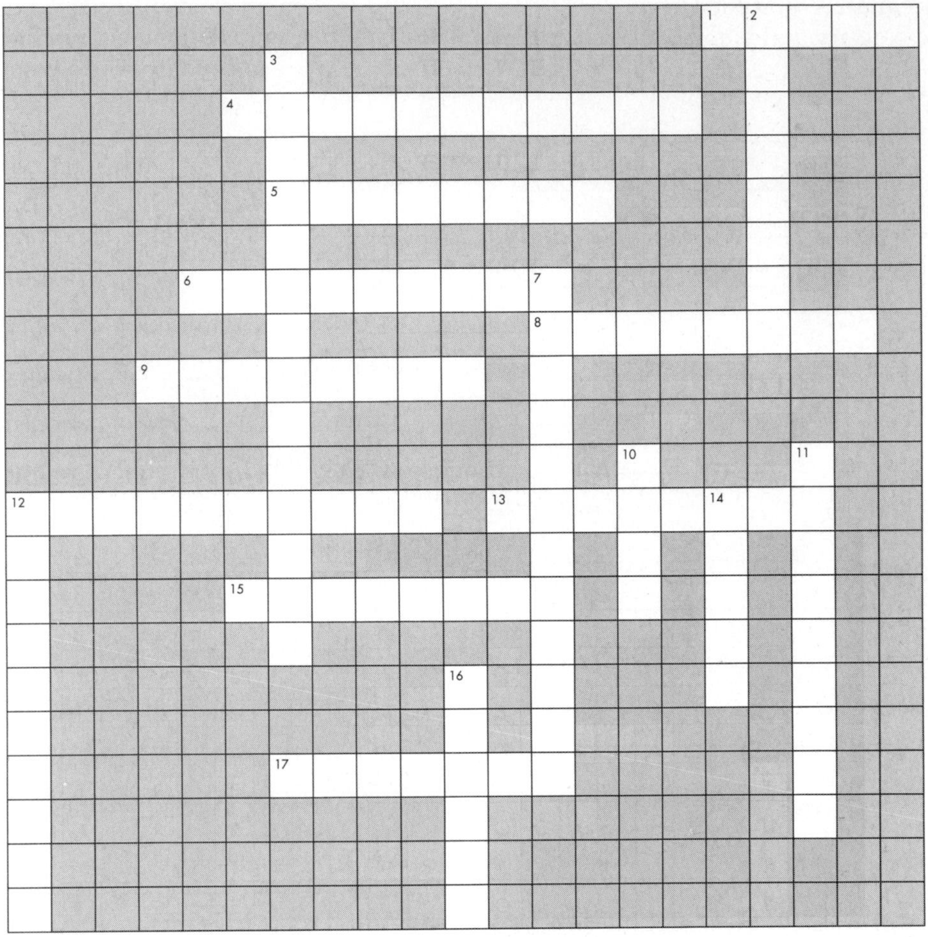
1
2
3
4
5
6
7
8
9
10
11
12
13
14
15
16
17

ACROSS CLUES

1. Infestation by mites
4. Study of skin
5. Absence of normal pigmentation
6. Outer layer of skin
8. Animal with hooves
9. Animal with a four-compartment stomach
12. Heat loss by fluid or air movement
13. Large tactile hair
15. Tube from which the hair grows
17. Raised hairs along the neck and back

DOWN CLUES

2. Loss of hair
3. Packing cells with fibrous protein
7. Sweat gland
10. Pad of a horse hoof
11. Meat-eating animal
12. Heat loss by direct contact
14. Secretion of sebaceous glands
16. Paleness of skin

Chapter 8 Answers

Exercise 1

1. stratum germinativum or basal layer, stratum spinosum or spiny layer, stratum granulosum or granular layer, stratum lucidum or clear layer, stratum corneum or horny layer
2. guard
3. horse
4. frog
5. albinism
6. top; under
7. circumoral
8. chestnut
9. polled
10. cyanosis

Exercise 2

1. C	6. J
2. B	7. G
3. I	8. D
4. F	9. E
5. H	10. A

Exercise 3

1. Primary hair papilla
2. Sebaceous gland
3. Duct of sweat gland
4. Secondary hair papilla
5. Arrector pili muscle
6. Epidermis
7. Dermis
8. Hypodermis
9. Primary hair shaft
10. Secondary hair shaft

Exercise 4

1. skin; fibers; tumor; a fibrous tumor of the skin
2. excessive; horny tissue; overgrowth of the horny layer of the epidermis
3. pus; skin; pus in the skin
4. nail or claw; cut out; declaw
5. self; graft; a graft in which donor and recipient are the same animal
6. no; sweat; inability to perspire
7. abnormal; keratin; abnormal keratinization of the skin
8. within; skin; within the skin (as opposed to *under* the skin, as in *subcutaneous*)
9. sebum; flow; skin; inflammation; skin inflammation with excessive sebum production

ANSWERS: CHAPTER 8 PUZZLE

																1 M	2 A	N	G	E
						3 K											L			
					4 D	E	R	M	A	T	O	L	O	G	Y		O			
						R											P			
						5 A	L	B	I	N	I	S	M				E			
						T											C			
				6 E	P	I	D	E	R	M	I	7 S					I			
						N						8 U	N	G	U	L	A	T	E	
			9 R	U	M	I	N	A	N	T		D								
						Z						O								
						A						R		10 F				11 C		
12 C	O	N	V	E	C	T	I	O	N		13 V	I	B	R	I	14 S	S	A		
O						I						F		O		E		R		
N					15 F	O	L	L	I	C	L	E		G		B		N		
D						N						R				U		I		
U										16 P		O				M		V		
C										A		U						O		
T						17 H	A	C	K	L	E	S						R		
I										L								E		
O										O										
N										R										

GLOSSARY

SKIN AND RELATED ANATOMIC TERMS

agouti (ă-gū'-tē): pattern of pigmentation in which several bands of light and dark pigment and black tips appear on individual hairs.
apocrine (ap'o-krin) *glands:* sweat glands, larger than eccrines, with a strong-smelling secretion, located throughout animal body.
arrector pili (pe'le): small muscle of skin that raises the hair.
cilia (sil'e-ah): plural form of *cilium.*
cilium (sil'e-um): eyelash.
corium (ko're-um): another term for *dermis.*
cornification (kōr-ni-fi-kā'-shŭn): conversion into keratin or horn.
derma (der'mah): skin.
dermis: inner, thicker layer of skin.
digitigrade (dij'-i-ti-grād): form of locomotion in which animal walks on its digits.
duct (dukt): tubelike passage, especially for excretions or secretions (also called *ductus*).
ductule (dukt'ūle): tiny duct.
eccrine (ek'rin) *glands:* ordinary sweat glands.
epidermis (ep″i-der'mis): outer layer of skin.
exocrine (ek'so-krin) *glands:* duct glands that empty secretions on skin surface (such as sweat glands).
hair bulb: expansion at proximal (root) end of hair.
hair follicle (fol'ĭ-k'l): tube in which hair grows.
hair shaft: portion of hair extending beyond surface of skin.
holocrine (hōl-ō-krin): wholly secretory. Sebaceous glands are holocrine glands in which the entire disintegrating cell is shed as a secretion.
hypodermis (hī-pō-der'-mis): subcutis.
keratin (ker'ah-tin): hard, protein constituent of hair, nails, epidermis, and horny tissues.
keratinization (ker'-ă-tun-ī-zā-shun): development of keratin.
melanin (mel'ah-nin): dark pigment of skin, hair, and other areas of body.
plantigrade (plan'-ti-grād): method of locomotion in which animal walks on phalanges, metacarpals (metatarsals), and carpal (tarsal) bones.
polled (pōld): individual animal of normally horned breed or breed of normally horned species that does not grow horns.
sebaceous (se-ba'shus) *gland:* secretes sebum that lubricates skin and hair.
sebum (se'bum): oily secretion of sebaceous glands.
stratum corneum: outer (horny) layer of epidermis.
stratum germinativum (jer″mĭ-na″-te'vum): innermost layer of epidermis (also called *basal* layer).
stratum granulosum: grainy layer of epidermis above basal layer; may not be present in thin skin (also called *granular* layer).
stratum lucidum (lu'sid-um): translucent layer of epidermis (also called *clear* layer), above the granular layer.
stratum spinosum (strat'-um spī-nō'-sum): layer of epidermis between stratum granulosum and stratum germinativum, marked by presence of prickle cells.
subcutaneous: located under skin.
subcutis (sub-kyū'-tis): subcutaneous tissue.
sudoriferous glands (su″dor-if'er-us): sweat glands.
supernumerary (su″per-nu'mer-ar″e): occurring in more than usual number.
topcoat (top'-cōt): outer coat of hair (overcoat).
undercoat (un'-der-cōt): hair growth below and partly concealed by main hair growth.
ungulate (un'-gū-lat): hoofed animal.
vibrissae (vī-bris'-ee): long, coarse, tactile hairs that grow from the muzzle and brow of most mammals, such as the whiskers of a cat.

DESCRIPTIVE TERMS

abscess (ab'-ses): localized accumulation of pus.
albinism: congenital defect in melanin development, causing lack of pigment in skin, hair, and eyes.
alopecia (al-ō-pē'-shē-ă): deficiency of hair or wool coat.
anhidrosis (an-hī-drō'-sis): abnormal reduction of sweating; common in horses in tropical climates, where affected animals show respiratory distress even at rest.
bleb: small blister.
bulla (bul'ah): large lesion filled with fluid (also called *blister* or *vesicle*).
cicatrix (sik-a'-triks): scar.

cicatrices (sik-a-tri'-sez): plural form of *cicatrix.*
cyanosis (si″ah-no'sis): bluish skin color caused by oxygen-starved hemoglobin in the blood.
dyskeratosis: abnormal alteration in keratinization.
ecchymosis (ek'ĭ-mo'sis): flat, circumscribed, reddish-purple spot caused by intradermal or submucous hemorrhages.
erythema: redness of skin caused by capillary congestion.
exanthema (ek-san'the'mah): any rash caused by fever or disease.
exfoliation: shedding or desquamation of horny layer of epidermis.
fissure: crack or groove.
hyperhidrosis: excessive sweating.
hyperkeratosis: overgrowth of horny layer of epidermis.
intradermal: within the tissues of the skin. An intradermal injection splits the layers of the skin, creating a bleb.
macula (mak'ū-lah): small, discolored spot on skin that can be seen but not felt.
nodule (nod'ūl): small, visible knot protruding above skin.
pallor: paleness of skin.
papule (pap'ul): small, rounded, solid elevation of skin.
pruritus (prū-rī'-tus): itching.
purpura (pur'pu-rah): group of conditions with purple-red or brown-red discolorations on epidermis, caused by hemorrhage into tissues (small ones are *petechiae,* large ones are *ecchymoses*).
pustule (pus'tūl): pus collected in hair follicle or pore.
scale: horny epithelial cells on epidermis or shed from it.
subcutaneous: beneath the skin. A subcutaneous injection is deposited into the areolar tissue below the dermis.

PATHOLOGIC CONDITIONS

Many eruptive diseases of the skin are symptoms of specific immune-system diseases (see Chapter 16.)

Inflammations and allergies

acne: inflammation of skin, caused by plugging of sebaceous glands, with development of papules and pustules. Canine and feline acne is commonly seen about the chin and lips.
allergic dermatitis (der″mah-tĭt'is): skin inflammation caused by allergy (also called *atopy*).
aphthous stomatitis (af'thus sto-mah-ti'tis): inflammation of mucous membranes of mouth, characterized by small, white, ulcerlike lesions (also called *canker sores* in primates).
contact dermatitis: caused by contact with various allergy-producing substances.
decubitus ulcer: skin surface lesion resulting from pressure on affected areas that results in defective circulation.
dermatitis (der″mah-ti'tis): inflammation of skin.
dermatocellulitis (der″mah-to-sel″u-li'tis): inflammation of skin and underlying connective tissue.
dermatosis (der″mah-to'sis): any skin disease, especially those not usually associated with inflammation.
discoid lupus erythematosus (DLE): autoimmune skin disease of dogs, characterized by depigmentation, erythema, scaling, erosions, ulcerations, and crusting, particularly on bridge of nose, face, and lips.
eczema (ek'zĕ-mah): general term for acute or chronic dermatitis.
exfoliative dermatitis: dermatitis with scaling, itching, loss of hair, and redness of skin, resulting from any of several abnormal skin conditions.
frostbite: tissue damage caused by exposure to extreme cold or by contact with chemicals that have a rapid freezing action.
herpes virus: affects primates, existing subclinically in one host, but can be deadly when transmitted to other hosts. For example, herpes virus B *(Herpesvirus simiae)* usually is innocuous in *Macaca* species but can cause fatal encephalitis and encephalomyelitis in humans.
parakeratosis: scaly dermatosis caused by overabundance of keratinocyte nuclei in horny layer of epidermis.
pemphigus vulgaris: autoimmune disease of dogs, characterized by shallow ulcerations of mucocutaneous junctions and oral mucosa.
petechia (plural, *petechiae*): pinpoint hemorrhage beneath skin, mucous membrane, or organ capsule.
pox: group of diseases caused by pox viruses. Lesions affect skin and range from erythema to papules or pustules.
seborrheic (seb″o-re'ik) *dermatitis:*

chronic, inflammatory dermatitis with yellowish, greasy scaling of skin, with or without *pruritus* (itching).

soremouth: virally caused dermatitis in which scabs form around lips and faces of sheep and goats; transmissible to humans (also called *contagious ecthyma* or *orf*).

urticaria (ur″tĭ-ka′re-ah): skin reaction, usually allergic, with wheals appearing on skin, accompanied by pruritus (also called *hives*).

wart: virus-caused, benign, small, tumorlike epidermal growth (also called *papillomatosis*).

wheal (wheel): round, smooth, slightly elevated lesion on skin, whiter or redder than surrounding area, which itches severely and usually is evidence of allergy.

Bacterial, fungal, and parasitic infections

acute moist dermatitis: superficial bacterial infection of skin caused by self-trauma, usually scratching, chewing, and licking (also called *hot spots*).

cellulitis: inflammation, usually bacterial, possibly purulent, especially involving loose subcutaneous tissue.

chiggers: infestation by mite larvae, causing severe itching and dermatitis.

cutaneous acariasis: infestation by mites (also called *mange*); varieties include red mange (also called *demodicosis*), caused by *Demodex* species; sarcoptic mange (also called *scabies*), caused by *Sarcoptes* species; and body mange, caused by *Psoroptes* species.

cutaneous blowfly myiasis: infestation by maggots; devitalized skin, skin covered by hair or wool, or skin wounds soiled by feces or urine are affected (also called *flystrike*).

dermatomycosis (der″mah-to-mi-ko′sis): fungal infection of the skin (also called *ringworm*).

ecthyma (ek-thi′mah): form of skin infection with shallow lesions and crusting caused by infectious agents.

flea bite dermatitis: inflammatory lesions caused by hypersensitivity to flea bites; self-trauma and secondary infection are common in dogs.

footrot: hoof disease commonly caused by *Fusobacterium* sp. in which severe dermatitis is spread from interdigital skin to deeper structures of the foot.

furunculosis (fu-rung″ku-lo′sis): persistent, consecutive occurrence of boils over period of time.

orf: viral dermatitis in which scabs form around lips and faces of sheep and goats; transmissible to humans (also called *contagious ecthyma* or *soremouth*).

paronychia (par″o-nik′e-ah): bacterial or viral inflammation of skin around nails or claws.

pediculosis: infestation by lice.

pyoderma: any purulent skin disease.

scabies: contagious skin disease caused by invasive mites, usually producing intense itching.

toxic epidermal necrolysis (TEN): acute exfoliative skin disease affecting dogs, cats, and monkeys; characterized by thick, epidermal necrosis and accompanied by erythema, vesicles, bullae, ulcers, fever, anorexia, and lethargy.

Oncology * know all

dermatofibroma (der″mah-to-fi-bro′mah): fibrous tumor of skin.

lipoma: benign tumor composed of mature fat cells.

malignant melanoma: rapidly growing, often ulcerated mass with tendency to metastasize; tumor cells may be pigmented.

mast cell tumor: benign local aggregation of mast cells that forms nodular tumor in skin; may become malignant.

sebaceous cyst: cyst of sebaceous gland plugged with sebum.

seborrheic keratosis: benign tumor of epidermis with many yellow or brown raised lesions on skin (also called *seborrheic wart*).

squamous cell carcinoma: type of carcinoma from squamous epithelium.

SURGICAL PROCEDURES

allograft (also called *homograft*): skin graft between genetically different individuals of same species.

autograft: skin graft that comes from patient's own body.

excisional biopsy: surgical incision to remove tissue of all or part of lesion and surrounding normal-appearing tissue.

heterograft (also called *xenograft*):

skin graft tissue transplanted between individuals of different species.

isograft: skin graft between individuals who are genetically identical, such as identical twins or animals from same inbred strain.

punch biopsy: sample of tissue obtained by use of punch.

skin graft: surgical procedure to transplant skin from one location to another.

DIAGNOSTIC TESTS

biopsy: removal of tissue for microscopic examination.

fungal culture: crusts of lesion and plucked hair are dropped into container of dermatophyte test medium or Sabouraud dextrose agar; container is loosely capped, incubated at room temperature, and observed daily for 2 weeks, noting growth and color changes. Positive identification can be made microscopically.

intradermal tests: several tests using injection of substances intradermally to observe reaction, including *PPD (purified protein derivative)* test for tuberculosis performed on human beings and *TB test* in which animals are tested for tuberculosis by injecting tuberculin intradermally and observing injection site for local swelling at 24, 36, and 72 hours after injection.

skin scrape: scalpel blade is used to scrape skin deeply while squeezing affected lesion, contents of scrape are examined microscopically for presence of mange mites.

tissue culture: epithelial cells, taken from body, grown in a medium for diagnostic or research purposes.

III

INTERNAL MECHANISMS OF THE BODY

Section III of LEARNING VETERINARY TERMINOLOGY consists of eight chapters that describe the internal workings of the body.

Chapter 9 presents the cardiovascular and lymphatic systems and their functions in the circulation of the blood and lymph in animals.

Chapter 10 discusses the respiratory system and its importance in providing the body with oxygen and eliminating waste gases from cell metabolism.

Chapter 11 deals with the gastrointestinal system and shows how differences in diet are reflected in species variations in structure and function of the digestive organs.

Chapter 12 presents the functions of the genitourinary system, beginning with the excretion of liquid waste and ending with some of the major species differences in the reproductive organs of both sexes.

Chapter 13 discusses the endocrine system and details the activity of the glands of internal secretion, which regulate body functions through chemical means.

Chapter 14 describes the nervous system and its functions in relaying information between the brain and the various body systems.

Chapter 15 describes the special senses, through which animals receive stimulation from the world around them.

Chapter 16 presents the immune system, which protects and defends the integrity of the body.

As in the previous sections, drawings in the chapters illustrate the principal parts of the anatomy in that particular chapter. Review questions are placed every few pages, with comprehensive exercises at the end of each chapter. The glossary for each system includes the words introduced in that chapter and other important words pertaining to that system.

9 The Cardiovascular and Lymphatic Systems

The transports of the body

CHAPTER OVERVIEW

This chapter explains the structures and functions of the heart, the various types of blood vessels, the characteristics of blood, and the mechanism of circulation. It also describes the lymphatic system and its relationship to circulation.

CARDIOVASCULAR SYSTEM

The cardiovascular system includes the heart, blood vessels, blood, and blood circulation.

The Heart

The heart (or cardiac muscle) is a hollow, cone-shaped muscular organ that is divided into four chambers and varies in size by species. Heart size is dictated by overall size of the animal (Figs. 9-1 and 9-2). The heart straddles the midline within the thoracic cavity, just dorsal to the sternum. The base of the heart is located craniodorsally, although the apex points ventrally and to the left. The apex is totally free within the pericardium. The heart is separated from the thoracic cavity wall by the lungs and pleura. The heart is a pump that circulates the blood throughout the body to nourish and to remove waste products from the tissues.

STRUCTURE OF THE HEART

The heart is covered by a saclike membrane, which has three layers:

- The *pericardium*—tough, fibrous external layer
- Two internal serous layers:
  - *Parietal* layer—lining the pericardium
  - *Visceral* layer (*epicardium*)—covering the surface of the heart

The space between the two layers of serous membrane is the *pericardial space,* which contains several drops of pericardial fluid.

The heart wall is composed of three layers. The outer layer is the visceral layer of membrane (epicardium), described earlier. The middle layer, the *myocardium,* is the heart (cardiac) muscle itself, and the innermost layer, the *endocardium,* lines the chambers of the heart and covers its valves.

CHAMBERS OF THE HEART

The heart is divided into a left and a right side. The hollow of the heart is divided into four chambers. Each cranial chamber is called an *atrium* (plural, *atria*), and each ventral chamber is called a *ventricle.* A wall called the *interatrial septum* divides the atria into right and left sides, and a similar wall, the *interventricular septum,* divides the ventricles into right and left sides. There is no

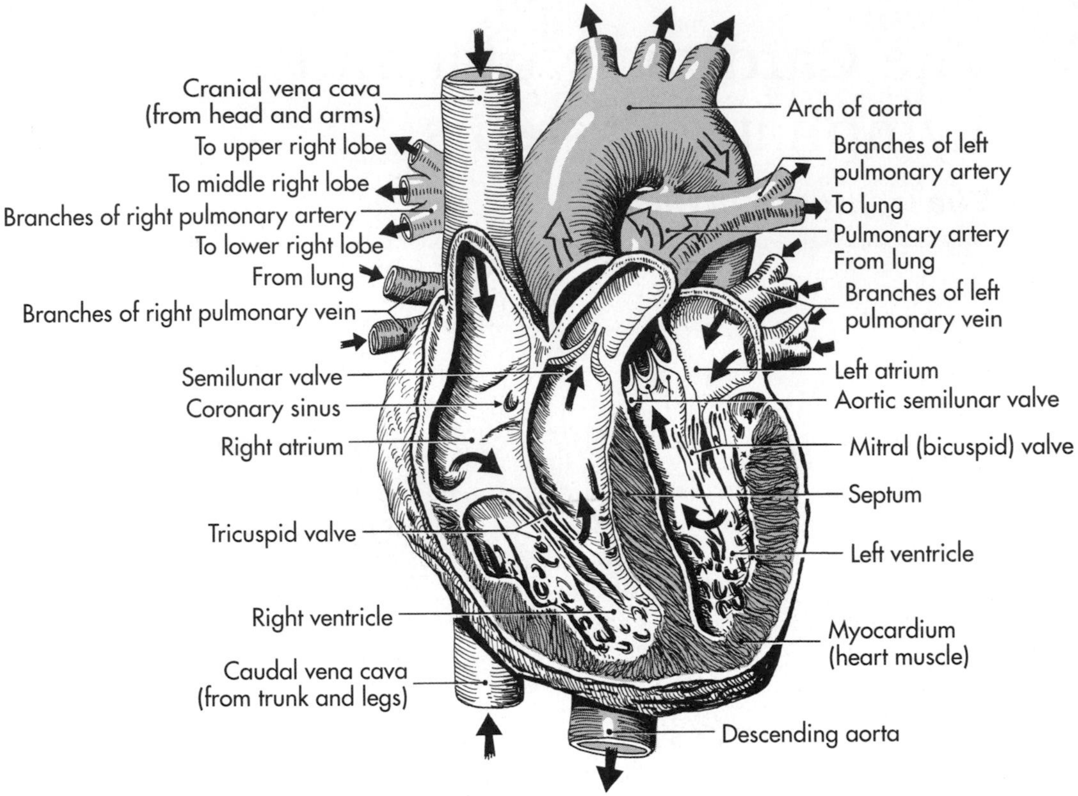
Cranial vena cava
(from head and arms)
To upper right lobe
To middle right lobe
Branches of right pulmonary artery
To lower right lobe
From lung
Branches of right pulmonary vein
Semilunar valve
Coronary sinus
Right atrium
Tricuspid valve
Right ventricle
Caudal vena cava
(from trunk and legs)
Arch of aorta
Branches of left
pulmonary artery
To lung
Pulmonary artery
From lung
Branches of left
pulmonary vein
Left atrium
Aortic semilunar valve
Mitral (bicuspid) valve
Septum
Left ventricle
Myocardium
(heart muscle)
Descending aorta

FIG. 9-1 Frontal section showing four chambers of heart and valves, openings, and major blood vessels. Arrows indicate direction of blood flow. (Branches of right pulmonary vein continue from right lung, behind heart, to enter left atrium.)

communication between the two sides. (See Fig. 9-1.)

The atria have thin walls and are the receiving chambers. The ventricles, which do the pumping, have thick walls. The right side of the heart receives blood from body tissues and sends it to the lungs to be oxygenated. The left side of the heart receives oxygenated blood from the lungs and sends it to the tissues. The walls of the left ventricle are thicker than the walls of the right ventricle because the left ventricle pumps blood to all the blood vessels of the body; the right ventricle pumps blood only to the lungs.

VALVES

Between the atria and ventricles are valves. These atrioventricular valves close to ensure that the blood flows in one direction and to prevent a backflow of blood into the atria. The left atrium and the left ventricle are separated by the *mitral* or *bicuspid* (two flaps) *valve.* The right atrium and the right ventricle are separated by the *tricuspid* (three flaps) *valve.* The *semilunar* (half-moon shaped) *valves,* which prevent a backflow of blood from the arteries into the ventricles, are located at the bases of the *pulmonary* artery and the *aorta* (Fig. 9-1).

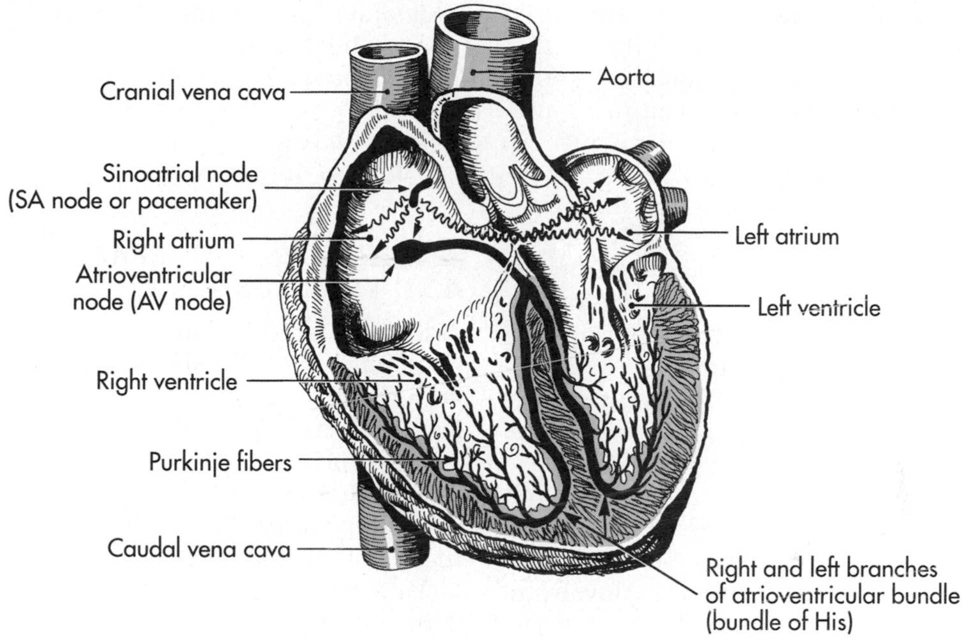
Cranial vena cava
Aorta
Sinoatrial node
(SA node or pacemaker)
Right atrium
Atrioventricular
node (AV node)
Left atrium
Left ventricle
Right ventricle
Purkinje fibers
Caudal vena cava
Right and left branches
of atrioventricular bundle
(bundle of His)

FIG. 9-2 Conduction system of heart. Sinoatrial node (pacemaker), located in wall of right atrium, sets basic heart rhythm.

CONDUCTION SYSTEM

The heart begins its pumping action in utero. This action depends on a conduction system consisting of the following:

The *sinoatrial node* (SA node)—called the *pacemaker,* consisting of cells in which electrical impulses originate, produce atrial contractions, and force blood into the ventricles.

The *atrioventricular node* (AV node)—consisting of conductile cells through which the electrical impulses continue down to.

The *atrioventricular bundle* (bundle of His), which continues on as the *Purkinje fibers,* which move the impulses on to stimulate ventricular contraction.

After a brief rest period, the entire process repeats itself (Fig. 9-2).

NERVE FUNCTION IN HEART ACTION

The *autonomic* nervous system has two divisions with opposite actions on the heart:

The *parasympathetic* division, mainly supplying the SA and AV nodes, slows the heart rate, reduces impulse conduction, and constricts the coronary arteries.

The *sympathetic* division, through the cardiac nerves, also acts on the SA and AV nodes to increase the heart rate and impulse conduction and dilate the coronary arteries. (See Chapter 14.)

CARDIAC CYCLE

The cardiac cycle includes the contraction *(systole)* and relaxation *(diastole)* of the atria and the ventricles. The heart chambers do not contract all at one time. The two atria contract in unison, and as they relax, the two ventricles contract. Similarly, as the ventricles relax, the atria contract, and the cycle is repeated.

When the atria contract, the blood is forced into the ventricles through the bicuspid and tricuspid valves. These valves open to allow the blood to pass from the atria to the ventricles, while the semilunar valves close to prevent blood from entering the aorta or the pulmonary artery.

When the atria relax, blood enters the atrial chambers from the pulmonary veins and venae cavae, and the ventricles contract. When the ventricles contract, the bicuspid and tricuspid valves close to prevent backflow to the atria, and the semilunar valves open to permit the blood to flow from the ventricles into the aorta and pulmonary artery.

When the ventricles relax, the semilunar valves close, the bicuspid and tricuspid valves open, the atria contract, and blood from the atria again starts to fill the ventricles, repeating the cycle.

Types of Blood Vessels

Animals have three major types of blood vessels: *arteries, capillaries,* and *veins.*

ARTERIES

Oxygenated blood is carried from the heart to all structures of the body by arteries, which are elastic tubes with thick walls composed of three layers:

Tunica intima (or intimal layer)—a lining of endothelium
Tunica media (or medial layer)—muscle layer
Tunica adventitia (or *tunica externa*)—the fibrous outer coat

ARTERIOLES, CAPILLARIES, AND VENULES

Arteries become smaller and smaller, branching and rebranching throughout the body, finally becoming *arterioles* (small arteries). The arterioles feed the blood into *capillaries,* which are billions of minute, very thin-walled vessels that communicate with other capillaries. The capillaries distribute the blood to the tissues. Other capillaries pick up the blood from the tissues and return it to *venules* (small veins), which pass the blood to the veins. The veins return the blood to the heart.

VEINS

The *veins* are hollow tubes, similar to the arteries, with thinner and less elastic walls, which transport blood back to the heart. The smallest veins *(venules)* collect blood from the capillaries, connect to larger veins, and finally join the venae cavae (plural of *vena cava*) to return the blood to the heart. Within venous channels are valves that help prevent backflow of blood. The flow of venous blood is also assisted by the alternate contraction and relaxation of the muscles of the limbs.

REVIEW A

1. The tough, fibrous external layer of the membrane covering the heart is called the ____________________. The outer surface of the heart itself is covered with a layer called the ____________________. The muscle of the heart is called ____________________. The chambers of the heart are lined with a layer called ____________________.
2. The two thin-walled receiving chambers of the heart are the ____________________. The thicker-walled chambers into which they feed are called ____________________.
3. The left atrioventricular valve is called the ____________________ valve, and the right is called the ____________________ valve. Backflow of blood from the arteries to the ventricles is prevented by the ____________________ valves.
4. The pacemaker of the heart is also called the ____________________ node. It produces electrical impulses that spread to the ____________________ node and ultimately through the ____________________ fibers to stimulate contraction of the ventricles.
5. Heart rate is influenced by the two branches of the autonomic nervous system. The parasympathetic division slows heart rate. The sympathetic division increases heart rate.
6. Small arteries are called arterioles, and small veins are called venules. The tiny vessels that connect them are called ____________________.

Blood

Blood is made up of about 60% liquid *(plasma)*, and 40% formed elements, which consist of *erythrocytes* (red cells), *leukocytes* (white cells), and *platelets* (thrombocytes). Blood transports oxygen from the lungs to the body tissues, collects carbon dioxide waste from the tissues, and brings it back to the lungs to be expelled. Blood distributes nutrients throughout the body, collects waste products of metabolism (such as urea, uric acid, and creatinine), and delivers them to the excretory organs for disposal. It carries hormones of the different ductless glands (such as the thyroid and parathyroid glands) to the cells, maintains the fluid content of the tissues, and serves as a temperature regulator for the body.

The average amount of blood contained in an adult animal varies by species. Blood volume usually is denoted as a percentage of body weight. Variations exist within a species with regard to size and health of the individual animal. Depending on the species, blood makes up 6% to 8% of total body weight.

Blood is extremely viscous and somewhat sticky, about five times as viscous as water. The color of blood varies from the bright red of oxygenated blood to the dark purple-red of deoxygenated blood. Blood is slightly alkaline and has a specific gravity slightly higher than that of water.

PLASMA

The clear, straw-colored, liquid portion of the blood is called blood plasma. It is approximately 90% water and 10% solutes. Protein makes up the major portion of the solutes. One of these, fibrinogen, is important in blood clotting. If it and other clotting elements are removed, the resulting liquid is called *serum*. Sheep, goats, dogs, and cats have very light-colored plasma. The plasma of cattle, horses, and rabbits is slightly darker. The coloration of plasma is due to the presence of carotene and bilirubin. Other solutes that are present in plasma, in much smaller amounts, include nutrients (lipids, glucose, and amino acids), end products of metabolism (urea, creatinine, uric and lactic acids), gases (oxygen and carbon dioxide), and hormones, enzymes, and antibodies.

BLOOD CELLS

All blood cells have their origin in undifferentiated stem cells, the *hemocytoblasts* (Fig. 9-3), which develop in the embryo. In young animals, blood cells are produced in almost all bone marrow, whereas in the adult, blood cells are produced in red bone marrow only. Proerythrocytes produce erythrocytes, myeloblasts produce granulocytes, lymphoblasts produce lymphocytes, monoblasts produce monocytes, and megakaryoblasts produce platelets. The logical progression through which the immature cells mature is shown in Figure 9-3.

Erythrocytes

At maturity, mammalian erythrocytes are extremely small, nonnucleated disks (Fig. 9-4). They contain *hemoglobin* (*heme*—iron; *globin*—protein), an iron-containing pigment that, in combination with oxygen, gives the blood its red color. Hemoglobin combines with oxygen in the lungs and distributes it to body cells; there the hemoglobin combines with carbon dioxide, which it carries to the lungs for disposal. The average life span of erythrocytes is about 120 days in dogs but varies widely among species. If iron is lacking in erythrocytes, there is a reduction of hemoglobin and the number of red cells, resulting in anemia.

Leukocytes

Leukocytes are much less numerous than erythrocytes, are colorless, and have nuclei (Fig. 9-4). They are divided into two groups:

- *Granulocytes*—originate in bone marrow, have lobed nuclei and cytoplasm that contains fine granules; and are classified according to staining characteristics:
  - *Neutrophils*—have red and blue staining granules and function mainly in *phagocytosis* (engulfing invading microorganisms)
  - *Eosinophils*—have orange or yellow acid dye-staining granules and detoxify foreign proteins from allergens or parasitic infections
  - *Basophils*—have purple, basic dye-staining granules; function not clear, but may prevent coagulation in blood vessels
- *Agranulocytes*—originate in lymphatic organs, with clear, nongranular cytoplasm and a round or horseshoe-shaped single nucleus:
  - *Lymphocytes*—have a rounded nucleus and function in phagocytosis and antibody formation
  - *Monocytes*—have a horseshoe-shaped nucleus and function mainly in phagocytosis

Platelets and Clotting Mechanism

Platelets (thrombocytes) originate in red bone marrow from *megakaryocyte* cells. Small pieces of the cell break off and become platelets, which function in the clotting mechanism.

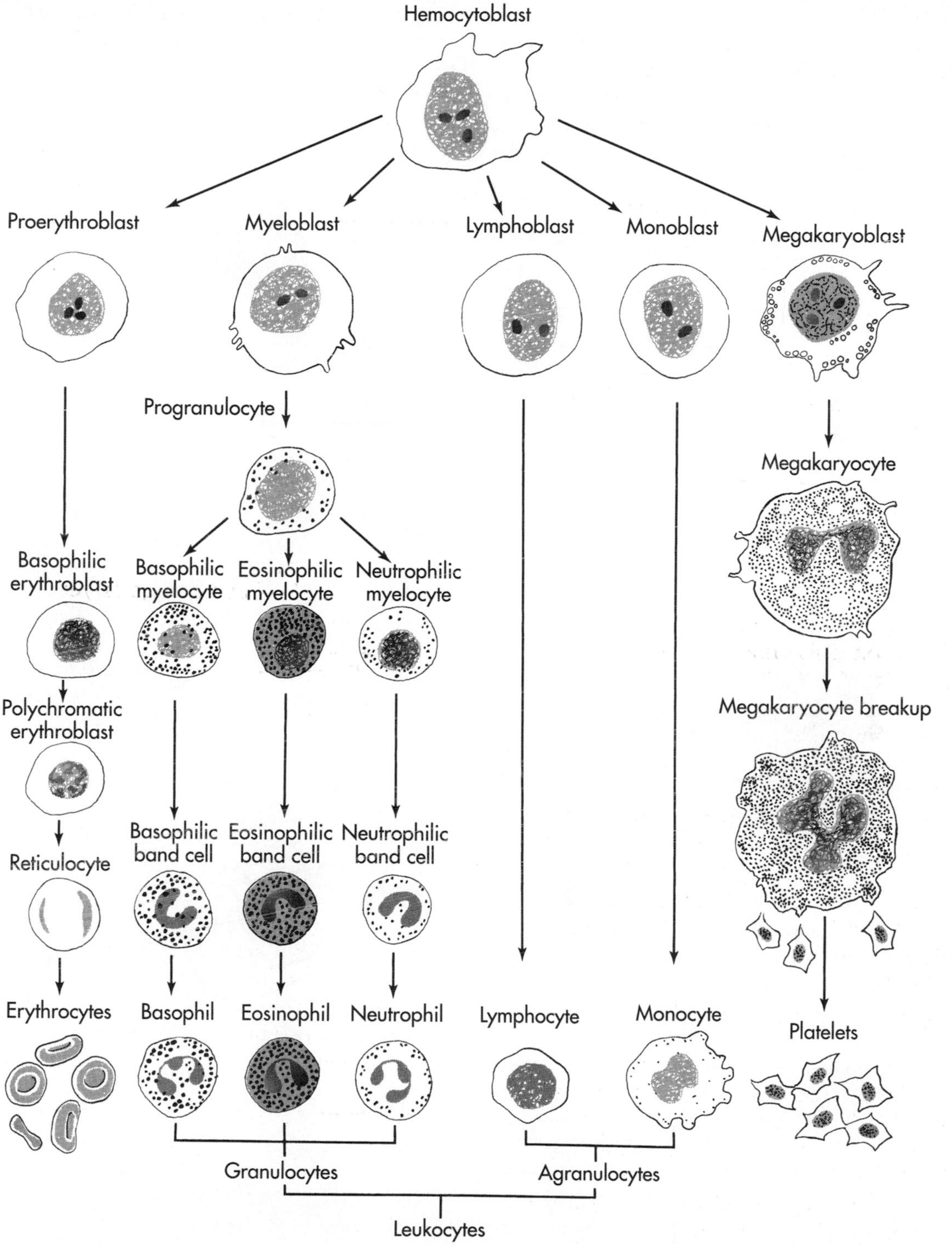

Hemocytoblast
Proerythroblast
Myeloblast
Lymphoblast
Monoblast
Megakaryoblast
Progranulocyte
Megakaryocyte
Basophilic erythroblast
Basophilic myelocyte
Eosinophilic myelocyte
Neutrophilic myelocyte
Polychromatic erythroblast
Megakaryocyte breakup
Reticulocyte
Basophilic band cell
Eosinophilic band cell
Neutrophilic band cell
Erythrocytes
Basophil
Eosinophil
Neutrophil
Lymphocyte
Monocyte
Platelets
Granulocytes
Agranulocytes
Leukocytes

FIG. 9-3 Hematopoiesis. All cells are derived from single progenitor cell, the hemocytoblast, which gives rise to progenitors of each cell type. (Redrawn from Seeley et al: *Anatomy and physiology,* St. Louis, 1989, Mosby.)

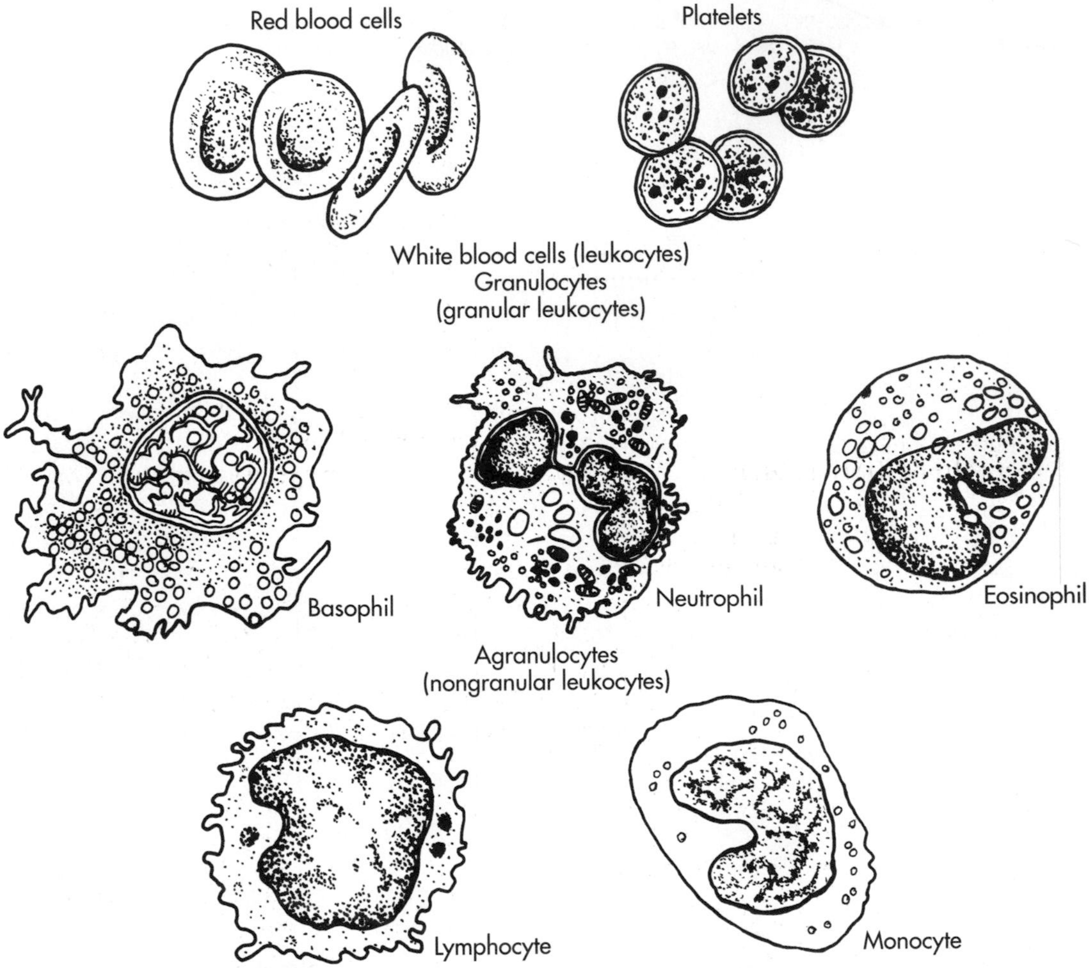
Red blood cells
Platelets
White blood cells (leukocytes)
Granulocytes
(granular leukocytes)
Basophil
Neutrophil
Eosinophil
Agranulocytes
(nongranular leukocytes)
Lymphocyte
Monocyte

FIG. 9-4 Typical mammalian white and red blood cells.

Clotting is the result of a chemical reaction. The platelets attach to the injured blood vessel and begin to release several substances that contract blood vessels and hasten clotting. *Prothrombin* and *fibrinogen* are proteins, made in the liver and present in blood plasma, that are necessary for clotting. Prothrombin is converted to *thrombin,* and thrombin changes fibrinogen to fibrin. Fibrin enmeshes the red blood cells, platelets, and plasma to form a clot and to close the wound. In all domestic animals with the exception of the cow and the horse, normally less than five minutes elapses from the onset of clot formation to actual clot formation. Clotting time varies from 2.5 minutes in sheep and dogs to 11.5 minutes in horses.

BLOOD GROUPING

Blood is grouped into major types or groups, named for the *antigens* (substances that stimulate the immune system to form antibodies) found on the membranes of red blood cells. The number of blood groups varies tremendously from species to species. The purpose of blood typing is to find a matching donor and recipient when performing transfusions so that blood is compatible, as well as to identify preferred breeding pairs of animals. Some animals must be blood typed before being registered by breed associations. For example, all thoroughbred horses must be blood typed before being registered.

ERYTHROLYTIC SYNDROMES

In some animal species there is a reaction of antibodies of the dam and the offspring. These conditions are similar to what is called the Rh factor in humans. Animals with these syndromes exhibit destruction of erythrocytes (RBCs). Other names for this disorder include *neonatal erythrolysis* and *isoimmune erythrolysis.* Horses and dogs exhibit neonatal erythrolysis by passing antibodies in their milk. Dogs who have multiple transfusions can have their blood sensitized by the donor's blood.

BLOOD PRESSURE

Blood pressure is the force exerted by the heart in pumping blood through the vessels of the body. *Systolic pressure* is produced by the blood pressing against the walls of the arteries during contraction of the ventricles of the heart. *Diastolic pressure* is produced by the blood pressing against the walls of the arteries during relaxation of the ventricles. Normal blood pressure in the average animal varies from species to species. The difference between the systolic and diastolic pressures is called *pulse pressure.* Diastolic pressure is considered more important medically because it shows the least amount of pressure to which the arterial walls are subjected. The condition in which the blood pressure is elevated is called *hypertension,* and low blood pressure is called *hypotension.*

The Pulse

The pulse is produced by the blood pumping out of the heart and into the aorta. This rhythmically increases and decreases the pressure on the walls of the aorta, which, because of their elasticity, expand as the blood enters and relax as it leaves. This rhythm is then transmitted from the aorta to surface arteries, where it is felt as the pulse.

REVIEW B

1. The liquid portion of blood is called ______________________. If the clotting elements are removed, it is called ______________________.
2. Blood makes up ______________________ to ______________________ of an animal's total body weight.
3. The undifferentiated stem cells from which all blood cells originate are called ______________________.
4. The scientific name for red blood cells is ______________________, and for white blood cells it is ______________________.
5. Of the two groups of white blood cells, the ones that originate in bone marrow are called ______________________. They are further classified by staining characteristics into three types: ______________________, ______________________, and ______________________.
6. White blood cells with nongranular cytoplasm are called ______________________. The two types are ______________________ and ______________________.
7. Blood platelets are also called ______________________. They originate in bone marrow from large multinucleated cells called ______________________.
8. In clotting, thrombin causes the blood protein ______________________ to change into ______________________.
9. Blood groups are named for the ______________________ that are found on the cell membranes of red blood cells.
10. Blood pressure rises and falls with each heartbeat. The higher pressure, produced during ventricular contraction, is called ______________________ pressure. The lower pressure is called ______________________ pressure. The difference between the two is called ______________________ pressure.

Circulation of the Blood

The blood circulates throughout the body in a closed vascular system. The basic circuit of the blood is known as *systemic circulation,* which includes a segment known as *portal circulation* and another circuit called *pulmonary circulation.*

SYSTEMIC CIRCULATION

Blood circulating from the left ventricle to the aorta, arteries, arterioles, capillaries, venules, and veins of the body and returning to the right atrium is known as systemic circulation.

PORTAL CIRCULATION

The circuit through the abdominal digestive organs is known as portal circulation. Blood from veins in the visceral walls and organs (gallbladder—except in rat and horse—pancreas, spleen, stomach, and intestines) is carried to the liver by the portal vein. The hepatic veins carry the blood from the liver to the caudal vena cava, which drains into the right atrium, where the blood begins the next circuit, pulmonary circulation.

PULMONARY CIRCULATION

Blood passes from the right atrium into the right ventricle, which contracts, forcing blood into the pulmonary artery, which has two branches, one to each lung. In the lung, the blood discharges carbon dioxide, is oxygenated, and then drains into the pulmonary veins, which empty into the left atrium.

Pulmonary veins are the only veins that carry oxygenated blood, which is a bright crimson color. All other veins carry waste products in the blood, making it a darker red color.

TRACING THE CIRCULATION

It takes about 1 minute for the blood to make a complete circuit of the body and return, always following the same pattern:

Left ventricle → arteries → arterioles → capillaries of body tissues → venules → veins → right atrium → right ventricle → pulmonary artery → arterioles of lung → lung capillaries → lung venules → pulmonary veins → left atrium → left ventricle (Fig. 9-5).

MAJOR BLOOD VESSELS OF CIRCULATION

The Arteries

The *aorta,* the largest artery in the body, originates from the left ventricle of the heart. The aortic valve, which is found between the aorta and the left ventricle, inhibits the backflow of blood from the aorta into the left ventricle. After leaving the heart, the aorta arches dorsally and then travels caudally, ventral to the thoracic vertebrae. It branches into other arteries that supply the head, neck, thoracic limbs, chest, and abdomen (abdominal aorta), finally dividing into arteries that supply the pelvic limbs (Fig. 9-6).

The major branches of the aorta include the following (Fig. 9-6):

- *Coronary* arteries, which supply the right and left sides of the myocardial muscle
- *Brachiocephalic (innominate)* artery, which divides into three large branches:
  - *Right subclavian* artery, supplying the right thoracic limb
  - *Right common carotid,* supplying the right side of the head
  - *Left common carotid,* supplying the left side of the head
- *Left subclavian artery,* supplying the left thoracic limb
  - The right and left subclavian arteries branch into the *axillary* and *brachial* arteries, which provide blood to the front legs.
- *Celiac* artery, supplying the liver, stomach, and spleen
- *Cranial mesenteric* artery, supplying the small intestine
- *Renal* arteries, supplying the kidneys
- *Ovarian* (or *testicular*) arteries, supplying the structures for which they are named
- *Caudal mesenteric* artery, supplying the large intestine

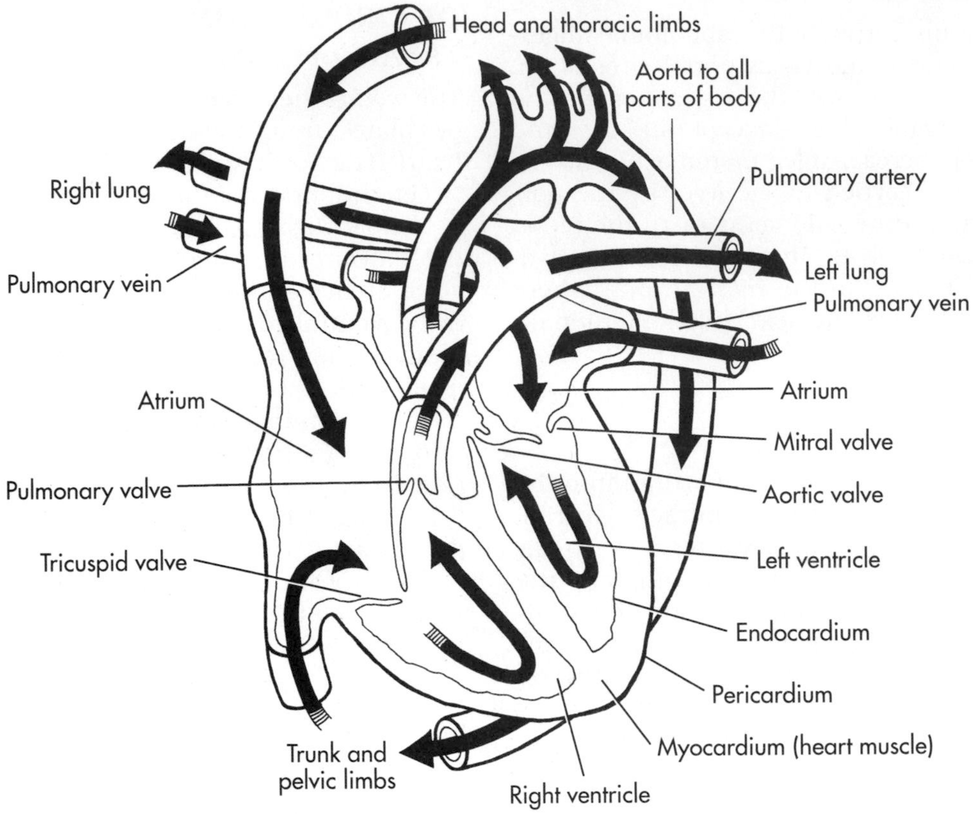
Head and thoracic limbs
Aorta to all parts of body
Right lung
Pulmonary artery
Pulmonary vein
Left lung
Pulmonary vein
Atrium
Atrium
Mitral valve
Pulmonary valve
Aortic valve
Tricuspid valve
Left ventricle
Endocardium
Pericardium
Trunk and pelvic limbs
Myocardium (heart muscle)
Right ventricle

FIG. 9-5 Circulation of blood through heart.

The aorta terminates in five branches:

- Right and left *external iliac* arteries, which continue outside the abdomen to become the *femoral* arteries, whose branches supply blood to the hind legs (they are one site for taking an animal's pulse)
- Right and left *internal iliac* arteries, supplying the pelvic wall and viscera
- *Caudal* artery, which supplies blood to the tail

The Veins

The previous section traced the blood from the heart through the arteries to the extremities. This section describes the return of the blood through the veins to the heart (Figs. 9-1 and 9-7).

The *pulmonary* veins are four veins that return the blood from the lungs to the left atrium of the heart and are the only veins that carry freshly oxygenated blood.

The systemic and portal veins return the blood to the heart from the rest of the body. Veins lying deep within the tissues are known as *deep* veins, whereas those close to the surface and sometimes visible through the skin are known as *superficial* veins. The major systemic veins as they are found in most species are as follows (Fig 9-7):

- *Internal jugular* veins—deep veins that drain the skull and brain and empty into the subclavians.
- *External jugular* veins—superficial veins that drain the blood from the head and neck and empty it into subclavian veins.

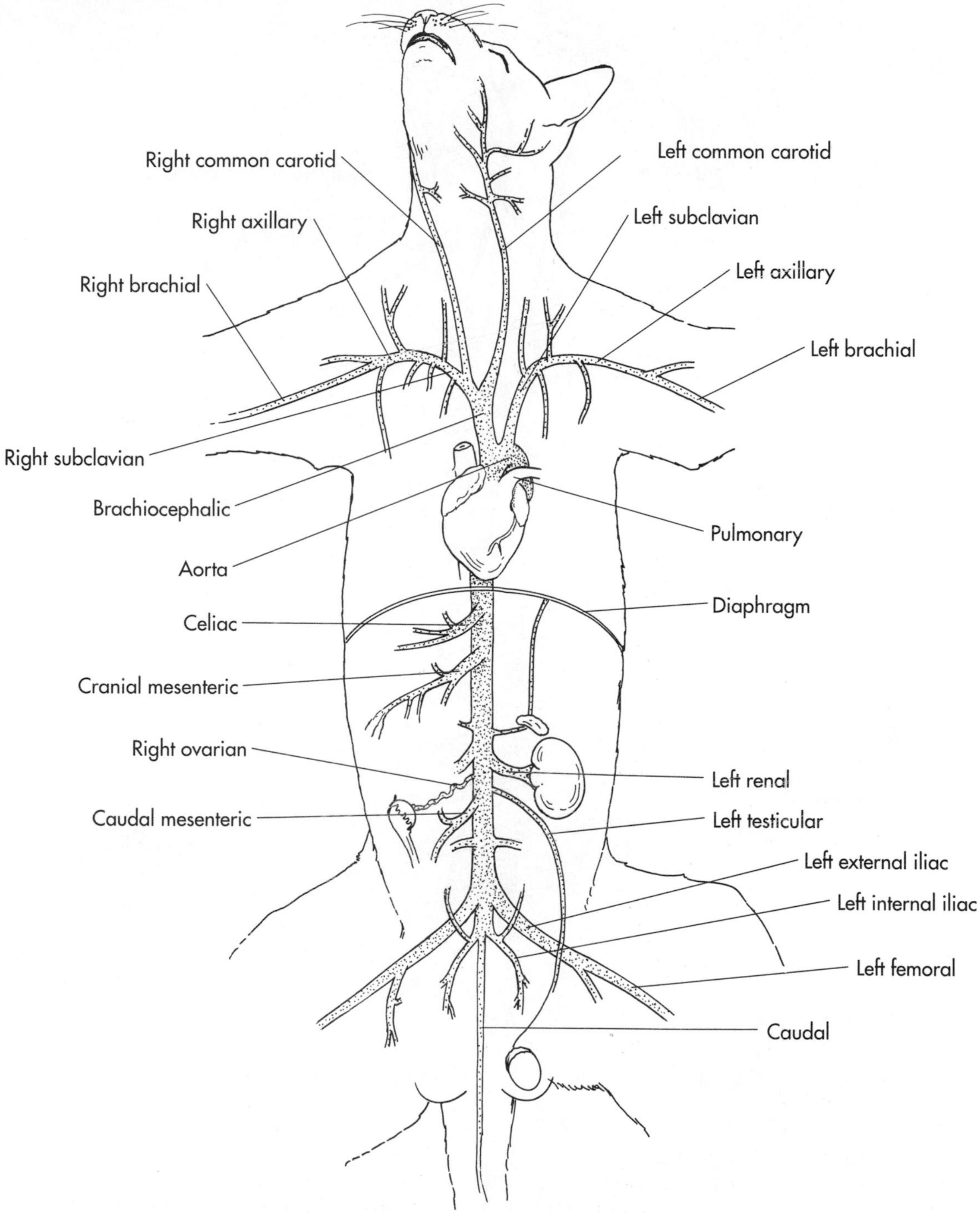
Right common carotid
Left common carotid
Right axillary
Left subclavian
Right brachial
Left axillary
Left brachial
Right subclavian
Brachiocephalic
Pulmonary
Aorta
Diaphragm
Celiac
Cranial mesenteric
Right ovarian
Left renal
Caudal mesenteric
Left testicular
Left external iliac
Left internal iliac
Left femoral
Caudal

FIG. 9-6 Major arteries in the cat.

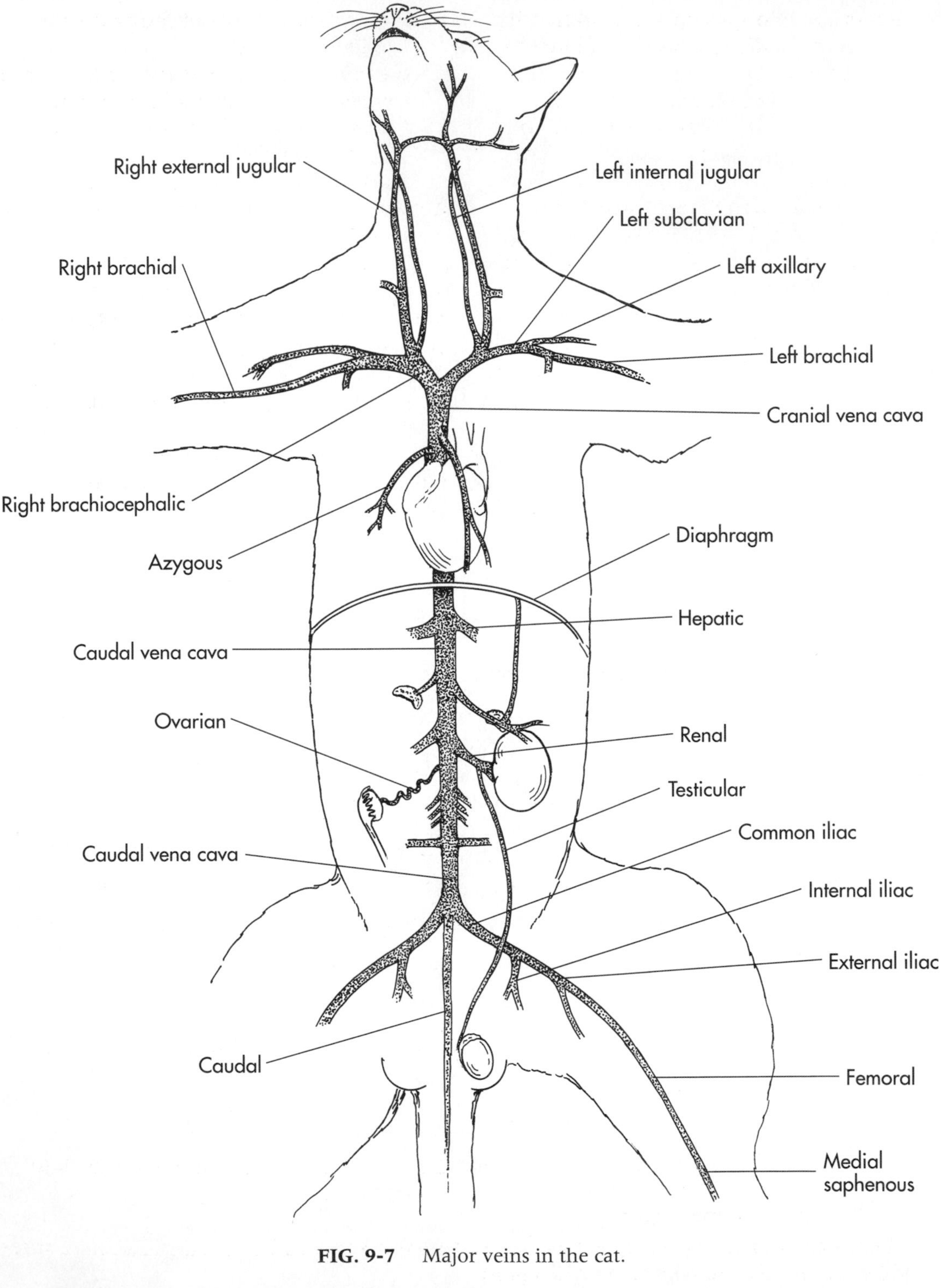
Right external jugular
Left internal jugular
Left subclavian
Right brachial
Left axillary
Left brachial
Cranial vena cava
Right brachiocephalic
Azygous
Diaphragm
Hepatic
Caudal vena cava
Ovarian
Renal
Testicular
Common iliac
Caudal vena cava
Internal iliac
External iliac
Caudal
Femoral
Medial saphenous

FIG. 9-7 Major veins in the cat.

Subclavian veins—deep veins originating from the *axillary, scapular,* and *thoracic* deep veins and the *cephalic* superficial vein. These empty into the *brachiocephalic* (or *innominate* veins) and from there into the *cranial vena cava.*

Azygous vein, which drains much of the chest wall and adjacent structures, also empties into the cranial vena cava, which ultimately delivers blood to the *right atrium.*

Major abdominal veins outside the portal circulation include the *renal, ovarian,* and *testicular* veins, which drain the kidneys, ovaries, and testicles, respectively.

The veins draining the pelvic limbs are both superficial and deep. Smaller veins of the feet and lower legs drain mainly into

Saphenous veins, which drain into

Femorals, veins of the thigh, which empty into

External iliacs, veins of the groin, which join

Internal iliacs (hypogastrics), veins forming

Common iliacs, which join to become the *caudal vena cava,* emptying into the *right atrium.*

The portal circulation involves the venous return from the digestive organs. Specific veins draining the blood from the stomach, intestine, spleen, pancreas, and gallbladder combine to form the *portal* vein. After entering the liver, the portal vein ramifies like an artery into tiny capillarylike sinusoids throughout the organ. The sinusoids in turn coalesce into larger and larger veins, culminating in the *hepatic* vein. The hepatic vein leaves the liver to empty into the *caudal vena cava,* which finally empties into the *right atrium.*

REVIEW C

1. The basic circuit of the blood, starting from the left ventricle, is known as the ____________ ____________ circulation. It includes a segment through the digestive organs and liver called the ______________________ circulation. The circuit of blood from the right ventricle and back to the heart is called the ______________________ circulation.
2. The only veins that carry oxygenated blood are the ______________________ veins. They carry blood from the ______________________ to the ______________________ .
3. The blood makes a complete circuit of the body in about ______________________ minute(s).
4. The largest artery in the body is the ______________________ .
5. The ______________________ arteries supply the myocardial muscle.
6. From its name you can tell that the brachiocephalic artery supplies the ______________________ and ______________________ .
7. The artery that supplies the kidney is the ______________________ artery.
8. The hepatic vein draws blood from the ______________________ and empties into the caudal ______________________ .
9. When the external iliac artery enters the leg it becomes the ______________________ artery, which can be used to take an animal's pulse.

The Lymphatic System

The lymphatic system is considered part of the circulatory system because it is made up of fluid called *lymph,* which comes from tissue fluids, and lymphatic vessels, which bring the lymph back to the blood. Lymph is an almost colorless fluid, rich in white blood cells, much like blood plasma in appearance and composition, and is circulated through the body by the lymphatic vessels. The organs of the lymphatic system include the lymph glands (nodes), spleen, tonsils, and thymus.

THE LYMPH VESSELS

The lymphatic vessels begin as lymphatic capillaries and form a vast network throughout the body. These capillaries join with slightly larger lymphatic vessels, which progressively repeat the process, forming larger and larger vessels. The lymphatic structure resembles that of veins, including valves, which prevent backflow of fluid. They collect the lymph and carry it toward the heart, eventually opening into the *thoracic duct* and *right lymphatic duct,* which in turn empty into the left and right subclavian veins, respectively. The lymph vessels collect proteins and water, which continually filter out of the blood into the tissue fluid and return to the blood.

The Lymph Glands

Along the course of the lymph vessels are numerous *lymph glands* or *nodes,* enclosed in fibrous capsules. These nodes vary in size from mere dots to larger, bean-sized and bean-shaped bodies, identified by their location (for example, cervical lymph nodes are in the neck). Superficial lymph nodes that are *palpable* (capable of being felt) in most species include the submandibular, prescapular, axillary, popliteal, and inguinal.

The lymph nodes act as filters to remove bacteria and other foreign bodies or particles, including malignant cells. They may be felt or even seen when they are inflamed or swollen by ingested bacteria and their toxins. If they are swollen and painful when palpated, an acute reaction is indicated. If they are swollen and lobulated and no pain is exhibited, a chronic condition is indicated. Another important function of the lymph glands is the manufacture of lymphocytes and monocytes. The lymphatic system is an extremely important part of the body's defense against infection.

THE SPLEEN

The spleen is a large, flattened, oval-shaped, glandlike organ, dark red in color, located in the left side of the abdominal cavity, just caudal to the diaphragm and behind the fundus of the stomach. (In ruminant animals, the spleen is displaced to the right by the rumen.) It is soft and pliable and is the largest structure of the lymphoid system. Its size varies in different species and at different times in the same species. The spleen enlarges during infectious diseases and decreases in size in old age.

The chief functions of the spleen are:

Hemopoiesis—the formation of lymphocytes, monocytes, and plasma cells

Phagocytosis—the removal and destruction of microorganisms, faulty platelets, and old erythrocytes and salvaging of globin and heme contents of the erythrocytes to be returned to the bone marrow and liver for later use

Storage area for blood in the splenic pulp

THE TONSILS

The tonsils are three pairs of small, round masses of lymphoid tissue that filter out bacteria and other foreign matter and play a part in forming lymphocytes:

The *palatine,* located at the back of the throat

The *lingual,* located at the root of the tongue

The *pharyngeal,* located at the back of the roof of the pharynx

THE THYMUS

The thymus is a grayish-pink structure of lymph tissue located in the mediastinum, cranial to the heart, extending into the neck in some species. The thymus plays an important part in the immune system (Chapter 16) by producing cells that destroy foreign substances and forming lymphocytes. Its maximum development, relative to body size, is in young animals, after which it begins to atrophy, so that it has almost disappeared by extreme old age.

REVIEW D

1. The fluid that circulates through the lymphatic capillaries is called ______________. It flows through progressively larger vessels as it moves toward the heart, eventually passing into the ______________ duct and the ______________ duct.
2. Palpable structures along the course of the lymph vessels that act as filters are called lymph ______________ or ______________.
3. The chief functions of the spleen are ______________, ______________, and ______________.
4. The three pairs of tonsils are named according to their location: the ______________ at the back of the palate, the ______________ at the root of the tongue, and the ______________ at the roof of the pharynx.
5. The grayish-pink structure of lymph tissue located just cranial to the heart is the thymus______________. It plays an important part in the immune______________ system.

Chapter 9 Answers

Review A

1. pericardium, epicardium, myocardium, endocardium
2. atria, ventricles
3. mitral (bicuspid), tricuspid, semilunar
4. sinoatrial (SA), atrioventricular (AV), Purkinje
5. autonomic, parasympathetic, sympathetic
6. arterioles, venules, capillaries

Review B

1. plasma, serum
2. 6%, 8%
3. hemocytoblasts
4. erythrocytes, leukocytes
5. granulocytes, neutrophils, eosinophils, basophils
6. agranulocytes, lymphocytes, monocytes
7. thrombocytes, megakaryocytes
8. fibrinogen, fibrin
9. antigens
10. systolic, diastolic, pulse

Review C

1. systemic, portal, pulmonary
2. pulmonary, lungs, heart
3. 1
4. aorta
5. coronary
6. front legs (arms), head
7. renal
8. liver, vena cava
9. femoral

Review D

1. lymph, thoracic, right lymphatic
2. nodes, glands
3. hemopoiesis, phagocytosis, blood storage
4. palatine, lingual, pharyngeal
5. thymus, immune

Chapter 9 EXERCISES

THE CARDIOVASCULAR AND LYMPHATIC SYSTEMS

Exercise 1: Fill in the blanks in the following statements:

1. The saclike membrane surrounding the heart is called the ______________________ .
2. The wall separating the left ventricle from the right is the ______________________ septum.
3. The atrioventricular valve with two flaps is the ______________________ , and the one with three flaps is the ______________________ .
4. In the systemic circulation oxygenated blood is carried away from the heart by blood vessels called ______________________ . They divide into smaller and smaller vessels called ______________________ and ultimately into the ______________________ , which distribute blood to the tissues. These in turn coalesce to form ______________________ , which join into larger and larger ______________________ , which return blood to the heart.
5. The red pigment in the erythrocytes is ______________________ . It consists of an iron-containing portion, ______________________ and a protein portion, ______________________ . The pigment combines with ______________________ in the lungs, which it exchanges for ______________________ in the tissues.
6. The process of engulfing invading microorganisms is called ______________________ . The granulocytes that do this are the ______________________ .
7. The largest structure of the lymphoid system is the ______________________ .

Exercise 2: Match the definitions in the right column with the terms in the left column by placing the appropriate letter in the blank space provided.

O	1. Cardiosclerosis	A. Decrease in lymphocytes
F	2. Angiosclerosis	B. Decrease in granulocytes
E	3. Erythropoiesis	C. Inner coat of blood vessel
G	4. Granulocytopoiesis	D. Decrease of erythrocytes
B	5. Granulocytopenia	E. Production of erythrocytes
D	6. Erythropenia	F. Hardening of walls of a vessel
J	7. Leukocytopenia	G. Production of granulocytes
A	8. Lymphocytopenia	H. Relaxation of heart
N	9. Tunica adventitia	I. An upper chamber of the heart
C	10. Tunica intima	J. Decrease of leukocytes
I	11. Atrium	K. Contraction of heart
K	12. Systole	L. A lower heart chamber
M	13. Sinoatrial node	M. Pacemaker
H	14. Diastole	N. External coat of blood vessel
L	15. Ventricle	O. Hardening of heart tissues and vessels

Exercise 3: Complete the following statements:

1. The blood vessel that carries blood from the heart to the lungs is called the ______________________ artery.
2. The large artery that carries blood from the heart to all parts of the body is the ______________________ .
3. The three large arteries branching from the brachiocephalic artery are the ______________________ , ______________________ and ______________________ .
4. The circulation from the abdominal digestive organs through the liver into the vena cava is called ______________________ circulation.
5. The arteries that supply the right and left sides of myocardial muscle are the ______________________ .
6. The two ducts in the lymphatic system that receive the lymph and empty into the subclavian veins are called ______________________ and ______________________ .
7. A ______________________ encloses lymph nodes.
8. There are ______________________ pairs of tonsils.
9. One function of tonsils is ____ .
10. Other than the lymphatic system, the thymus plays a part in the ______________________ system.

Exercise 4: The arrows in Fig. 9-8 trace the flow of blood through the heart. The heart chambers, membranes, and vessels are labeled with letters; the heart valves are labeled with numbers. In the blanks provided, write the name of the structures opposite the appropriate number or letter.

1. ________________________________
2. ________________________________
3. ________________________________
4. ________________________________

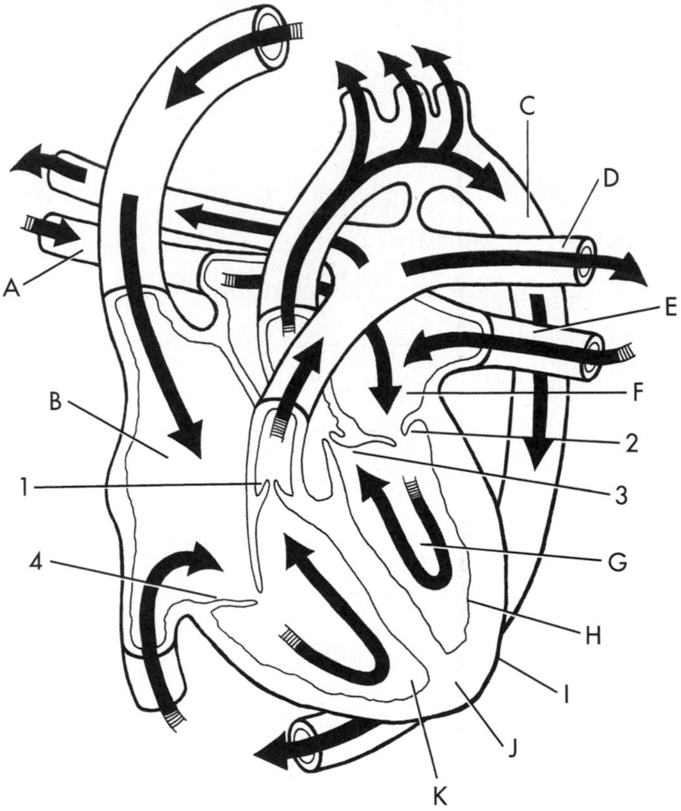
A
B
C
D
E
F
G
H
I
J
K
1
2
3
4

FIG. 9-8 Circulation of blood through heart.

A. ________________________________

B. ________________________________

C. ________________________________

D. ________________________________

E. ________________________________

F. ________________________________

G. ________________________________

H. ________________________________

I. ________________________________

J. ________________________________

K. ________________________________

Exercise 5: Using the list of terms, identify each structure in Fig. 9-9 by writing its name in the corresponding blank.

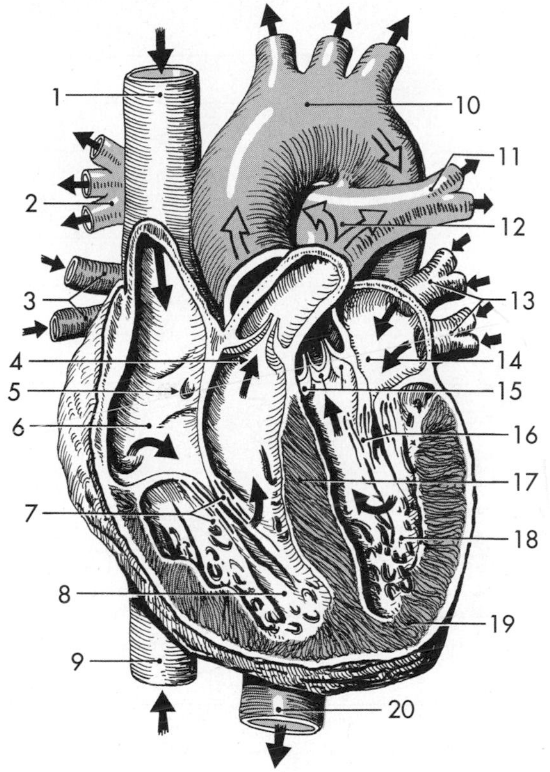
1
2
3
4
5
6
7
8
9
10
11
12
13
14
15
16
17
18
19
20

Aortic semilunar valve
Branches of right pulmonary vein
Left ventricle
Septum
Right atrium
Branches of left pulmonary artery
Coronary sinus
Mitral (bicuspid) valve
Cranial vena cava
Arch of aorta
Branches of left pulmonary vein
Descending aorta
Myocardium
Tricuspid valve
Pulmonary artery
Branches of right pulmonary artery
Caudal vena cava
Right ventricle
Semilunar valve
Left atrium

FIG. 9-9 Frontal section showing the four chambers of the heart and the valves, openings, and major blood vessels. Arrows indicate directions of the blood flow. (The two branches of the right pulmonary vein continue from the right lung, behind the heart, to enter the left atrium.)

1. ____________________
2. ____________________
3. ____________________
4. ____________________
5. ____________________
6. ____________________
7. ____________________
8. ____________________
9. ____________________
10. ____________________
11. ____________________
12. ____________________
13. ____________________
14. ____________________
15. ____________________
16. ____________________
17. ____________________
18. ____________________
19. ____________________
20. ____________________

Exercise 6: Give the meaning of the components in the following words, and then define the word as a whole. Before reaching for your medical dictionary, check the glossary at the end of the chapter.

1. Hemocytoblast

   hemo ______________________

   cyto ______________________

   blast ______________________

   ____

2. Lymphadenoma

   lymph ______________________

   aden ______________________

   oma ______________________

   ____

3. Pericarditis

   peri ______________________

   card ______________________

   itis ______________________

   ____

4. Endocarditis

   endo ______________________

   card ______________________

   itis ______________________

   ____

5. Hematemesis

   hemat ______________________

   emesis ______________________

   ____

6. Neonatal erythrolysis

   neo ______________________

   natal ______________________

   erythro ______________________

   lysis ______________________

   ____

7. Leukocytopoiesis

   leuko ______________________

   cyto ______________________

   poiesis ______________________

   ____

8. Cardiomyopathy

   cardio ______________________

   myo ______________________

   pathy ______________________

   ____

9. Polymorphonuclear leukocyte

   poly ______________________

   morpho ______________________

   nuclear ______________________

   leuko ______________________

   cyte ______________________

   ____

10. Megakaryocyte

    mega ______________________

    karyo ______________________

    cyte ______________________

    ____

CHAPTER 9 PUZZLE

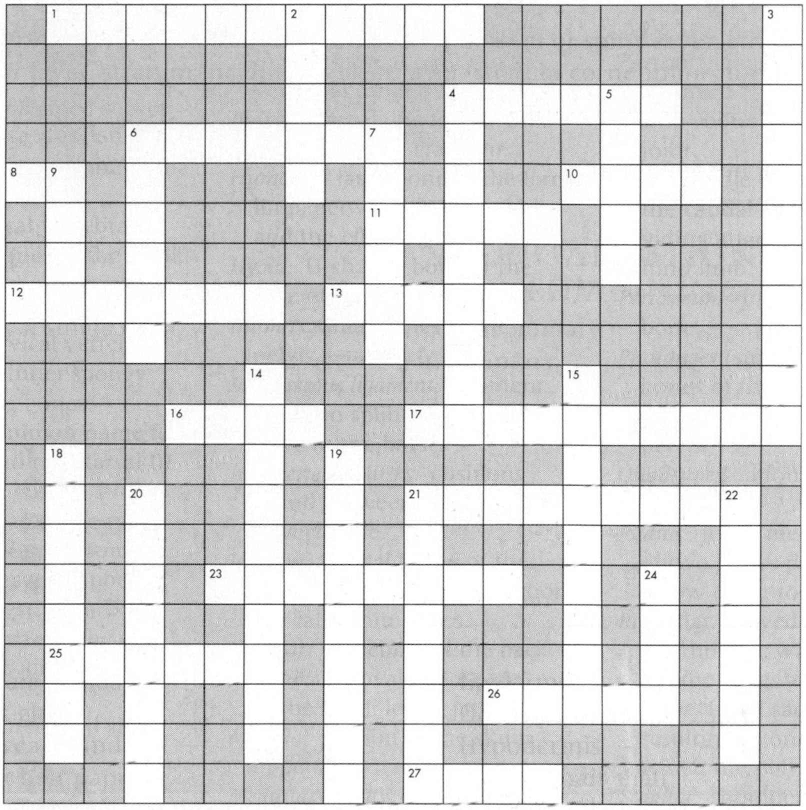

ACROSS CLUES

1. Small blood vessels
4. Segment of circulation
6. Three pairs of lymphoid tissue
8. Two blood types of cats
10. Aortic branch called aortic ____
11. Fluid carried by lymphatic system
12. Very small veins
13. Major type of blood vessel
16. Lower border of heart
17. Heart muscle
21. Another term for thrombocytes
23. Innermost membrane covering heart
25. Heart valve with two flaps
26. Number of heart wall layers
27. Right ventricle pumps blood to this organ

DOWN CLUES

2. Upper heart chambers
3. External layer of heart covering
4. Part of systemic circulation
5. Largest artery
6. Source of lymphocyte formation
7. Lymphatic glandlike organ
9. Upper border of heart
14. Lower heart chambers
15. The sinoatrial node
18. Basic blood circuit
19. This valve separates right atrium and ventricle
20. Relaxation part of cardiac cycle
21. Middle layer of heart covering
22. Contraction part of cardiac cycle
24. Iron

Chapter 9 Answers

Exercise 1

1. pericardium
2. interventricular
3. bicuspid, tricuspid
4. arteries, arterioles, capillaries, venules, veins
5. hemoglobin, heme, globin, oxygen, carbon dioxide
6. phagocytosis, neutrophils
7. spleen

Exercise 2

1. O	6. D	11. I
2. F	7. J	12. K
3. E	8. A	13. M
4. G	9. N	14. H
5. B	10. C	15. L

Exercise 3

1. pulmonary
2. aorta
3. right subclavian, right common carotid, left common carotid
4. portal
5. right and left coronaries
6. thoracic duct, right lymphatic duct
7. fibrous capsule
8. three
9. playing a part in leukocyte formation, filtering out bacteria and foreign matter
10. immune

Exercise 4

1. pulmonary valve
2. mitral valve
3. aortic valve
4. tricuspid valve

A. pulmonary vein
B. atrium
C. aorta
D. pulmonary artery
E. pulmonary vein
F. atrium
G. left ventricle
H. endocardium
I. pericardium
J. myocardium
K. right ventricle

Exercise 5

1. cranial vena cava
2. branches of right pulmonary artery
3. branches of right pulmonary vein
4. semilunar valve
5. coronary sinus
6. right atrium
7. tricuspid valve
8. right ventricle
9. caudal vena cava
10. arch of aorta
11. branches of left pulmonary artery
12. pulmonary artery
13. branches of left pulmonary vein
14. left atrium
15. aortic semilunar valve
16. mitral (bicuspid) valve
17. septum
18. left ventricle
19. myocardium
20. descending aorta

Exercise 6

1. blood; cell; embryonic state of development; primitive blood cell
2. lymph; gland; tumor; tumor of the lymph glands
3. around; heart; inflammation; inflammation of the membrane surrounding the heart
4. inside; heart; inflammation; inflammation of the tissue lining the inside of the heart
5. blood; vomiting; vomiting of blood
6. new; born; red cell; breakdown; destruction of the red blood cells in the newborn
7. white; cell; production; production of white blood cells
8. heart; muscle; disease; disease of the heart muscle
9. many; form; nucleus; white; cell; white blood cell with multishaped nucleus (synonym for *neutrophil*)
10. large; nucleus; cell; cell with large nucleus (source of blood platelets)

ANSWERS: CHAPTER 9 PUZZLE

	1 C	A	P	I	L	L	2 A	R	I	E	S								3 P
							T												E
							R				4 P	O	R	T	5 A	L			R
			6 T	O	N	S	I	L	7 S		U				O				I
8 A	9 B		H				A		P		L			10 A	R	C	H		C
	A		Y						11 L	Y	M	P	H		T				A
	S		M						E		O				A				R
12 V	E	N	U	L	E	S		13 V	E	I	N	S							D
			S						N		A								I
						14 V					R			15 P					U
				16 A	P	E	X			17 M	Y	O	C	A	R	D	I	U	M
	18 S					N		19 T						C					
	Y		20 D			T		R		21 P	L	A	T	E	L	E	T	22 S	
	S		I			R		I		A				M				Y	
	T		A		23 V	I	S	C	E	R	A	L		A		24 H		S	
	E		S			C		U		I				K		E		T	
	25 M	I	T	R	A	L		S		E				E		M		O	
	I		O			E		P		T		26 T	H	R	E	E		L	
	C		L			S		I		A								E	
			E					D		27 L	U	N	G						

GLOSSARY

CARDIOVASCULAR AND LYMPHATIC SYSTEM RELATED ANATOMIC TERMS

Heart

aortic valve: semilunar valve that prevents backflow of blood from aorta to heart.

apex (a'peks): rounded tip of heart, pointing left and downward.

atrial appendage: ear-shaped continuation of left and right upper part of atria.

atrioventricular node: located in right atrium near lower portion of interatrial septum and composed of small mass of atypical cardiac muscle tissue (also called *AV node*).

atrioventricular valves: valves between atria and ventricles of heart (left valve is *bicuspid* or *mitral* valve and right valve is *tricuspid* in some species).

atrium (a'tre-um): left or right upper chamber of heart.

bundle of His: band of specialized cardiac muscle fibers that arise in atrioventricular node and branch down on both sides of interventricular septum, transmitting atrial contraction rhythm to ventricles (also called *atrioventricular bundle*).

chordae tendineae (kor'de ten″din'e-e): tendinous strings resembling cords that extend from cusps of atrioventricular valves to papillary muscles of heart.

conus arteriosus (ko'nus ar-te″re-o'sus): upper, anterior angle of right ventricle where pulmonary artery begins (also called *infundibulum of the heart*).

cor: heart.

coronary arteries and veins: blood vessels of heart.

cusp: leafletlike segment of cardiac valve.

diastole (di-as'to-le): relaxation stage of heart action.

ductus arteriosus: blood vessel present in fetal circulation that connects pulmonary artery to descending aorta.

endocardium: endothelial membrane lining chambers of heart.

epicardium: outermost serous layer covering heart.

foramen ovale (fo-ra'men o″vah'le): opening between atria in fetal heart, normally closed after birth.

interventricular: between ventricles.

myocardium: thick middle muscle layer of heart wall.

pacemaker: sinoatrial node, which initiates heartbeat and regulates its rate.

pericardium: external layer of membrane covering heart.

pulmonary valve: valve at base of pulmonary artery (also called *semilunar valve*).

Purkinje fibers: specialized cardiac muscle fibers that are involved in impulse-conducting system of heart.

semilunar valves: the half-moon–shaped valves at base of pulmonary artery and aorta.

sinoatrial node: see *pacemaker.*

systole (sis'tole): contraction stage of heart action.

valves: membranous structures in passages that close to prevent reflux of contents.

Blood

antibody: protein substance formed in lymphoid tissue that interacts with specific antigen to protect body.

antigen: substance that triggers formation of specific antibodies, which react against antigen.

basophil (ba'so-fil): cell that stains with basic dyes.

capillary: small blood vessel that connects arterioles with venules, forming vast network throughout body.

eosinophil (e″o-sin'o-fil): cell that stains readily with orange or yellow acid eosin dyes.

erythrocyte (e'rith'ro-sīt): red blood cell.

erythropoiesis (e-rith″ro-poi-e'sis): red blood cell production.

granulocyte (gran'u-lo-sīt): cell containing granules (leukocytes with cytoplasmic granules of neutrophils, basophils, or eosinophils).

granulocytopoiesis (gran″u-lo-si″to-poi-e'sis): production of granulocytes.

hematopoiesis (hem″ah-to-poi-e'sis): production of red blood cells (also called *hemopoiesis*).

heme: insoluble, nonprotein, iron-containing portion of hemoglobin.

hemoglobin: iron-containing red pigment (heme) that combines with protein substance (globin), giving blood its red color.

heparin (hep'ah-rin): anticoagulant substance.

leukocyte (lu″ko-sīt): white blood cell.

leukocytopoiesis: leukocyte production (also called *leukopoiesis*).
lymphocyte (lim'fo-sīt): clear, nongranular leukocyte with single, round nucleus that functions in phagocytosis and antibody formation.
lymphopoiesis (lim″fo-poi-e'sis): production of lymphocytes.
macrocyte (mak'ro-sīt): abnormally large erythrocyte.
megakaryocyte (meg″ah-kar'e-o-sīt): giant cell of bone marrow that produces mature blood platelets.
monocyte: phagocytic, mononuclear white blood cell (leukocyte).
monocytopoiesis (mon″o-si″to-poi-e'sis): formation of monocytes.
neutrophil (nu'tro-fil): neutral dye-staining granular leukocyte containing lobed nucleus (also called *polymorphonuclear leukocyte*).
phagocytosis (fag″o-si-to'sis): ingestion and destruction of microorganisms, cells, and foreign matter.
plasma: liquid portion of blood.
plasmocyte: plasma cell.
platelet: disklike, nonnucleated element in blood, originating in red bone marrow and necessary for blood coagulation (also called *thrombocyte*).
prothrombin: factor in blood plasma that converts to thrombin and is part of blood-clotting mechanism.
reticulocyte (re-tik'u-lo-sit″): immature red blood cell, which shows basophilic reticulum (network) under vital staining.
serum: blood plasma without the clotting elements.
sinusoid (si'nus-oid): large, variable, anastomosing, terminal blood vessel with reticuloendothelium lining, found in organs such as liver and spleen.
thrombin: activated prothrombin; changes fibrinogen to fibrin.
thrombocyte: blood platelet.
thromboplastin (throm″bo-plas'tin): substance in blood and body tissue that aids in converting prothrombin to thrombin.
tunica: outer covering or lining of organ or body part.
tunica adventitia: fibrous elastic outer covering of blood vessels.
tunica intima: inner coat of blood vessel.
tunica media: middle coat of blood vessel.
vas: vessel.

Arteries

aorta (a-or'tah): largest artery in body and main trunk of entire arterial system.
aortic arch: the first section of the aorta, where it makes a 180-degree curve from its initial craniodorsal direction to a caudal direction.
arteriole (ar-te're-ol): tiny arterial branch.
axillary (ak'si-lar″e): branch of subclavian artery that distributes to axilla and forelimb.
brachial (bra'ke-al): axillary artery branch distributing to forelimb.
brachiocephalic (innominate) (brak″e-o-se-fal'ik): aortic arch branch distributing to head, neck, and right forelimb.
carotids (kah-rot'ids): right and left common carotids, originating from brachiocephalic artery, distributing to right and left sides of head.
celiac trunk: branch of abdominal aorta distributing to stomach, liver, pancreas, spleen, and duodenum.
colic: distributes to colon.
coronary: left and right arteries distributing to left and right sides of myocardial muscle (atria and ventricles).
femoral: branch of external iliac artery that distributes to external genitalia, hind leg, and lower abdominal wall.
iliac (il'e-ak): the *common* iliac artery and its branches distribute to the pelvis, abdominal wall, hind legs, and reproductive organs.
mesenteric: cranial and caudal branches of the abdominal aorta distributing respectively to lower half of colon and rectum and to small intestine and proximal half of colon.
nutrient: any artery that supplies blood to bone marrow (also called *medullary* artery).
ovarian: branch of abdominal aorta that distributes to ovaries, uterine tube, and ureters.
pulmonary: only arteries in body that carry nonoxygenated blood, which is delivered to lungs for oxygenation.
renal: branch of abdominal aorta that distributes to kidneys, adrenals, and ureters.
subclavian: two arteries distributing to neck, forelimbs, thoracic wall, spinal cord, brain, and meninges.
testicular: branch of abdominal aorta that supplies testicles

and associated structures (also called *spermatic artery*).

thoracic: three arteries (lateral, superior, and internal) distributing respectively to pectoral muscles and mammary glands; axillary area of chest wall; and diaphragm, structures of mediastinum, and anterior thoracic wall.

ulnar: brachial artery branch distributing to foreleg.

Veins

axillary: basilic and brachial vein continuation to subclavians.

azygos (az'ĭ-gos): three veins of trunk that empty into superior vena cava.

brachiocephalic (innominate) (brak"e-o-sĕ-fal'ik): left and right branches unite to form cranial vena cava.

cardiac: veins of heart, including coronary veins (also called *venae cordis*).

cephalic (se-fal'ik): superficial veins of front leg.

common iliac: large veins draining blood from pelvis and hind leg, joining to form caudal vena cava.

cutaneous: small subcutaneous veins draining into deep veins.

femoral: major vein draining hind leg.

hepatic: veins that drain liver.

iliac: external and internal; join with saphenous to form common iliac vein.

intercostal: veins that accompany intercostal arteries.

jugular: three pairs of veins (anterior, internal, and external) serving head and neck.

lingual: veins serving tongue, area below tongue and mandibular glands, and floor of mouth.

mesenteric: intestinal veins emptying into portal vein.

plexus: network of nerves, lymph, or blood vessels.

portal: carries blood from digestive system to liver.

pulmonary: four veins returning oxygenated blood from lungs to left atrium of heart.

renal: veins of kidney.

saphenous (sah-fe'nus): superficial vein running over lateral surface of hock (and on medial surface in cats).

subclavian: main veins of upper extremity, joining internal jugulars to form two brachiocephalic veins.

venae cavae: two large veins that return blood to heart: cranial from head, neck, chest, and thoracic extremities and caudal from abdominal viscera, pelvis, and pelvic extremities.

Lymphatics

cisterna chyli (sis-ter'nah): origin of thoracic duct and saclike reservoir for lymph collection.

hilum: depression where vessels and nerves enter spleen.

lymphatic duct: channel conducting lymph, referring chiefly to right lymphatic duct and left lymphatic or thoracic duct.

lymphatic glands (nodes): glandlike masses of lymphatic tissue varying in size from dots to bean-sized bodies, identified by their locations along course of lymphatic vessels.

lymphatic vessel: channel for conveying lymph.

lymph follicle (fol'ĭ-k'l): saclike collector of lymphoid substances, chiefly beneath mucous surfaces.

sinusoids: sinuslike capillaries with specialized function.

spleen: largest lymphoid system structure, flattened, oval-shaped, glandlike organ located in upper left side of abdominal cavity.

splenic pulp: white splenic pulp is sheath of lymphatic tissue that surrounds arteries of spleen; red splenic pulp is lymphatic tissue permeated with sinusoids filled with blood.

thoracic duct: left lymphatic duct draining left side of body above and entire body below diaphragm.

thymus gland: grayish-pink structure of lymph tissue in mediastinum that has function in immune system.

tonsils: three pairs of small, round masses of lymphoid tissue.

PATHOLOGIC CONDITIONS

Inflammations and infections

arteritis (ar"te-ri'tis): inflammation of artery.

bacteremia: bacteria in blood.

carditis: inflammation of heart.

endarteritis: inflammation of tunica intima of artery.

endarteritis obliterans: endarteritis with narrowing and closure of arterial lumen (passage space within tube).

endocarditis (en"do-kar-di'tis): inflammation of endocardium.

erythrocytosis: abnormal increase in red blood cells.

leukocytosis: temporary increase in number of leukocytes in blood, caused by inflammation, infection, or hemorrhage.

lymphadenitis (lim-fad″ĕ-ni′tis): inflammation of lymph nodes.
lymphangitis (lim″fan-ji′tis): inflammation of one or more lymphatic vessels.
myocarditis (mi″o-kar-di′tis): inflammation of heart muscle.
panarteritis: inflammatory arterial disease involving all layers of arterial wall.
periarteritis: inflammation of adventitia (outer layer) of artery.
pericarditis (per″ĭ-kar′dit′is): inflammation of pericardium.
phlebitis (fle-bi′tis): inflammation of vein, with thrombus formation, accompanied by pain and edema.
polyarteritis: inflammatory condition of arterial system with many destructive lesions.
septicemia (sep″ti-se′me-ah): general systemic blood infection caused by presence of pathogenic microorganisms or their toxins (also called *blood poisoning*).
thrombophlebitis: inflammation of vein with clot formation.

Hemorrhages and related conditions

epistaxis (ep″ĭ-stak′sis): nosebleed.
hemarthrosis (hem″ar-thro′sis): presence of blood in joint.
hematemesis (hem″at-em′ĕ-sis): vomiting of blood.
hematocele (hem″ah-to-sēl″): blood in cavity or cyst.
hematoma (hem″ah-to″mah): blood, usually clotted, accumulated in tissue, organ, or space due to blood vessel wall break.
hematometra (hem″ah-to-me′trah): accumulation of blood in cavity of uterus.
hematomyelia (hem″ah-to-mi-e′le-ah): bleeding into spinal cord.
hematopericardium (hem″ah-to-per″ĭ-kar′de-um): escape of blood into pericardium (also called *hemopericardium*).
hematoperitoneum (hem″ah-to-per″ĭt-to-ne′um): escape of blood into peritoneum.
hematuria: blood in urine.
hemothorax: accumulation of blood in pleural cavity.
melena: passing of tarry stools due to presence of digested blood.
petechial hemorrhages (pe-te′ke-al): small pinpoint hemorrhages in skin or mucous membranes.
postpartum hemorrhage: hemorrhage after parturition.

Anemias

anemia: reduction in red blood cells.
aplastic anemia: anemia resulting from bone marrow disease or destruction.
deficiency anemia: anemia caused by lack of necessary nutrients.
hemolytic anemia: anemia resulting from erythrocyte destruction.
hypochromic microcytic anemia: anemia in which erythrocytes are smaller than normal and contain abnormally low amounts of hemoglobin.
macrocytic: anemia in which erythrocytes are enlarged.

Leukemias

This is a limited list of leukemias. Refer to a medical dictionary for a more detailed list with definitions.

aleukemic leukemia: leukemia in which white blood cell count is normal or below normal.
leukemia (lu-ke′me-ah): malignant, progressive disease, marked by abnormal increase in leukocyte production and decrease in erythrocytes and platelets, causing anemia and vulnerability to infection and hemorrhage classified by (1) acute or chronic type, (2) cell type involved (myeloid, lymphoid, or monocytic), and (3) increase or nonincrease of abnormal cells.
lymphatic leukemia: leukemia combined with hyperplasia and overactivity of lymphoid tissue (also called *lymphocytic* and *lymphoid leukemia*).
monocytic leukemia: leukemia in which monocytes are predominant white blood cells.
myeloblastic leukemia: leukemia in which myeloblasts are predominant white blood cells.
stem cell leukemia: leukemia that is difficult to type because prevailing cell is too immature and may be lymphoblasts, myeloblasts, or monoblasts.

Hereditary, congenital, and developmental disorders

hemophilia (he″mo-fil′e-ah): hereditary disease of dogs in which there is deficiency in clotting of blood.
patent ductus arteriosus: duct between left pulmonary artery and descending aorta in fetus that closes normally at birth.
pulmonary stenosis: narrowing of passage between pulmonary artery and right ventricle.

tetralogy of Fallot (fal-o'): group of four cardiac anomalies, including pulmonary stenosis, dextroposition of aorta, interventricular septal defect, and marked hypertrophy of right ventricle (also called *Fallot's tetrad*).

von Willebrand's disease: clotting disorder found in Dobermans, German shepherds, and certain other breeds.

Other abnormalities

agranulocytosis (ah-gran"u-lo-si-to'sis): disease characterized by decrease in granulocytes.

aneurysm: blood-filled, saclike formation caused by localized dilation of blood vessel wall (usually artery) or heart.

angina: refers to any condition with attacks of suffocating, paroxysmal pain.

angina pectoris (an-ji'nah pec'toris): severe, paroxysmal chest pain in humans, usually radiating from the cardiac area of the chest to the left shoulder and down the left arm.

angiomegaly (an"je-o-meg'ah-le): enlargement of blood vessel.

angionecrosis (an'je-o-nekro'sis): necrosis (death) of blood vessel walls.

angiosclerosis: sclerosis (hardening) of blood vessel walls.

angiostenosis: narrowing of vessels.

aortic insufficiency: blood from aorta flows back to the left ventricle because of malfunctioning of semilunar valve of aorta.

arrhythmia (ah-rith'me-ah): irregular rhythm of the heartbeat.

arteriosclerosis (ar-te"re-o-skle-ro'sis): classification of diseases of arteries, marked by thickening of walls of arteries and loss of their elasticity.

arteriospasm (ar-te're-o-spazm): spasm of artery.

arteriostenosis (ar-te"re-o-ste-no'sis): narrowing of diameter of artery.

atherosclerosis (ath"er-o-skle-ro'sis): type of arteriosclerosis marked by formation of plaques containing cholesterol and lipids within intima of large and medium-sized arteries.

bradycardia: slow heartbeat.

cardiac arrest: abrupt stopping of cardiac function and absence of arterial blood pressure.

cardiac hypertrophy: enlargement of heart.

cardiac murmur: abnormal heart sound.

cardiomegaly (kar"de-o-meg'ah-le): enlargement of heart.

cardiomyopathy: heart muscle disease found in cats.

carotenemia: presence of carotene in blood, sometimes producing a jaundicelike coloring.

congestive heart failure: prolonged inability of heart to pump and maintain blood flow adequately, resulting in impaired circulation, edema throughout body, and blood backed up in veins leading to heart.

cor pulmonale: cardiac condition caused by pulmonary hypertension resulting from disease of lungs or their blood vessels.

cyanosis: bluish color of skin and mucous membranes caused by reduced amounts of oxygen in blood.

embolism (em'bo-lizm): blocking of blood vessel by obstruction, such as blood clot, air bubble, fat globule, tissue, bacteria clump, or amniotic debris, carried by blood flow.

erythrocytosis (e'rith"ro-si-to'sis): increase of red blood cells in circulation.

erythropenia: deficiency of erythrocytes (also called *erythrocytopenia*).

fibrillation: arrhythmia with uncoordinated, irregular contractions of heart muscle affecting atria or ventricles.

granulocytopenia (gran"u-lo-si"to-pe'-ne-ah): decrease of granulocytes in blood (also called *granulopenia*).

granulcytosis: unusually large number of granulocytes in blood.

heart block: partial or complete interference with the conduction of cardiac electrical impulses.

hemangiectasis (hem"an-je-ek-tah-sis): dilation of blood vessels (also called *angiectasis*).

hematocytopenia (hem"ah-to-si"to-pe'ne-ah): deficiency in elements of blood cells.

hematocytosis: increase in elements of blood.

hematopenia: decrease in blood.

hemaglobinemia (he"mo-glo'bĭ-ne'meah): free hemoglobin in blood plasma.

hypertension: high blood pressure.

hypotension: low blood pressure.

infarct: area of tissue that is damaged or necrotic because of an insufficient blood supply resulting from obstruction to circulation.

ischemia: local, temporary deficiency of blood supply to area of body caused by obstruction in blood vessel supplying area.

leukopenia (leukocytopenia): reduction in amount of white blood cells.

lymphadenitis: lymph node inflammation.

lymphadenopathy: disease of lymph nodes.

lymphangiectasis (lim-fan″je-ek′tah-sis): swelling of vessels of lymphatics.

lymphedema (lim″fe-de′mah): swelling caused by blockage of lymphatics.

lymphocytopenia: decrease of lymphocytes in blood.

lymphocytosis: excess of lymphocytes in blood.

lymphorrhea: discharge of lymph from cut or torn lymph vessel.

lymphostasis (lim-fos′tah-sis): obstruction to lymph flow.

mitral insufficiency: most common cause of congestive heart failure in dogs.

mitral valve prolapse (MVP): protrusion of mitral valve into left atrium, causing backflow of blood caused by incomplete closure.

monocytopenia: decrease of monocytes in blood.

monocytosis: increase of monocytes in blood.

neutropenia: decrease of neutrophils in blood (also called *neutrocytopenia*).

occlusion: obstruction of blood vessel, which may be caused by thrombus or embolus.

palpitation: rapid action or tachycardia of heart.

paroxysmal tachycardia (par″ok-siz′mal): sudden onset of rapid heartbeat, beginning and ending abruptly.

phlebangioma: aneurysm of vein.

phlebectasia (fleb″ek-ta′ze-ah): swelling of vein or veins or varicosity (also called *phlebectasis*).

phlebostenosis: narrowing of the walls of vein.

polycythemia: increase of erythrocytes in blood.

pulmonary edema: edema of lungs symptomatic of congestive heart failure.

reticulocytopenia (re-tik″u-lo-si″to-pe′ne-ah): decrease in amount of reticulocytes in blood (also called *reticulopenia*).

splenomegaly: enlargement of spleen.

thrombocytopenia (throm″bo-si″to-pe′ne-ah): decrease in platelets in blood.

thrombosis: formation, presence, or development of blood clot or thrombus.

thrombus: blood clot obstructing blood vessel.

thymopathy: any disease of thymus.

thymus hyperplasia: enlarged thymus.

vasoconstriction (vas″o-kon-strik′shun): narrowing of blood vessels.

vasodilation: expansion of blood vessels.

vasospasm: blood vessel spasm causing narrowing in its diameter.

Oncology

hemangioma: benign tumor caused by cluster of newly formed blood vessels.

hemangiosarcoma: malignant tumor of vascular tissue.

lymphangioma (lim-fan″je-o′mah): tumor made up of newly formed lymph channels and spaces.

lymphangiosarcoma: malignant tumor of lymph vessels.

lymphoma: lymphoid tissue tumors, usually malignant.

lymphomatosis (lim″fo-mah-to′sis): development of multiple lymphomas in body.

lymphosarcoma (lim″fo-sar′ko-mah): malignant neoplasm of lymphoid tissue.

Surgical procedures

anastomosis (ah-nas″to-mo′sis): creation of passage between two vessels.

angioplasty (an′je-o-plas″te): repair of vessel.

angiorrhaphy (an″je-or′ah-fe): suture of vessel.

arteriectomy: excision of section of artery.

arterioplasty (ar-te″re-o-plas′te): repair of artery.

arteriorrhaphy (ar-te″re-or′ah-fe): suture of artery.

arteriotomy: incision of artery.

artificial cardiac pacemaker: device (implanted or external) used in place of defective sinoatrial node to supply electrical impulses to heart.

cardiac prosthesis: artificial replacement of cardiac tissue, such as plastic valves and patches or plastic tubular grafts for diseased arteries.

cardiocentesis (kar″de-o-sen-te′sis): surgical puncture or incision of heart.

cardiotomy (kar″de-ot′o-me): surgical incision of heart.

lymphadenectomy (lim-fad″e-nek′to-me): excision of lymph node.

open heart surgery: surgical procedures involving prolonged manipulation inside heart, with heart detached from systemic circulation and heart-lung machine replacing its function.

splenectomy: removal of spleen.

splenorrhapy: repair of spleen.

splenotomy: incision of spleen.

thrombectomy (throm-bek'to-me): excision of thrombus from blood vessels.

thymectomy: removal of thymus.

venipuncture: puncture of vein to draw blood.

Laboratory tests and procedures

abdominal aortography: X-ray studies of abdominal aorta and other vessels, using contrast medium.

activated partial thromboplastin time: blood test to screen for coagulation disorders and various clotting factors.

angiocardiogram: contrast medium injected to study heart and its vessels by use of X ray.

angiogram: contrast medium injected into blood vessels and X ray taken (used to study vessels throughout body).

blood culture: sample of blood incubated in growth medium to determine type of organism causing infection.

bone marrow aspiration: insertion of needle into bone to obtain samples of bone marrow for analysis to diagnose disorders involving red and white blood cells by evaluating them as to appearance, numbers, development, and presence of infection.

cardiac catheterization: passage of a small catheter into heart via vein to inject dye for X-ray purposes, to record pressure, and to discover anomalies of heart.

coagulation tests: tests of blood plasma and serum to determine clotting ability.

complete blood count (CBC): tests to determine number of red and white cells, hematocrit, and hemoglobin percentage in blood.

Coombs's test: test to determine presence of antibodies against red blood cells.

differential blood count: percentages of leukocytes in blood sample.

echocardiography (cardiac ultrasound examination): use of high-frequency sound waves to visualize heart for assessing valvular heart disease and overall heart function.

electrocardiograph (ECG or EKG): instrument that produces graphic record of electrical currents of heart.

erythrocyte sedimentation rate: measure of rate at which red blood cells settle in unclotted blood, used as an indication of presence of inflammatory diseases and infections.

glucose tolerance test: measurement of blood sugar levels at specific intervals after fasting patient's intake of glucose, used to determine effectiveness of sugar metabolism.

hematocrit: procedure or apparatus for determining erythrocytic volume in whole blood.

hemogram: written record of differential blood count.

hemolysis: rupture of red cells with release of hemoglobin.

prothrombin time: test to determine time necessary for clot formation in plasma, which provides measure of activity of various coagulation factors.

reticulocyte count: measure of reticulocytes as percentage of all red cells.

10 Respiratory System

CHAPTER OVERVIEW

In this chapter the various parts of the respiratory system are presented and the process of respiration is reviewed and illustrated. The respiratory system's interaction with the circulatory system is also described.

STRUCTURES AND FUNCTIONS

The organs of the respiratory system include the nose, pharynx, larynx, trachea, bronchi, and lungs. The thorax and the diaphragm serve as accessory structures. The process of respiration generally involves the *inspiration* (inhalation) of air that contains oxygen (O_2) for use by the cells of the body and the *expiration* (exhalation) of carbon dioxide (CO_2), which is a waste product from the cells of the body. The respiratory system depends on the circulatory system to complete the respiratory cycle. Oxygen is inhaled by the lungs and is transported via the blood to all parts of the body. The cellular waste product carbon dioxide is collected by the blood and brought back to the lungs to be exhaled.

The Nose

The *nose* (*naso* and *rhino* mean nose) is the part of the respiratory system that acts as an entrance for air and an exit for carbon dioxide. A *ciliated* epithelial mucous membrane (mucosa) lines the nose and much of the respiratory tract. It serves as a filter for dust and other foreign matter. The nose warms and moistens the entering air and has *olfactory* (sense of smell) receptors located in the nasal mucosa.

The nostrils *(nares)* are paired external openings to the airways. The nostrils vary in pliability and expandability between species. The horse has pliable and expandable nostrils. Expandability is essential for this species. Because mouth breathing is not characteristic in the horse, this expandability accommodates the increased need for oxygen when running. The pig, conversely, has a rigid nostril formation.

The Pharynx

The *pharynx* (throat) is a musculomembranous, saclike structure (Fig. 10-1). The upper portion is attached to the base of the skull, and the lower portion unites with the esophagus. The pharynx communicates with the nasal chambers, mouth, larynx, and eustachian tubes. The pharynx is divided into three parts: the *nasopharynx* (opening into the back of the nasal chambers and into the eustachian tubes), the *oropharynx* (opening into the back of the mouth), and the *laryngopharynx* (opening into the larynx and esophagus).

The pharynx is used by the respiratory and digestive tracts as a passageway for air and food. Depending on the species, it may also have a role in vocalization.

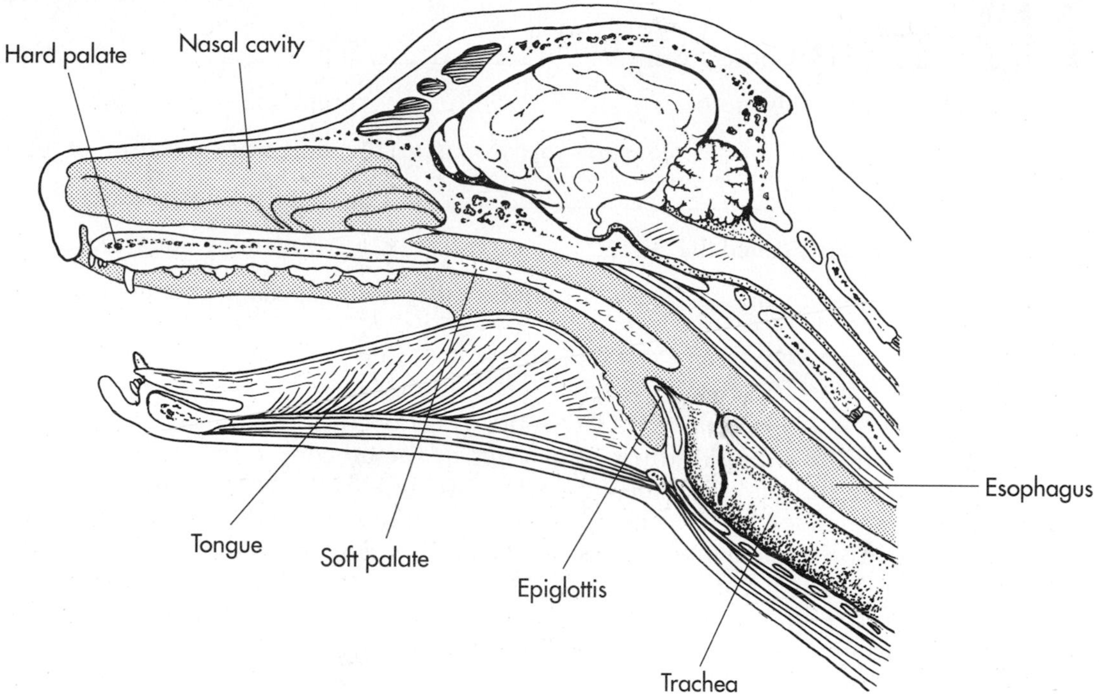
Hard palate
Nasal cavity
Esophagus
Tongue
Soft palate
Epiglottis
Trachea

FIG. 10-1 Cross-section of the upper respiratory tract of the dog.

The Larynx

The *larynx* is commonly called the voice box and is located just below the pharynx. It also serves as a passageway for air. The *epiglottis,* a lidlike cartilaginous structure, prevents foods from entering the airway during swallowing. It plays an important role as the main organ of sound in mammals. Air, passing through the *glottis* during expiration, causes a vibration, producing the sound. In birds, the organ of sound is the *syrinx,* which is located where the trachea divides to form the bronchi.

REVIEW A

1. Two word forms meaning nose are ________________ and ________________.
2. The sense of smell depends on the ________________ receptors.
3. The pharynx is divided into three parts, according to the adjacent structure of each: ________________, ________________, and ________________.
4. The voice box is properly called the ________________. The opening into this structure is called the ________________. The lidlike structure that helps prevent food from entering is the ________________.

The Trachea

The *trachea* (windpipe) is a tube formed of smooth muscle with numerous C-shaped rings of cartilage embedded in the muscle tissue (Fig. 10-2). The cartilaginous rings prevent collapse of the structure. The trachea stretches from the larynx to the bronchi and is lined with mucous membrane.

The Bronchi

The lower end of the trachea separates into smaller airways called the right and left *primary bronchi.* The bronchi, like the trachea, are lined with a ciliated mucous membrane and have C-shaped cartilaginous rings in their walls. The rings become complete as the bronchi enter the lungs. The two primary bronchi enter the lungs, one to the right lung and one to the left. The bronchi then divide into smaller branches called the *secondary bronchi,* which branch into *bronchioles.* These continue to branch into smaller and smaller bronchioles, which finally become *alveolar ducts.* The alveolar ducts have *alveolar sacs* at their termination. The walls of the alveolar sacs are composed of many alveoli, which are minute, squamous, epithelium-lined spaces that allow the lungs to achieve their main function of oxygen and carbon dioxide exchange.

As the bronchioles get smaller, the cartilage rings begin to disappear. There are no rings in the alveolar ducts, sacs, or alveoli. The structure of the bronchi and their bronchioles resembles an upside-down tree, hence the term *bronchial tree.*

The *lungs* are the primary structures of the respiratory system. They are paired structures that occupy almost the entire thoracic cavity. Each lung contains millions of minute alveoli and blood capillaries lining its membranes. (There are probably more than 300 million alveoli in a pair of human lungs.) The lungs are encased in a serous membranous sac called the *visceral pleura.* The thoracic cavity that houses the lungs is lined with another serous membrane called the *parietal pleura.* These pleural membranes reduce friction during respiration. The space between the two membranes is called the *pleural cavity* or *potential space.*

The functions of the lung are the distribution of air to the alveoli and the exchange of gases. This latter function is a cooperative effort of the alveoli and the blood capillaries.

The Thorax

The *thoracic* (chest) *cavity* is lined with a layer of serous membrane similar to that covering the lungs. This membrane allows the lubrication of both surfaces during respiration. The membrane is divided into three parts:

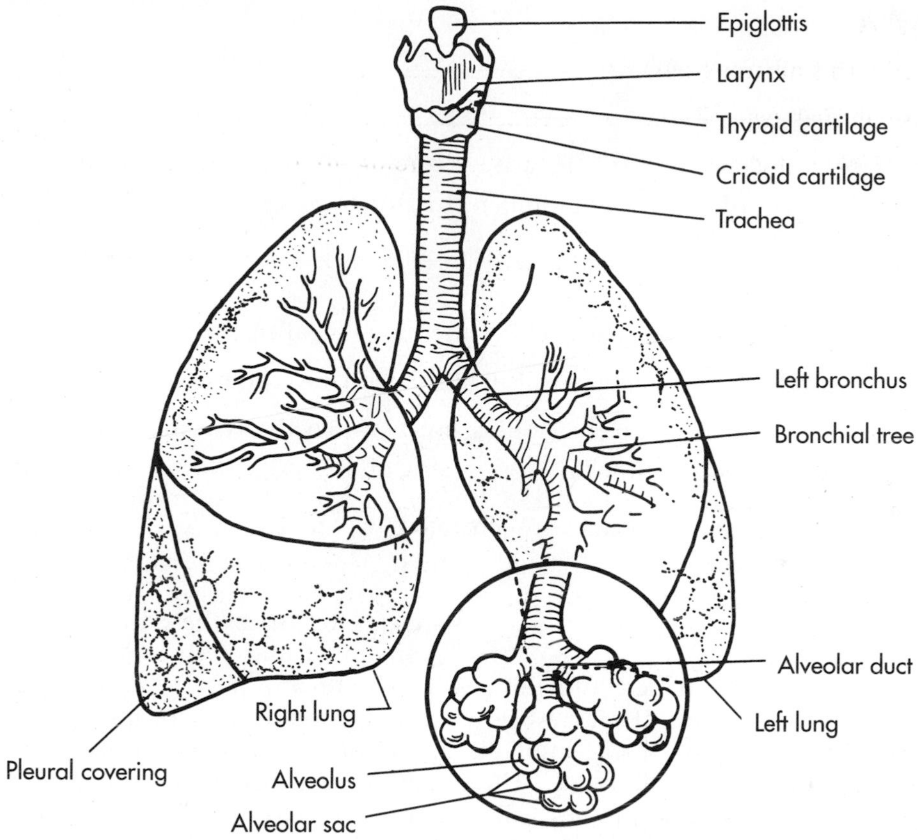
Epiglottis
Larynx
Thyroid cartilage
Cricoid cartilage
Trachea
Left bronchus
Bronchial tree
Alveolar duct
Left lung
Right lung
Pleural covering
Alveolus
Alveolar sac

FIG. 10-2 Lower respiratory tract, including an alveolus.

the right pleural cavity, the left pleural cavity, and the mediastinum. The *mediastinum* contains the heart, thymus, esophagus, trachea, bronchi, nerves, various arteries, veins, and lymphatic vessels and nodes.

The Diaphragm

The *diaphragm* is a dome-shaped musculomembranous partition separating the thoracic and abdominal cavities. It attaches to the lumbar vertebrae, lower ribs, and sternum. It is the chief muscle of respiration. During inspiration, the diaphragm contracts, flattens, and lowers, which increases the capacity of the thoracic cavity. This expansion allows the lungs to fill with air and expand. On expiration, the diaphragm relaxes and returns to its original position.

REVIEW B

1. The windpipe is properly called the ______________________. At its lower end it divides into right and left ______________________. They in turn divide into ______________________, which branch into progressively smaller ______________________.
2. The alveolar ducts of the lungs terminate in structures called ______________________, whose walls are composed of many ______________________ where gaseous exchange takes place.
3. The serous membranous sac that encloses the lungs is called the ______________________ pleura. The inside of the thoracic wall is lined with the same type of membrane, called the ______________________ pleura. The space between the two membranes is called the ______________________.
4. The thoracic and abdominal cavities are separated by the ______________________.

THE PROCESS OF RESPIRATION

The respiratory cycle is divided into three parts: *inspiration* (inhalation of air), *expiration* (exhalation of air), and *rest* (the interval between inspiration and expiration). The time interval of the respiration cycle varies depending on the species.

Respiration involves oxygen being passed throughout the body by the circulation and carbon dioxide wastes returning via the blood to the lungs to be exhaled. The bright red color of arterial blood results from the mix of oxygen and hemoglobin being carried to the tissues. The dark red venous blood indicates that very little oxygen is present in the blood returning from the tissues.

The amount of oxygen retained by the tissues depends on need. Tissues do not store oxygen, and they do not take more oxygen than is needed. Increased activity of any tissue calls for more oxygen. During strenuous exercise, the use of oxygen may be more than doubled. Significant increases in the amount of blood supplied to the muscles results in an increased amount of oxygen consumed and carbon dioxide discharged.

The flow of air into and out of the lungs depends entirely on changes in the capacity of the thoracic cavity. Inspiration and expiration are strictly in accordance with the pressure differences between the atmosphere and the air in the lungs. These pressure differences are caused by the expansion or contraction of the thoracic boundaries (Table 10-1).

Tidal volume (TV)—the volume of air inspired or expired during ordinary respiration.

Inspiratory reserve volume (IRV) or complemental air—the maximum volume of air that can be forcibly inspired in addition to tidal air. The same principle applies to expiration.

Expiratory reserve volume (ERV) or *supplemental air*—the volume of air that can be forcibly expelled in addition to the tidal air. No matter how forcibly an animal exhales, some air always remains trapped in the alveoli because the intrathoracic pressure is be-

Table 10-1 RESPIRATORY TERMS

Stage of respiration	Applicable terms
Ordinary inhalation	Tidal volume
Additional inhalation	Inspiratory reserve volume or complemental air
Ordinary exhalation	Tidal volume
Additional exhalation	Expiratory reserve volume or supplemental air
Forcible exhalation	Residual volume
Total lung collapse	Minimal volume
Largest volume	Vital capacity; total of inspiratory and expiratory reserves plus tidal air

low the atmospheric (normal air) pressure.

Residual volume (RV)—the volume of trapped air in the alveoli.

Minimal volume—the small amount of air left in the alveoli after a total lung collapse. This happens when the intrathoracic pressure rises to equal the atmospheric pressure (as in pneumothorax).

Vital capacity (VC)—the largest volume of air that can be moved in and out of the lungs. It is the sum of the total of inspiratory and expiratory reserve volumes plus the tidal air.

The respiratory center in the brain controls the movements of respiration. The nerves from the brain that pass down the chest wall and diaphragm to control respiration are as follows:

Vagus nerve—originates in the brain; sends branches to the larynx, heart, bronchi, esophagus, stomach, liver, and abdomen.

Phrenic nerve—originates in the cervical spine, passes to the diaphragm.

Thoracic nerve—originates in the thoracic spinal cord; these are the nerves of the muscles of the thorax.

In summary, during inspiration, the thoracic cavity enlarges in all directions. The diaphragm contracts and descends, the ribs elevate, and air is drawn into the lungs. During expiration, there is a relaxation of the inspiratory muscles, and the thoracic framework resumes its original position. As the lungs contract, the diaphragm relaxes upward toward the thoracic cavity.

REVIEW C

1. The respiration cycle is divided into three parts: ____________________, ____________________, and ____________________.
2. The amount of air inhaled during ordinary respiration is called ____________________.
3. The air trapped in the alveoli is called ____________________.
4. The respiratory center is in the ____________________.
5. The small amount of air left in the alveoli after a total lung collapse is called ____________________.

Chapter 10 Answers

Review A

1. naso, rhino
2. olfactory
3. nasopharynx, oropharynx, laryngopharynx
4. larynx, glottis, epiglottis

Review B

1. trachea, primary bronchi, secondary bronchi, bronchioles
2. alveolar sacs, alveoli
3. visceral, parietal, pleural cavity or potential space
4. diaphragm

Review C

1. inspiration (inhalation), expiration (exhalation), rest
2. tidal volume
3. residual volume
4. brain
5. minimal volume

Chapter 10 EXERCISES

RESPIRATORY SYSTEM

Exercise 1: Complete the following statements.

1. Respiration generally involves the acts of ________________ and ________________.
2. The organs of the respiratory system are ________________, ________________, ________________, ________________, ________________, and ________________.
3. Two functions of the pharynx are ________________ and ________________.
4. Two functions of the larynx are ________________ and ________________.
5. The function of the tracheal rings is to ________________.
6. The structure that separates the lungs from each other and divides the thoracic cavity into two parts is the ________________.

Exercise 2: Match the term in the right column with the correct definition or statement in the left column by placing the appropriate letter in the blank space provided.

H	1. Air sacs of the lung	A. Diaphragm
G	2. Branch of the trachea going to each lobe of the lung	B. Oxygen
d	3. Warms and moistens entering air	C. Carbon dioxide
C	4. Odorless, colorless gas formed in tissues and excreted by the lungs	D. Mucous membrane
J	5. Conveys both food and air	E. Bronchiole
F	6. Potential space between the parietal and visceral pleural membranes	F. Pleural cavity
A	7. Muscular and membranous partition that separates the thoracic cavity from the abdominal cavity	G. Bronchus
D	8. Epithelial lining of the nose	H. Alveoli
E	9. Small branch of the bronchial tree extending from secondary bronchi	I. Nose
B	10. Gas present in air; necessary for survival	J. Pharynx

Exercise 3: Using the following list of terms, identify each part in Fig. 10-3 by writing its name in the corresponding blank.

~~tongue~~
epiglottis
~~trachea~~
hard palate
~~nasal cavity~~
soft palate
~~esophagus~~

1. ______________________
2. ______________________
3. ______________________
4. ______________________
5. ______________________
6. ______________________
7. ______________________

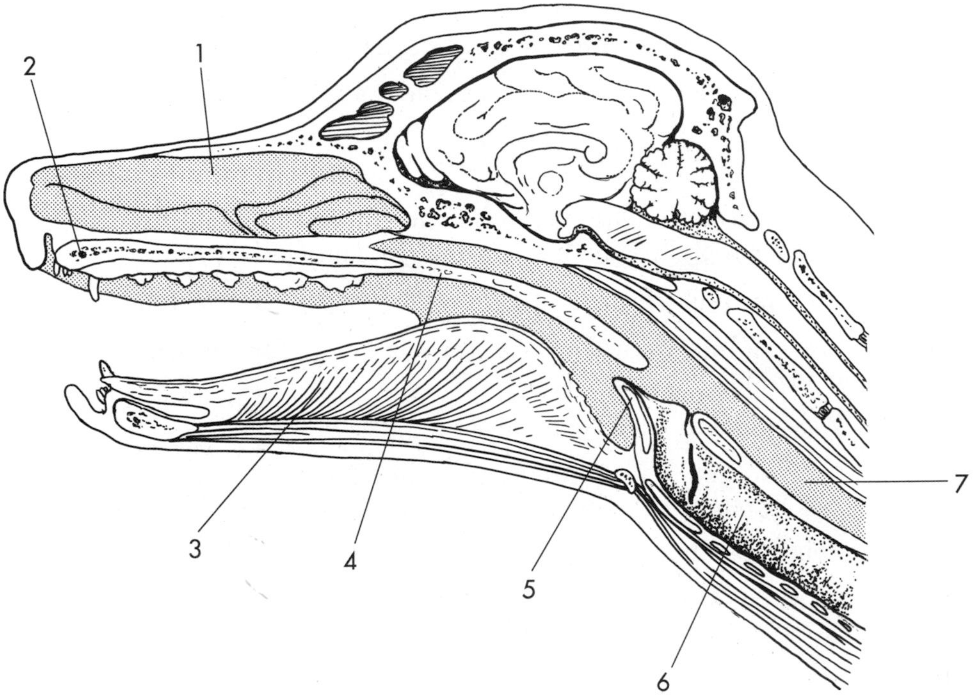
1
2
3
4
5
6
7

FIG. 10-3

Exercise 4: Name the structures in Fig. 10-4 identified by the following numbers:

1. ____________________ 7. ____________________
2. ____________________ 8. ____________________
3. ____________________ 9. ____________________
4. ____________________ 10. ____________________
5. ____________________ 11. ____________________
6. ____________________ 12. ____________________

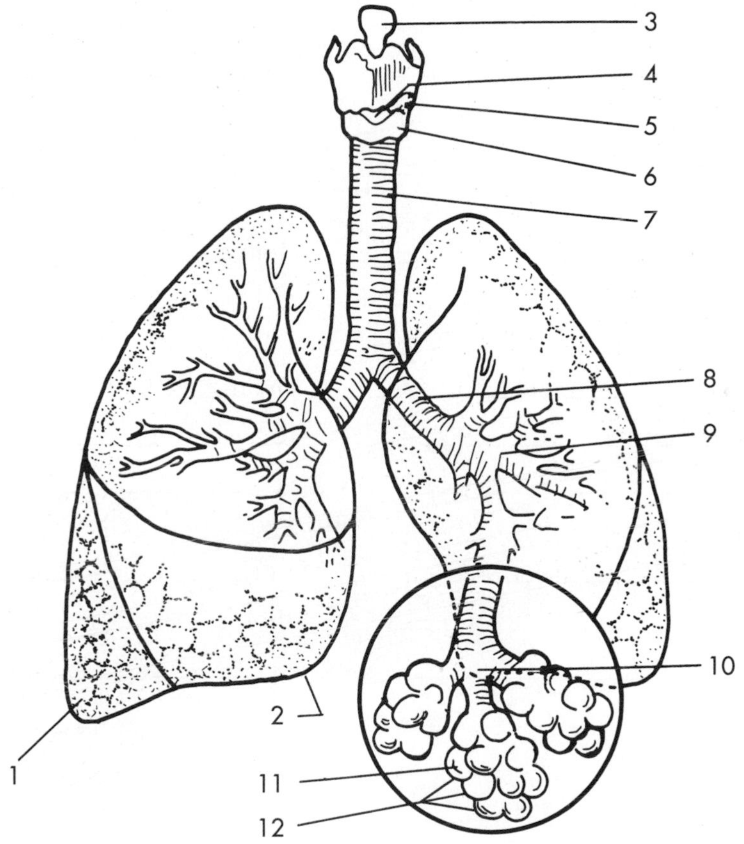
3
4
5
6
7
8
9
10
2
1
11
12

FIG. 10-4

Exercise 5: Give the meaning of the components in the following words and then define the word as a whole.

1. Nasopharyngitis

   naso ______________________

   pharyng ______________________

   itis ______________________

   ____

2. Rhinitis

   rhin ______________________

   itis ______________________

   ____

3. Pneumothorax

   pneumo ______________________

   thorax ______________________

   ____

4. Tracheobronchitis

   tracheo ______________________

   bronch ______________________

   itis ______________________

   ____

5. Bronchostenosis

   broncho ______________________

   sten ______________________

   osis ______________________

   ____

6. Bronchiectasis

   bronchi ______________________

   ectas ______________________

   is ______________________

   ____

7. Tracheostenosis

   tracheo ______________________

   sten ______________________

   osis ______________________

   ____

8. Pharyngostomy

   pharyngo ______________________

   stomy ______________________

   ____

9. Chylothorax

   chylo ______________________

   thorax ______________________

   ____

10. Pyothorax

   pyo ______________________

   thorax ______________________

   ____

CHAPTER 10 PUZZLE

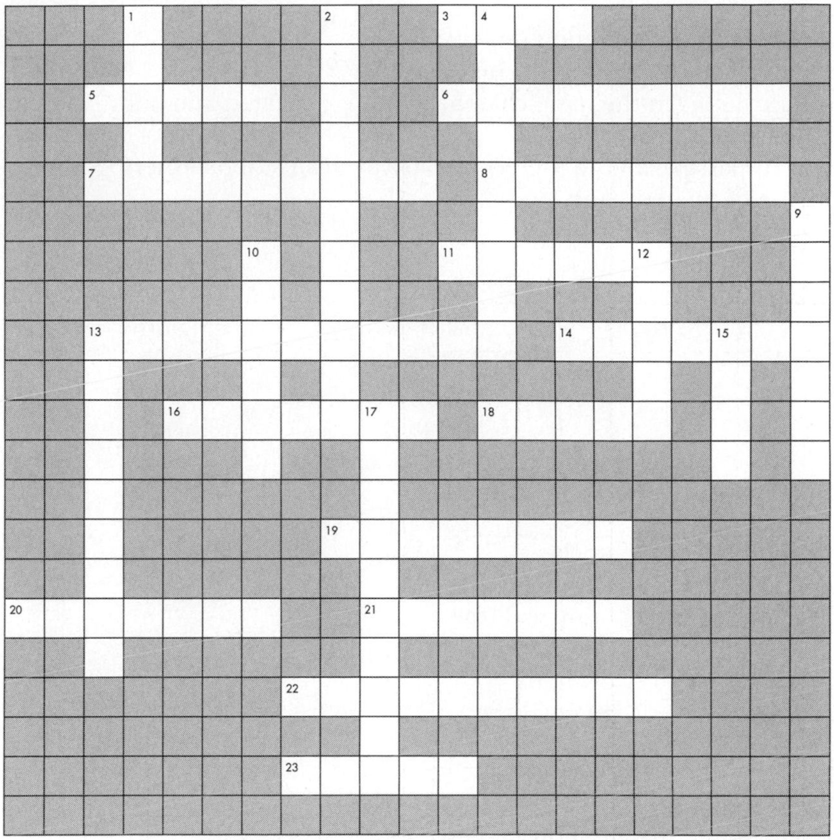
1
2
3
4
5
6
7
8
9
10
11
12
13
14
15
16
17
18
19
20
21
22
23

ACROSS CLUES

3. Interval between inspiration and expiration
5. Volume of air normally inhaled or exhaled
6. Musculomembranous partition
7. Space between pleural cavities
8. Of the chest cavity
11. Gas needed by body tissues
13. Small bronchi branches
14. A nerve controlling respiration
16. Difficult breathing
18. A nerve controlling respiration
19. Pleural sac encasing lungs
20. Throat
21. Minute air spaces in lungs
22. Leaf-shaped, lidlike cartilage
23. Cessation of breathing

DOWN CLUES

1. Combining form for nose
2. Process involving inspiration and expiration
4. Nosebleed
9. Windpipe
10. Membrane lining respiratory tract
12. Nostrils
13. Upside-down tree structure
15. Combining form for nose
17. Exhalation

Chapter 10 Answers

Exercise 1

1. inspiration (inhalation), expiration (exhalation)
2. nose, pharynx, larynx, trachea, bronchi, lungs
3. to communicate between the nasal chambers, mouth, larynx, and eustachian tubes; as a passageway for food and air
4. to provide an air passage and to protect the airway against food entering during swallowing
5. prevent collapse of the structure
6. mediastinum

Exercise 2

1. H
2. G
3. I
4. C
5. J
6. F
7. A
8. D
9. E
10. B

Exercise 3

1. nasal cavity
2. hard palate
3. tongue
4. soft palate
5. epiglottis
6. trachea
7. esophagus

Exercise 4

1. pleural covering
2. right lung
3. epiglottis
4. larynx
5. thyroid cartilage
6. cricoid cartilage
7. trachea
8. left bronchus
9. bronchial tree
10. alveolar duct
11. alveolus
12. alveolar sac

Exercise 5

1. nose; pharynx; inflammation; inflammation of nose and pharynx
2. nose; inflammation; inflammation of nose or nasal passages
3. air; chest; air in pleural cavity
4. trachea; bronchi; inflammation; inflammation of trachea and bronchi
5. bronchi; narrowing; condition; narrowing of bronchi
6. bronchus; dilate; state or condition; dilatation of the bronchi
7. trachea; narrowing; condition; narrowing of the trachea
8. pharynx; surgical opening; surgical opening into the pharynx
9. milky fluid (chyle); chest; presence of chyle in pleural cavity
10. pus; chest; pus in pleural cavity

ANSWERS: CHAPTER 10 PUZZLE

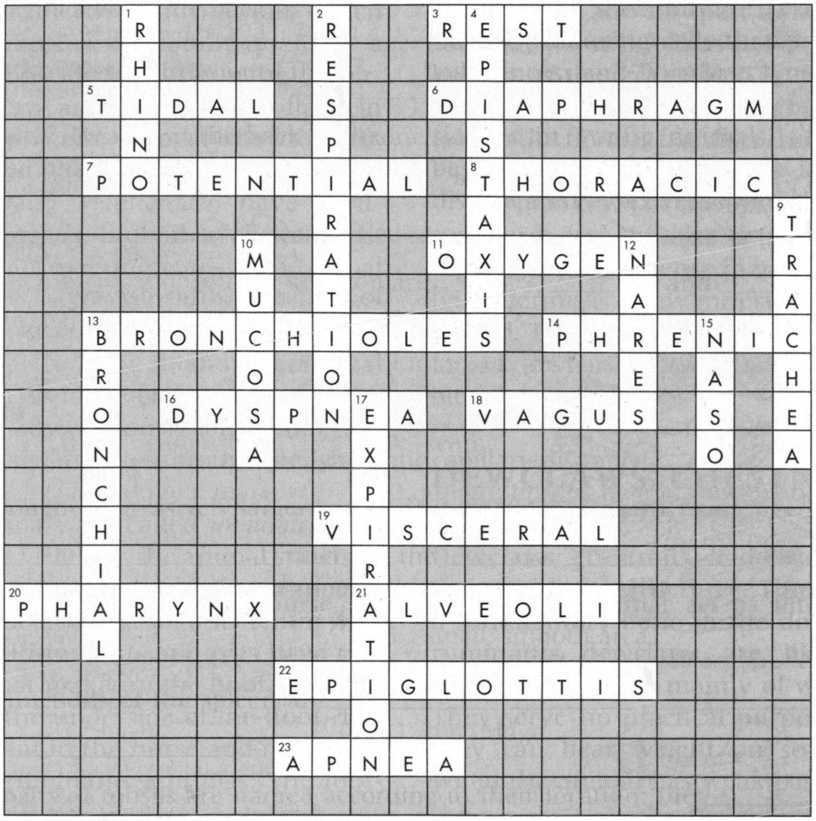
1 RHINO
2 RESPIRATION
3 REST
4 EPISTAXIS
5 TIDAL
6 DIAPHRAGM
7 POTENTIAL
8 THORACIC
9 TRACHEA
10 MUCOSA
11 OXYGEN
12 NARES
13 BRONCHIOLES
13 BRONCHIAL
14 PHRENIC
15 NASO
16 DYSPNEA
17 EXPIRATION
18 VAGUS
19 VISCERAL
20 PHARYNX
21 ALVEOLI
22 EPIGLOTTIS
23 APNEA

GLOSSARY

RESPIRATORY SYSTEM RELATED ANATOMIC TERMS

alveolar ducts: connecting passages between bronchioles and alveolar sac.

alveoli (al-ve'o-lie): plural form of *alveolus.*

alveolus (al-ve'o-lus): air cell of lungs.

arytenoid (ar-ret'te-noid) *cartilage:* one of paired laryngeal cartilages that provides attachment for muscles that adduct and abduct vocal cord.

bronchi (brong'kie): plural form of *bronchus.*

bronchial tree: trachea, bronchi, and bronchioles.

bronchiole (brong'ke-ol): small branch of secondary bronchus.

bronchioli (brong'ke-ol-lie): plural form of *bronchiole.*

bronchus (brong'kus): branch of trachea going to each lobe of lung.

carbon dioxide (CO_2): odorless, colorless gas formed in tissues as waste product and expelled by lungs.

cilia (sil'e-ah): plural form of *cilium.*

cilium (sil'e-um): tiny, hairlike process on epithelial tissue that filters out foreign matter.

complemental air: inspiratory reserve volume.

cricoid cartilage: cartilage of larynx.

diaphragm (di'ah-fram): musculomembranous partition that separates thoracic cavity from abdominal cavity.

ductus arteriosus (duk'tus ar-te"re-o'sus): fetal blood channel from pulmonary artery to aorta.

epiglottis (ep"i-glot'is): leaf-shaped, lidlike cartilaginous structure covers entrance to larynx.

ethmoid sinus: air spaces in ethmoid bone that open into nasal cavity.

expiration or *exhalation:* breathing out; expelling air from lungs.

expiratory reserve volume or *supplemental air:* amount of air that can be forcibly expelled beyond that exhaled during ordinary respiration.

frontal sinuses: air spaces in frontal bone communicating with nasal cavity.

glottis (glot'is): space between true vocal cords, helping to produce vocal sound.

hilus of lung: depression on mediastinal surface of each lung for entry of bronchi, blood vessels, and nerves.

inspiration or *inhalation:* breathing of air into lungs.

inspiratory reserve volume or *complemental air:* amount of air that can be forcibly inhaled beyond that inhaled during ordinary respiration.

laryngopharynx: the part of pharynx below upper edge of epiglottis, opening into larynx and esophagus (also called *hypopharynx*).

larynx (lar'inks): musculocartilaginous structure at top of trachea and below root of tongue and hyoid bone, housing vocal cords (also called voice box).

maxillary sinuses: two air spaces in maxilla, communicating with middle opening of nasal cavity on each side.

mediastinum: space in thorax between two pleural sacs, containing such structures as heart and blood vessels.

minimal volume: air remaining in alveoli of collapsed lung.

mucous membrane: epithelial lining of respiratory tract.

nares (na'rez): pleural form of *naris.*

naris (na'riz): nostril.

nasal septum: membranous, skeletal partition between nasal cavities.

nasopharynx (na"zo-fahr'inks): the part of pharynx above soft palate of mouth, opening into nose.

obligate nasal breather: able to breathe only through nasal passages (for example, horses).

oropharynx (o"ro-fahr'inks): the part of pharynx between soft palate and upper edge of epiglottis.

oxygen (O_2): element in air necessary for life, used by all cells of body.

parietal pleura: lining of thoracic cavity.

pharynx: airway between nasal chambers, mouth, and larynx; also passageway for food.

phrenic (fren'ik) *nerve:* nerve of diaphragm.

pleura (ploor'ah): serous membrane encasing lungs, lining thoracic cavity, and enclosing pleural cavity (potential space).

pleural cavity: potential space between parietal and visceral layers of pleura.

residual volume: air remaining in lungs after forced expiration.

respiration: process involving inspiration and expiration, distribution of oxygen to cells of body, and removal of carbon dioxide from these cells.

retropharynx: back part of pharynx.

sphenoid sinuses: spaces in sphenoid bone, opening to nasal cavity.

supplemental air: expiratory reserve volume.

tidal volume: air inhaled in ordinary respiration.

trachea: cartilaginous, muscular tube, extending from larynx to bronchi; also called *windpipe.*

tracheal rings: horseshoe-shaped rings of cartilage embedded in muscle tissue of trachea.

turbinates: papery, scroll-like bones that support mucous membranes of nose.

vagus (va'gus) *nerve:* nerve extending from brain to pharynx, larynx, and thoracic and abdominal viscera (*vagus* means wandering).

vestibule: front part of nostrils and nasal cavity.

visceral pleura: serous sac covering lungs.

vital capacity: largest amount of air that can be moved in and out of lungs; sum total of inspiratory and tidal air.

vocal cords: two pairs of membranous bands in larynx.

windpipe: trachea.

PATHOLOGIC CONDITIONS

Inflammations and infections

The following conditions affect primarily the lungs.

bronchiectasis (brong"ke-ek'tah-sis): chronic dilation of bronchi or bronchioles as consequence of obstruction or inflammation.

bronchiolitis (bron ke-o-li'tis): inflammation of bronchioles.

bronchitis (brong-ki'tis): inflammation of bronchial membranes.

bronchopneumonia (brong"ko-nu-mo'neah): inflammation of lungs originating in terminal bronchioles.

chronic respiratory disease (CRD), murine respiratory mycoplasmosis, or *chronic murine pneumonia:* disease of mice and rats, caused by *Mycoplasma pulmonis* and characterized by dyspnea, nasal discharge, head tilt, and incoordination.

coccidioidomycosis (kok-sid"e-oi"do-mi-ko'sis): several forms of respiratory fungal infection caused by *Coccidiodes immitus* (also known as *valley fever, desert fever,* and *San Joaquin Valley fever*).

epiglottitis (ep"i-glot-ti'tis): inflammation of epiglottis (also called *epiglottiditis*).

exercise-induced pulmonary hemorrhage (EIPH) or *bleeder:* blood found in lungs of 60% of horses after racing; less than 1% of these horses bleed from nostrils.

herpes virus: family of viruses, including causative agents of infectious bovine rhinotracheitis, equine viral rhinopneumonitis, feline rhinopneumonitis, canine herpes virus respiratory, infectious laryngotracheitis (birds), and Marek's disease (birds).

histoplasmosis (his'to-plaz-mo'sis): systemic fungal respiratory infection caused by inhaling *Histoplasma capsulatum* spores.

influenza: acute, contagious respiratory disease transmitted by airborne viral droplet infection.

laryngeal hemiplegia or *roaring:* unilateral paralysis of larynx causing exercise intolerance and loud stertor (snoring) at exercise in horses.

laryngitis (lar"in-ji'tis): inflammation of mucous membranes of larynx.

pharyngitis: inflammation of mucous membranes of pharynx.

pleurisy: inflammation of pleura.

pleurocarditis: inflammation of pleura and pericardium.

pleuropneumonia (ploor'o-nu-mo'ne-ah): pleurisy with pneumonia.

pneumonia (nu-mo'ne-ah): inflammation and congestion of lung.

pneumopleuritis: pleurisy with presence of air in pleural cavity.

psittacosis (sit-ah-ko'sis): respiratory fungal infection of birds, zoonotic in that it can be transferred to humans through contact with infected birds (also called *parrot fever*).

Q fever: febrile rickettsial respiratory infection caused by *Coxiella burneti.*

rhinitis: inflammation of nasal mucous membranes.

snuffles: upper respiratory disease of rabbits caused by *Pasteurella multocida* characterized by purulent nasal and ocular discharge, which cakes insides of forepaws; sneezing and coughing seen; pneumonia common.

tracheitis (tra"ke-i'tis): inflammation of membrane lining trachea.

tracheobronchitis: inflammation of membranes lining trachea and bronchi (called *kennel cough* in dogs).

tuberculosis: infectious disease of cattle caused by *Mycobacterium bovis;* may cause bronchopneumonia.

Other conditions and diseases

allergic rhinitis: any allergic response of nasal mucosa.

apnea: cessation of breathing.

asphyxia: condition resulting from lack of oxygen.

asthma (az'ma): disease marked by recurring attacks of paroxysmal shortness of breath, wheezing, and coughing.

atelectasis (at'e-lek'tah-sis): collapse of lung or incomplete expansion of lung at birth.

broncholithiasis (brong"ko-li-thi'ah-sis): stone in part of tracheobronchial tree.

bronchospasm (brong'ko-spazm): spasm of muscles of walls of bronchi.

chronic obstructive pulmonary disease (COPD): general term for pulmonary obstructive diseases with breathing difficulties, such as chronic bronchitis and emphysema. Heaves (in horses) is a specific example.

cyanosis: bluish discoloration of skin and mucous membranes caused by excessive concentration of reduced hemoglobin in blood.

dyspnea (disp-ne'ah): difficulty in breathing.

emphysema (em"fi-se'mah): chronic pulmonary condition marked by abnormal increase in size of air spaces in lungs, caused by alveolar dilation or destructive changes in alveolar walls.

epistaxis (ep"i-stak'sis): nosebleed.

hemopneumothorax: blood and air in pleural cavity.

hemoptysis (he-mop'ti-sis): spitting of blood.

hemothorax: blood in pleural cavity.

hiccup: involuntary, spasmodic contraction of diaphragm causing characteristic sounds in breathing (also called *hiccough*).

hydropneumothorax: collection of fluid and air in pleural cavity.

hydrothorax: fluid in pleural cavity.

hyperpnea (hi"perp-ne'ah): abnormal increased respiration.

hyperventilation: abnormally prolonged, rapid, deep breathing.

laryngospasm (lah-ring'go-spazm): spasmodic closing of larynx.

laryngostenosis (lah-ring"go-ste-no'sis): narrowing of larynx.

nasopharyngeal spasm: reverse sneeze.

pneumothorax: air in pleural cavity.

pulmonary edema: serous fluid accumulation in air sacs and tissues of lung.

pulmonary fibrosis: progressive, usually fatal fibrosis of walls of alveoli of lungs (also called *diffuse interstitial pulmonary fibrosis*).

purring: semiautomatic, cyclic, controlled respiration involving alternating activity of diaphragm and intrinsic laryngeal muscles in cats; occurs when content, sick, or sleeping.

pyothorax: collection of pus in pleural cavity (also called *empyema*).

rales (rahlz): abnormal breathing sounds heard in lungs.

tracheostenosis (tra"ke-o-ste-no'sis): narrowing of trachea.

SURGICAL PROCEDURES

cordectomy (kor-dek'to-me): excision of all or part of vocal cord (debarking).

intubation: insertion of tube into airway to clear it of obstruction, named for location of insertion (for example, oral, nasal, endotracheal).

laryngoscope (lah-ring'go-skop): instrument for examining larynx.

laryngostomy (lar"ing-gos'to-my): creating permanent opening in larynx through neck.

pneumocentesis (nu"mo-cen-te'sis): puncture of lung for aspirating fluid.

tracheostomy: creation of artificial opening into trachea through neck (also called *tracheotomy*).

LABORATORY AND EXAMINATION PROCEDURES

auscultation: listening to sounds within the body.

bronchoscopy (brong'ko-sko-pee): examination of bronchi by means of bronchoscope (fiberoptic flexible tube or endoscope inserted through mouth or trachea).

chest X ray: examination to determine presence of lung disease.

endoscopy: examination using endoscope (flexible tube with light and refracting mirrors) to examine larynx and esophagus.

laryngoscopy: examination of larynx and upper trachea using laryngoscope (an endoscope) to detect tumors and other abnormalities.

lung scan: visualization procedures involving intravenous

injection of radioactive material to diagnose pulmonary abnormalities.

magnetic resonance imaging (MRI): noninvasive method of scanning body by use of electromagnetic field and radio waves; provides visual images on computer screen and magnetic tape recordings (also called *nuclear magnetic resonance).*

percussion: use of light, sharp taps to chest surfaces to detect abnormalities by sound produced.

throat culture: incubation, in growth medium, of material taken form throat surfaces to determine presence and type of infection.

11 Gastrointestinal Tract

CHAPTER OVERVIEW

In this chapter, the gastrointestinal (GI) system and its various parts and functions are described and explained with illustrations.

STRUCTURES AND FUNCTIONS

The organs of the GI system, commonly called the digestive or alimentary tract, form a tubelike passage through the body cavities. They extend from the mouth to the anus by way of the pharynx, esophagus, stomach, and intestines. The main functions of this system are in the prehension, transport, and breakdown of food and the absorption of nutrients. The GI system also carries waste materials to be eliminated from the body. Food usually is chewed to some extent in the mouth. It is swallowed by way of the pharynx and esophagus, passing through the neck and thorax into the abdomen, where it is received by the stomach. Generally, in nonruminating mammals, the stomach partially digests the food before it is passed on to the small intestine for further digestion and absorption. *Ruminants* are animals that regurgitate and remasticate food. This process allows fermentation of the food by bacteria and protozoa, which digest cellulose and produce energy for the body. The remaining ingesta moves from the small intestine to the large intestine, where it is retained until excreted through the anus.

The movement of contents through the digestive tract is aided by *peristalsis*, an involuntary, wavelike movement. This movement is produced by circular and longitudinal muscle fibers of the tubular structures.

The digestive tract in all mammals generally has the same parts (mouth, teeth, tongue, pharynx, esophagus, stomach, small intestine, large intestine) with accessory organs (salivary glands, liver, pancreas). The order in which these organs occur also remains the same in all mammals. The length, size, and function of the parts vary in accordance with the natural diet of the species. Special adaptations such as those seen in the cecum and the rumen have occurred over time for survival of each species. Animals are classified according to their natural diets are as follows:

Carnivores (for example, cats) eat meat.
Omnivores (for example, pigs) eat both meat and plants.
Herbivores (for example, cows) eat plants.

The Mouth

LIPS

Lips (*labia* means lips) form the entrance to the mouth. They are covered with a thin skin on the outside, and in some species, *tactile hairs* border the lips. Mucous membranes on the inside of the lips extend to cover the surfaces of the oral cavity. The lips of sheep, goats, and horses are soft and flexible and aid in picking up food. Lips of cattle and hogs are stiff and immobile and do little more than close the mouth. Rats have lips that come together behind their incisors to permit them to chew through materials such as concrete without ingesting any of the matter. Llamas and other members of the camelidae have deeply split upper lips that allow them to graze close to the ground without disturbing the roots of the plants that grow so sparsely in their native habitat. Large *conical papillae* (cone-shaped, finger-like projections) are found projecting inward on the mucosa of the lips of ruminants to prevent food from escaping from the mouth during chewing.

ORAL CAVITY

The oral cavity is formed by the arch of the upper and lower jaws and is bounded by the lips and cheeks. It contains the gums *(gingivae),* the teeth (*dento* and *donto* refer to teeth), and the tongue. The structure forming the roof of the mouth is the palate, which is divided into the hard and soft palates. The *hard palate* is a rigid bony structure covered with mucous membrane. It contains transverse ridges formed by thickening of this membrane. The *soft palate* is a partition between the mouth and nasopharynx. It is composed of muscle tissue and is covered with mucous membrane.

The oral cavity serves as a food receptacle and the location where the food particle size is broken down (this is not normally the case in birds or reptiles).

CHEEKS

The cheeks are formed by buccinator muscles and a subcutaneous pad of fat called the *buccal pad.* The muscles keep the food between the teeth during chewing. The elastic tissue of the mucous membrane of the cheeks keeps the lining from forming folds that otherwise could be bitten during chewing.

TONGUE

The tongue is composed of skeletal muscle tissue with fibers pointing in three directions and covered by mucous membrane. It keeps food between the teeth during chewing and aids in swallowing by exerting pressure against the hard palate. In ruminants, there is a prominence of thickened mucosa on the dorsal surface of the tongue, which is called the *lingual torus.* A thin mucous membrane, the *lingual frenulum,* anchors the underside of the tongue to the floor of the mouth.

The small elevations on the sides and upper surface of the tongue are called *papillae,* which are of three types categorized by their appearance: *filiform* (threadlike), *fungiform* (mushroomlike), and *vallate* (rim-shaped). Both the fungiform and vallate contain the taste buds.

The tongue can be used for food prehension as well as for licking and grooming. It can also be used in a ladle function to lap up liquids. It is believed that some animals can determine through taste whether the food to be eaten is poisonous.

GINGIVAE OR GUMS

The gingivae consist of mucous membranes with supporting fibrous tissue. They cover the surfaces of the *maxilla* and *mandible* (jawbones). Richly vascular but poorly innervated, the gums form a collar around each tooth.

TEETH

The numbers of *deciduous* (baby teeth) and permanent teeth vary with the species and the natural diet of the animal. Teeth perform a variety of functions in animals, including the cutting and grinding of food and as a defense mechanism (biting). The deciduous teeth found in most species fall out and are replaced by permanent teeth. Rodents and rabbits are unique in that they have one set of teeth that grows continuously throughout the animal's life.

Carnivores have *brachydont* (short-crowned) teeth, with a structure similar to that of humans. Each tooth has a *crown* (the part projecting from the gumline), a *neck* (located in the gumline), and a *root* (which firmly fixes the tooth in the bony *alveolus,* or socket; Fig. 11-1). The crown is encased in *enamel,* the hardest substance in the body, and the root in *cementum,* which is bonelike. *Dentin,* the third calcified tissue of the tooth, underlies both enamel and cementum. It makes up the bulk of the tooth. Inside the dentin is the *pulp cavity,* a small space that contains nerves and blood vessels supplying the tooth. The *periodontal ligament,* a tough, fibrous tissue, connects the cementum to the bone of the alveolus. The term *periodontium* includes the periodontal ligament and its connections in the cementum and surrounding alveolar bone.

The teeth of the herbivores are *hypsodont* (long-crowned) and do not have a well-defined neck. The enamel-covered portion of the tooth extends well below the gumline. With age, the tooth continues to erupt as it wears. Furthermore, the enamel layer is

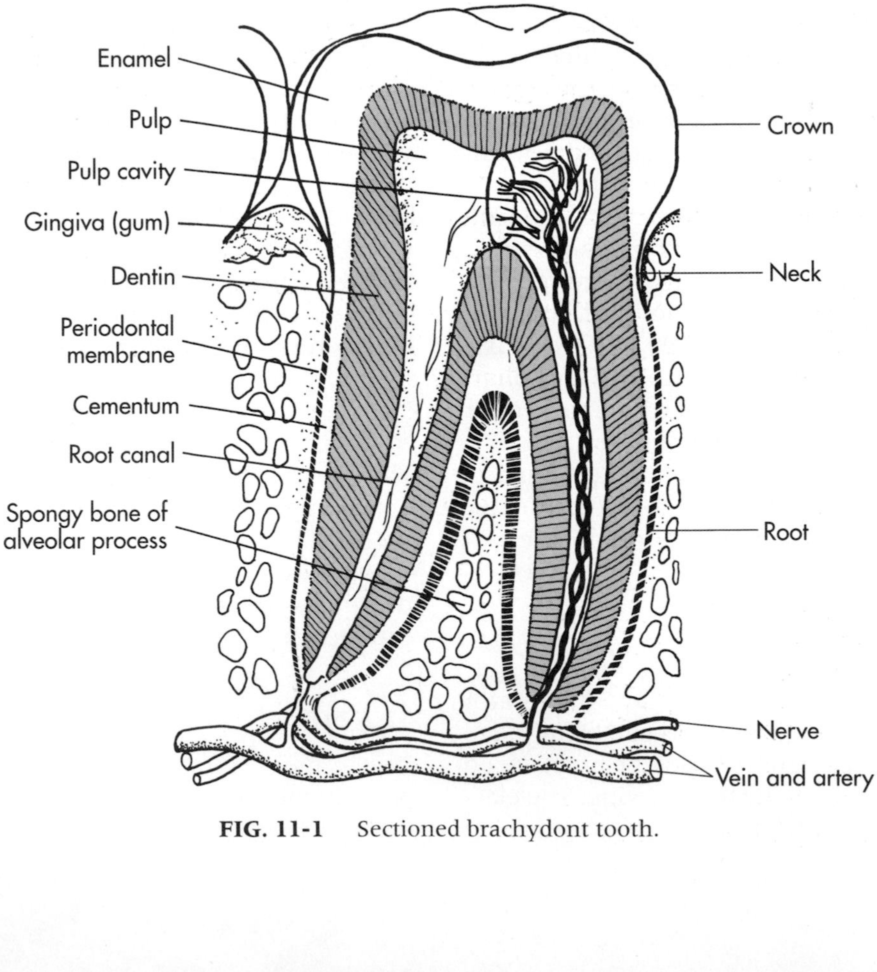
Enamel
Pulp
Pulp cavity
Gingiva (gum)
Dentin
Periodontal membrane
Cementum
Root canal
Spongy bone of alveolar process
Crown
Neck
Root
Nerve
Vein and artery

FIG. 11-1 Sectioned brachydont tooth.

enfolded with the other hard layers during development. As a result the *occlusal* surface of the tooth shows ridges of enamel interspersed with segments of cementum and dentin. Because of this folding, the incisors of horses show longitudinal grooves on the sides and cups on the occlusal surfaces that can be used to estimate an animal's age.

The front teeth are called the *incisors* and are designated in a dental formula by the letter *I.* These teeth are used primarily for shearing or cutting grasses or forage. They can also be used for defense. In ruminants, the upper incisors are absent and are replaced with a *dental pad.* The *canines,* designated by the letter *C,* are also called fangs, eyeteeth, or tusks. They are used for tearing and are especially prominent in carnivorous species. These teeth can also be used for defense. The cheek teeth, also called *premolars,* designated by the letter *P,* and *molars,* designated by the letter *M,* are used to grind food into a size that can be swallowed easily. The premolars are caudal to the canines and rostral to the premolars.

Dental formulas are written to indicate the number and type of teeth found on one side of the mouth. The numerator represents the teeth in the upper jaw, and the denominator represents the teeth in the lower jaw. The numbers are then doubled to represent the total number of teeth. Typical dental formulas include the following:

$$\text{cattle } 2\left(\mathrm{I}\,\frac{0}{4}\;\mathrm{C}\,\frac{0}{0}\;\mathrm{P}\,\frac{3}{3}\;\mathrm{M}\,\frac{3}{3}\right) = 32$$

(note the absence of upper incisors and canines)

$$\text{dogs } 2\left(\mathrm{I}\,\frac{3}{3}\;\mathrm{C}\,\frac{1}{1}\;\mathrm{P}\,\frac{4}{4}\;\mathrm{M}\,\frac{2}{3}\right) = 42$$

The surfaces of the teeth are named as follows:

Lingual—surface of the tooth next to the tongue
Buccal—surface of the tooth next to the cheek
Labial—surface of the tooth next to the lips
Occlusal—chewing or biting surface

SALIVARY GLANDS

The salivary glands in animals are composed of three pairs of well-defined glands and a variety of minor saliva-secreting tissues or glands. The primary salivary glands are the *parotid, mandibular,* and *sublingual.* Some of the minor glands or tissues include labial, buccal, lingual, and palatine. The dog also has a salivary gland near the eye called the zygomatic gland. The serous fluid secreted by these glands is called *saliva.* The chief functions of saliva are to dissolve or lubricate food to facilitate swallowing and, in some species, to initiate carbohydrate digestion. The smell, sight, or thought of food can cause saliva secretion in some species, whereas in others, particularly ruminants, salivary flow can be continuous.

REVIEW A

1. The involuntary wavelike movement of contents through the digestive tract is called ______________.
2. Meat-eating animals are called ______________, plant-eating animals are ______________, and animals that eat both are ______________.
3. Two word forms meaning tooth or teeth are ______________ and ______________.
4. The underside of the tongue is anchored to the floor of the mouth by a membrane called the ______________.
5. The small elevations on the upper surface of the tongue are called ______________. The names of three types of these, based on their shape, are ______________, ______________, and ______________.
6. Baby teeth are properly called ______________. Short-crowned and long-crowned teeth are called ______________ and ______________, respectively.
7. The three calcified tissues of the teeth are ______________, ______________, and ______________.
8. The fibrous tissue that connects the tooth to the alveolus is the ______________.
9. Teeth generally are divided into four types, although some may be missing in certain species. The four types, from front to rear, are ______________, ______________, ______________, and ______________.

The Pharynx

The pharynx, a musculomembranous saclike structure, is further described in Chapter 10. It acts as a common passageway for air and food in all species. It works by mechanical and reflex action by closing off the airway during swallowing. The pharynx opens into mouth and nasal cavities, eustachian tubes, and larynx.

The Esophagus

The esophagus is a narrow muscular tube from the pharynx through the diaphragm to the stomach. The lumen of the tube normally is closed but dilates as needed for passage of food.

Swallowing

There are three phases to the act of swallowing. Only the first is voluntary; the other two are instinctive reflexes. The voluntary phase is the passing of food from the mouth into the pharynx. This is followed by the second (reflex) phase, which passes the food into the stomach from the esophagus. When the food enters the pharynx, all other openings are blocked to ensure its passage into the esophagus. This is achieved by the tongue pressing against the hard palate to close off the oral cavity. The stimulation of the act of swallowing also creates a momentary respiratory suspension that helps prevent food from passing into the respiratory tract. This is an involuntary reflex action and is part of the second phase of swallowing. The third phase of swallowing takes place in the esophagus, where the food is propelled by muscle contraction (peristalsis) through the *cardiac sphincter* into the stomach.

The Nonruminant Stomach (Simple Stomached, Monogastric)

In nonruminants, the stomach (*gastro* refers to stomach) is a musculomembranous structure located just caudal to or below the left side of the diaphragm (see Fig. 11-2). The stomach is subdivided into three sections:

Fundus—the rounded section above the esophageal opening
Body—the middle section
Pylorus—the lower, small end

SPHINCTER MUSCLES

The ringlike muscles that contract to close an opening are called sphincter muscles. The *cardiac sphincter* muscle is located between the esophagus and the stomach. It relaxes to allow food to enter the stomach and contracts while digestion is taking place. It prevents the stomach contents from reflux. The *pyloric sphincter* muscle is located between the pylorus of the stomach and the duodenum. It contracts to prevent the stomach contents from escaping during digestion and then relaxes to allow the contents to enter the duodenum on completion of the gastric digestive process.

GASTRIC COATS AND GLANDS

The stomach wall is made up of four coats: an outer serous coat; a muscular coat consisting of circular, longitudinal, and oblique fibers; a submucous coat; and mucous lining coat. The muscles of the stomach walls allow expansion when food enters and allow the mixing and churning of these foods during the digestive process. Scattered throughout the mucosa of the stomach are innumerable microscopic, tubular, gastric glands. The gastric juice produced by these glands contains enzymes, mucin, and hydrochloric acid. The food in the stomach mixes with these secretions, forming a partially digested semiliquid called *chyme*, which is passed on to the small intestine for further digestion.

The Ruminant Stomach

The true stomach of the ruminant is preceded by three chambers or *diverticula*, where food is soaked and subjected to digestion by microorganisms. (See Fig. 11-2.) Regurgitation and remastication of the food assist fermentation by breaking down the food into smaller particles, which are then acted on by microorganisms. The four chambers are the reticulum, rumen, omasum, and abomasum. The first three chambers ferment the food, which in turn supplies energy to the animal.

The phase "chewing the cud" or *rumination* is the remastication of regurgitated fluid reticular contents. The *cud* is brought back into the mouth for remastication through a series of physiological actions. The regurgitated reticular contents are compressed at the back of the tongue, and the fluid portion is swallowed immediately. The solid material is brought into the mouth and chewed for about 1 minute and then reswallowed. Animals who are frightened or offered food may stop rumination temporarily.

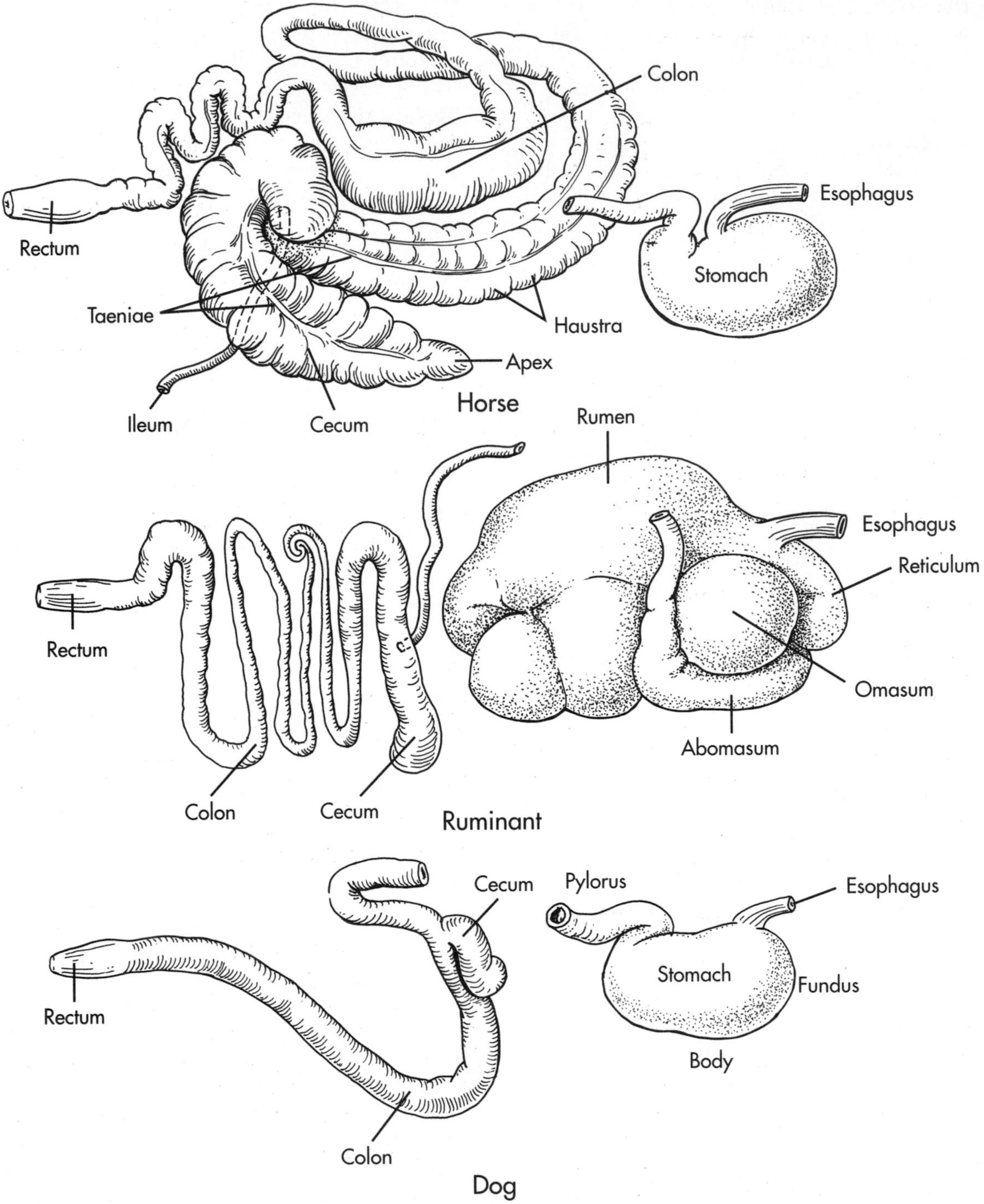
Colon
Esophagus
Rectum
Stomach
Taeniae
Haustra
Apex
Ileum
Cecum
Horse
Rumen
Esophagus
Reticulum
Rectum
Omasum
Abomasum
Colon
Cecum
Ruminant
Cecum
Pylorus
Esophagus
Stomach
Fundus
Rectum
Body
Colon
Dog

FIG. 11-2 Comparison of three gastrointestinal tracts. (Most of the small intestines omitted for clarity.)

THE RETICULUM

The *reticulum* (also called the honeycomb) is the most cranial chamber and lies almost in apposition to the heart. It is lined with mucous membrane that contains numerous intersecting ridges, resulting in a honeycomb appearance. It is in this chamber, with its location near the heart, where *hardware disease* (traumatic reticulitis) caused by perforation by foreign objects such as wire or nails may be a problem.

THE RUMEN

The *rumen* (also called the *paunch*) is a large, muscular sack that extends from the diaphragm to the pelvis and fills almost the entire left side of the abdominal cavity and makes up about 20% of the animal's total weight. It is divided into two sections: the ventral sac and the dorsal sac. The rumen is lined with mucous membrane, with the most ventral parts of both sacs having numerous papillae up to 1 cm long.

THE OMASUM

The *omasum* is round and is lined with mucous membrane and studded with short, blunt papillae. These papillae grind the roughage before it enters the abomasum for further digestion. Contractions of the omasum squeeze the fluid out of the ingesta and grind the solids, which then move into the abomasum.

THE ABOMASUM

The *abomasum* is the true stomach in the ruminant. It is the first glandular portion of the ruminant digestive system that secretes digestive enzymes to further break down the food particles. The abomasum opens into the small intestine by way of the pylorus.

REVIEW B

1. The ______________________ acts as a passageway for both food and air.
2. The entrance to the stomach from the esophagus is through the ______________________ sphincter, and the exit is through the ______________________ sphincter.
3. The simple stomach is divided into three parts: the ______________________, the ______________________, and the ______________________.
4. The four chambers of the ruminant stomach are the ______________________, ______________________, ______________________, and ______________________.
5. "Chewing the cud" is properly called ______________________.

Digestive Process

The ingested food is liquefied by reaction from the digestive enzymes and passes into the duodenum. The chyme moves through the jejunum and ileum by means of the peristaltic waves and is further digested and absorbed. When the ileum empties into the colon, the contents contain both water to be absorbed by the large intestine and waste to be eliminated from the body.

Abdominal Cavity

The stomach and the large and small intestines are enclosed in the space between the diaphragm and pelvis. The abdomen is lined with a serous membrane called the *peritoneum.* The *mesentery,* a fold of the peritoneum, connects a portion of the intestines to the dorsal abdominal wall, and the *visceral peritoneum* covers all or part of the many visceral organs and helps to hold them in place. The *omentum,* a double fold of the peritoneum, attaches to the stomach, connecting it to the abdominal viscera.

SMALL INTESTINE

The small intestine (*entero* refers to intestines) occupies a large portion of the abdomen and is divided into three parts:

Duodenum—attaches to the pyloric end of the stomach (abomasum in ruminants) and receives the pancreatic and common bile ducts (depending on species), which empty into it. Digestion and absorption take place here in species where extensive fermentation is not needed.

Jejunum—the middle section of the small intestine, held in place by the mesentery; vigorous peristaltic waves rapidly move fluid contents into the ileum.

Ileum—the longest portion of the small intestine and the location in which most of the food absorption takes place.

The intestinal digestive juice containing mucus and many enzymes of digestion is stimulated to flow by a hormone called *secretin.* It is produced by the intestinal glands when the chyme reaches the small intestine. The digestive process is completed in the small intestine, and the digested food is then absorbed through the intestinal walls into the blood by the *villi* (countless thread-like projections in the mucous membrane lining the small intestine; see Fig. 11-3). These villi are sloughed off when a dog contracts canine parvovirus.

LARGE INTESTINE

The large intestine is divided into the cecum, colon, and rectum (Fig. 11-2). The contents of the terminal part of the ileum enter the large intestine at the cecum in the horse, at the colon in the dog, or at the cecum and colon in the ruminant and pig. The natural diet of the species determines the extent of development of the large intestine. Fermentation occurs to some extent in the large intestine of all species but especially in herbivores. The forestomachs in ruminants function as fermentation vats, whereas the cecum and colon provide fermentation for simple-stomached herbivores.

Cecum—first part of the large intestine. It forms a dilated pouch (dual pouches in some species) that joins the colon. As a result of the fermentation process, this structure is larger in herbivores than in carnivores. Further digestion by fermentation occurs in species such as rabbits and horses, which have enlarged caeca and colons. The primary function of the cecum is to break down fibrous materials. The vermiform (wormlike) appendix or process is a narrow, tube-shaped projection attached to the ce-

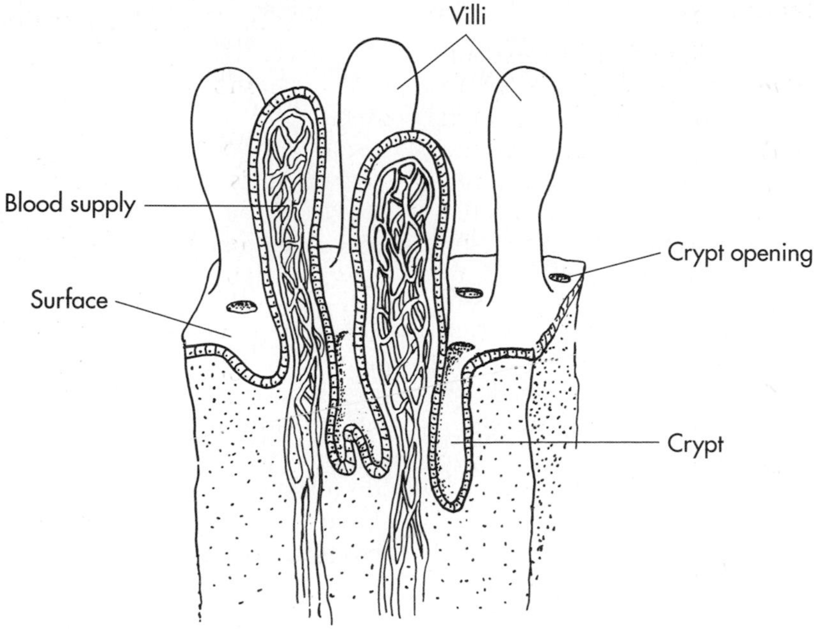
Villi
Blood supply
Surface
Crypt opening
Crypt

FIG. 11-3 Intestinal villi.

cum. In humans, this process, known as the appendix, often is surgically removed because of inflammation.

Colon—divided into three sections: ascending, transverse, and descending. All animals have a transverse and descending; however, the arrangement between the transverse colon and the cecum varies between species.

The cecum and colon of the pig, horse, and rabbit appear sacculated because of longitudinal bands of muscle called *taenia.* The term *haustra* is used when identifying the sacculations.

Rectum—the section of the descending colon located within the pelvis. It dilates to store feces until their expulsion through the anus. The *anus* is the termination of the digestive tract and is composed of both smooth and striated muscle. Species such as the rabbit demonstrate *coprophagy* as a normal physiological activity. Rabbits have two forms of feces: day feces, the normal excreted waste product, and night feces, a nutrient-rich source of vitamins. The moist night feces are ingested directly from the anus and provide the rabbit with essential nutrients.

PANCREAS

The *pancreas* is an elongated gland located near the first part of the duodenum. It serves as both an *exocrine* (secreting into ducts) and *endocrine* (ductless secreting) gland. The exocrine cells secrete pancreatic juice containing enzymes necessary for digestion. These juices are collected within the pancreas and transferred into the duodenum. In sheep and goats, the pancreatic duct empties directly into the common bile duct. The islets of Langerhans are groups of endocrine cells that secrete insulin and glucagon, which have opposing roles in carbohydrate metabolism.

LIVER

The liver (*hepat* refers to liver), the largest gland in the body, is classified as an exocrine gland. It is always located immediately caudal to the diaphragm and more to the right side in ruminants. The liver normally is soft and pliable and should have a reddish-brown color as a result of numerous blood vessels. The four major functions of the liver are as follows:

- Secreting bile for use in digestion
- Providing essential steps in the metabolism of proteins, fats, and carbohydrates
- Filtering and destroying foreign matter and neutralizing toxins
- Storing iron, glycogen, and vitamins A, B_{12}, and D

GALLBLADDER

The main function of the gallbladder (*cholecyst* means gallbladder) is to store the concentrated bile deposited by the hepatic and cystic ducts. The stored bile is then expelled into the duodenum during digestion (*chol* and *chole* mean bile). The rat and the horse do not have gallbladders. These two species have a large amount of hepatic bile flowing continuously into the duodenum.

REVIEW C

1. The serous membrane lining the abdomen is the pertitoneum ______. The fold of this tissue that connects the intestines to the dorsal abdominal wall is the messentry ______.
2. The word root for *intestine* is entero ______.
3. The small intestine is divided into three parts: du ______, ______, and ileum ______.
4. Food is absorbed through fingerlike projections in the small intestine called ______.
5. The large intestine is divided into three parts: ______, ______, and ______.
6. The ingestion of night feces by rabbits is called coprophagy ______.
7. The organ with both exocrine and endocrine functions is the ______.
8. The word root for *liver* is hepat ______.

Chapter 11 Answers

Review 1

1. peristalsis
2. carnivores, herbivores, omnivores
3. dento, donto (also odonto)
4. lingual frenulum
5. papillae; filiform, fungiform, vallate
6. deciduous; brachydont, hypsodont
7. enamel, cementum, dentin
8. periodontal ligament
9. incisors, canines, premolars, molars

Review B

1. pharynx
2. cardiac, pyloric
3. fundus, body, pylorus
4. rumen, reticulum, omasum, abomasum
5. rumination

Review C

1. peritoneum, mesentery
2. entero
3. duodenum, jejunum, ileum
4. villi
5. cecum, colon, rectum
6. coprophagy
7. pancreas
8. hepat

Chapter 11 — EXERCISES

GASTROINTESTINAL TRACT

Exercise 1: Number the order of the structures in the ruminant digestive system (a structure may be included more than once).

__1__ lips

____ duodenum

____ cecum

__2__ tongue

__15__ rectum

____ rumen

____ reticulum

____ pharynx

____ esophagus

____ abomasum

____ ileum

____ jejunum

____ colon

____ mouth

__16__ anus

____ omasum

Exercise 2: Complete the following statements.

1. *Labia* means __lips__ .
2. The partition between the mouth and nasopharynx is the __pharaynx__ .
3. The buccal pad is found in the __cheeks__ .
4. The upper and lower jawbones are called the __mandiuable__ and __maxialbe__ , respectively.
5. The three parts of a brachydont tooth are the __crown__ , the __neck__ , and the __root__ .
6. The bony socket holding a tooth is called the __alveoli__ .

7. The calcified layer that immediately surrounds the pulp cavity of a brachydont tooth is the ______________________ .
8. The tooth surface next to the tongue is the ______________________ surface; the surface next to the cheek is the ______________________ surface. The chewing surface is called the ______________________ surface.
9. The ______________________ salivary gland is under the tongue.
10. The word root for stomach is ______________________ .
11. The semiliquid passed into the small intestine from the stomach is called ______________________ .
12. In ruminants the "honeycomb" is the ______________________ , the "paunch" is the ______________________ , and the "true stomach" is the ______________________ .
13. The longitudinal muscle bands on the cecum of the horse are called ______________________ . The sacculations they produce are called ______________________ .
14. The cholecyst is commonly called the ______________________ . Its function is to store ______________________ . Two species that lack this structure are the ______________________ and the ______________________ .

Exercise 3: Match the term in the right column with the correct definition or statement in the left column and place its letter in the space provided.

B 1. Rigid bony structure in the roof of the mouth

a 2. Partition between the mouth and nasopharynx

E 3. Long-crowned teeth found in herbivores

F 4. Musculomembranous tube from pharynx to stomach

M 5. Lower left margin of the surface of the stomach

P 6. The "true stomach" of the ruminant

L 7. Very hard substance that covers the exposed part of the tooth

C 8. Chief substance of the tooth surrounding pulp

g 9. Semifluid material produced by gastric digestion of food

O 10. Threadlike projections that cover the mucosa of the small intestine

D 11. Front teeth of either jaw

H 12. Broad teeth used in grinding

I 13. Fibrous tissue attaching tooth root to alveolus

Q 14. Portion of rumen affected by hardware disease

G 15. Ringlike muscle that contracts to close an opening

A. Soft palate
B. Hard palate
C. Dentin
D. Incisors
E. Hypsodonts
F. Esophagus
G. Sphincter
H. Molars
I. Periodontium
J. Chyme
K. Lesser curvature
L. Enamel
M. Greater curvature
N. Uvula
O. Villi
P. Abomasum
Q. Reticulum

Exercise 4: Multiple choice.

1. The peritoneal fold that attaches the intestine to the posterior abdominal wall is the
   a. Mesentery
   b. Lesser curvature
   c. Omentum
2. The dilated intestinal pouch that joins the colon below the juncture of the ileum and colon is the
   a. Jejunum
   b. Cecum
   c. Duodenum
3. *Vermiform* is a name given to the
   a. Cecum
   b. Appendix
   c. Rectum
4. The word root for bile is
   a. Chole
   b. Chyle
   c. Chyme
5. Hypsodont teeth wound be found in a
   a. Cat
   b. Cow
   c. Dog
6. The involuntary, wavelike movement of the gastrointestinal tract is called
   a. Peristalsis
   b. Gastritis
   c. Alimentary
7. The bonelike connective tissue covering the root and neck of a tooth is called
   a. Periodontium
   b. Enamel
   c. Cementum

Exercise 5: Give the meaning of the components in the following words, and then define the word as a whole. Check the glossary at the end of the chapter if you need help.

1. Xerostomia

   xero dry

   stom mouth

   ia condition

   dryness of mouth

2. Colonoscopy

   colono colon

   scopy examing

   act of examing colon

3. Gastroenteritis

   gastro stomach

   enter intestine

   itis inflammation

   ____

4. Abdominocentesis

   abdomino __________

   centesis __________

   ____

5. Hepatitis

   hepat liver

   itis inflammation

   inflammation of the liver

6. Abomasopexy

   abomaso __________

   pexy __________

   ____

7. Cheilitis

   cheil __________

   itis ~~[illegible]~~ inflammation

   ____

8. Sialoadenitis

   sialo __________

   aden __________

   itis inflammation

   ____

9. Proctitis

   proct __________

   itis inflammation

   ____

10. Achlorhydria

    a __________

    chlor __________

    hydr __________

    ia condition

    ____

11. Glossitis

    gloss tongue

    itis inflammation

    ____

12. Gingivitis

    gingiv gums

    itis inflammation

CHAPTER 11 PUZZLE

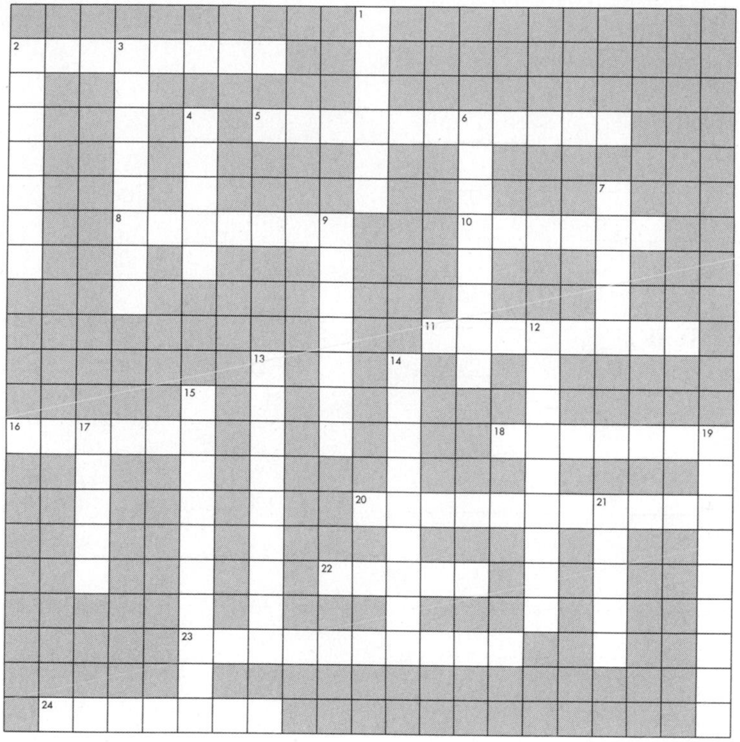

ACROSS CLUES

2. Small elevations on tongue
5. Terminal function of the GI tract
8. Connects stomach to other visceral organs
10. Prefix meaning intestines
11. First portion of small intestine
16. Surface of tooth against the cheek
18. Middle portion of small intestine
20. Involuntary wavelike motion
22. Semifluid stomach contents after digestion
23. Method of obtaining nutrients during digestion
24. Common opening for digestive and respiratory systems

DOWN CLUES

1. Hardest material in the body
2. Opening between stomach and small intestine
3. Chisel-shaped front teeth
4. Portion of ruminant stomach called the paunch
6. Tooth socket in jaw bone
7. Exposed surface of the tooth
9. Upper jaw bone
12. Act of breaking down food particles for use by the body
13. Tubular muscle that extends from pharynx to stomach
14. Term for gallbladder
15. Tract that extends from mouth to anus
17. Blind pouch portion of large intestine
19. Attaches intestines to abdominal wall
21. Lips

Chapter 11 Answers

Exercise 1

1	lips
17	duodenum
20	cecum
3, 10	tongue
22	rectum
14	rumen
6, 13	reticulum
4, 8, 11	pharynx
5, 7, 12	esophagus
16	abomasum
19	ileum
18	jejunum
21	colon
2, 9	mouth
23	anus
15	omasum

Exercise 2

1. lips
2. palate
3. cheek
4. maxilla, mandible
5. crown, neck, root
6. alveolus
7. dentin
8. lingual, buccal, occlusal
9. sublingual
10. gastro
11. chyme
12. reticulum, rumen, abomasum
13. taeniae, haustra
14. gallbladder, bile, horse, rat

Exercise 3

1. B	6. P	11. D
2. A	7. L	12. H
3. E	8. C	13. I
4. F	9. J	14. Q
5. M	10. O	15. G

Exercise 4

1. a
2. b
3. b
4. a
5. b
6. a
7. c

Exercise 5

1. dry; mouth; condition; dryness of the mouth (caused by insufficient saliva production)
2. colon; act of examining; act of examining the colon
3. stomach; intestine; inflammation; inflammation of stomach and intestine
4. abdomen; surgical puncture to remove fluid; surgical puncture of abdomen to remove fluid
5. liver; inflammation; inflammation of the liver
6. abomasum; fixation; surgical fixation of abomasum (to prevent recurrence of displacement)
7. lip; inflammation; inflammation of the lip
8. saliva; gland; inflammation; inflammation of a salivary gland
9. rectum; inflammation; inflammation of the rectum
10. without; green; water; condition; lacking green water (in the stomach) is the literal meaning; the word is used to indicate lack of acid in the stomach
11. tongue; inflammation; inflammation of the tongue
12. gums; inflammation; inflammation of the gums

ANSWERS: CHAPTER 11 PUZZLE

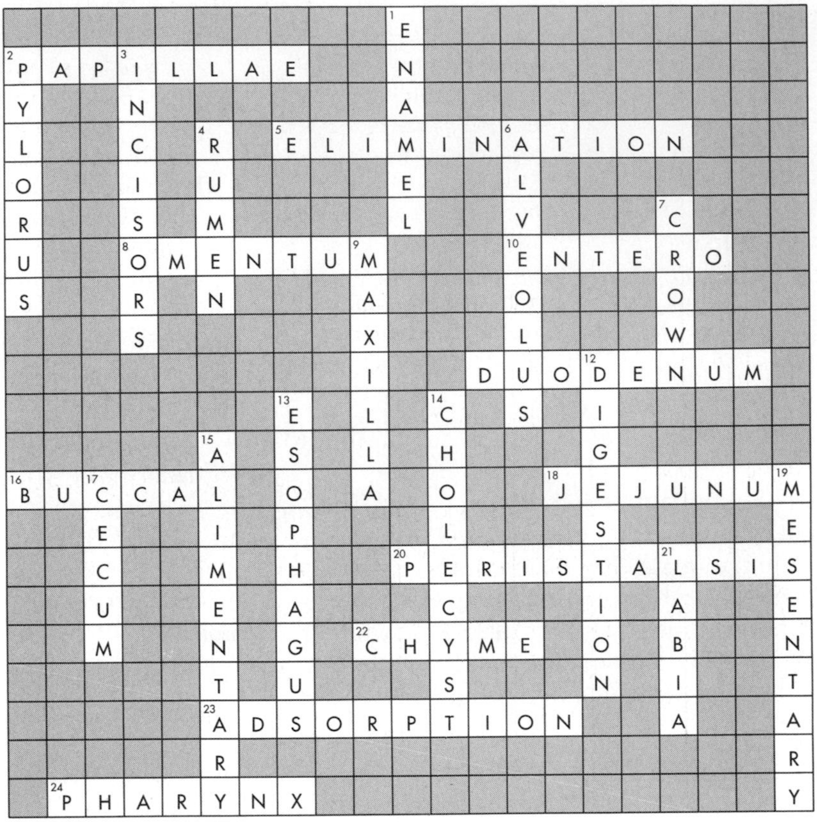
1 ENAMEL
2 PAPILLAE
2 PYLORUS
3 INCISORS
4 RUMEN
5 ELIMINATION
6 ALVEOLUS
7 CROW
8 OMENTUM
9 MAXILLA
10 ENTERO
DUODENUM
12 DIGESTION
13 ESOPHAGUS
14 CHOLECYST
15 ALIMENTARY
16 BUCCAL
17 CECUM
18 JEJUNUM
19 MESENTARY
20 PERISTALSIS
21 LABIA
22 CHYME
23 ADSORPTION
24 PHARYNX

GLOSSARY

GASTROINTESTINAL SYSTEM

abomasum: true stomach of ruminant digestive system.

alimentary or *digestive tract:* passage from mouth to anus.

alveolus (al-ve'o-lus): tooth socket in the maxilla and mandible (also refers to air sac of lung).

ampulla (am-pul'lah): sac-shaped dilation of canal or tube.

anus: distal opening of alimentary tract.

appendix: any appendage, especially vermiform appendix attached to cecum.

bile: secretion of liver that aids in digestion.

biliary: pertaining to bile.

brachydont: short-crowned tooth with enamel covering the crown.

buccal surface of tooth: surface of tooth next to cheek.

cecum (se'kum'): blind pouch portion of large intestine for fermentation of food.

celiac (se'le-ak): pertaining to abdomen.

cementum: bonelike connective tissue that covers the roots of brachydont teeth.

cholecyst (ko'le-sist): gallbladder.

choledochus (ko-led'o-kus): common bile duct.

chyle (kīl): milky fluid conveyed by lymphatic vessels from intestine after digestion into circulation.

chyme (kīm): semifluid contents of stomach after digestion.

colon: part of large intestine extending from cecum to rectum.

common bile duct: duct formed by junction of cystic and hepatic ducts.

coprophagia (coprophagy): oral ingestion of fecal material.

cud: bolus containing fiber, other food particles, rumen liquid, and flora; regurgitated by ruminants.

deciduous: shed at a specific stage of development.

dentin: connective tissue surrounding tooth pulp that is covered by enamel on exposed tooth and by cementum on part implanted in jaw.

diastema: interdental space between incisors, canines, and cheek teeth.

duodenal glands: glands in submucous layer of duodenum.

duodenum (du"o-de'num): first portion of small intestine, extending from pylorus of stomach to jejunum.

enamel: hard, white substance (hardest in the body) covering dentin of crown part of tooth.

esophagus (e-sof'ah-gus): musculomembranous canal that extends from pharynx to stomach.

filiform: threadlike.

flexure (flek'sher): bend, fold, or curved part of structure.

fungiform: mushroom-shaped.

gallbladder: organ located on undersurface of liver; stores bile.

gastric glands: glands of stomach that secrete digestive chemicals.

gingivae (jin'ji-vie): gums of mouth.

hypsodont: long-crowned tooth found in herbivores that has enamel extending below the gumline and invaginated into longitudinal grooves of the tooth; a distinct neck is lacking.

ileocecal valve: mucous membrane folds between ileum and cecum; prevent reflux from colon into ileum (also called *ileocolic valve*).

ileum: distal portion of small intestine, extending from jejunum to cecum.

incisor (in-si'zer): any one of front teeth of either jaw.

islets of Langerhans (lahng'er-hanz): irregular, microscopic formations of cells in pancreas; secrete insulin and glucagon.

jejunum (je-joo'num): portion of small intestine that extends from duodenum to ileum.

labia (la'be-ah): lips.

lingua (ling'gwah): tongue.

liver: large, dome-shaped organ in upper part of abdomen under diaphragm.

mesentery (mes'en-ter"e): peritoneal fold that attaches intestine to dorsal abdominal wall.

omasum: third and smallest compartment of rumen.

omentum: fold of peritoneum overlying stomach and other visceral organs.

oropharynx: section of pharynx that lies between soft palate and epiglottis.

palate: roof of mouth separating oral cavity from nasal cavity.

pancreas: long, irregularly shaped gland located in the mesentery of the duodenum; secretes pancreatic juice into the duodenum (exocrine function) and hormones into the blood (endocrine function).

parotid salivary gland: large salivary gland located near ear.

peptic glands: glands of mucous membrane of simple stomach that secrete acid and pepsin.

peristalsis (per″i-stal′sis): wavelike movement by which alimentary tract propels its contents.

peritoneum (per″i-to-ne′um): serous membrane lining abdominal cavity, with part covering viscera and holding them in place.

pharynx: musculomembranous opening into nasal cavities, mouth, larynx, and esophagus.

pylorus: distal opening of stomach through which stomach contents enter duodenum.

regurgitation: backward flow as in casting up of food.

reticulum: smallest, most cranial portion of ruminant stomach; also called honeycomb.

rugae (roo′guy): wrinkles or folds appearing on surface of mucous membrane of simple stomach when muscular coat contracts.

rumen: largest of compartments of forestomach of ruminants; serves as fermenting vat.

rumination: includes regurgitation, remastication, ensalivation, and reswallowing of partially digested food.

saliva (sah-li′vah): clear secretion of salivary glands containing digestive enzymes.

salivary glands: oral cavity glands that secrete saliva.

secretin: hormone produced by glands of duodenum that stimulates secretion of pancreatic juice.

sphincter (sfingk′ter): ringlike muscle that closes natural opening.

stomach: musculomembranous digestive pouch at distal end of esophagus.

sublingual salivary glands: smallest of salivary glands; located beneath tongue on either side.

submandibular and submaxillary salivary glands: salivary glands below angle of lower jaw on either side.

tongue: freely moving muscular organ of taste, located in floor of mouth; aids in prehension, mastication, grooming, swallowing, sound articulation, and other functions, depending on species.

vallate: rim-shaped.

villi: threadlike projections covering mucosa of small intestine; aid in absorption of digested matter.

PATHOLOGIC CONDITIONS

Inflammations, infections, and toxic conditions

actinobacillosis (wooden tongue): disease of cattle infected with *Actinobacillus lignieresi,* which causes localized, firm swelling of tongue.

actinomycosis (lumpy jaw): disease of cattle infected with *Actinomyces bovis,* causing periostitis of jaws with soft tissue reaction.

ancylostomiasis (an-si-lo-sto-mi′ah-sis): infection with hookworm, member of genus *Ancylostoma.*

anusitis: inflammation of anus.

aphthous (af′thus) *stomatitis:* ulcer of mucous membranes of mouth.

ascariasis (as″kah-ri′ah-sis): infection with parasitic intestinal roundworms of genus *Ascaris.*

bovine virus diarrhea/mucosal disease (BVD/MD): contagious disease of cattle.

cheilitis (ki-li′tis): inflammation of lip.

cholangiolitis (ko-lan″je-o-li′tis): bile duct inflammation.

cholecystitis (ko″le-sis-ti′tis): inflammation of gallbladder.

colic: severe abdominal pain.

colitis: inflammation of colon.

colitis X: rapidly fatal colitis of horses causing profuse diarrhea and profound dehydration, sometimes occurring in outbreaks; cause unknown.

cysticercosis (sis″ti-ser-ko′sis): infection with tapeworm larvae of genus *Cysticercus.*

displaced abomasum: chronic disease of recently calved cows when abomasum becomes trapped under rumen.

distomiasis (dis″to-mi′ah-sis): infection with trematode worm of genus *Fasciola.*

diverticulitis (di″ver-tik-u-li′tis): inflammation of one or more diverticula (pockets) in intestine.

duodenitis: inflammation of duodenum.

dysentery (dis′en-ter″ee): any of a number of disorders that involve inflammation of intestines, particularly colon.

enteritis (en″ter-i′tis): inflammation of intestines, particularly small intestine.

enterocolitis (en″ter-o-ko-li′tis): inflammation of colon and small intestine.

enterogastritis (en″ter-o-gas-tri′tis): inflammation of intestines and stomach (also called *gastroenteritis*).

esophagitis (e-sof″ah-ji′tis): inflammation of esophagus.

gastric dilation and volvulus (bloat): seen most often in large-breed dogs; cause unclear, but aerophagia and overeating are factors.
gastritis: inflammation of stomach.
giardiasis (je″ar-di′ah-sis): parasitic infection of intestinal tract caused by protozoa *Giardia lamblia.*
gingivitis (jin″ji-vi′tis): inflammation of gums.
glossitis (glos-si′tis): inflammation of tongue.
hepatitis (hep″ah-ti′tis): inflammation of liver caused by toxic or viral causes.
herpes (her′pez) *simplex:* virus causing sores of fever blister in humans and primates and fatal disease in owl monkeys and tree shrews.
ileitis (il″e-i′tis): inflammation of ileum.
Johne's disease (paratuberculosis): chronic wasting disease of cattle caused by *Mycobacterium paratuberculosis.*
oxyuriasis: infestation of *Oxyuris* nematodes causing intense perianal itching in horses.
pancreatitis (pan″kre-ah-ti′tis): inflammation of pancreas.
peritonitis (per″i-to-ni′tis): inflammation of peritoneum.
pinworm: any oxyurid, especially noted in horses, rabbits, hamsters, and mice.
Potomac horse fever: highly fatal enterocolitis disease caused by *Ehrlichia risticii,* characterized by high fever, leukopenia, and acute diarrhea.
proctitis: inflammation of rectum.
salmonellosis: highly contagious zoonotic disease of all animal species caused by *Salmonella* bacteria; may cause acute or chronic enteritis and other symptoms; of particular importance to people involved in food hygiene.
scours: diarrhea caused by dietary changes, nutritional deficiency, or parasites.
shigellosis: acute, highly fatal septicemia of very young foals caused by *Actinobacillus equuli* with characteristics of diarrhea, fever, prostration, and dyspnea.
sialoadenitis (si″al-ad″e-ni′tis): inflammation of salivary glands.
strongyle: any roundworm in family *Strongylidae.*
strongyloidiasis (stron″ji-loi-di′ah-sis): infection with intestinal roundworm of genus *Strongyloides;* not to be confused with *Strongylus.*
traumatic reticulitis (hardware disease): ingestion of foreign objects, which settle in reticulum, causing digestive problems and possible complications of peritonitis as a result of perforation of reticulum or pericarditis because of pericardium perforation.
trichuriasis (trik″u-ri′ah-sis): infection with an intestinal parasite of genus *Trichuris.*
verminous colic: colic resulting from an abundance of parasites, usually small strongyles.
wet tail (proliferative ileitis, regional enteritis): disease of hamsters, thought to be associated with *Campylobacter jejuni;* symptoms of diarrhea and dehydration.

Hereditary, congenital, and developmental disorders

atresia (ah-tre′ze-ah): occlusion or nonexistence of normal body opening or tubular formation; may occur in anus, bile duct, or esophagus.
cleft palate: incomplete closure in midline of palate.
harelip: cleft upper lip, so called because of resemblance to normal rabbit appearance.
megacolon: abnormality of cats and dogs associated with loss of muscle function and dilation of colon.

Other abnormalities

achalasia (ak′ah-la′ze-ah): failure to relax of smooth muscle fibers of GI tract.
achlorhydria (ah″klor-hi′dre-ah): absence of hydrochloric acid in gastric secretions.
anorexia: lack of appetite.
ascites (ah-si′tez): accumulation of fluid in abdominal cavity.
cachexia (kah-kek′se-ah): generalized poor nutrition.
calculi: plural form of *calculus.*
calculus: formation of stone.
cholelithiasis (ko″le-li-thi′ah-sis): gallstones.
chylous ascites (ki′lus ah-si′tez): accumulation of chyle in peritoneal cavity resulting from thoracic duct obstruction.
cirrhosis (sir-ro′sis): liver disease with progressive destruction of liver cells.
colic: acute, paroxysmal abdominal pain.
constipation: sluggish bowel with difficult or incomplete evacuation.
crepitus (krep′i-tus): flatulent discharge from bowel.
cribbing (crib-ing): vice of horses in which solid object is grasped with incisor teeth, neck is arched and pulled back and air is swallowed.
dental caries: destruction of enamel, dentin, or cementum

of tooth resulting in tooth decay and cavities.
diarrhea: frequent discharge of abnormally liquid feces.
diverticulosis (di″ver-tik″u-lo′sis): presence of pouches in intestines protruding through intestinal wall.
dyspepsia: indigestion.
emesis: vomiting.
enterolith (en′ter-o-lith): stone in intestines.
eructation: belching.
fecalith (fe′kah-lith): stonelike fecal mass.
fistula: abnormal opening between two organs or between a hollow organ and body surface, commonly found in GI system.
gastralgia: pain in stomach.
gastrolith: stone in stomach.
halitosis: bad breath.
hemoperitoneum (he″mo-per″i-to-ne′um): escape of blood into peritoneal cavity.
hepatomegaly: enlarged liver.
hernia: protrusion of organ or part through its normal containing structures (also called *rupture*).
hydrops (hi′drops): abnormal accumulation of fluid in tissues or body cavity (also called *dropsy*).
hyperchlorhydria (hi″per-klor-hi′dre-ah): excessive hydrochloric acid in gastric secretion.
hypercholia: excessive bile secretion.
hyperglycemia (hi″per-gli-se′me-ah): abnormally high concentration of glucose in blood.
hyperinsulinism (hi″per-in′su-lin-izm): excessive pancreatic insulin secretion.
hypersplenism (hi″per-splen′ism): abnormally increased hemolytic function of spleen.
hypervitaminosis: condition caused by excessive ingestion of vitamins, especially A and D.
hypochlorhydria: deficiency of hydrochloric acid in stomach.
hypoglycemia (hi″po-gli-se′me-ah): low blood glucose level.
hypovitaminosis: disease caused by deficiency of one or more essential vitamins.
icterus: jaundice; yellow discoloration of skin, sclera, mucous membranes, and excretions.
ileus (il′e-us): obstruction of intestines with colic, vomiting, fever, and dehydration.
incontinence of feces: inability to control fecal evacuation.
intussusception (in″tus-sus-sep′shun): prolapse of portion of intestine into lumen of immediately adjacent portion.
jaundice (jawn′dis): icterus; yellowish tinge of skin, sclerae, and other tissues, with deposits of bile pigments in excretions.
malocclusion: failure of proper closure of jaws because of malposition of teeth.
mucocele (mu′ko-seel): cyst or polyp containing mucus.
nausea: sick sensation often resulting in vomiting.
obstipation: extreme constipation caused by intestinal obstruction.
phytobezoar (fi″to-be′zor): gastric mass composed of vegetable matter.
pica (pi′ka): licking or eating foreign materials.
polydipsia: extreme thirst.
polyphagia: ravenous eating.
proctalgia: pain in or near rectum and anus.
proctoptosis (prok″top-to′sis): rectal prolapse.
pruritus ani: chronic, intense itching of anal region.
pylorospasm: spasm of pylorus of stomach.
rickets: disorder caused by deficiency of vitamin D intake, chiefly affecting calcification of bones with resulting bending and deformation of bones.
scurvy: disease resulting from vitamin C (ascorbic acid) deficiency; primates and guinea pigs susceptible.
splenomegaly: enlarged spleen.
stenosis: narrowing of opening or passage.
tenesmus (te-nez′mus): painful, ineffective straining to defecate or urinate.
trichobezoar: hair ball.
ulcer: lesion on surface of mucous membrane or skin caused by disintegration of inflamed necrotic tissue.
volvulus: intestinal obstruction caused by twisting of bowel.
vomiting: forcible expulsion of gastric contents through mouth.
xerostomia: dryness of the mouth caused by insufficient secretion of saliva.

ONCOLOGY

cholangioma (ko-lan″je-o′mah): bile duct tumor.
dentigerous cyst (den-tij′er-us): cyst containing tooth or teeth.
epulis: any tumor of gingivae such as abscess or gumboil.
hepatoma (hep″ah-to′mah): malignant tumor of liver (also called *hepatocarcinoma*).
odontoma (o-don-to′mah): tumor of dental tissue.

polyp: small, tumorlike growth on mucous membrane surface, especially throat or intestines.

SURGICAL PROCEDURES

abdominocentesis (ab-dom″i-no-sen-te′sis): paracentesis of abdominal cavity (also called *celiocentesis*).
abomasopexy: fixation of abomasum to correct displacement.
cecostomy: creation of artificial opening into cecum.
celiotomy: incision into the abdomen (same as laparotomy).
cheiloplasty (ki′lo-plas″te): repair of lip.
cholecystectomy: excision of gallbladder.
colostomy: formation of artificial opening into colon from surface of body.
enteropexy: fixation of intestine to abdominal wall.
enterostomy (en″ter-os′to-me): creation of opening into intestine through abdominal wall.
enterotomy: incision into intestine.
esophagotomy: incision into esophagus.
exteriorize: transpose internal organ to outside of body.
gastrectomy: total or partial excision of stomach.
gastropexy: fixation of stomach.
gastroplasty: repair of stomach.
gastrostomy (gas-tros′to-me): creation of opening into stomach.
gastrotomy: incision into stomach.
hernioplasty: repair of hernia.
herniorrhaphy (her″ne-or′ah-fe): suture or repair of hernia.
laparotomy: incision into the abdomen (same as celiotomy).
pancreatectomy: surgical removal of all or part of pancreas.
paracentesis: surgical puncture of cavity for fluid aspiration.
pharyngotomy: incision into pharynx.
proctopexy: fixation of prolapsed rectum to adjacent tissues.
rumenotomy: incision into the rumen.

LABORATORY TESTS AND PROCEDURES

biopsy: insertion of needle to obtain sample of tissues in organs such as liver to detect abnormalities and diseases.

Blood tests

amylase: pancreatic enzyme elevated in disease of pancreas or salivary glands.
bromsulphalein: injected and found retained in blood over specified time period.
insulin test: to determine amount of insulin secreted by pancreas after fasting and again after receiving glucose.
lactic dehydrogenase isoenzymes: pattern of distribution is diagnostic for liver disease.
liver function tests: to determine damage or disease, normal enzymes or injected chemicals are measured for elevation or retention in blood serum.
total alkaline phosphatase: increased levels indicate liver disease.
transaminases: alanine aminotransferase (formerly known as SGPT), liver specific for dogs, cats, and primates; aspartate aminotransferase (formerly known as SGOT), not organ specific but will increase with liver damage and must be run with other enzyme tests.

Endoscope examinations

colonoscopy: examination of colon.
endoscope: tubelike device with light and refracting mirrors that is used to examine internal body areas for abnormalities and to remove tissue samples and small growths.
esophagoscopy: examination of esophagus.
gastroscopy: examination of stomach and upper GI tracts.
protoscopy: examination of anus and rectum.

Radiologic studies

barium enema: studies using contract media to visualize colon and rectum.
gastrointestinal series: X-ray studies of esophagus, stomach, and small intestine, after swallowing contrast medium such as barium; large intestine is visualized by use of barium enema.
X-ray scans: X-ray studies of liver, spleen, and pancreas to detect tumors or other abnormalities.

Stool tests

combined fatty acids test: to determine ability to digest fat.
parasites test: microscopic examination of fecal matter to detect parasitic infection.
stool culture: fecal matter incubated in growth media to detect presence of microorganisms.

trypsin activity: reduction indicates disease of exocrine portion of pancreatic function.
urobilinogen: metabolic product that decreases in liver and gallbladder diseases.

Urine tests

amylase: elevated in pancreatitis.
inulin clearance: rate of excretion of inulin indicates presence of liver disease.
oral glucose tolerance test: measurable level of sugar present indicates metabolic disorder.
qualitative glucose: present in metabolic disease such as diabetes.

12 The Genitourinary System

Animal reproduction and the processing of liquid wastes

CHAPTER OVERVIEW

The genitourinary system includes the reproductive and urinary systems of both sexes. This chapter presents the basic terminology needed for understanding the structures and functions of this system.

THE URINARY SYSTEM

The organs that produce and excrete the waste substance urine from the body are the two *kidneys,* which filter the blood and remove waste products of metabolism in the form of urine; two *ureters,* which carry the urine from the kidneys; a *bladder,* which receives and stores the urine; and a *urethra,* which excretes the urine from the body. These organs are common to both sexes, with essentially the same structures.

Kidneys

The kidneys (Fig. 12-1) of most domesticated animals are bean-shaped organs.* *Nephro* and *reno* refer to kidney. The kidneys are located on both sides of the vertebral column dorsally beneath the parietal peritoneum and ventral to the first few lumbar vertebrae. Kidneys are *retroperitoneal:* they are situated outside the peritoneal cavity. *Renal fasciae* (fibrous tissue) connecting to other structures, in conjunction with heavy encapsulating pads of fat surrounding the kidneys, hold them in place. Each kidney has a concave depression, the *hilus,* on its medial margin, for entry of blood vessels, nerves, and its ureter.

KIDNEY COMPOSITION AND STRUCTURE

The kidneys are dark reddish-brown in color, with the exception of the cat's, which are yellowish-red. They are solid organs except for the *renal sinus,* the space into which the hilus opens. Cross-sectioning of the kidneys shows it to be composed of an external *cortex* and an internal *medulla.*

The renal sinus (except in the bovine) contains the *renal pelvis,* blood vessels, nerves, and fat. The renal pelvis, a funnel-shaped reservoir that occupies most of the renal sinus, is made up of the major and minor *calyces,* irregular saclike structures that collect the urine from all portions of the kidney. The broad portion of the renal pelvis lies within the renal sinus. Its apical portion passes out through the hilus to unite with the *ureter,* the outlet tube of the kidney, extending to the bladder.

Cone-shaped structures called *medullary pyramids,* which make up the medulla, stud the walls of the renal sinus, with their *bases* facing the cortex and their narrow ends, the *papillae,* extending into the renal pelvis calyces, where the urine collects through ducts

*Some species, such as cattle, have lobulated kidneys; the horse's right kidney is heart shaped rather than bean shaped.

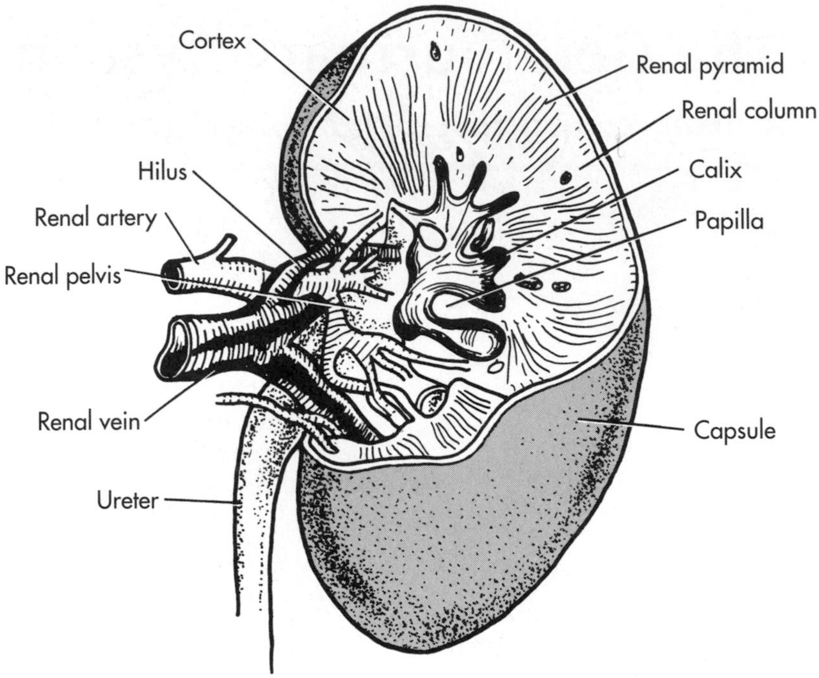
Cortex
Renal pyramid
Renal column
Calix
Papilla
Hilus
Renal artery
Renal pelvis
Renal vein
Capsule
Ureter

FIG. 12-1 Structure of the kidney.

in the papillae. Cattle, lacking a renal pelvis, have calyces that empty urine directly in the ureter. The cortex extends between the pyramids, forming the *renal columns.*

The Functional Unit of the Kidney

The *nephron* is the functional unit of the kidney, consisting of the *renal corpuscle* and the *renal tubule.* There are about 1 million nephrons in the kidney. The renal corpuscle consists of a double-walled, cup-shaped structure called the *glomerular* or *Bowman's capsule,* which contains a twisted cluster of capillary channels called the *glomerulus,* forming a rounded body. The renal tubule is divided into the *proximal convoluted tubule,* the *descending limb of the loop of Henle,* the *ascending limb of the loop of Henle,* the *distal convoluted tubule,* and the *collecting tubule* (Figs. 12-2 and 12-3).

The renal corpuscles and the attached proximal convoluted tubules into which they drain lie in the cortical portion of the kidney, with the tubules making up the largest part of the renal cortex. The *loop of Henle* follows the proximal convoluted tubule and is divided into a descending and an ascending limb, lying for the most part within the renal medulla. The distal convoluted tubule resembles the proximal convoluted tubule in structure, except that it is much shorter when uncoiled and drains into the collecting tubules, which convey the urine to the renal pelvis by way of the papillary ducts of the pyramids.

Kidney Functions

The main function of the kidneys is to filter waste materials from the blood and excrete them in the urine. The waste products in-

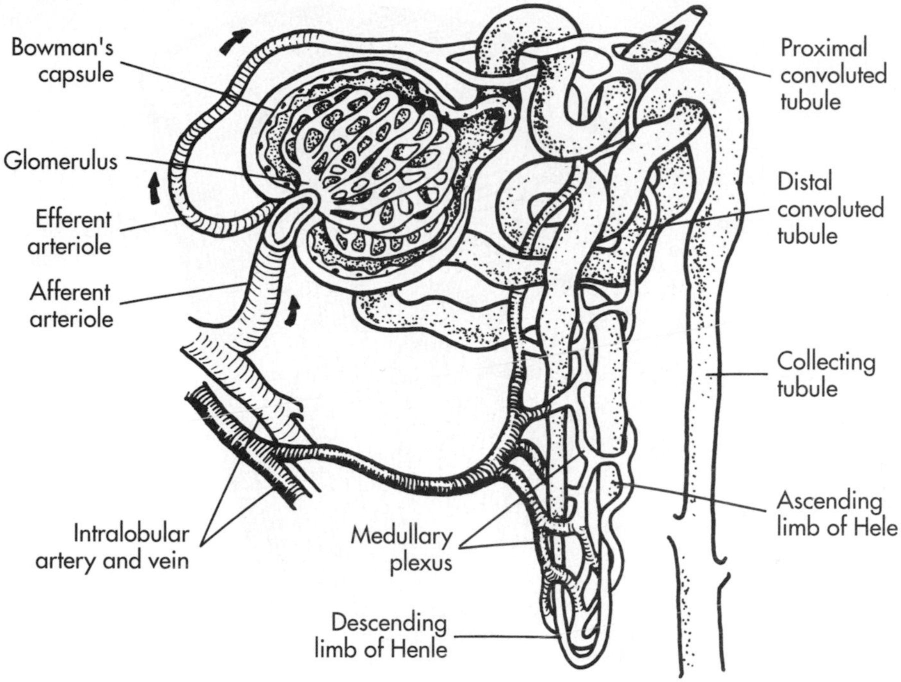
Bowman's capsule
Glomerulus
Efferent arteriole
Afferent arteriole
Intralobular artery and vein
Medullary plexus
Descending limb of Henle
Proximal convoluted tubule
Distal convoluted tubule
Collecting tubule
Ascending limb of Hele

FIG. 12-2 The nephron, the functional unit of the kidney.

clude nitrogenous wastes from the breakdown of proteins, toxic substances, mineral salts, excess glucose, and water (both ingested water and that produced during metabolism). In the blood-filtering process, water and solutes from blood in the glomeruli pass through the capillaries and the glomerular walls into the tubules. The tubules select substances needed by the body and return them to the blood.

The speed at which the blood filters through the kidneys is affected by the blood pressure. If the systemic blood pressure drops, as in shock, it may cause blood filtration to slow to a point where the kidneys stop functioning. Similarly, if the systemic pressure is too high, kidney damage may result, causing a loss of substances that normally would have been reabsorbed for use by the body.

The kidneys affect the rate of secretion of some hormones, synthesize other hormones, and maintain the pH of the blood so that it does not become too acid or too alkaline.

THE URETERS

The *ureters,* one from each kidney, are muscular tubes extending from the renal pelvis of the kidney caudal to the urinary bladder. The walls of the ureters are made up of an outer fibrous tissue layer, two center layers of smooth muscle, and a mucous membrane lining. The ureters enter the neck of the bladder at the *trigone.* Because the ureters enter the bladder obliquely, the flow of urine back to the kidney is effectively controlled by a natural valve.

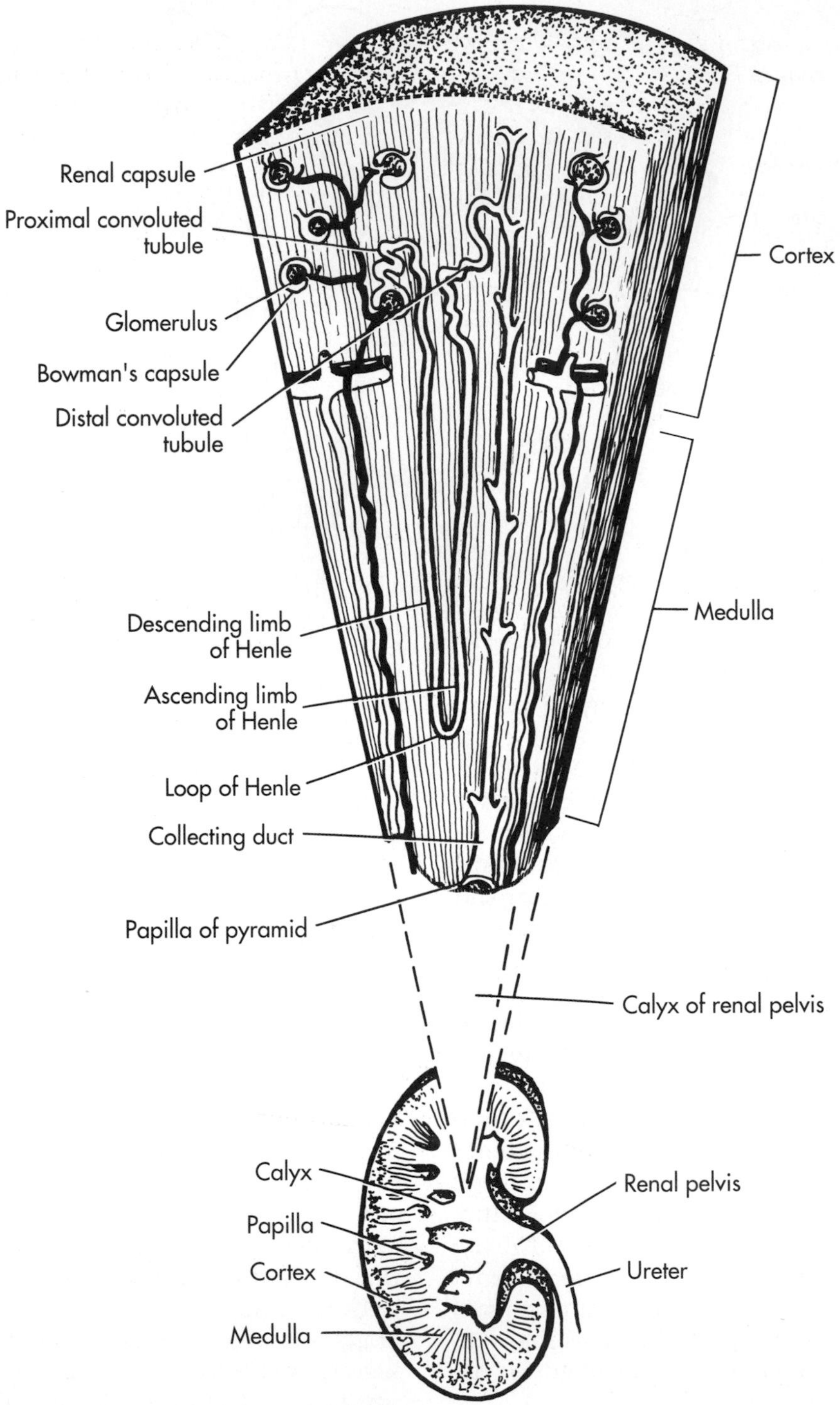
Renal capsule
Proximal convoluted tubule
Glomerulus
Bowman's capsule
Distal convoluted tubule
Cortex
Medulla
Descending limb of Henle
Ascending limb of Henle
Loop of Henle
Collecting duct
Papilla of pyramid
Calyx of renal pelvis
Calyx
Papilla
Cortex
Medulla
Renal pelvis
Ureter

FIG. 12-3 Magnification showing renal corpuscles, proximal and distal convoluted tubules, and loops of Henle and collecting tubules.

Urine enters the bladder by way of the ureters on an average of every 10 to 30 seconds (which varies with the species), in spurts rather than in a continuous flow. The spurts are produced by the action of successive peristaltic waves, beginning in the renal pelvis and passing caudally throughout the extent of the ureters. Situated at the bladder entrance is a ureteral orifice, which opens for 2 to 3 seconds, then closes until a succeeding peristaltic wave opens it again, preventing urine from flowing back to the ureters during bladder contraction.

THE URINARY BLADDER

The *urinary bladder* is an extremely elastic, musculomembranous sac lying in the pelvis, formed of three layers of smooth muscle tissue lined with mucous membrane. The size and position of the bladder in the pelvis vary depending on the amount of urine it contains. It contains two openings to receive urine from the two ureters and another opening into the urethra, through which urine is excreted. The neck of the bladder, which unites with the urethra, contains a *sphincter muscle,* which controls the flow of urine into the urethra. The bladder has two functions: to serve as a storage place for urine and to excrete urine through the urethra.

The amount of urine a bladder holds varies between species and with water intake, but a large amount usually creates a desire to empty the bladder. The contraction of the bladder and the relaxation of the internal and external sphincter muscles are involuntary actions except in animals that are conditioned to voluntarily control the external sphincter muscle. The voiding of urine from the bladder is called *micturition.* The act of preventing or concluding voiding is learned and voluntary in more intelligent forms of animal life.

THE URETHRA

The *urethra* is a membranous, tubular canal that carries urine from the bladder to the exterior of the body.

In the female, the urethra varies in length by species, extending from the neck of the bladder to the exterior of the body. The exterior opening of the urethra, called the *urinary meatus,* is located between the vagina and clitoris directly cranial to the vulva. In the female, the only function of the urethra is urination.

The male urethra varies in length by species and penile anatomic structure and is narrower than in the female. This anatomic difference makes the male more prone to blockages from *urolithiasis* (stone formation in the urinary tract). It extends from the neck of the bladder, through the accessory sex glands, between the fascia connecting the pubic bones, and through the penis. The male urethra is divided into three sections: *prostatic, membranous,* and *cavernous.* The exterior opening of the urethra in the male is also called the *urinary meatus.* In males, the urethra serves a dual function, carrying both urine and reproductive organ secretions.

CHARACTERISTICS OF NORMAL URINE

Normal urine in most species is clear, pale amber in color with a characteristic odor. Horses, rabbits, hamsters, and a few other animals normally have cloudy urine. Urine is approximately 95% water, containing many dissolved substances such as nitrogenous wastes, electrolytes, toxins, pigments, hormones, and at times some abnormal substances such as glucose, albumin, or blood.

The average urinary output in a 24-hour period varies by species, temperature, water intake, and type of work the animal is performing. The normal range of pH varies with species and diet. Carnivore urine is acidic, whereas that of herbivores is basic. Thus herbivores have a higher pH than do carnivores.

REVIEW A

1. Two word roots meaning kidney are ________________ and ________________ .
2. To say that the kidneys are retroperitoneal means ______________________________ .
3. The ________________ is the functional unit of the kidney.
4. The cluster of capillary channels within Bowman's capsule is called the ________________ .
5. The tubular structures that carry urine from the kidneys to the bladder are the ________________ . The tube from the bladder to the urinary meatus is the ________________ .
6. The male urethra is divided into three sections: ________________ , ________________ , and ________________ .

> **THERIOGENOLOGY**
>
> The word *theriogenology* is from the combining forms *therio-* (pertaining to beasts), *-gen* (that which generates), and *-ology* (science or study). Theriogenologists study the normal anatomy and physiology of the reproductive tracts of animals and the pathology and diseases of those organs. Unlike gynecology (*gyneco-*, woman) in human medicine, theriogenology deals with both sexes.

MALE REPRODUCTIVE ORGANS

The basic male reproductive organs *(gonads)* are the *testes*. The accessory organs are ducts, glands, and supporting structures. The ducts are the *epididymides* (singular, *epididymis*), *vasa deferentia* (singular, *vas deferens*), *ejaculatory ducts*, and *urethra*. The accessory sex glands are not all present in all species but may include the *seminal vesicles, prostate, bulbourethral (Cowper's)*, and *coagulating glands*. The *penis, scrotum*, and *spermatic cords* function as primary structures (Figs. 12-4, 12-5, and 12-6).

The Testes

The *testes* or *testicles* are a pair of egg-shaped glands in most species, normally located in a saclike structure called the *scrotum*. Their size, shape, and location vary from species to species. Each testicle is enclosed in a fibrous white capsule called the *tunica albuginea*. The interior of the testicle is divided into numerous conical lobules or compartments, each containing a mass of coiled *seminiferous tubules* and *interstitial cells (cells of Leydig)*. The seminiferous tubules join into a cluster from which several ducts emerge and enter the head of the *epididymis*.

The testes have two functions: producing *spermatozoa* (sperm cells) and secreting hormones. The sperm cells are produced by the

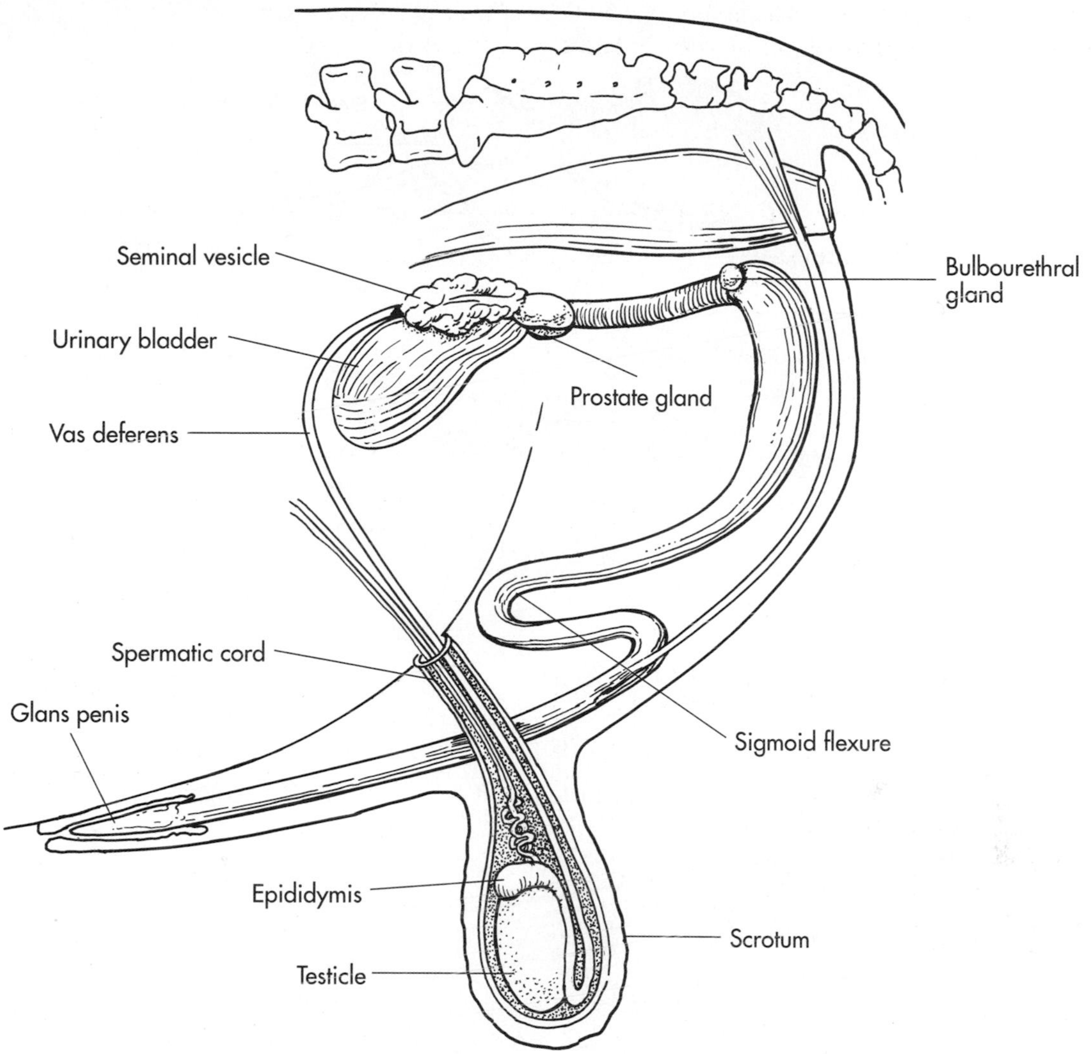
Seminal vesicle
Urinary bladder
Vas deferens
Prostate gland
Bulbourethral gland
Spermatic cord
Glans penis
Sigmoid flexure
Epididymis
Scrotum
Testicle

FIG. 12-4 Reproductive system of the bull.

seminiferous tubules. The chief hormone *testosterone* is secreted by the cells of Leydig, which are specialized interstitial cells. Testosterone has several functions. It induces and maintains male secondary sex characteristics, such as the massive head and shoulders of bulls, the crest of the withers on stallions, tusks on boars, and horns on certain breeds of rams. It also influences muscle and bone growth, with male animals generally having less subcutaneous fat and *marbling* (fat distribution in lean meat) of the muscle. This anatomic characteristic of males makes their meat less tender and juicy. A surgical procedure called *castration* (removal of testicles) is performed on all

A

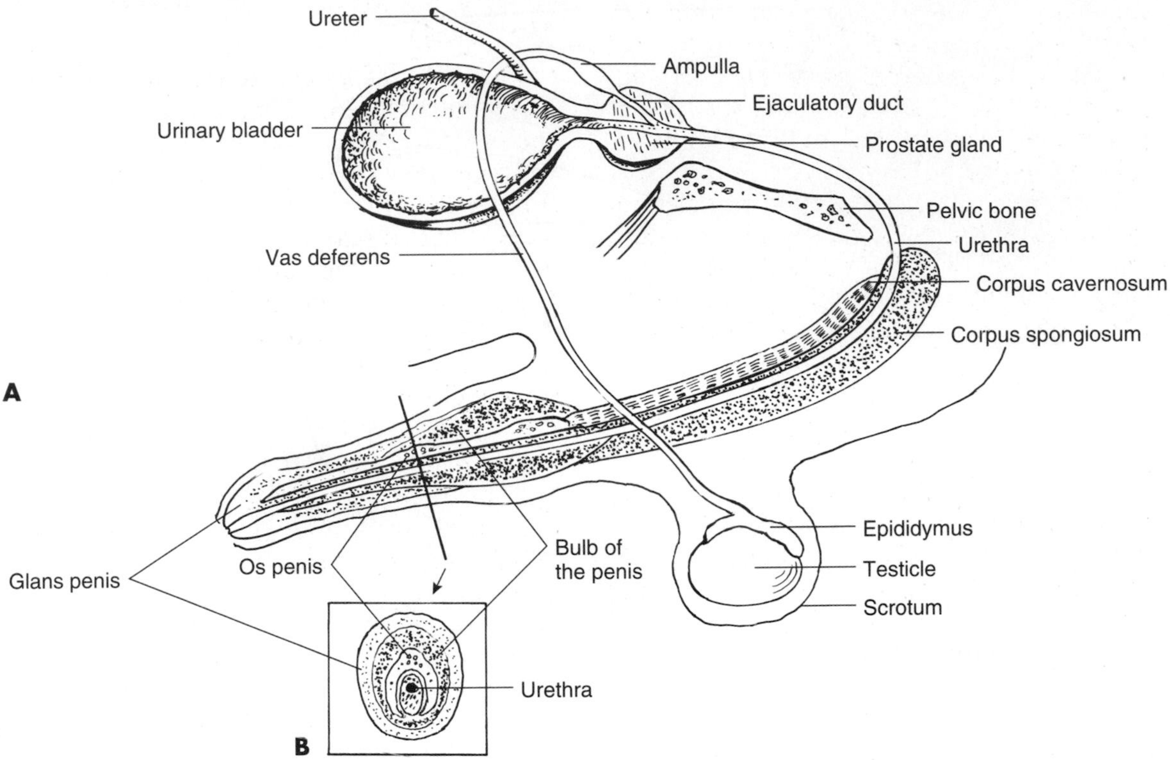
Ureter
Ampulla
Ejaculatory duct
Urinary bladder
Prostate gland
Pelvic bone
Urethra
Vas deferens
Corpus cavernosum
Corpus spongiosum
Epididymus
Testicle
Scrotum
Glans penis
Os penis
Bulb of the penis
Urethra

B

FIG. 12-5 Reproductive system of the male dog. **A,** Modified midsagittal section. **B,** Cross-section of the penis.

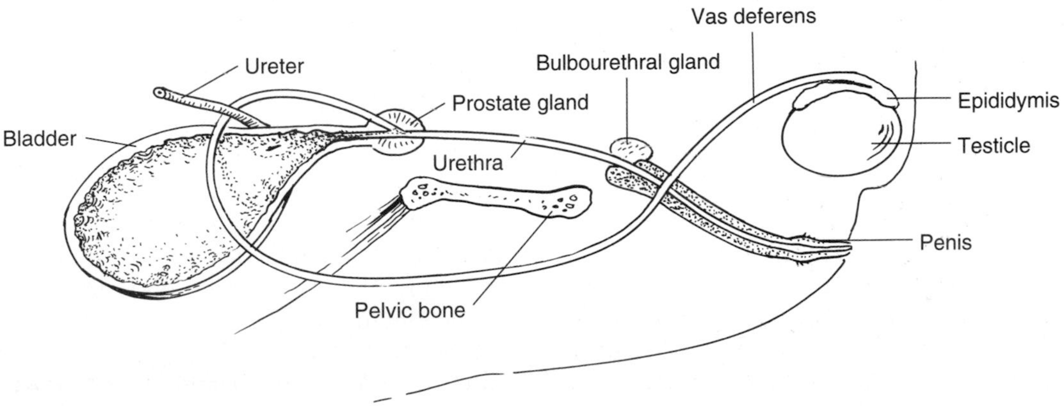
Vas deferens
Ureter
Bulbourethral gland
Epididymis
Prostate gland
Bladder
Testicle
Urethra
Penis
Pelvic bone

FIG. 12-6 Reproductive system of the tomcat.

male animals intended for meat production to eliminate the source of testosterone production after sexual maturity. Castration enables the animal to accumulate subcutaneous fat and marbling of the meat similar to that of the female. Testosterone has an influence on general as well as fluid and electrolyte metabolism. It also has an excitatory effect on kidney tubule reabsorption and suppresses anterior pituitary secretion of gonadotropins.

Epididymis

The *epididymides* (singular, *epididymis*), a pair of tightly coiled, tubelike structures, lie along the caudal border and parallel to the long axis of the testis. The epididymides act as a place for sperm to mature, store sperm before ejaculation, and secrete a small portion of the seminal fluid (semen).

Vas Deferens (Ductus Deferens)

The *vasa deferentia* are a pair of muscular tubes with diameters that vary by species. They are a continuation of the tail of the epididymis and extend from the epididymis up through the inguinal canal. Each epididymis is encased by the *spermatic cord.* On entering the abdominal cavity, they travel to the bladder and connect with the seminal vesicle duct and form the *ejaculatory duct.* The *vas deferens* moves the sperm from the tail of the epididymis to the ejaculatory duct.

Ejaculatory Ducts

The *ejaculatory ducts* are two short tubes formed by the joining of the vas deferens with the ducts of the seminal vesicles. They pass through the prostate gland and extend to the urethra.

Vesicular Glands (Seminal Vesicles)

The *vesicular glands* are two twisted pouches lying along the dorsal and caudal surface of the bladder, ventral to the rectum. *Seminal vesicles* is the term used to describe the structure in a stallion, and *vesicular glands* describes the anatomic structures in most other animals. They are lacking in the dog and cat. They secrete the mucid, liquid part of the semen and also prostaglandins.

Prostate Gland

The *prostate* is composed of smooth muscle and glandular tissue, walnut-shaped in the dog and the stallion and more diffuse in other animals. It surrounds the pelvic urethra, and its ducts open into the urethra. The prostate secretes a viscous, alkaline substance that makes up most of the seminal fluid and gives semen its characteristic odor. The alkalinity protects the sperm from acid if it is present in the urethra of the male and vagina of the female and increases its motility.

Bulbourethral Glands

The *bulbourethral (Cowper's) glands* are two rounded glands located caudal to the seminal vesicles on either side of the membranous part of the pelvic urethra and connected to it by a duct. They are found in most male animals and are particularly large in the boar. The dog does not possess bulbourethral glands. These glands secrete and produce seminal fluid with a similar action to the prostate secretion.

Spermatic Cords

The *spermatic cords* are formed of white, fibrous tissue, encasing the vas deferens, blood and lymph vessels, and nerves. They are located between the tail of the epididymis within the scrotum and the abdominal cavity in the inguinal canals.

Scrotum

The *scrotum* is a pendulous, saclike, skin-covered structure (Figs. 12-4 and 12-5) that houses the testicles and is normally suspended in the inguinal region of most animals. The scrotum of the boar, cat (Fig. 12-6), and stallion is not pendulous and is located just ventral to the anus. It is separated into two sacs internally by the *scrotal septum,* each containing one testis, one epididymis, and the first segment of the spermatic cord. The scrotum houses the testicles and maintains their temperature. The scrotum is considered a thermoregulatory structure.

Penis

The *penis* is made up of three rounded masses of cavernous (erectile) tissue encased in a heavy fibrous capsule. The *glans penis* (Fig. 12-4), which is the terminal end of the penis, varies from species to species and serves the purpose of stimulation. The stallion has a slight bulge at the cranial end, whereas the ram has a free end of the urethra that protrudes cranially past the glans. The bull and the ram have a helmet-shaped glans. The glans penis of the dog has two structures: a bulged cranial end and a midportion bulbus, which surrounds a bone called the *os penis* (Fig. 12-5). The terminal cranial end of the boar's penis is twisted like a corkscrew and lacks a glans.

The penis of the stallion and the dog (Fig. 12-5) is composed of almost all erectile tissue and very little connective tissue. Erection is achieved by blood engorgement of the erectile tissue. The penis of the bull, ram, and boar is composed of almost all connective tissue and very little erectile tissue. These animals achieve an erection by the straightening of the *sigmoid* (S-shaped) *flexure* (Fig. 12-4). Erection is achieved in a way very similar to forcing water under high pressure through a coiled garden hose. The penis contains the urethra, which carries both reproductive tract secretions and urine, and is the organ through which sperm is introduced into the female.

REVIEW B

1. Spermatozoa are produced in the ______________ tubules. These tubules coalesce to enter the head of the ______________, which sits like a cap over the testicle.
2. Testosterone is secreted by the cells of ______________, which are specialized ______________ cells of the testes.
3. The ______________ is the tubular structure that moves sperm from the tail of the epididymis to the ejaculatory duct. The latter structure enters the urethra surrounded by the ______________ gland.
4. The prostate is present in almost all male mammals. The other accessory male sex glands are ______________, ______________, and ______________, one or more of which may be absent in some species.
5. The bone in the dog's penis is called the ______________.
6. The S-shaped part of the bull's penis is called the ______________. bull, ram, boar

FEMALE REPRODUCTIVE ORGANS

The basic female reproductive organs (gonads) are a pair of *ovaries*. The accessory organs consist of an internal group of structures, which include a pair of *oviducts* (*uterine* or *fallopian tubes*); a *uterus,* consisting of two uterine horns and a body of the uterus; a *cervix;* and a *vagina*. The external structures include the *vulva* and *mammary glands* (Figs. 12-7 and 12-8).

Ovaries

The adult ovaries are two almond-shaped glands in most species, located caudal to the left and right kidneys and on each side of the uterus. The size of the ovaries varies from species to species and sometimes even within species. Each ovary is connected to the uterus by a ligament. The open end of each oviduct is suspended over the corresponding ovary but not directly attached to it.

STRUCTURE

A single layer of epithelial cells forms the ovarian surface. The interior consists primarily of a network of connective tissue in which are embedded countless numbers of microscopic formations, called *follicles,* containing *ova* (female sex cells) in different stages of development.

FUNCTIONS

The functions of the ovaries are ovulation and hormonal secretion. The ova develop in the ovaries, and when an ovum matures, it is expelled (ovulated) by the ovary to be caught up by the infundibulum of the oviduct over that ovary.

Estrogen and *progesterone* are the ovarian hormones. Estrogen is also produced in the adrenal cortex (male and female), the testes (male), and the fetal-placental unit (during gestation) and has a variety of functions in both sexes. Ovarian estrogen has several functions. It induces development of female

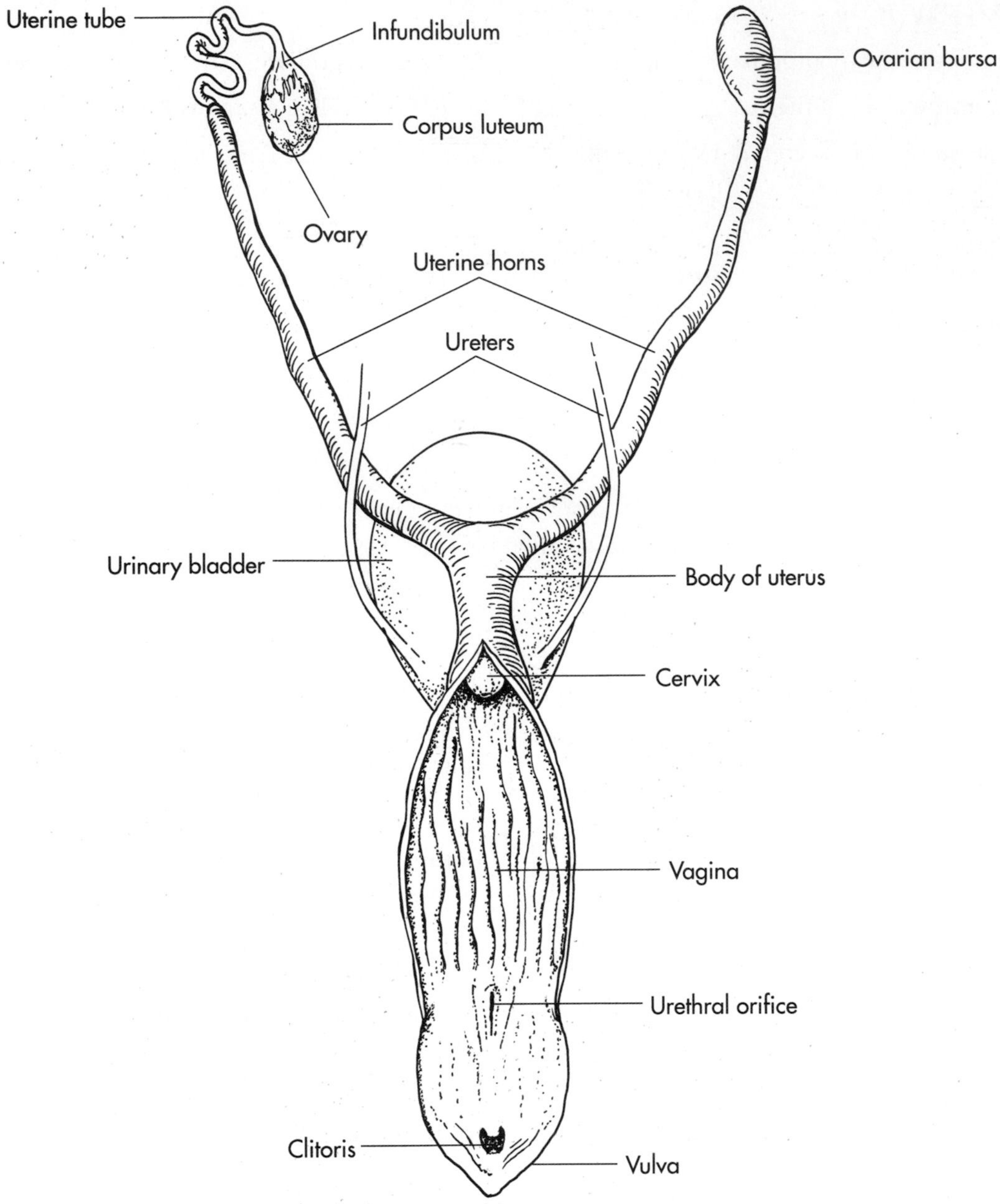
Uterine tube
Infundibulum
Ovarian bursa
Corpus luteum
Ovary
Uterine horns
Ureters
Urinary bladder
Body of uterus
Cervix
Vagina
Urethral orifice
Clitoris
Vulva

FIG. 12-7 Reproductive system of the bitch.

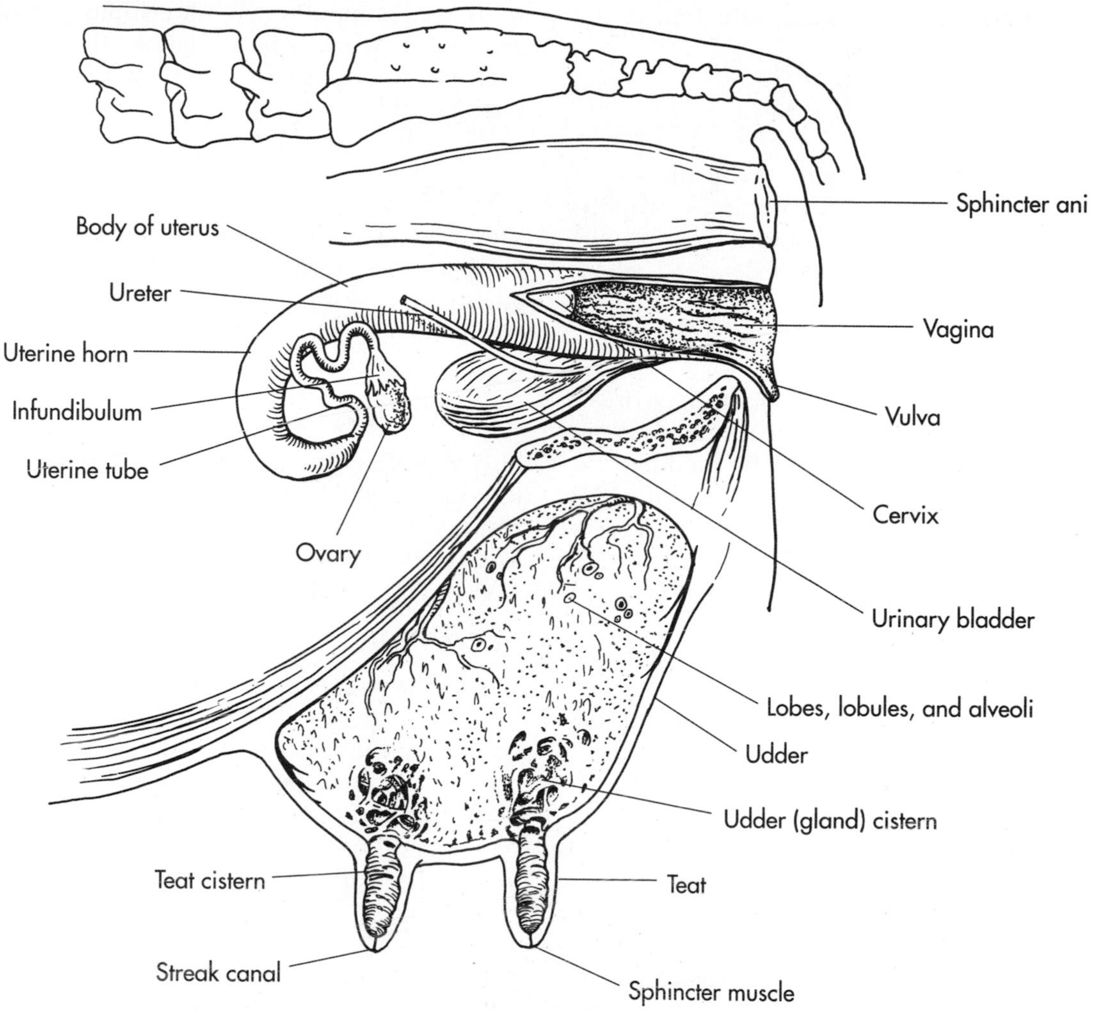
Sphincter ani
Body of uterus
Ureter
Vagina
Uterine horn
Infundibulum
Vulva
Uterine tube
Cervix
Ovary
Urinary bladder
Lobes, lobules, and alveoli
Udder
Udder (gland) cistern
Teat cistern
Teat
Streak canal
Sphincter muscle

FIG. 12-8 Cross-section of the reproductive system of a cow, showing the udder.

secondary sex characteristics and cyclic changes in the uterus in preparation for implantation and developmental support of a fertilized ovum and eventual fetus. Progesterone, which is produced in the adrenal cortex and in the *corpus luteum* of the ovary and the placenta, also prepares the uterus to receive and nurture the fertilized ovum and has an effect on the female secondary sex characteristics.

Oviducts or Uterine (Fallopian) Tubes

There are two *oviducts,* consisting of an inner, ciliated, mucous membrane layer; a middle, smooth muscle layer; and an outer layer of serous tissue. The proximal end of each oviduct is attached to the uterine horn. The ovarian end, the *infundibulum,* is funnel shaped, with fringed, fingerlike processes called *fimbria.* The fimbriated ends are suspended adjacent to but not attached to the ovaries.

FUNCTION

The oviducts act as ducts to the uterus for the ova produced by the ovaries. Normally, *fertilization* (ovum and sperm cell union) takes place in the oviduct.

Uterus

The *uterus* is a thick-walled, hollow organ (*metro* and *hystero* refer to the uterus) lying in the pelvic cavity dorsal to the bladder and ventral to the rectum. Anatomically, the uterus is made up of a body *(corpus)*, a cervix *(neck)*, and two horns *(cornus)*. There are wide species variations in the size and shape of both the uterine horns and body.

The uterine walls are formed of three layers. The inner lining is a specialized epithelial mucous membrane called the *endometrium*. The middle layer, the *myometrium*, is formed of layers of smooth muscle extending diagonally, crosswise, and lengthwise. The external layer, the *perimetrium*, is an extension of the parietal peritoneum serous membrane, covering the uterus. The perimetrium is continuous with the band of peritoneum commonly known as the *broad ligament*. The broad ligament supports the internal genitalia.

FUNCTIONS

The uterus has several functions. During estrus, it prepares for the possible acceptance of a developing fetus. The endometrium develops specialized structures for attachment of the placenta to the uterine wall. These specialized structures vary by species. It also produces uterine milk, which is necessary to nourish the embryo before implantation. During pregnancy, the uterus maintains and supports the developing fetus. When an animal is in labor, the myometrium contracts to move the fetus into the birth canal.

Cervix

The *cervix* is continuous cranially with the body of the uterus and caudally with the vagina. It is normally located just dorsal to the bladder and ventral to the rectum.

STRUCTURE

The cervix is composed of smooth muscle that is arranged in a ringlike fashion, called a sphincter muscle. Its shape and muscular arrangement vary with the species.

FUNCTION

The cervix prevents foreign bodies from entering the uterus during gestation, possibly contaminating the fetus and resulting in abortion. It is usually tightly closed to prevent invasion except during estrus, when it relaxes and dilates to allow sperm to enter for fertilization. During pregnancy, the cervix is filled with a mucus plug, which acts as a physical barrier and keeps out foreign bodies. The cervix releases the mucus plug and dilates at the time of parturition to allow the fetus to pass into the birth canal.

Vagina

The *vagina* is located caudal to the cervix and cranial to the vulva. It extends from the cervix of the uterus to the external genitalia.

Structure

The vagina is an extremely elastic tube of circular smooth muscle, lined with a mucous membrane. It varies in size by species and age. Before sexual maturity and breeding, the external vaginal orifice may be partly or completely occluded by a fold of mucous membrane called the *hymen*. This structure is often unnoticed in domestic animals.

FUNCTIONS

The *vagina* acts as a sheath to accept the penis during copulation and to receive the semen of ejaculation. It also provides passage out of the body for uterine secretions and acts as the birth canal to move the neonate to the exterior during parturition.

Vulva

The *vulva* (external genitalia), sometimes called the lips of the vagina, consists of the vaginal orifice, vestibular glands, clitoris, hymen, and urethral orifice. Unlike humans, domestic animals possess simple lips *(labia)* of the vulva instead of both major and minor labia. The outer lips in conjunction with the anus and hair growth pattern form the *escutcheon*. The vulva is located ventral to the anus.

The *clitoris* is an organ formed of erectile tissue covered by stratified squamous epithelium and is located in the ventral portion of the vulva. The clitoris and the glans penis of the male have the same embryonic origin. Many sensory nerve endings converge into the clitoris, creating an organ of stimulation. The urethral orifice is found where the vagina and vulva join and is sometimes accompanied by a vestigial hymen, which is located just cranial to the urethral orifice. The hymen in some young animals can interfere with copulation and must be removed surgically.

Mammary Glands

The mammary glands are the milk-producing glandular structures located along the entire ventral surface of litter-bearing animals. Animals used for milk production have mammary glands located in the inguinal region, with either two or four functional teats. Mammary gland development is controlled by estrogen and progesterone, two hormones secreted by the ovaries and corpus luteum.

STRUCTURE

Each mammary gland is composed of connective and adipose tissue in lobes and lobules with milk-secreting cells *(alveoli)* around a duct. The individual ducts join with others to form larger ducts or an *udder cistern*. The udder cistern, located dorsally to the base of the teat, transports the milk at the time of milk letdown into the teat cistern and to the exterior through the sphincter muscle located at the most ventral end of the teat (Fig. 12-8).

FUNCTION

The mammary glands produce milk for the feeding of the neonate and, in the case of cows and goats, for human consumption. Milk production is stimulated by the lactogenic hormone *prolactin*, which is produced by the anterior lobe of the pituitary gland. Milk letdown or the emptying of milk-secreting tissue is caused by the hormone *oxytocin*, released by the posterior lobe of the pituitary gland. Oxytocin release is stimulated by the suckling action of the neonate or by the pulsation and vacuum action of a milking machine.

REVIEW C

1. Three different names for the tube that carries ova to the uterus are ____________________, ____________________, and ____________________. The funnel-shaped open end of this structure is called the ____________________.
2. Two word roots meaning uterus are ____________________ and ____________________.
3. The body of the uterus is called the ____________________, and the two horns are the ____________________.
4. The muscle layer of the uterus is the ____________________, and the inner lining is the ____________________.
5. The structure between the vagina and the uterus is the ____________________. Its name literally means ____________________.

THE ESTROUS CYCLE

In domestic animals, secondary sex characteristics begin to develop, and the ability to reproduce sexually is achieved at puberty. Puberty varies between and within species. Puberty can be accelerated or delayed by nutrition, hormones, climate, and heredity.

The onset of the estrous cycle occurs at puberty and normally continues for the life of the animal. Unlike humans, animals do not go through menopause and can become pregnant very late in life. Sexual maturity brings about ovarian development, which includes the production of ova, ovulation, and the production of *corpora lutea* (singular, *corpus luteum*). Each of these occurrences causes changes to other structures of the reproductive system.

The female reproductive system undergoes cyclical changes at regular intervals. These intervals vary greatly between species. The estrous cycle is under the control of hormones produced by both the ovaries and the anterior lobe of the pituitary. Even though there are great variations in the length of the cycle, each animal follows the same basic pattern. Species variations are noted during different phases of the cycle. The purpose of the estrous cycle is to prepare the uterus to receive a fertilized ovum.

At the beginning of each cycle, ova within follicles in the ovaries begin to develop. One or more follicles (depending on the species) continue to develop until they reach what is called *graafian follicle* or ripened follicle size. One or more graafian follicles rupture *(ovulation)*, and the ovum is expelled from the ovary to the uterine tube. Most animals are considered spontaneous ovulators, with ovulation occurring cyclically. Some animals such as the cat, rabbit, ferret, llama, and mink are considered reflex or induced ovulators. In these species, ovulation occurs only after copulation. Ovulation usually occurs during estrus, when the animal is said to be *in heat*. The ruptured follicle grows larger, filling with a yellow lipoid material, and becomes the *corpus luteum* (yellow body). The corpus luteum secretes progesterone. If fertilization occurs, the corpus luteum continues to secrete progesterone and prevents future estrous cycles during pregnancy. If fertilization does not take place, the corpus luteum and its secretions diminish, forming a *corpus albicans* (white body). The reduced levels of hormone production lead to a new estrous cycle.

Stages of Estrous Cycle

Domestic animals have an estrous cycle that is divided into four phases or periods: *proestrus, estrus, metestrus, diestrus,* and in some species *anestrus.*

PROESTRUS

Proestrus (building-up phase) is the period before desire. During this phase, follicle-stimulating hormone (FSH) is secreted by the anterior lobe of the pituitary gland and causes follicles to develop within the ovary. FSH stimulates the ovary to release increased amounts of estrogen, which causes changes in the vagina, uterus, vulva, oviducts, and ovaries. All these changes prepare the reproductive tract for pregnancy.

ESTRUS

Estrus is the period of sexual desire. During this phase and in some cases right after, *ovulation* (release of ova) occurs. FSH levels decrease, and luteinizing hormone (LH) increases, causing the ripened (graafian) follicles to rupture (ovulation).

METESTRUS

Metestrus (postovulatory phase) is the period after desire. During this phase, the corpus luteum forms and produces progesterone. Amounts of estrogen decrease during this period. Progesterone is responsible for proper implantation and for maintaining pregnancy. If pregnancy does not occur, the corpus luteum decreases in size to a *corpus albicans,* thus decreasing the amounts of progesterone. The cycle continues. Metestrus can logically be followed by pregnancy, a false pregnancy, diestrus, or anestrus.

DIESTRUS AND ANESTRUS

Diestrus is the period after metestrus. This is a short inactive phase before the onset of the next proestrus in polyestrous animals.

Anestrus is a phase of sexual inactivity and ovarian quiescence that is normal in certain animals. Seasonally polyestrous species such as sheep are in anestrus between the seasons when they undergo sexual activity. Species such as dogs, which are in estrus only twice a year, have long periods of anestrus between cycles. In animals that normally cycle continuously, such as the dairy cow, anestrus usually is abnormal.

Pregnancy

Pregnancy is the period of time between conception and parturition. At conception, the ovum normally is penetrated by one sperm cell while it is in the uterine tube. After fertilization, the fertilized ovum begins to form a rounded mass of cells and slowly moves from the uterine tube to the uterus, where it develops a placenta and attaches *(implantation)* to the endometrial lining of the uterus. The inner cells of the rounded mass form the embryo and its *amnion,* the thin, clear sac filled with amniotic fluid in which the embryo and fetus float. The outer cells of the rounded cell mass *(chorion)* help to form the placenta, along with the endometrium of the uterus. Species variations exist as to how and where the fetus attaches. Until implantation, the developing organism is called an *embryo.* After implantation and until parturition, the developing organism is called a *fetus.*

The placenta is the only connection between the *dam* and the developing fetus. Although the maternal and fetal circulations are independent of each other, the placenta carries nutrients, oxygen, and antibodies from the maternal blood to that of the fetus. Fetal metabolic waste is carried back to the maternal blood for disposal via the placenta. The placenta secretes estrogen, progesterone, and relaxin. Human placentas produce human chorionic gonadotropin (HCG), and the mare placenta produces pregnant mare serum (PMS). These hormones stimulate ovarian secretions of estrogen and progesterone.

Gestation periods vary between and within species. Some examples of average normal gestation periods are bovine, 280 days; equine, 336 days; caprine and ovine, 150 days; porcine, 114 days or 3 months, 3 weeks, and 3 days; and canine and feline, approximately 63 days.

REVIEW D

1. Ovulation involves the rupture of the ________________ follicle. If this process occurs cyclically, without the presence of the male, the animal is a ________________ ovulator. Animals that ovulate only after copulation are called ________________ ovulators.
2. An animal in heat is in the ________________ phase of the estrous cycle. The phase immediately before this is ________________; the stage immediately after it is ________________. The final phase is known as ________________, although some species (e.g., the dog) also have an anestrus phase.
3. The color of the corpus luteum is ________________ and the corpus albicans is ________________.
4. Before implantation the fertilized ovum is called a(n) ________________. After implantation it is called a(n) ________________.
5. Implantation is the attachment of the placenta to the ________________.

Chapter 12 Answers

Review A

1. nephro, reno
2. they are situated outside the peritoneal cavity
3. nephron
4. glomerulus
5. ureters, urethra
6. prostatic, membranous, cavernous

Review B

1. seminiferous, epididymis
2. Leydig, interstitial
3. vas deferens, prostate
4. vesicular (seminal vesicles), bulbourethral (Cowper's), coagulating
5. os penis
6. sigmoid flexure

Review C

1. uterine tube, oviduct, fallopian tube; infundibulum
2. metro, hystero
3. corpus, cornus
4. myometrium, endometrium
5. cervix, neck

Review D

1. mature (ripened, graafian), spontaneous, induced
2. estrus, proestrus, metestrus, diestrus
3. yellow, white
4. embryo, fetus
5. endometrium

Chapter 12 — EXERCISES

THE GENITOURINARY SYSTEM: ANIMAL REPRODUCTION AND THE PROCESSING OF LIQUID WASTES

Exercise 1: Complete the following statements.

1. The concave depression in the medial margin of the kidney is the ____________________.
2. Sectioning of the kidney shows it to be composed of an external ____________________ and an internal ____________________.
3. The voiding of urine from the bladder is called ____________________, or urination.
4. The flow of urine from the bladder into the urethra is controlled by a ____________________ muscle.
5. From its name you would expect the color of the tunica albuginea to be ____________________.
6. Surgical removal of the testes is called ____________________.
7. The short tube formed by the joining of the vas deferens with the duct of the vesicular glands is known as the ____________________.
8. The end of the uterine tube nearest the ovary is called the ____________________. It is edged with fingerlike processes called ____________________.
9. Fertilization usually takes place in the ____________________; implantation takes place in the ____________________.
10. The ovarian hormones are ____________________ and ____________________.

Exercise 2: Using the terms below, identify the parts in Fig. 12-9 by placing the part name in the corresponding blank.

~~Cortex~~	~~Renal artery~~	~~Ureter~~
Renal pyramid	Calix (calyx)	Capsule
~~Hilus~~	Renal pelvis	Papilla
Renal column	~~Renal vein~~	

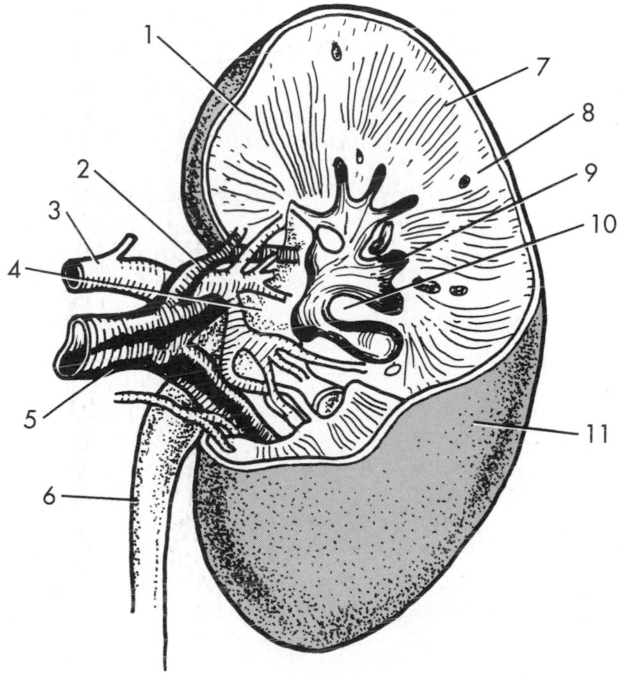
1
2
3
4
5
6
7
8
9
10
11

FIG. 12-9 Structure of the kidney.

1. Cortex
2. hilus
3. renal ~~vein~~ artery
4.
5. renal ~~artery~~ vein
6. ureter
7.
8.
9.
10.
11.

Exercise 3: Complete the following statements.

1. The male hormone ______________________ is produced by the ______________________ cells of the testes.
2. A renal tubule is divided into a proximal and distal ______________________, a descending and ascending ______________________, and the ______________________.
3. The outer end of the penis is called the ______________________.
4. The testicles of the tomcat are (dorsal, ventral) to the penis. (Circle correct answer.)
5. The milk-secreting cells are in the ______________________ of the lobules of the mammary gland. (Clue: The same name is used for the small sacs of the lungs.)
6. The lactogenic hormone ______________________ stimulates milk production, and the hormone ______________________ stimulates milk letdown.
7. Ovulation usually occurs during or shortly after the ______________________ phase of the estrous cycle.
8. The age at which female animals begin their estrous cycles is called ______________________.
9. The seminiferous tubules produce ______________________.
10. The body of the uterus leads from the ______________________ to the ______________________.
11. The membrane that surrounds the ovary and uterine tube of the bitch is called the ______________________. (See Fig. 12-7.)

Exercise 4: Using the following terms, identify each structure in Fig. 12-10 by writing its name in the corresponding blank.

Bladder	Prostate gland	Spermatic cord
Bulbourethral gland	Seminal vesicle	Testicle
Epididymis	Sigmoid flexure	Vas deferens
Glans penis		

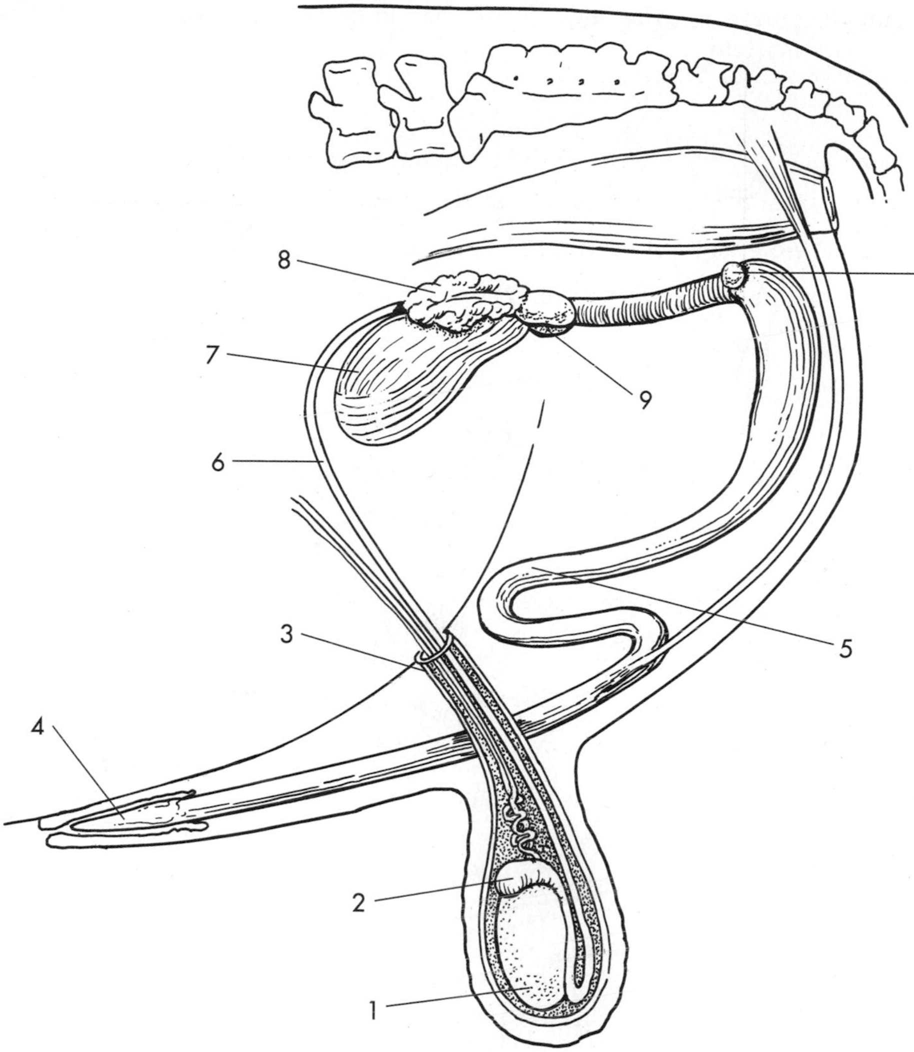
8
7
6
9
10
3
4
5
2
1

FIG. 12-10 Reproductive system of the bull.

1. testicle
2. epididymis
3. Spermatic cord
4. glans penis
5. Sigmoid flexure
6. vas deferens
7. bladder
8. seminal vesicle
9. prostate gland
10. bulbourethral gland

Exercise 5: Using the following terms, identify each part in Fig. 12-11 by writing the appropriate name in the blank to the right.

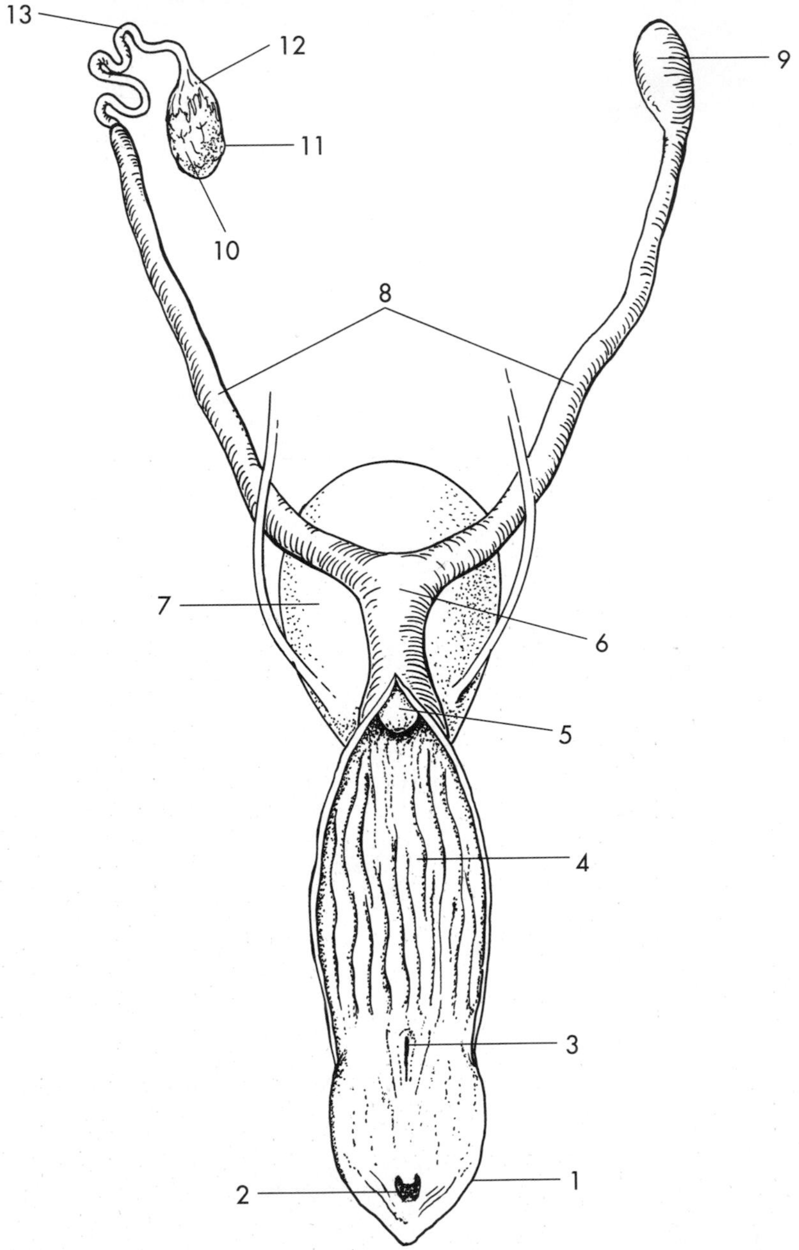
13
12
9
11
10
8
7
6
5
4
3
2
1

FIG. 12-11 Reproductive system of the bitch.

Corpus luteum
Uterine tubes (oviducts)
Clitoris
Cervix
Ovary
Vagina
Uterine horns
Vulva
Body of uterus
Infundibulum
Urinary bladder
Ovarian bursa
Urethral orifice

1. Vulva
2. Clitoris
3. urethral orifice
4. vagina
5. Cervix
6. body of uterus
7. urinary bladder
8. uterine horns
9. ovarian bursa
10. ovary
11. Corpus luteum
12. infundibulum
13. uterine tubes (oviducts)

Exercise 6: Using the following terms, identify each part in Fig. 12-12 by placing its name in the corresponding blank to the right.

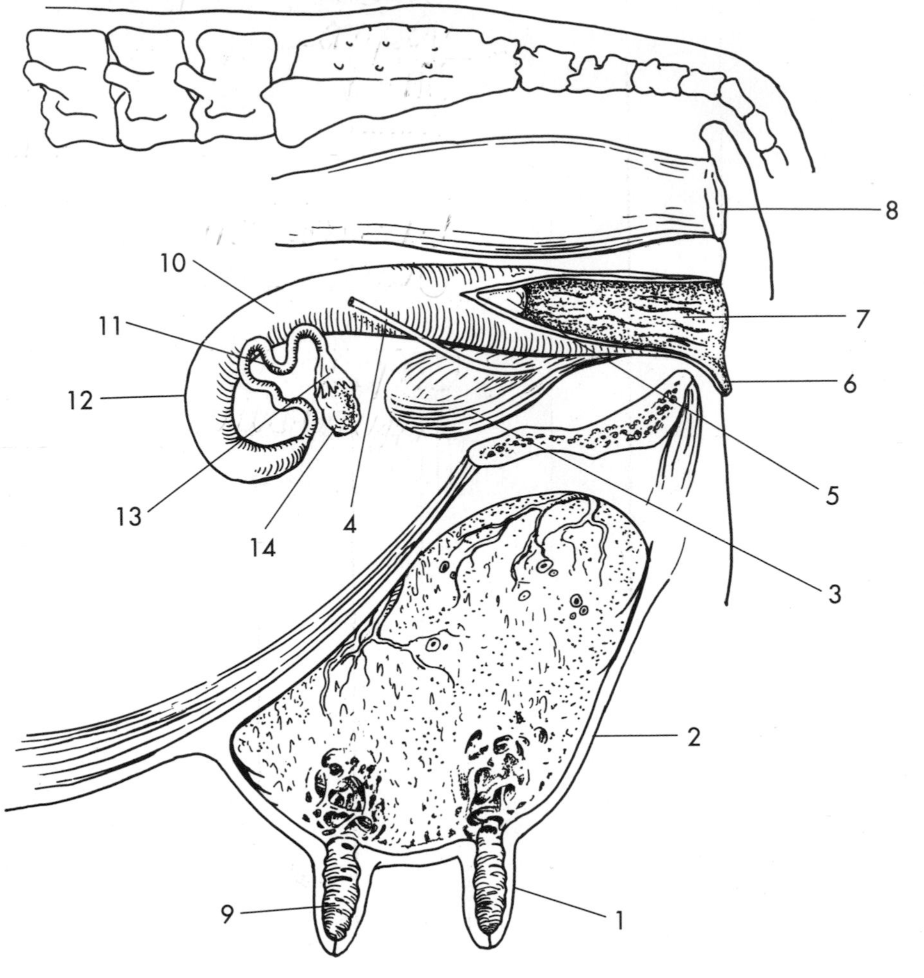
8
10
7
11
6
12
5
13
4
14
3
2
9
1

FIG. 12-12 Cross-section of the reproductive system of a cow, showing the udder.

~~Urinary bladder~~	1.	teat cistern
~~Body of uterus~~	2.	udder
~~Cervix~~	3.	urinary bladder
~~Uterine horn~~	4.	~~Sphincter ani~~ ~~ut~~ ureter
~~Teat~~	5.	cervix
~~Udder~~	6.	vulva
~~Sphincter ani~~	7.	vagina
~~Vulva~~	8.	Sphincter ani
~~Vagina~~	9.	teat
~~Ovary~~	10.	body of uterus
~~Ureter~~	11.	oviduct
~~Teat cistern~~	12.	uterine horn
~~Oviduct~~	13.	infundibulum
~~Infundibulum~~	14.	ovary

Exercise 7: Match the terms in the right column with the definitions or statements in the left column by placing the appropriate letter in the blank space provided.

B	1. Pouches just above the prostate whose duct unites with the vas deferens to form the ejaculatory duct Seminal vesicles	A. Vas deferens
A	2. Pair of tubes encased by spermatic cords vas deferens	B. Seminal vesicles
M	3. Male gland producing spermatozoa testis	C. Semen
E	4. Specialized interstitial cells that secrete the male sex hormone (testosterone) and are responsible for secondary sex characteristics leydig's cells	D. Spermatozoa
D	5. Sperm cells of the male spermatozoa	E. Leydig's cells
L	6. Reproductive cells of the female Ova	F. Endometrium
G	7. Where fertilization takes place Oviduct/uterine tube	G. Oviduct/uterine tube
F	8. Mucous membrane lining of the uterus endometrium	H. Corpus luteum
N	9. Early or developing stage of any organism embryo	I. Fimbria/infundibulum
C	10. Secretion discharged by male reproductive organ Semen	J. Endocervix
K	11. Developing animal after implantation fetus	K. Fetus
I	12. Fringelike processes at ends of uterine (fallopian) tubes fimbria/infundibulum	L. Ova
J	13. Interior of cervix endocervix	M. Testis
P	14. S-shaped curve of bull penis sigmoid flexure	N. Embryo
H	15. Yellow body that forms on ovary to produce progesterone Corpus luteum	O. Vulva
O	16. External female genitalia vulva	P. Sigmoid flexure
Q	17. Elastic muscular tube caudal to cervix, extending to body exterior Vagina	Q. Vagina

Exercise 8: Give the meaning of the components in the following words and then define the word as a whole. Check the glossary at the end of the chapter if you need help.

1. Pyuria

   py ______

   ur ______

   ia ______

   ______

2. Cystitis

   cyst ______

   itis inflammation

   ______

3. Colpotomy

   colpo ______

   tomy Inscision

   ______

4. Endometritis

   endo ______

   metr utures

   itis inflamation

   ______

5. Vasectomy

   vas ______

   ectomy Sx remove

   ______

6. Theriogenology

   therio ______

   gen ______

   ology Study of

   ______

7. Episiotomy

   episio ______

   tomy inocion

   ______

8. Cystotomy

   cysto ______

   tomy inocion

   ______

9. Ovariohysterectomy

   ovario Overies

   hyster utures

   ectomy Sx remove

   ______

10. Balanitis

    balan ______

    itis inflammation

    ______

11. Pyelonephritis

    pyelo ______

    nephr Kidney

    itis Inflammation

    ______

12. Urolithiasis

    uro ______

    lith ______

    iasis ______

    ______

CHAPTER 12 PUZZLE

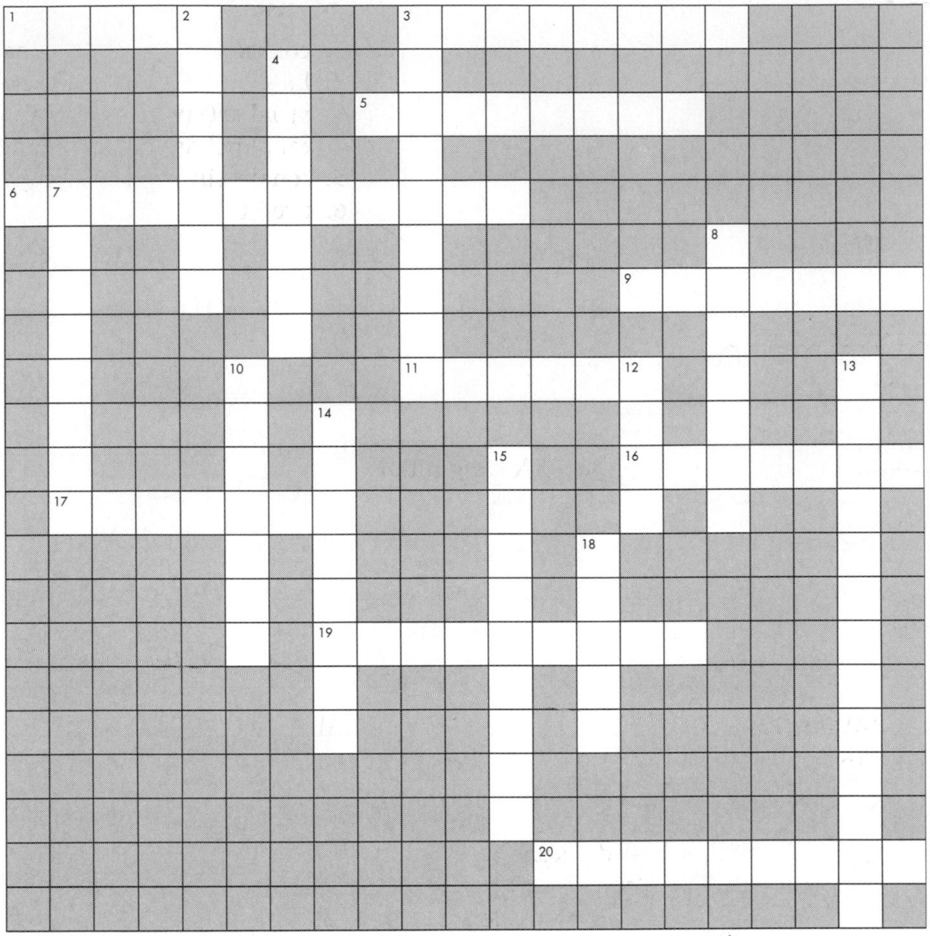
1
2
3
4
5
6
7
8
9
10
11
12
13
14
15
16
17
18
19
20

ACROSS CLUES

1. Concave depression on kidney
3. Fingerlike processes
5. Female stimulatory organ
6. Male sex hormone
9. Stores urine
11. Root meaning kidney
16. Tubes carrying urine to storage
17. Functional unit of kidney
19. Primary male reproductive organs
20. Rupture of graafian follicle

DOWN CLUES

2. S-shaped flexure of bull penis
3. Uterine tube(s)
4. Tube that excretes urine
7. Female sex hormone
8. Where urine collects
10. Primary female reproductive organs
12. Female sex cell
13. Union of ovum and sperm
14. Fluid in which fetus floats
15. Minute formations embedded in ovary
18. Female external genitalia

Chapter 12 Answers

Exercise 1

1. hilus
2. cortex, medulla
3. micturition
4. sphincter
5. white
6. castration
7. ejaculatory duct
8. infundibulum, fimbriae
9. uterine tube, uterus
10. estrogen, progesterone

Exercise 2

1. cortex
2. hilus
3. renal artery
4. renal pelvis
5. renal vein
6. ureter
7. renal pyramid
8. renal column
9. calix (calyx)
10. papilla
11. capsule

Exercise 3

1. testosterone, interstitial (Leydig's)
2. convoluted tubule, loop of Henle, collecting tubule
3. glans penis
4. dorsal
5. alveoli
6. prolactin, oxytocin
7. estrus
8. puberty
9. sperm
10. cervix, cornus (horns)
11. ovarian bursa

Exercise 4

1. testicle
2. epididymis
3. spermatic cord
4. glans penis
5. sigmoid flexure
6. vas deferens
7. bladder
8. seminal vesicle
9. prostate gland
10. bulbourethral gland

Exercise 5

1. vulva
2. clitoris
3. urethral orifice
4. vagina
5. cervix
6. body of uterus
7. urinary bladder
8. uterine horns
9. ovarian bursa
10. ovary
11. corpus luteum
12. infundibulum
13. uterine tubes (oviducts)

Exercise 6

1. teat
2. udder
3. urinary bladder
4. ureter
5. cervix
6. vulva
7. vagina
8. sphincter ani
9. teat cistern
10. body of uterus
11. oviduct
12. uterine horn
13. infundibulum
14. ovary

Exercise 7

1. B	7. G	13. J
2. A	8. F	14. P
3. M	9. N	15. H
4. E	10. C	16. O
5. D	11. K	17. Q
6. L	12. I	

Exercise 8

1. pus; urine; condition; pus in the urine
2. bladder; inflammation; inflammation of the urinary bladder
3. vagina; incision; surgical incision into the vagina
4. inner; uterus; inflammation; inflammation of the lining of the uterus
5. vessel; cutting out; cutting out the vas deferens
6. beasts; origin; study; study of animal reproduction
7. vulva; incision; surgical incision into the vulva
8. bladder; incision; surgical incision into the bladder
9. ovary; uterus; cutting out; surgical removal of ovaries and uterus (spaying operation)
10. glans penis; inflammation; inflammation of the penis
11. pelvis; kidney; inflammation; inflammation of the pelvis of the kidney
12. urine; stone; condition; presence of stones in the urine

ANSWERS: CHAPTER 12 PUZZLE

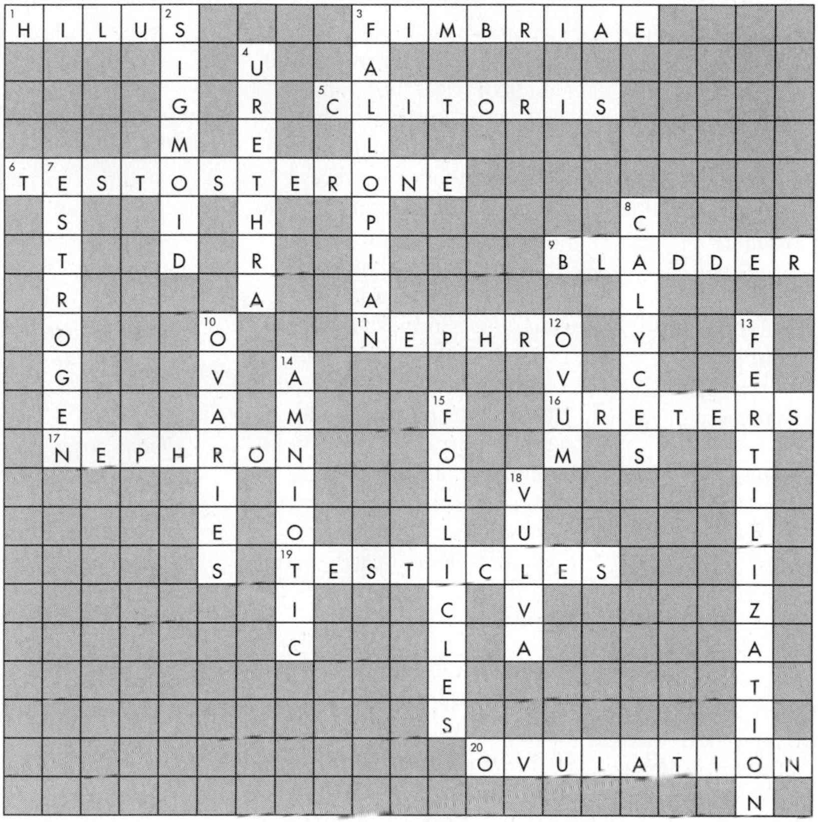
1 HILUS
2 SIGMOID
3 FIMBRIAE
3 FALLOPIA
4 URETHRA
5 CLITORIS
6 TESTOSTERONE
7 ESTROGEN
8 CALYCES
9 BLADDER
10 OVARIES
11 NEPHRO
12 OVUM
13 FERTILIZATION
14 AMNIOTIC
15 FOLLICLES
16 URETERS
17 NEPHRON
18 VULVA
19 TESTICLES
20 OVULATION

GLOSSARY

URINARY TRACT ORGANS AND RELATED ANATOMIC TERMS

bladder: elastic musculomembranous sac for storing urine.

Bowman's capsule: glomerular capsule of kidney containing cluster of capillary channels (glomerulus).

calix or *calyx* (ka'liks): urine-collecting, irregular, saclike structures of renal pelvis.

collecting tubules: terminal collection passages that carry urine to renal pelvis.

distal convoluted tubules: portion of convoluted tubules between Henle's loop and collecting tubules.

glomeruli: plural form of *glomerulus.*

glomerulus: coils of capillaries within Bowman's capsule.

Henle's loop: U-shaped turn in convoluted tubule of kidney, located between proximal and distal ends, with both ascending and descending limbs.

hilus: concave depression on medial margin of kidney through which ureters, blood vessels, and nerves enter.

kidneys: paired abdominal organs that filter blood and produce urine.

nephron (nef'ron): functional and structural unit of kidney, including renal corpuscle and renal tubule.

renal corpuscle: glomerulus and Bowman's capsule.

renal cortex (kor'teks): outer part of kidney, extending between renal pyramids to form renal columns.

renal medulla: inner part of kidney composed of conical structures, called renal pyramids.

renal papillae: narrow, conical ends of renal pyramids.

renal pelvis: reservoir that collects urine, made up of major and minor calices.

renal pyramid; see renal medulla.

renal sinus: kidney cavity containing renal pelvis, blood vessels, nerves, and fat.

renal tubule: minute tubule of kidney that secretes, collects, and transports urine and forms part of functional unit, the nephron.

uresis: normal passage of urine.

ureter: tube that carries urine from kidney to bladder.

urethra: tube that carries urine from bladder to surface of body.

PATHOLOGIC CONDITIONS OF THE URINARY TRACT

Inflammations and infections

balanitis (bal″ah-ni'tis): inflammation of glans penis.

cystitis: bladder inflammation.

glomerulonephritis (glo-mer″u-lo-nĕ-fri'tis): kidney disease with inflammation of glomeruli.

nephritis (nĕ-fri'tis): inflammation of kidneys.

perinephritis (per″ĭ-nĕ-fri'tis): inflammation of tissues surrounding kidney.

pyelitis (pi″ĕ-li'tis): inflammation of kidney pelvis.

pyelonephritis (pi″ĕ-lo-nĕ-fri'tis): inflammation of kidney pelvis caused by infection (also called *nephropyelitis*).

ureteritis (u″re-ter-i'tis): inflammation of ureter.

urethritis (u″re-thri'tis): inflammation of urethra.

urethrocystitis (u-re″thro-sis-ti'tis): inflammation of urethra and bladder.

Hereditary, congenital, and developmental disorders

epispadias (ep″ĭ-spa'de-as): urethral opening on dorsum of penis (*spadias* refers to cleft).

hypospadias (hi″po-spa'de-as): urethra opens on undersurface of penis or on perineum.

renal ectopia: displaced kidney.

Other abnormalities

albuminuria: presence of albumin and other proteins in the urine.

anuria: lack of urine being excreted (also called *anuresis*).

azotemia (az″o-te'me-ah): presence of urea or other nitrogenous elements in blood.

cylindruria (sil″in-droo're-ah): presence of cylindric casts in urine.

dysuria: painful or difficult urination.

hematuria: presence of blood in urine.

hydronephrosis (hi″dro-nĕ-fro'sis): distension of kidney caused by obstruction of ureter.

incontinence (in-kon'tĭ-nens): inability to control urination.

isosthenuria (cye-sos'then-ur'-ia): fixed specific gravity of urine.

nephrolith (nef'ro-lith): kidney stone.

nephrolithiasis (nef″ro-li-thi'ah-sis): condition characterized by presence of kidney stones (renal calculi).

nephrosis (nĕ-fro'sis): any disease of kidney.

oliguria: scanty urine output.
phosphaturia (fos″fat-u′re-ah): excess of phosphates excreted in urine.
pollakiuria: abnormally frequent urination.
polyuria: excretion of an abnormally large quantity of urine.
pyelonephrosis (pi″ĕ-lo-nĕ-fro′sis): any disease of kidney pelvis.
pyuria: pus in urine.
renal colic: pain resulting from passage of calculus in kidney or ureter.
renal infarction: ischemia of kidney because of thrombus or embolus.
retention: keeping within body a substance that is usually excreted, such as urine.
uremia: disturbed kidney function in which products of protein metabolism are found in blood and produce toxic condition.
urinary calculus (kal′ku-lus): stone or concretion in kidney, ureter, or bladder.
urolithiasis (you′-roe-lith-eye″-a-sis): formation of calculi (stones) in the urinary tract.

SURGICAL AND OTHER PROCEDURES

cystectomy: total or partial resection of bladder.
cystolithectomy (sis″to-lĭ-thek′to-me): removal of stone by incising urinary bladder (also called *cystolithotomy*).
cystoplasty: plastic repair of bladder.
cystostomy: creation of opening into bladder.
cystotomy: incision into urinary bladder.
lithotripsy: use of shock waves to crush kidney stones as substitute for surgical removal.
nephrectomy (ne-frek′to-me): excision of kidney.
nephrotomy (ne-frot′o-me): incision into kidney.
ureterostomy (u″re-ter-os′to-me): creation of permanent passage through which ureter can discharge its contents.
ureterotomy: incision of ureter.
urethroplasty: plastic repair of urethra for wound or defect.
urethrostomy: creation of opening passage into urethra to relieve stricture.
urethrotomy: cutting of urethra to relieve stricture.

LABORATORY TESTS AND PROCEDURES FOR THE URINARY SYSTEM

catheterized urine specimen: obtaining urine specimen under sterile conditions to check for microorganisms in urinary system.
concentration test: determines kidney's ability to concentrate and dilute urine.
creatinine test: urine test for elevation of creatinine, a protein waste product present in kidney function disturbance.
cystogram: X-ray study of bladder.
cystoscope: fiberoptic endoscope to examine interior of bladder.
hemoglobin: urine test to determine presence of hemoglobin in urine, indicating abnormal condition or disease of genitourinary tract.
intravenous pyelogram: X-ray record of kidneys and urinary tract after intravenous injection of dye substance.
renal angiography and arteriography: X-ray studies of blood vessels surrounding kidneys, renal artery, and related blood vessels, after injection of contrast media.
renal scan: X-ray scan using intravenous injection of radioactive substance to determine size, shape, and exact location of kidneys and to diagnose abnormalities.
retrograde pyelogram: X-ray record of kidneys and urinary tract, using injection of contrast medium directly into bladder.
total volume: measurement of urine excreted in 24-hour period to evaluate kidney function.

MALE REPRODUCTIVE ORGANS AND RELATED ANATOMIC TERMS

bulbourethral glands: glands located on either side of urethra whose alkaline secretion has protective function for sperm (also called *Cowper's glands*).
ejaculatory ducts: two short tubes formed by joining of vas deferens and ducts of seminal vesicles, which pass through prostate and extend to the urethra.
epididymides: plural form of *epididymis.*
epididymis (ep″ĭ-did′ĭ-mis): pair of tightly coiled tubelike structures that secrete part of semen, serve as storage areas for sperm before ejacula-

tion, and provide passageways for sperm from testes to the body surface.

glans penis: slight bulge at distal end of penis.

Leydig's cells (li'digz): specialized interstitial cells that secrete male sex hormone testosterone.

penis: male sex organ, containing urethra, which carries both reproductive tract secretions and urine to body surface.

prepuce (pre'puse): retractible, double fold of skin covering glans penis.

prostate: gland surrounding urethra, secreting thick, alkaline substance that makes up part of seminal fluid.

scrotum (skro'tum): saclike, skin-covered structure, hanging from perineal area, containing testes, epididymides, and part of spermatic cords.

semen: secretion discharged by male reproductive organs, containing spermatozoa.

seminal vesicles: two twisted pouches lying along dorsal surface of bladder, ventral to rectum, which secrete liquid part of semen and prostaglandins.

seminiferous tubules (se″mĭ-nif'er-us): coiled tubules within testes that produce sperm cells.

Sertoli's cells (ser″to'lēz): cells in testis that support and nourish sperm germ.

sigmoid flexure: S-shaped flexure of penis of bull, ram, and boar.

spermatic cords: white, fibrous tissue encasing vas deferens, blood and lymph vessels, and nerves.

spermatid (sper'mah-tid): germ cell developing into a spermatozoon (also called *spermatoblast*).

spermatozoa: plural form of *spermatozoon.*

spermatozoon (sper″mah-to-zo'on): male reproductive (sperm) cell.

testis (tes'tis): egg-shaped male gland (also called *testicle*) that produces spermatozoa and secretes hormones (*orchis* refers to testis).

vas deferens: excretory duct of testis that joins epididymis with ejaculatory duct (also called *ductus deferens*).

FEMALE REPRODUCTIVE ORGANS AND RELATED TERMS

anestrus: a normal interval of ovarian quiescence and sexual inactivity in species such as the dog that do not cycle continuously. Anestrus is abnormal in polyestrous species such as the cow.

cervix (ser'viks): neck of uterus.

clitoris (kli'to-ris): small mound of erectile tissue similar to the male penis.

corpora: plural form of *corpus.*

corpus (kor'pus): body.

corpus albicans: the white scar tissue resulting from the regression of a corpus luteum.

corpus luteum (lu'te-um): yellow body formed by graafian follicle that has discharged its ovum (*luteum* means yellow).

diestrus: a short period of sexual quiescence between two estrus periods during which the uterus is prepared for a fertilized ovum.

ectopic pregnancy (ek-top'ik): fertilized ovum implanted outside uterus, most commonly in uterine tube (*ectopic* means out of normal position).

endocervix: mucous membrane lining cervical canal or opening of cervix into uterus.

endometrium (en-do-me'tre-um): mucous membrane lining uterus.

estrous cycle: the recurring set of physiological and behavioral changes that take place from one period of estrus to another.

estrus: the periodic state of sexual excitement that immediately precedes ovulation, during which the female is most receptive to mating (also called *heat period, being in heat*).

fallopian tubes: see uterine tubes.

fimbria (fim'bre-ah): fringe-like processes at ends of uterine tubes over ovaries.

graafian (graf'e-an) *follicles:* mature ovarian follicles.

hymen: fold of mucous membrane partially blocking vaginal orifice.

infundibulum: funnel at end of uterine tube (oviduct) that catches ovum.

mammary glands: milk-producing organs of mammals.

metestrus: the period of sexual inactivity that follows estrus, during which the corpus luteum forms.

myometrium (mi-o-me'tre-um): middle, muscular coat of uterus.

os: mouth; *internal os* is opening from cervix into cervical canal; *external os* is opening from cervical canal into vagina.

ova: plural form of *ovum.*

ovary: female gland that produces ova or eggs.
oviducts: see uterine tubes.
ovum: female reproductive cell (the plural is *ova*).
proestrus: the period immediately before estrus, characterized by development of the endometrium and ovarian follicles.
uterine tubes: pair of tubes extending from the uterus to the ovary on each side, which pick up and convey expelled ova to the uterus (also called *fallopian tubes* or *oviducts*).
uterus: thick-walled, hollow organ in pelvic cavity of female that houses and nourishes embryo and fetus.

PREGNANCY AND RELATED ANATOMIC TERMS

amnion (am'ne-on): membrane containing fetus floating in amniotic fluid.
chorion (ko're-on): outermost layer of placenta.
cyesis (si-e'sis): pregnancy (*cyema* means embryo).
decidua (de-sid'u-ah): mucosa of uterus thrown off after birth.
ectoderm: outer of three germ layers of embryo.
embryo: early developing stage of organism.
endoderm: innermost of three germ layers of the embryo.
fetus: developing offspring.
gravid (grav'id): pregnant.
lactiferous ducts (lak-tif'er-us): ducts that carry the milk secretions of udder to and through teats.
mesoderm: middle of three germ layers of embryo, lying between ectoderm and endoderm.
neonate: newborn.
omphalus (om'fah-lus): *see umbilicus.*
parturition (par"tu-rish'un): process of giving birth.
placenta (plah-sen'tah): vascular fetal organ within uterus that connects fetus to mother by way of umbilical cord for exchange of nutrients, oxygen, antibodies, and waste products.
presentation: presenting part of fetus at birth.
pseudocyesis: false pregnancy.
umbilical cord: communication channel between placenta and fetus.
umbilicus (um-bil'ĭ-kus): scar that marks site of connection of umbilical cord in the fetus (also called *omphalus* or *navel*).
zygote (zi-gōt): fertilized ovum.

PATHOLOGIC CONDITIONS OF THE MALE AND FEMALE REPRODUCTIVE SYSTEMS

Inflammation and infections

cervicitis: inflammation of mucous membrane tissues of uterine cervix.
endometritis (en'do-me-tri'tis): inflammation of endometrium.
epididymitis: inflammation of epididymis.
mastitis (mas"ti"tis): inflammation of mammary gland.
metritis (me-tri'tis): inflammation of uterus.
oophoritis (o"of-o-ri'tis): ovarian inflammation.
oophorosalpingitis (o-of'o-ro-sal"pin-ji'tis): inflammation of ovary and uterine tube.
orchitis: inflammation of testicles.
prostatitis: inflammation of prostate gland.
pyometra (pi"o-me'trah): collection of pus in the uterine cavity.
pyosalpinx (pi"o-sal'pinks): accumulation of pus in uterine tube.
salpingitis (sal"pin-ji'tis): uterine tube inflammation.
seminal vesculitis: seminal vesicle inflammation.
theriogenology: the branch of veterinary science that deals with the anatomy, physiology, pathology, and diseases of the reproductive tracts of animals.
vaginitis: inflammation of vagina.
vulvitis: inflammation of vulva.

Hereditary, congenital, and developmental disorders

anorchism (an-or'kizm): absence of one or both testes.
atresia of vagina (ah-tre'za-ah): absence of vaginal opening.
cryptorchism (krip-tor'kizm): testes do not descend into scrotum (also called *cryptorchidism*).
ectopia of testis: one or both testes misplaced in other location.
hermaphroditism (her-maf"ro-di'tizm): having both ovarian and testicular tissue.
hypoplasia of cervix: underdevelopment of cervix.
ovotestis: gonad that contains both ovarian and testicular tissue *(see hermaphroditism).*
polyorchism: presence of more than two testes.

pseudohermaphroditism: presence of gonads of one sex, with physical characteristics of both sexes.
rudimentary uterus: underdeveloped or imperfectly developed uterus.
supernumerary: more than normal number, referring to such structures as teats, ovaries, and uterine tubes.

Other abnormalities

aspermatogenesis (ah-sper″mah-to-jen′ĕ-sis): failure to develop spermatozoa.
aspermia (ah-sper′me-ah): failure to form or emit semen.
corpus hemorrhagicum: blood clot in corpus luteum or blood in ovarian follicle.
hydrocele: collection of fluid in testis.
lactation: secretion of milk.
leukorrhea (lu″ko-re′ah): whitish discharge from vagina.
oligospermia (ol″i-go-sper′me-ah): diminished amount of spermatozoa in semen.
parovarian cyst: cyst located beside ovary.
phimosis (fi-mo′sis): constriction of skin of prepuce over glans penis.
prolapse of uterus: protrusion of uterus through vaginal orifice (cast wethers in the cow).
prostatic hypertrophy: enlargement of prostate.
spermaturia (sper″mah-tu′re-ah): discharge of semen in urine.
spontaneous abortion: premature discharge of embryo or nonviable fetus from uterus.
sterility: inability to reproduce.

SURGICAL PROCEDURES

abortion: termination of pregnancy.
cesarean section: surgical incision through abdominal and uterine walls for delivery of neonate.
colpotomy: surgical incision of vaginal wall.
embryotomy (em″bre-ot′o-me): cutting up of dead fetus for removal from uterus.
episioplasty (e-piz′e-o-plas″te): repair of vulva.
episiorrhaphy (e-piz″e-or′ah-fe): repair of torn vulva or episiotomy.
episiotomy: incision of vulva to prevent tearing on delivery of neonate.
fetomy: cutting apart fetus for removal.
hymenotomy: incision of hymen.
hysterectomy: removal of uterus.
mastotomy: incision of the mammary gland (also called *mammotomy*).
orchidorrhaphy: surgical fixation of undescended testicle into scrotum (also called *orchiopexy*).
orchiectomy (or″ke-ek′to-me): excision of one or both testes; also called *orchidectomy.*
ovariectomy (o″va-re-ek′to-me): excision of one or both ovaries (also called *oophorectomy*).
ovariohysterectomy (o-va-re-o-his″ter-ek′to-me): removal of uterus and ovaries (also called *oophorohysterectomy*).
panhysterectomy (pan″hist-er-ek′to-me): complete removal of uterus and cervix.
prostatectomy (pros″tah-tek′to-me): removal of all or part of prostate gland.
vasectomy: excision of all or part of vas deferens.
vasotomy: incision into vas deferens.

13 The Endocrine System

The chemical stimulators

CHAPTER OVERVIEW

This chapter describes the ductless glands (pituitary, thyroid, parathyroids, adrenals, pineal, pancreas, ovaries, and testes) that constitute the endocrine system. The structure and function of the glands and their secretions are detailed narratively and in chart form.

THE ENDOCRINES

The complex activities of the body are controlled by the endocrine and central nervous systems. The central nervous system acts directly and instantaneously, whereas the action of the endocrine system is more subtle, discharging its secretions slowly into the circulatory system and influencing target organs.

The endocrine system (Fig. 13-1) is made up of ductless glands of internal secretion, so called because they have no ducts to carry away their secretions and depend on the capillaries and, to a certain extent, the lymph vessels, for this function. The secretions of these glands are called *hormones* (which means to rouse or set in motion). Although most hormones are excitatory in function, some are inhibitory.

The secretion of hormones is controlled by a feedback mechanism. The presence and amount of a hormone and any substances released by tissue excited by that hormone regulate further secretion of that hormone by its gland. This feedback loop ensures that the right amount of the hormone, no more and no less, maintains the proper balance of bodily functioning.

Pituitary Gland

The *pituitary gland* or *hypophysis,* despite all its important functions, is a small organ. It has been called the "orchestra leader" and "master gland" because it exerts control over all other glands.

STRUCTURE

The pituitary gland lies protected within the sphenoid bone in a saddle-shaped depression called the *sella turcica.* It is further protected by an extension of the *dura mater* (membrane covering the brain) called the *pituitary diaphragm.* A stemlike portion of the pituitary gland, the *pituitary stalk,* extends through the diaphragm and provides a connection (the *infundibulum*) to the hypothalamus portion of the brain, located on the underside.

The pituitary gland actually is made up of two separate glands with different embryonic origins and functions: the *anterior lobe* or *anterior pituitary gland (adenohypophysis)* develops as an upgrowth from the embryonic pharynx, and the *posterior lobe* or *posterior pituitary gland (neurohypophysis)* as a downward extension of the brain (Fig. 13-2).

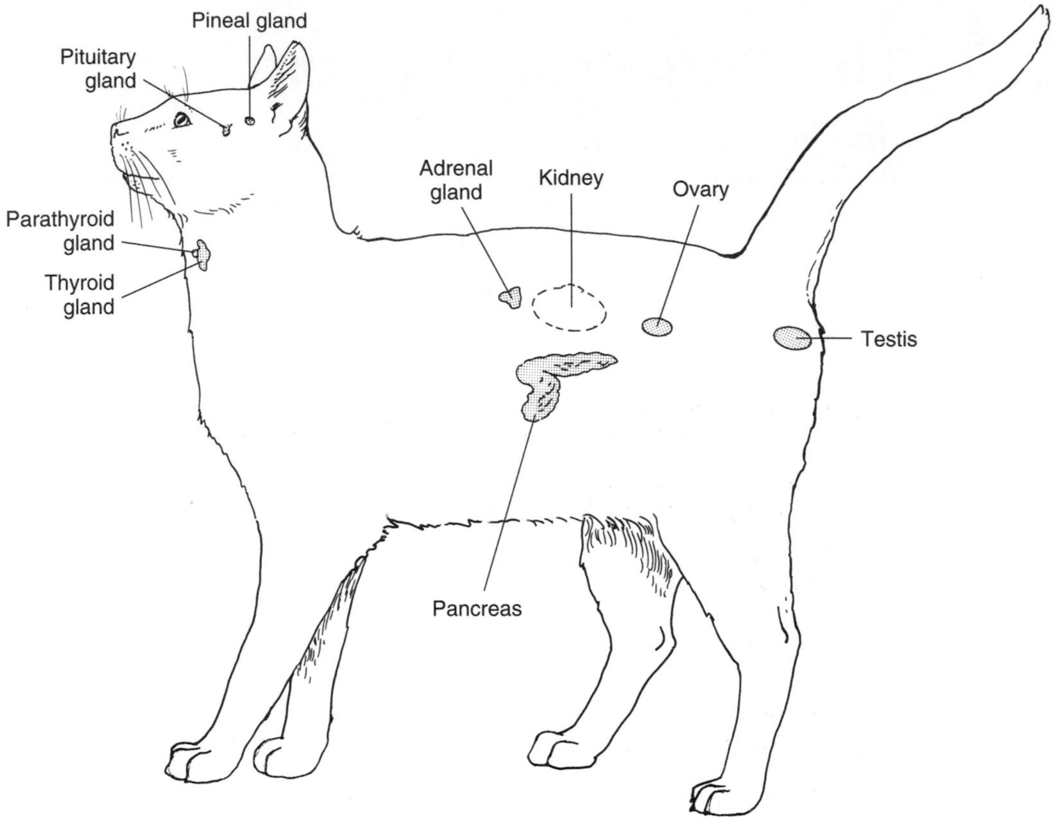
Pineal gland
Pituitary gland
Parathyroid gland
Thyroid gland
Adrenal gland
Kidney
Ovary
Testis
Pancreas

FIG. 13-1 Relative location of the endocrine glands in the cat.

Functions of the Anterior Lobe

The master role is played by the anterior lobe, with its numerous anterior pituitary hormones influencing the actions of other endocrines. This internal regulation is further coordinated by the action of hypothalamic releasing factors on the anterior lobe controlling the release of six major types of anterior pituitary hormones (Table 13-1).

Somatropin (GH), the growth hormone, promotes bodily growth of both bony and soft tissues. (*Somato* means body, *tropin** means nourishment.)

*The root *-trop* means turning, or affinity. The hormones ending in *-tropin* or *-tropic* can also be spelled *-trophin* or *-trophic,* a root meaning nourishment.

A *thyrotropic* (thyroid-stimulating) *hormone (TSH)* of the anterior pituitary lobe influences the thyroid gland and causes secretion of the thyroid hormone.

Two *gonadotropic hormones* influence the ovarics and testes and are necessary for the proper development and function of the reproductive system:

Follicle-stimulating hormone (FSH)—stimulates the growth of mature graafian follicles and the secretion of estrogen in the female and the development of the seminiferous tubules and sperm cells in the male.

Luteinizing hormone (LH)—stimulates the formation of the corpus lutrum and secretion of estrogen and progester-

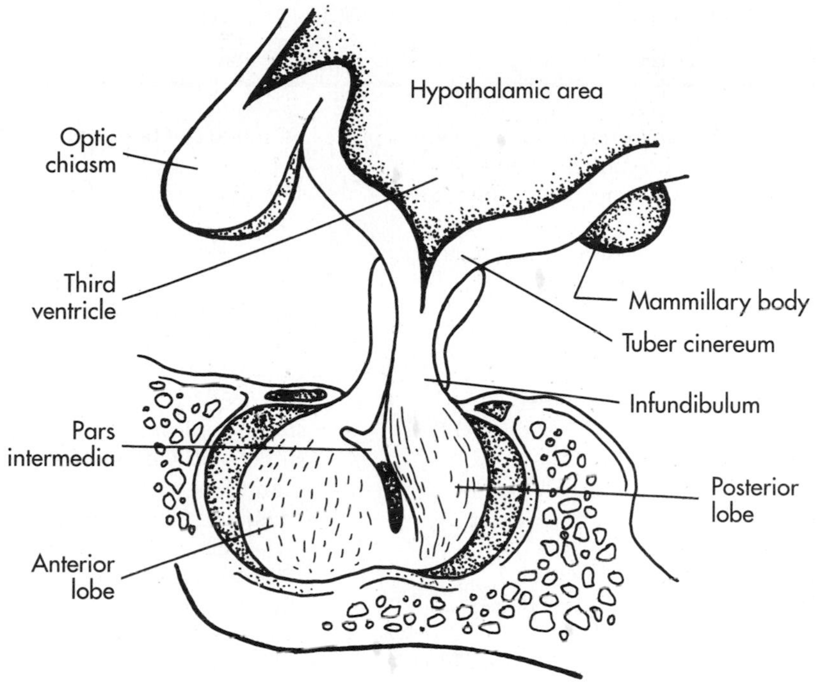
Hypothalamic area
Optic chiasm
Third ventricle
Mammillary body
Tuber cinereum
Infundibulum
Pars intermedia
Posterior lobe
Anterior lobe

FIG. 13-2 Pituitary gland and brain structures in proximity.

one in the female; *interstitial cell-stimulating hormone (ICSH)* stimulates development and secretion of testosterone in the interstitial cells of the testes of the male.

Prolactin or *lactogenic hormone* is responsible for mammary gland development during pregnancy and, as its name implies, for milk production.

Adrenocorticotropic hormone (ACTH) or *adrenocorticotropin* influences growth of the adrenal glands and stimulates the adrenal cortex to synthesize and release corticosteroids. ACTH also appears to have a relationship to skin pigmentation.

Melanocyte-stimulating hormone (MSH), the last of the anterior pituitary hormones, stimulates formation of melanin pigment in the skin and hair. The effect of MSH on feather pigmentation is unclear. MSH is also involved in the ability of some vertebrates to undergo chameleonlike color changes by aggregating or dispersing pigmented epidermal granules.

Functions of the Posterior Lobe

The posterior lobe of the pituitary gland secretes two hormones that are made in the hypothalamus and passed through the infundibulum into the posterior lobe, where they are secreted into the circulation. The first of these, an *antidiuretic hormone (ADH), vasopressin,* limits the development of large volumes of urine by stimulating water reabsorption by the distal and collecting tubules of the kidneys. The second hormone, *oxytocin,* stimulates both the ejection (letdown) of milk into the mammary ducts and contraction of the pregnant uterus during parturition.

Table 13-1 THE ENDOCRINE GLANDS AND THEIR HORMONES

Gland	Hormone	Function
Pituitary		
Anterior lobe	somatotropin (GH; growth hormone)	promotion of bone and soft tissue growth
	thyrotropic hormone (TSH)	stimulates thyroid gland production of thyroid hormone
	follicle-stimulating hormone (FSH)	stimulates ovarian follicle growth stimulates estrogen secretion in ovaries stimulates development of seminiferous tubules in testes stimulates development and production of sperm cells
	luteinizing hormone (LH)	stimulates formation of corpus luteum stimulates ovarian secretion of estrogen and progesterone stimulates development of testes interstitial cells stimulates testes secretion of testosterone
	lactogenic hormone (prolactin)	stimulates mammary gland development and milk production
	adrenocorticotropin (ACTH)	stimulates adrenal cortex to synthesize and release corticosteroids affects skin pigmentation
	melanocyte-stimulating hormone (MSH)	stimulates formation of melanin pigment in skin and hair
Posterior lobe	antidiuretic hormone (ADH; vasopressin)	stimulates water reabsorption by kidney tubules
	oxytocin	stimulates milk letdown and uterine contractions in pregnancy
Thyroid	thyroid hormone (thyroxine, triiodothyronine)	regulates growth, development, and metabolism
	calcitonin	promotes calcium absorption in bones and reduced concentration in blood
Parathyroid	parathyroid hormone	regulates phosphorus content of blood and bones increases calcium concentration in blood and reduction in bones
Adrenal		
Cortex	mineralocorticoids (aldosterone)	regulation of sodium and potassium
	sex hormones (androgen and estrogen)	in conjunction with ovaries and testes regulates growth of bones and musculature and secondary sex characteristics
	glucocorticoids (cortisol and corticosterone)	metabolism of carbohydrates, fats, and proteins lymphatic functions, antibody formation, recovery from injury and inflammation

Table 13-1 THE ENDOCRINE GLANDS AND THEIR HORMONES—cont'd

Gland	Hormone	Function
Adrenal—cont'd		
Medulla	epinephrine (adrenaline) and norepinephrine (noradrenaline)	stimulates sympathetic nervous system responses, especially fight-or-flight reaction
Pineal	melatonin	important in many species for timing of reproductive and other behavior; involved in circadian rhythms
Pancreas		
Islets of Langerhans	insulin	regulates use and storage of carbohydrates reduces glucose in blood
	glucagon	increases glucose in blood
	pancreatic polypeptide (PP)	production of glucagon and gastric juices functions in digestion and metabolism
Gonads		
Ovaries	estrogenic hormones (estradiol, estrone)	promotes secondary sex development and estrus after puberty
Testes	testosterone	promotes secondary sex development after puberty

Thyroid

The thyroid glands are paired bilateral glands located near the trachea below the larynx. The thyroid may be felt slightly and may even be visible as a swelling in some diseases of the gland, especially in feline hyperthyroidism.

STRUCTURE

The thyroid glands are soft, highly vascular, paired masses, brownish-red in color, consisting of tiny sacs or follicles that are filled with a gelatinous yellow fluid called *colloid.* The colloid contains the hormone secreted by the thyroid. This hormone is stored in the colloid and passed into the capillaries to be sent to the tissues as needed. Although lymph vessels drain some of the hormones, most is carried away by the capillaries. The hormone secreted by the thyroid is under the control of the anterior pituitary lobe.

FUNCTIONS

The main function of the thyroid is the secretion of two iodine-laden hormones, *thyroxine* (T_4) and *triiodothyronine* (T_3), which together are called *thyroid hormone.* This hormone is high in iodine and vital for growth and metabolism. Through variations in the activity of the gland, the hormone alters the metabolic rate in accordance with changing physiologic demands. Growth and differentiation of tissue during development are also regulated by the thyroid hormone.

Iodine is the essential element of the thyroid hormone. Most disorders of the thyroid are caused by overproduction or underproduction of the thyroid hormone and its iodine-containing substance. The iodine in the thyroid hormone is combined with a protein in the blood, which is then called *protein-bound iodine (PBI)*. However, when the hormone enters the tissue, the separate components become unbound from the protein.

A secondary function of the thyroid gland is the secretion of *calcitonin*, which produces a decrease in the concentration of calcium in the blood, helping to maintain the balance of calcium necessary for a variety of bodily processes. This balance is achieved in conjunction with the functioning of the parathyroid glands.

In birds, thyroid hormone is also important in molting and other behavior linked to changes in daylight.

REVIEW A

1. The secretions of the endocrine glands are called ______________________ .
2. The "master gland" is the ______________________, also called the hypophysis. It is connected to the hypothalamus of the brain by the ______________________, a word meaning funnel.
3. The anterior lobe of the hypophysis is called the ______________________ because of its glandular nature. The posterior lobe develops from nerve tissue and so is called the ______________________ .
4. Growth hormone is also called ______________________ .
5. The full name of the gonadotropin that stimulates follicle development in the female and sperm growth in the male is ______________________ . The other gonadotropin is called ______________________ in the female and ______________________ in the male.
6. ACTH stands for ______________________ . ADH stands for ______________________ .
7. Iodine is an essential part of the hormone produced by the ______________________ gland.

Parathyroid Glands

The *parathyroids* (*para* means alongside of or next to) are small, smooth, shiny, round glands. There are usually two on each side, in close proximity to the thyroid gland and embedded in its posterior surface.

STRUCTURE

The parathyroid glands are composed of large, round cells of two types: *chief* cells (also called *principal* cells), which are believed to produce *parathyroid hormone (PTH)*, and *oxyphil* cells, whose function is unclear. The blood supply of the parathyroid glands is from the inferior thyroid artery, and their functional activity is controlled by a hormone of the anterior lobe of the pituitary gland.

FUNCTIONS

Parathyroid hormone, secreted by the glands, regulates the calcium and phosphorus content of the blood and bones. The regulation of calcium content is very important in certain tissue activities such as blood formation and coagulation, milk production, and maintenance of normal neuromuscular excitability.

Parathyroid hormone increases blood calcium concentration. This mechanism is antagonistic (opposite) to that of the hormone calcitonin from the thyroid gland. These two hormones together maintain calcium balance.

Adrenal Glands

The *adrenal (suprarenal) glands* are small organs located close to the kidney.

STRUCTURE

The adrenal glands are composed of two distinct parts: the outer portion, or *cortex,* and the *medulla,* each with different functions. The cortex is indispensable to life, but the medulla is not. The cortex makes up the bulk of the gland and is divided into three zones: *zona glomerulosa* (outer), *zona fasciculata* (middle), and *zona reticularis* (inner).

FUNCTIONS

All known adrenal hormones of the cortex are classified as steroids based on their chemical structure. Many can be manufactured synthetically. They are classified as follows:

Mineralocorticoids—secreted by the outer zone, which are concerned with the regulation of sodium and potassium and their excretion; the principal one is *aldosterone,* which maintains electrolyte and water balance by acting on the blood sodium concentration.

Glucocorticoids—secreted mainly by the middle zone, including *cortisol (hydrocortisone)* and *corticosterone;* the glucocorticoids affect all cells in the body, but their general effect is in the metabolism of carbohydrates, fats, and proteins, resistance to stress, antibody formation, lymphatic functioning, and recovery from injury and inflammation.

Sex hormones—secreted in small amounts by the inner zone of the adrenal cortex in some species; these hormones are produced not only by the adrenals but also by the testes in the male and the ovaries in the female; *androgens* and *estrogens* are responsible for secondary sex characteristics and for reproductive behavior. The presence of *adrenocorticotropin (ACTH),* a pituitary hormone, in the blood supply is necessary for the anatomic integrity and functioning of the adrenal cortex in secreting androgens and cortisol.

The adrenal medulla secretes *epinephrine (adrenaline)* and *norepinephrine (noradrenaline).* Epinephrine in particular aids the body in meeting stressful situations such as defense, flight, attack, or pursuit. By stimulating or boosting the sympathetic nervous system, epinephrine aids in coping with stress. The effects of these secretions include increases in heartbeat, blood pressure, blood glucose level, and blood clotting rate.

Pineal Gland

The *pineal gland* or *body (epiphysis cerebri),* which derives its name from its resemblance to a pinecone, is a small, firm, oval body located near the base of the brain. Although exact functions have not been established, it secretes *melatonin,* which is believed to inhibit ovarian function and secretion of the pituitary luteinizing hormone. Melatonin probably is related to the circadian rhythms of the body. (See Chapter 14.)

Pancreas

The pancreas, as part of the gastrointestinal system, is described in Chapter 11. Specialized cells of the pancreas, called the *islands* (or *islets*) *of Langerhans*, secrete *insulin, glucagon,* and *pancreatic polypeptide (PP)* into the circulation.

Insulin is necessary for the use and storage of carbohydrates and acts to decrease blood glucose levels, whereas glucagon acts to increase them. The level of glucose in the blood also depends on the action of many of the other endocrine secretions, such as the pituitary growth hormone, epinephrine, ACTH, and the glucocorticoids. All these endocrine secretions increase glucose. The thyroid hormone decreases glucose. Pancreatic polypeptide plays a role in producing glucagon and gastric juices and has been identified as having additional functions in digestion and metabolism.

Gonads

The male and female gonads, as parts of the genitourinary system, are described in Chapter 12. As endocrine glands, the female ovaries and the male testes produce hormones important to the functioning of the reproductive system. These glands become active at puberty under the influence of the anterior pituitary lobe and produce the secondary sex characteristics and reproductive behavior. Table 13-1 and the glossary contain descriptions of the gonadal hormones.

REVIEW B

1. The action of parathyroid hormone on blood calcium is antagonistic to the action of the hormone ____________ from the ____________ gland.
2. The name adrenal tells you that the gland is ____________ the kidney. The name *suprarenal* tells you that it is ____________ the kidney. (The latter name is less appropriate for quadrupeds than the former.)
3. The outer portion of the adrenal gland is called the ____________ and lends part of its name to several hormones. Name at least two of them: ____________, ____________.
4. The inner portion of the adrenal gland is called the ____________. Its hormones, ____________ and ____________, are responsible for the fight-or-flight reaction.
5. Melatonin is the hormone of the ____________ gland, which is located in the ____________.
6. The specialized cells of the pancreas that secrete insulin are the islets of ____________. The islets also secrete ____________ and ____________ into the circulation.

Chapter 13 Answers

Review A

1. hormones
2. pituitary, infundibulum
3. adenohypophysis, neurohypophysis
4. somatotropin
5. follicle-stimulating hormone, luteinizing hormone, interstitial cell-stimulating hormone
6. adrenocorticotropic hormone, antidiuretic hormone
7. thyroid

Review B

1. calcitonin, thyroid
2. near, above
3. cortex; mineralocorticoids, glucocorticoids, cortisol, hydrocortisone, or cortisol
4. medulla, epinephrine (adrenaline), norepinephrine (noradrenaline)
5. pineal, brain
6. Langerhans, glucagon, pancreatic polypeptide

Chapter 13 **EXERCISES**

THE ENDOCRINE SYSTEM: THE CHEMICAL STIMULATORS

Exercise 1: For each hormone, write the abbreviation for the endocrine gland that produces it.

Endocrine Glands	
Adrenal cortex	AC
Adrenal medulla	AM
Anterior pituitary	AP
Ovaries	Ov
Pancreas	Pan
Parathyroid	Par
Pineal	Pin
Posterior pituitary	PP
Testes	Tes
Thyroid	Thy

Hormones

1. ADH ___PP___
2. Adrenaline ___AM___
3. Adrenocorticotropin ___AP___
4. Aldosterone ___AC___
5. Calcitonin ___Thy___
6. Corticosterone ___AC___
7. Epinephrine ___AM___
8. Follicle-stimulating hormone ___AP___
9. Glucagon ___Pan___
10. Glucocorticoids ___AC___
11. Growth hormone ___AP___
12. Insulin ___Pan___
13. Lactogenic hormone ___AP___
14. Luteinizing hormone ___AP___
15. Melanocyte-stimulating hormone ___AP___
16. Melatonin ___Pin___
17. Norepinephrine ___AM___
18. Oxytocin ___PP___
19. Prolactin ___AP___
20. Somatotropin ___AP___
21. Thyrotropic hormone ___AP___
22. Thyroxine ___Thy___
23. Triiodothyronine ___Thy___
24. TSH ___AP___
25. Vasopressin ___PP___

Exercise 2: Match the hormone in the right column with its function in the left column by placing the appropriate letter in the blank space provided.

H	1. Affects the circadian rhythms of animals	~~A. ACTH~~
B	2. Lowers blood calcium levels	~~B. Calcitonin~~
L	3. Promotes bone and soft tissue growth in young animals	~~C. Epinephrine~~
D	4. Promotes secondary sex development of female animals	~~D. Estrogens~~
J	5. Raises blood calcium levels	~~E. FSH~~
I	6. Regulates sodium and potassium levels in blood	~~F. Insulin~~
F	7. Regulates use and storage of carbohydrates	~~G. LH~~
G	8. Stimulates development of interstitial cells of testes	~~H. Melatonin~~
M	9. Stimulates hormone production by thyroid gland	~~I. Mineralocorticoids~~
K	10. Stimulates mammary gland development	~~J. Parathyroid hormone~~
A	11. Stimulates release of corticosteroids by adrenal cortex	~~K. Prolactin~~
E	12. Stimulates estrogen secretion by ovaries	~~L. Somatotropin~~
C	13. Stimulates sympathetic nervous system responses	~~M. TSH~~
N	14. Stimulates water reabsorption by kidney tubules	~~N. Vasopressin~~

Exercise 3: Using the following list of terms, identify each part in Fig. 13-3 by writing the name in the corresponding blank.

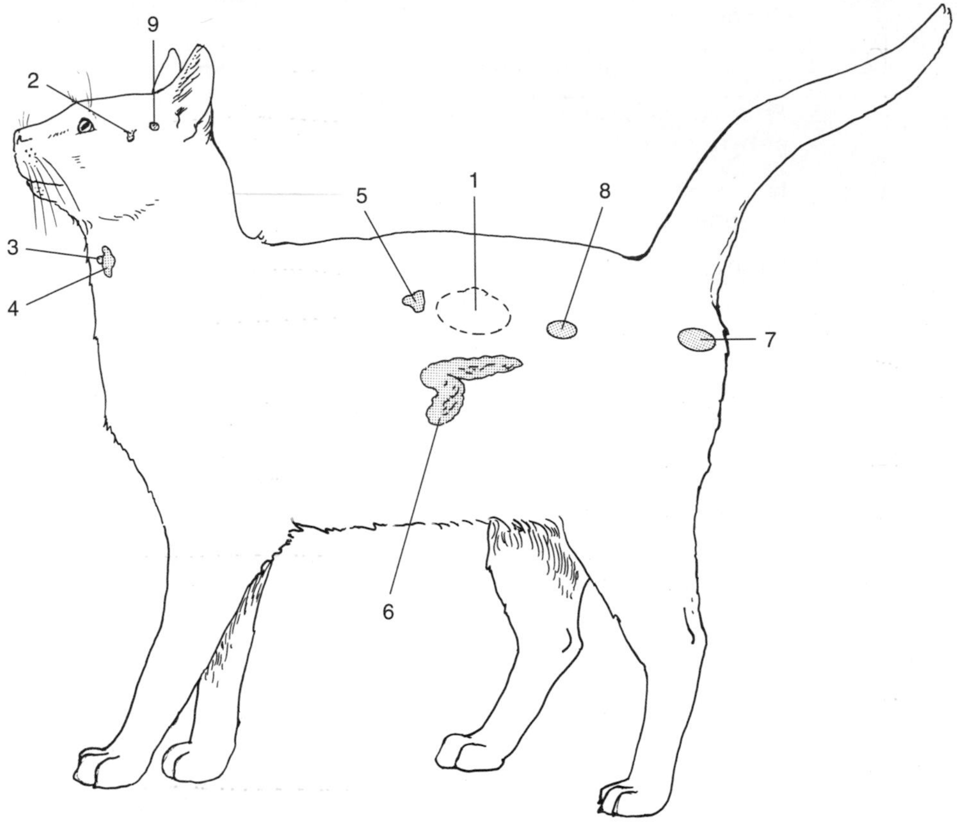
9
2
1
5
8
3
4
7
6

FIG. 13-3 Relative location of the endocrine glands in the cat.

~~Adrenal gland~~	1. ________________
~~Ovary (female)~~	2. ________________
~~Kidney~~	3. ________________
~~Thyroid gland~~	4. ________________
~~Pineal gland~~	5. ________________
Pituitary gland (hypophysis)	6. ________________
Parathyroid glands	7. ________________
~~Testis (male)~~	8. ________________
Pancreas	9. ________________

Exercise 4: Give the meaning of the components in the following words, and then define the word as a whole. Check the glossary at the end of the chapter if you need help.

1. Adrenalopathy
   adrenalo adrenals
   pathy disease
   ______

2. Euthyroid
   eu normal
   thyroid thyroid
   ______

3. Hypothyroidism
   hypo dehydration
   thyroid thyroid
   ism Condition
   ______

4. Hypoadrenocorticism
   hypo dehydration
   adreno adrenals
   cortic Cortex
   ism Condition
   ______

5. Hypogonadism
   hypo dehydration
   gonad gonad
   ism Condition
   ______

6. Hyperthyroidism
   hyper excessive
   thyroid thyroid
   ism Condition
   ______

7. Adrenal hyperplasia
   hyper excessive
   plasia growth
   ______

8. Thyrotoxicosis
   thyro thyroid
   toxic poison
   osis Condition
   ______

9. Polyuria
   poly excessive
   ur urine
   ia Condition
   ______

10. Thyroidectomy
   thyroid thyroid
   ectomy cutting out
   ______

CHAPTER 13 PUZZLE

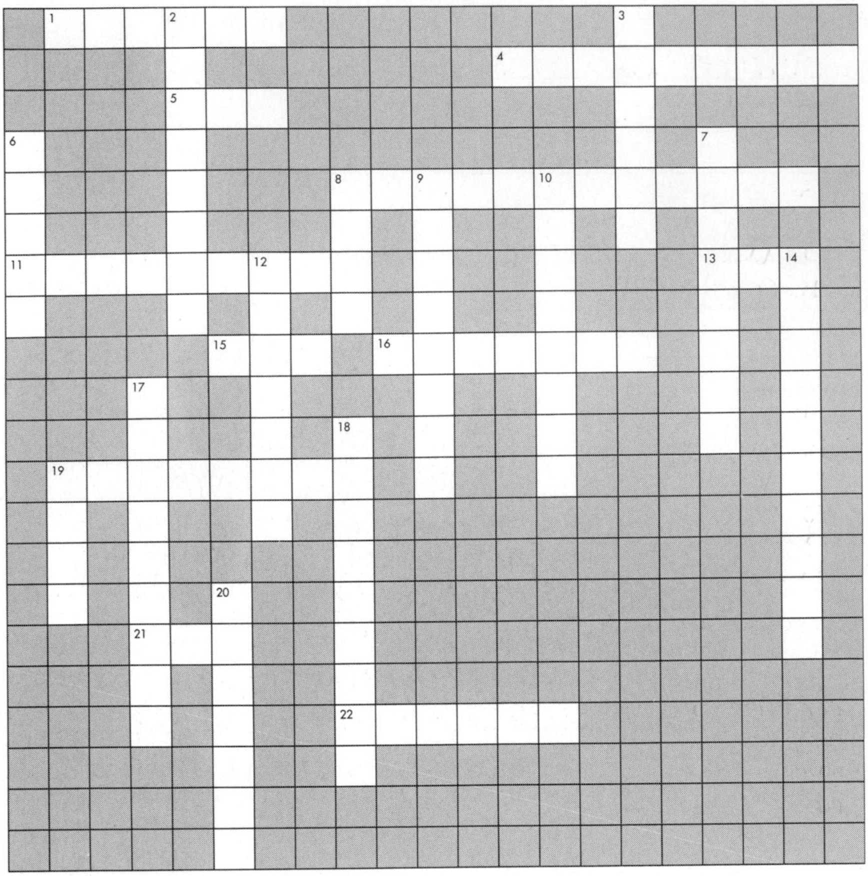
1
2
3
4
5
6
7
8
9
10
11
12
13
14
15
16
17
18
19
20
21
22

ACROSS CLUES

1. Gland resembling pine cone
4. Pituitary gland
5. Abbreviation for *thyrotropic hormone*
8. Female sex hormone
11. A lobe of pituitary
13. Abbreviation for *melanocyte-stimulating hormone*
15. Abbreviation for *follicle-stimulating hormone*
16. Fluid filling thyroid sacs
19. A lobe of the pituitary
21. Principal cells of parathyroid
22. Element of thyroid hormone

DOWN CLUES

2. Female sex hormone
3. Outer portion of adrenals
6. This and capillaries carry hormones throughout body
7. Secretions of ductless glands
8. Means alongside or next to
9. Stimulates uterine contraction
10. All cortical adrenal hormones
12. Secretion of pancreas
14. Pituitary gland
17. Master gland
18. Hormone of milk production
19. Abbreviation for *adrenocorticotropin*
20. Gland in neck

Chapter 13 Answers

Exercise 1

1. PP
2. AM
3. AP
4. AC
5. Thy
6. AC
7. AM
8. AP
9. Pan
10. AC
11. AP
12. Pan
13. AP
14. AP
15. AP
16. Pin
17. AM
18. PP
19. AP
20. AP
21. AP
22. Thy
23. Thy
24. AP
25. PP

Exercise 2

1. H
2. B
3. L
4. D
5. J
6. I
7. F
8. G
9. M
10. K
11. A
12. E
13. C
14. N

Exercise 3

1. kidney
2. pituitary gland (hypophysis)
3. parathyroid glands
4. thyroid gland
5. adrenal gland
6. pancreas
7. testis (male)
8. ovary (female)
9. pineal gland

Exercise 4

1. adrenals; disease; any disease of the adrenal glands
2. normal; thyroid; normal-functioning thyroid gland
3. deficient; thyroid; condition; decreased function of the thyroid gland
4. deficient; adrenal gland; cortex; condition; decreased function of the adrenal cortex
5. deficient; gonad; condition; decreased function of the gonads
6. excessive; thyroid; condition; excessive secretion by the thyroid gland
7. excessive; growth; excessive growth of adrenal tissue
8. thyroid; poison; condition; poisoning caused by excess secretion of the thyroid gland
9. excessive; urine; condition; excessive production of urine
10. thyroid; cutting out; surgical removal of the thyroid gland

ANSWERS: CHAPTER 13 PUZZLE

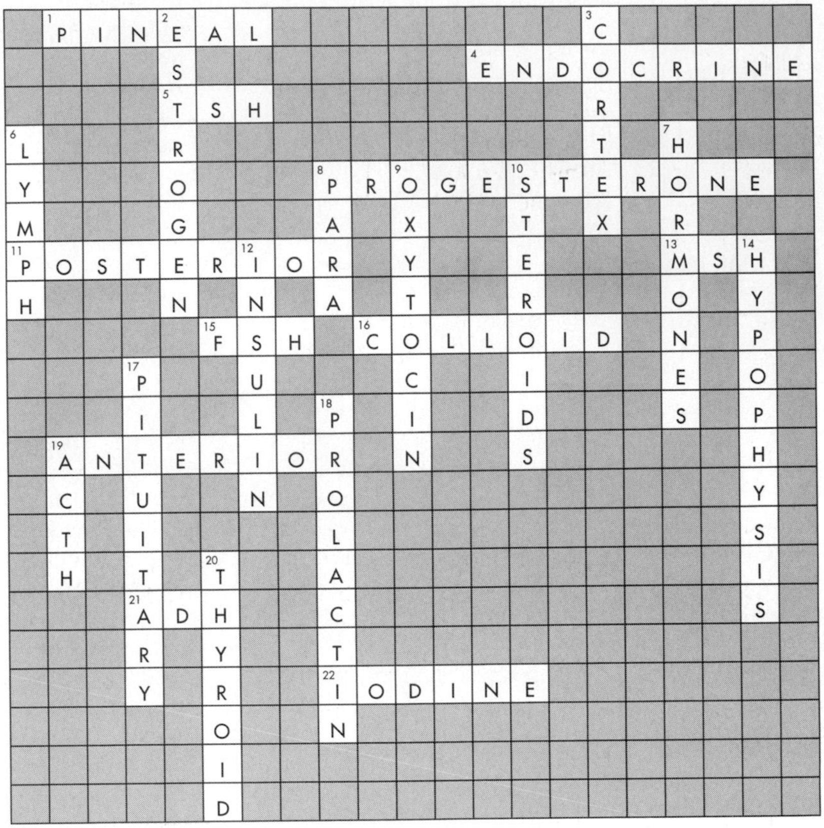
1 PINEAL
2 ESTROGEN
3 CORTEX
4 ENDOCRINE
5 TSH
6 LYMPH
7 HORMONES
8 PROGESTERONE
8 PARA
9 OXYTOCIN
10 STEROIDS
11 POSTERIOR
12 INSULIN
13 MSH
14 HYPOPHYSIS
15 FSH
16 COLLOID
17 PITUITARY
18 PROLACTIN
19 ANTERIOR
19 ACTH
20 THYROID
21 ADH
22 IODINE

GLOSSARY

ENDOCRINE GLANDS, HORMONES, AND RELATED ANATOMIC TERMS

acidophil (ah-sid'o-fil): acid-staining cell of anterior lobe of pituitary gland; secretes growth and lactogenic hormones.

adenohypophysis (ad"e-no-hi-pof'i-sis): anterior lobe of pituitary gland (hypophysis), as distinguished from posterior lobe (neurohypophysis).

adrenal glands: glands located near kidney (also called *suprarenal glands*).

adrenaline (ad-ren'ah-lin): adrenal medulla hormone, which stimulates smooth muscle, cardiac muscle, and glands, to assist body in meeting stress (also called *epinephrine*).

adrenalopathy (ad-re"nal-op'ah-the): any adrenal gland pathology (also called *adrenopathy*).

adrenocorticotropin (ACTH) (ad-re"no-kor"ti-ko-trop'in): hormone of anterior pituitary gland that promotes growth and development of adrenal cortex and stimulates cortex to secrete glucocorticoids (also spelled *adrenocorticotrophin*).

androsterone (an-dros'ter-ōn): androgen or male sex hormone secreted by adrenal gland.

antidiuretic hormone (ADH): hormone secreted by posterior pituitary that stimulates water reabsorption by distal and collecting kidney tubules (also called *vasopressin*).

basophils: basic-staining cells of anterior lobe of pituitary which secrete thyrotropin, a thyroid-stimulating hormone (TSH), adrenocorticotropin (ACTH), follicle-stimulating hormone (FSH), luteinizing hormone (LH), and melanocyte-stimulating hormone (MSH).

chorionic gonadotropin: hormone secreted by cells of placental chorion.

chromophobe (kro'mo-fōb): non-staining cell of anterior pituitary lobe.

colloid (kol'oid): gelatinous substance in follicles of thyroid gland that contain hormone secreted by thyroid.

cortex (kor'teks): outer portion of adrenal gland that secretes mineralocorticoids, glucocorticoids, androgens, and some estrogens.

corticosterone (kor"ti-kos'ter-ōn): adrenocortical glucocorticoid hormone.

cortisol (kor'tĭ-sol): adrenocortical glucocorticoid hormone (also called *hydrocortisone*).

estrogenic hormones: ovarian hormones (estradiol and estrone) that influence cycle of changes (estrus) in female genital tract.

euthyroid (u-thi'roid): normally functioning thyroid gland.

follicle-stimulating hormone (FSH): anterior pituitary hormone that stimulates growth of ovarian follicles and secretion of estrogen in the female and development of seminiferous tubules and sperm cells in male.

glucocorticoid: group of adrenocortical steroids that are concerned with protein, fat, and carbohydrate metabolism and aid body in resisting stress.

gonadotropic hormones: pituitary hormones that influence gonads.

hormone: chemical substance secreted by endocrine gland.

hypophysis cerebri (hi-pof'ĭ-sis): another name for pituitary gland.

infundibulum (in"fun-dib'u-lum): funnel-shaped passage with neural tracts from hypothalamus of brain to pituitary gland.

iodine (i-o'dīn): essential element of thyroid hormone.

islands of Langerhans (lahng'er-hanz): specialized pancreatic cells secreting insulin, glucagon, and pancreatic polypeptide (PP) into circulation.

luteinizing hormone (LH): anterior pituitary hormone that stimulates formation of corpus luteum and progesterone in female and development and secretion of testosterone in interstitial cells of testes.

medulla: inner portion of adrenal glands producing epinephrine and norepinephrine.

mineralocorticoid: adrenocortical steroid that affects sodium and potassium balance.

neurohypophysis: posterior lobe of pituitary gland.

norepinephrine: hormone secreted by adrenal medulla (also called *noradrenaline*).

oxyphil (ok'se-fil): cell in parathyroid glands.

oxytocin (ok"se-to'sin): hormone of posterior lobe of pituitary gland that stimulates uterine contractions during parturition.

parathyroid hormone: parathyroid gland secretion that regulates calcium and phosphorus content of blood and bones.

parathyroids: glands, normally two on each side, behind or embedded in thyroid gland.

pineal body: small gland located near base of brain.

pituicyte (pĭ-tu'ĭ-sīt): fusiform cell of posterior lobe of pituitary gland.

pituitary gland (pĭ-tu'ĭ-tār"e): master gland attached to base of brain that exercises control over other endocrine glands.

progesterone: hormone produced by corpus luteum, whose function is to prepare uterus to receive fertilized ovum by causing growth and development of uterine endometrial lining.

prolactin: pituitary hormone responsible for mammary gland development and milk production in pregnancy.

somatotropin (so"mah-to-tro'pin): growth hormone (GH) secreted by acidophils and anterior pituitary gland (also called *somatotrophin*).

suprarenals: adrenal glands.

testosterone: masculinizing hormone of testis that induces and maintains secondary sex characteristics.

thyroid (thi'roid): large gland situated on the front part of neck just below larynx.

thyrotropin (thi'rot'ro-pin): thyroid-stimulating hormone (TSH) of anterior pituitary gland that promotes growth and development of thyroid gland and stimulates it to secrete thyroxine and triiodothyronine, the two major hormones of thyroid gland (also called *thyrotrophin*).

thyroxine (thi-rok'sin): one of two iodine-laden hormones making up thyroid hormone, whose main function is to regulate metabolic rate and processes of growth and tissue differentiation (also called T_4).

triiodothyronine (tri"i-o"do-thi'ro-nēn): second of two hormones that make up thyroid hormone, containing less iodine than thyroxine but having the same functions (also called T_3).

vasopressin: antidiuretic hormone (ADH) of posterior pituitary.

PATHOLOGIC CONDITIONS OF THE ENDOCRINE SYSTEM

acromegaly (ak"ro-meg'ah-le): disease caused by pituitary hypersecretion of growth hormone after completion of bone development, characterized by enlargement of bones of the front and rear feet and face.

Addison's disease: life-threatening condition of adrenal insufficiency characterized by severe weakness, low blood pressure, anorexia, digestive disturbance, bradycardia, and altered sodium-potassium balance.

adrenal cortical carcinomas: malignant, metastasizing tumors of adrenal cortex, which produce Cushing's syndrome.

adrenalitis: inflammation of adrenal glands.

adrenocortical hyperfunction: overfunctioning of adrenal cortex.

adrenocortical hypofunction: underfunctioning of adrenal cortex.

anorexia (an"o rek'se-ah): lack or loss of appetite; symptom in some endocrine disorders.

basophilic adenoma: pituitary gland tumor whose cells stain with basic dyes.

cachexia (kah-kek'se-ah): general ill health and malnutrition, which may be symptomatic of some endocrine disorders.

chromophobic adenoma (kro'mo-fōb-ik): benign tumor of pituitary gland, whose cells resist staining with dyes.

Cushing's syndrome: pituitary basophilism, with excessive secretion of adrenocortical hormone, characterized by potbellied appearance, alopecia, increased thirst and urination, muscle wasting and thin skin (also called *hyperadrenocorticism*).

diabetes insipidus (di"ah-be'tēz in"sip'ĭ-dus): metabolic disorder characterized by polyuria and excessive thirst resulting from insufficient production of antidiuretic hormone (ADH).

diabetes mellitus: metabolic disease caused by absolute or relative lack of insulin; signs include increased thirst and urination and sugar in urine *(glucosuria).*

goiter (goi'ter): enlargement of thyroid.

hyperparathyroidism: hyperfunction of parathyroid gland of primary type resulting from neoplasms or unknown causes and secondary type because of metabolic disorder, producing calcium imbalance in bodily systems, with osteoporosis and deposition of calcium in tissues.

hyperthyroidism: overproduction of thyroid hormone, especially common in older cats.

hypogonadism: developmental disorder caused by inadequate secretion of pituitary gonadotropins, resulting in sexual immaturity and decreased functional activity of gonads in males and females.

hypoparathyroidism: insufficiency of parathyroid glands, which may be familial or because of excision, disease, or injury of thyroid or parathyroid glands, resulting in hypocalcemia, with increased bone density resulting from decreased bone resorption.

hypothyroidism: underfunction of thyroid gland.

parathyroid tetany: muscular cramps and spasms, resulting from hypocalcemia because of excision of or injury to parathyroids.

polydipsia: excessive thirst; symptom of diabetes.

polyuria: excessive urination; symptom of diabetes.

testicular tumors: seminoma, Sertoli's cell tumor (estrogen-secreting) and interstitial cell tumor (androgen secreting), usually benign tumors of testes; more common in cryptorchid testicles.

tetany: muscle spasm and cramp; symptom of hypoparathyroidism.

thyroid adenoma: benign tumor of thyroid gland; may occur in cats with hyperthyroidism.

thyroiditis: inflammation of thyroid gland.

thyrolytic: pertaining to substances destructive to thyroid gland.

thyropathy: any disease or disorder of thyroid gland.

SURGICAL PROCEDURES

adrenalectomy (ad-re″nal-ek′to-me): excision of adrenal glands.

hypophysectomy (hi″po-fiz-ek′to-me): excision of hypophysis or anterior pituitary gland.

parathyroidectomy: excision of parathyroid gland.

thyroidectomy: excision of thyroid gland.

LABORATORY TESTS AND PROCEDURES OF THE ENDOCRINE SYSTEM

ACTH (adrenocorticotropic hormone) stimulation test: test of adrenocortical function.

cortisol test: blood plasma test to measure levels of cortisol to detect diseases of adrenal glands.

dexamethasone suppression test: test of adrenocortical function.

estrogen receptor test: test to determine whether hormonal treatment will be used in cancer treatment by measuring response of cancer to estrogen.

protein-bound iodine (PBI) test: test of thyroid function in which blood protein-bound iodine is measured to estimate amount of available thyroid hormone in peripheral blood.

radioactive iodine uptake (RAIU) or thyroid^{131}I uptake test: thyroid function evaluated by introducing radioactive iodine orally or intravenously during selected time period and measuring its absorption by thyroid with counter.

thyroid hormone tests: triiodothyronine (T_3) thyroxine (T_4) thyroxine-binding globulin (TBG): group of blood tests to determine thyroid hormone levels and diagnose disorders of the thyroid.

thyroid scan: intravenous injection of radioactive substance for organ imaging to detect abnormalities in size, shape, location, and function of thyroid gland.

thyroid stimulation test: anterior pituitary thyroid-stimulating hormone (TSH) injected to determine whether thyroid problems result from pituitary or thyroid dysfunction.

thyroid ultrasonography: noninvasive procedure to detect cysts and tumors of thyroid by directing ultrasonic pulses at gland that are reflected back for display on oscilloscope.

14 The Nervous System

The central processing unit

white → myelonated (fatcovered)
gray → nerve cell bodies

CHAPTER OVERVIEW

This chapter explores the structure and functions of the nervous system, both central and peripheral, including the brain, spinal cord, and nerves.

SYSTEM CHARACTERISTICS

The nervous system has been compared with a computer system, with the brain acting as the central processing unit, relaying messages by way of the spinal cord, through nerve fibers. Nerves radiate to every structure in the body to provide connections for input and output data. Sensory nerves bring impulses or information from the various body systems, whereas motor nerves carry impulses from the central coordinating point to muscles or glands.

CNS & cerebrospinal system

The nervous system is divided into the *central nervous system (CNS),* which includes the brain and spinal cord, and the *peripheral nervous system (PNS),* which is composed of the cranial nerves, spinal nerves, autonomic nerves, and ganglia.

NERVE STRUCTURE AND FUNCTION

Nervous system cells are called *neurons.* All neurons are similar in that they have a cell body (or *soma*) and at least two processes: one *axon* and one or more *dendrites.* The cell body has a nucleus, which is responsible for maintaining the life of the whole nerve cell. The dendrites branch extensively, like tiny trees, conducting nerve impulses toward the cell body. The axon is a single process that extends out from the cell body and ends in a fine spreading branch called a *terminal twig.* A neuron's axon carries impulses away from the cell body. Axons vary in length and diameter and often have side branches called *axon collaterals* (Fig. 14-1).

The threadlike dendrites and axons are also called *nerve fibers.* Bundles of these fibers found together are called *nerves.* Groups of neuron cell bodies within the brain or spinal cord are called *nuclei,* whereas those outside are called *ganglia* (the singular is *ganglion*). A bundle of neuron fibers within the brain or spinal cord is known as a *tract.*

Nerve fibers are of different types. Some are myelinated, with a coat of white fatty material called a *myelin sheath* surrounding them. The myelin sheath is interrupted along the length of a fiber at regularly spaced intervals, known as *nodes of Ranvier.* Myelinated fibers are found mainly in the central nervous system. Some fibers have only a thin layer of myelin and are called *nonmyelinated.* Nonmyelinated fibers are found especially in the autonomic nervous system. Peripheral myelinated and nonmyelinated nerves have a continuous tubelike membrane covering called the *neurilemma* or *Schwann's sheath* (Fig. 14-2). There are axon fibers that have no sheath, found in the central nervous system and within organs.

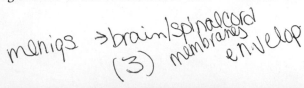

menigs → brain/spinalcord (3) membranes envelop

The nerve cells and their gossamer filaments are held together and supported by a specialized type of tissue called *neuroglia.* Neuroglial cells have many processes or branches that form a dense network between neurons. They are divided into four main types: *astrocytes* (*astro* means star), *microglia, oligodendroglia,* and *Schwann cells.* Astrocytes cover the surfaces of the capillaries of the brain and together with the walls of the capillaries form the *blood-brain barrier.* The blood-brain barrier regulates the passage of nutritive and chemical molecules to the brain neurons. Microglia are phagocytic cells that fight infection and help in healing. Oligodendroglia aid in holding nerve fibers together and forming the myelin sheath in the central nervous system. Schwann cells, which are only found outside the central nervous system, form the neurilemma and a thin layer of myelin around nerve fibers.

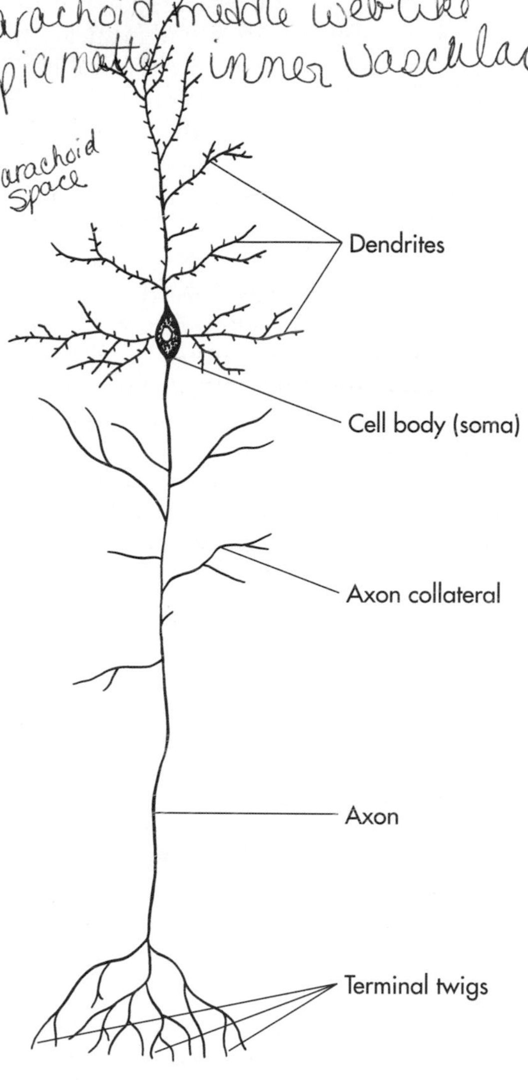
Dendrites
Cell body (soma)
Axon collateral
Axon
Terminal twigs

FIG. 14-1 A typical neuron, showing the cell body, dendrites, and axons.

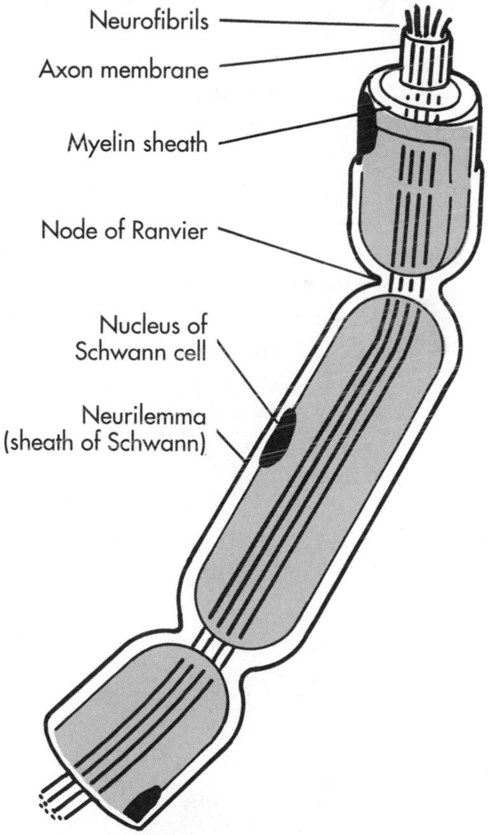
Neurofibrils
Axon membrane
Myelin sheath
Node of Ranvier
Nucleus of Schwann cell
Neurilemma (sheath of Schwann)

FIG. 14-2 Diagram of a nerve and its coverings.

Neurons are divided into *sensory* (or *afferent*), *motor* (or *efferent*), and *connector* (or *interneuron*) neurons. In sensory neurons, the dendrites are connected to receptors (eyes, ears, and other sense organs), and the axons are connected to other neurons. The receptors change information from external sources, such as light waves or sound vibrations, into electrical impulses. In motor neurons, the dendrites are connected to other neurons and the axons to affecters (muscles and glands). In connector neurons, the dendrites and axons are connected to other neurons (Fig. 14-3).

Normally, impulses pass in only one direction. Sensory neurons conduct impulses from the sense organs to the spinal cord and brain. Motor neurons conduct impulses from the brain and spinal cord to muscles and glands. The impulses are essentially the same in all types of neurons. The initiating stimulus of the impulse in one section of a nerve fiber causes a similar reaction in the next connecting section. This chain reaction continues until the impulse reaches the end of the nerve fiber. Nerve impulses differ only in terms of the body part affected: an impulse created by light rays entering the eye may result in vision, an impulse received in the ear may result in hearing, other impulses may result in muscle movement, and still others may result in glandular secretions.

The point at which an impulse is transmitted from the axon of one neuron to the dendrite of another is a microscopic space called a *synapse*. There is no physical contact of neurons at the synapse. The electrical impulses from one neuron to the next neuron do not directly jump the synapse but instead cause release of a chemical at the synapse. The *neurotransmitter* chemical is released from vesicles in the axon terminal to activate other impulses in the dendrites of connecting neurons (Fig. 14-4).

Injury to nervous tissue elicits responses by neurons and neuroglia. If the injury is severe, cell death occurs. Neurons are so specialized that they have lost the power to reproduce new cells. When an axon is severed, that part distal to the cell body dies. A new axon may gradually grow and restore the nerve, but such regeneration occurs only in the peripheral nervous system. Once a connection is broken within the central nervous system, it is broken forever. Other nerve structures may take over the functions of the injured nerves.

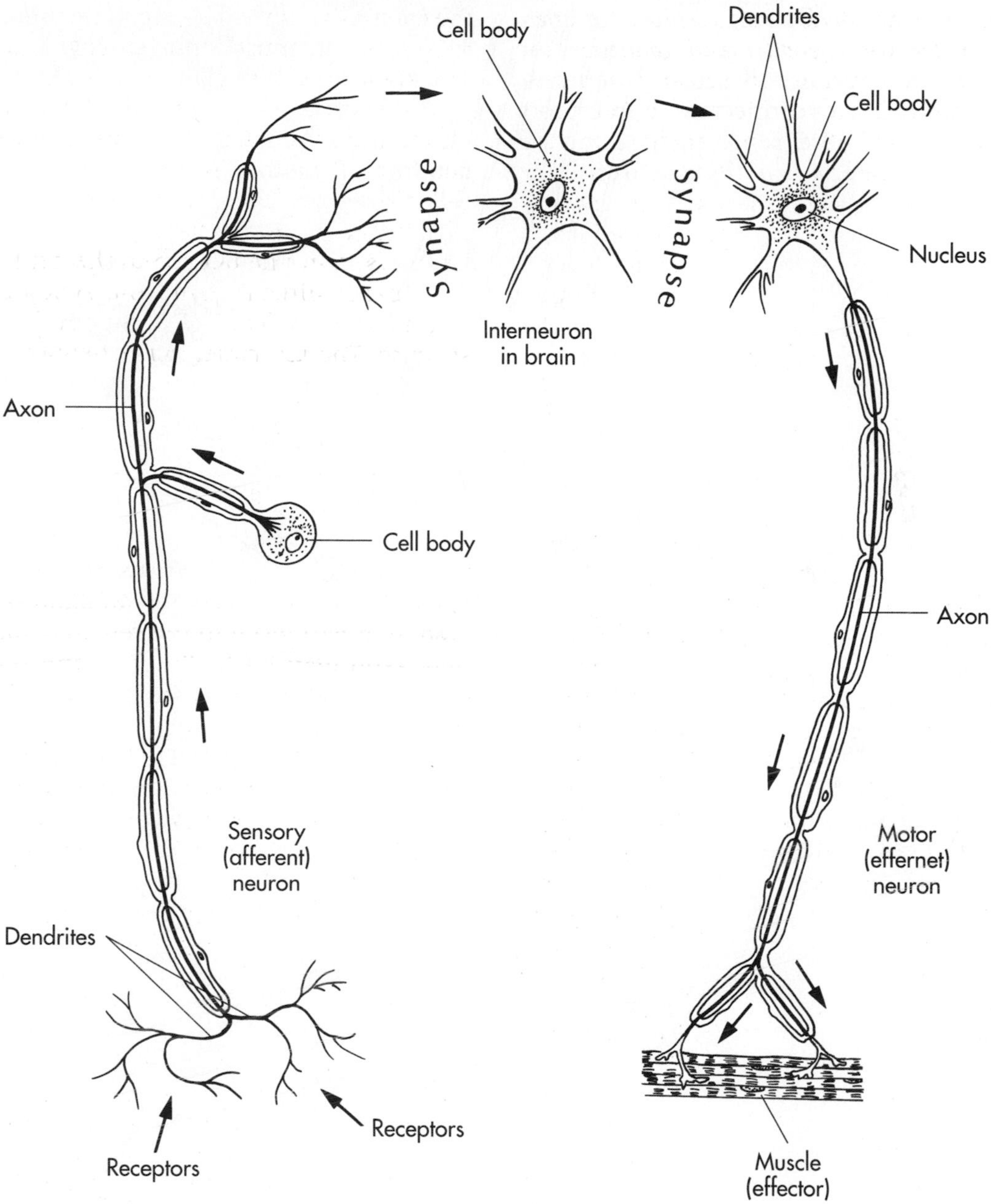
Cell body
Dendrites
Cell body
Synapse
Synapse
Nucleus
Interneuron
in brain
Axon
Cell body
Axon
Sensory
(afferent)
neuron
Motor
(effernet)
neuron
Dendrites
Receptors
Receptors
Muscle
(effector)

FIG. 14-3 Types of neurons involved in a reflex arc.

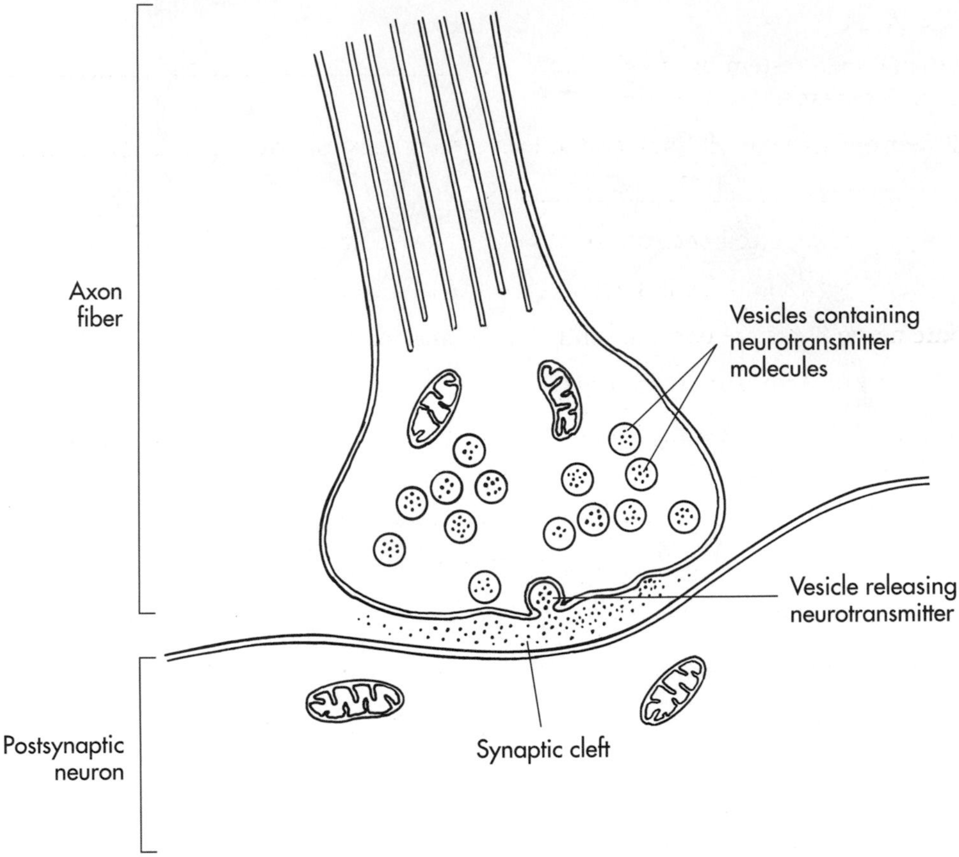
Axon
fiber
Vesicles containing
neurotransmitter
molecules
Vesicle releasing
neurotransmitter
Postsynaptic
neuron
Synaptic cleft

FIG. 14-4 Components of the synapse.

REVIEW A

1. The nervous system is divided into the ________________ and ________________ nervous systems.
2. All neurons have a cell body and at least two processes: one ____________________ and one or more ____________________ .
3. Groups of neuron cell bodies *within* the brain and spinal cord are called ________________ .
4. Groups of neuron cell bodies *outside* the brain and spinal cord are called ________________ .
5. Some nerve fibers are covered with a white fatty material called ____________________ .
6. The sheath of Schwann is also called the ________________ .
7. The ____________________ regulates the passage of nutritive and chemical molecules to the brain neurons.
8. Neurons are divided into ____________________ or afferent, ____________________ or efferent, and ____________________ or interneuron neurons.
9. Receptors change information from external sources such as light waves into electrical ____________________ .
10. The microscopic space over which an impulse is transmitted is called a/an ______________ .

CENTRAL NERVOUS SYSTEM

The central nervous system includes the brain and spinal cord. This system is also called the *cerebrospinal system*. The brain lies in the cranial cavity. The spinal cord lies within the spinal cavity, extending from the *foramen magnum*, an opening in the occipital bone of the head, down through the vertebral column. The brain and spinal cord are both protected from injury by the skeletal system: the brain by the bones of the skull, the spinal cord by the vertebrae.

The central nervous system contains both white and gray matter. The white color is created by the myelinated fibers of the bundles of axons and dendrites. The gray color is created by the masses of nerve cell bodies.

The Meninges

The meninges (*meninx* means membrane; the plural is *meninges*) are three membranes that envelop the central nervous system, separating the brain and spinal cord from the body cavities. The meninges are composed predominantly of white, fibrous connective tissue, giving support and protection to the brain and spinal cord.

The *dura mater*, the outermost layer, is the hardest, toughest, and most fibrous of the three. The *arachnoid* (*arachno* means spider), the middle membrane, is much less dense and is weblike in appearance. The *pia mater*, the innermost, thin, compact membrane that is closely adapted to the surface of the brain and spinal cord, is very vascular and supplies the blood for the central nervous system tissue.

The space between the dura mater and the arachnoid is known as the *subdural space.* Between the arachnoid and the pia mater is another space, the *subarachnoid space* (Fig. 14-5). Inflammation of the meninges is called *meningitis.* Meningitis most often involves the arachnoid and pia mater or the *leptomeninges,* as they are sometimes called.

The Brain

The brain is the greatly enlarged part of the central nervous system, containing about 100 billion neurons. The brain in the dog and cat is a highly evolved structure but is less well developed than in more specialized mammals, such as primates. The canine brain is more immature than the human brain at birth, but maturation of cerebral function proceeds at a higher rate. A 1-month-old puppy has near-adult development of the central nervous system.

The divisions of the brain are the *forebrain,* the *midbrain,* and the *hindbrain* (Fig. 14-6, *A*).

THE FOREBRAIN

The *telencephalon* and *diencephalon* together are called the *forebrain.* The telencephalon includes the *cerebrum,* the *corpora striata,* and the *rhinencephalon* (or *olfactory brain*). The diencephalon includes the *thalamus,* the *epithalamus,* and the *hypothalamus* (Fig. 14-6, *B*).

The Telencephalon

The cerebrum, the largest part of the brain, is divided into two hemispheres called the *cerebral hemispheres,* which occupy most of the brain cavity. The outer surface, or *cervical cortex,* is made up of gray matter, beneath which is white matter, which forms the central portion of the brain. As the brain develops, the cerebral hemispheres increase greatly in size in relation to the rest of the brain. As the gray matter ~~of the cortex increases in amount, the surface of each cerebral hemisphere~~ is thrown into ~~folds called~~ *gyri* (the singular is *gyrus*) or *convolutions.* The gyri are separated from each other by furrows called *sulci* (the singular is *sulcus*), with deeper furrows called *fissures.*

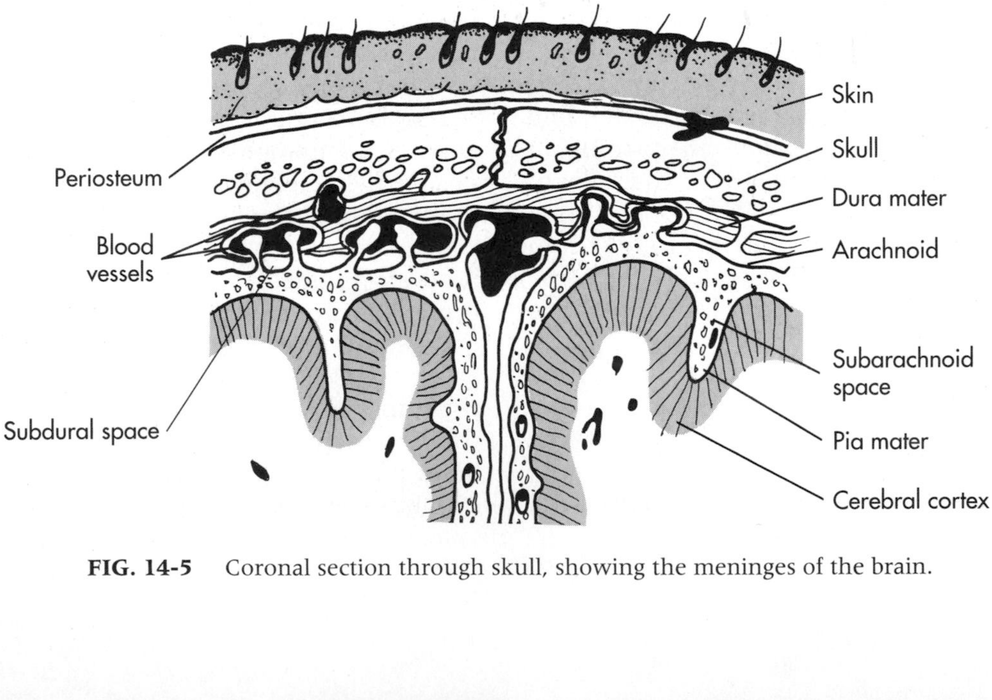
Skin
Skull
Periosteum
Dura mater
Blood vessels
Arachnoid
Subarachnoid space
Subdural space
Pia mater
Cerebral cortex

FIG. 14-5 Coronal section through skull, showing the meninges of the brain.

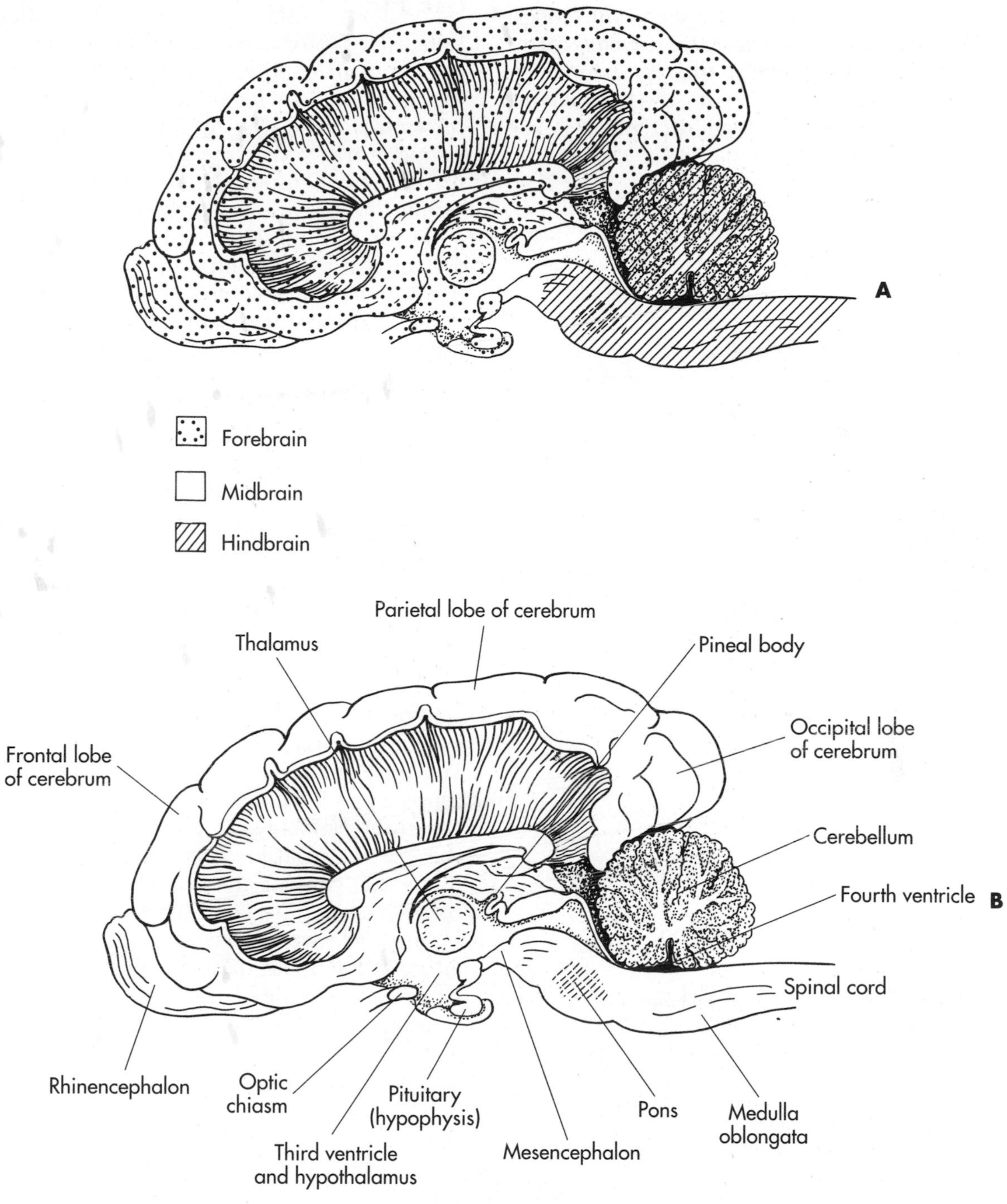
A
Forebrain
Midbrain
Hindbrain
Parietal lobe of cerebrum
Thalamus
Pineal body
Frontal lobe of cerebrum
Occipital lobe of cerebrum
Cerebellum
Fourth ventricle
B
Spinal cord
Rhinencephalon
Optic chiasm
Pituitary (hypophysis)
Third ventricle and hypothalamus
Mesencephalon
Pons
Medulla oblongata

FIG. 14-6 **A,** Sagittal section of the brain showing major divisions. **B,** Sagittal section of the brain showing major structures.

The cerebral cortex is divided into lobes: *frontal, temporal, parietal,* and *occipital,* corresponding to the bones in the region in which they are located (Fig. 14-7). The frontal lobe, the most anterior of all the lobes, is the center for voluntary movement. It is often called the motor area, containing areas for control of gross, fine, and complicated muscle movements. The parietal lobe collects, recognizes, and organizes sensations of pain, temperature, touch, position, and movement. The temporal lobe contains the centers for awareness and correlations of auditory stimuli. The occipital lobe forms the posterior extremity of each cerebral hemisphere. It involves visual perception and visual memory and plays a role in eye movements.

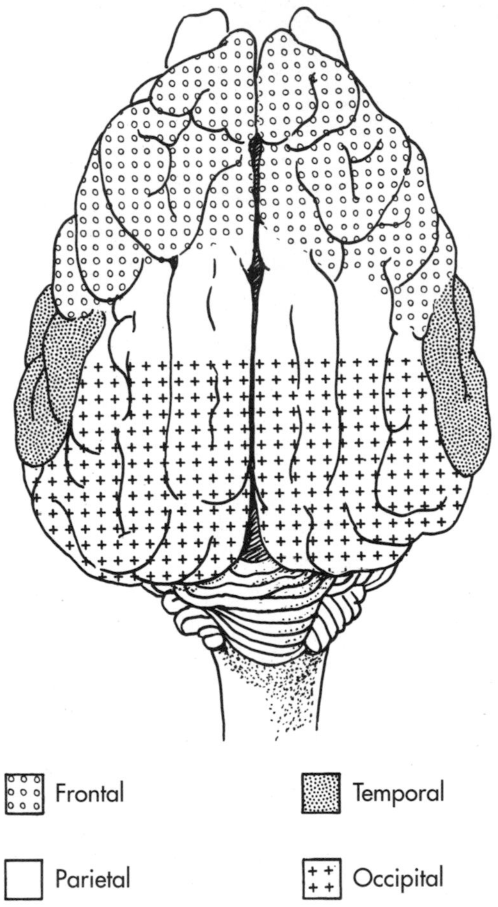
Frontal
Temporal
Parietal
Occipital

FIG. 14-7 Dorsal view of the brain showing lobes of the cerebral cortex.

The left hemisphere of the cerebrum controls the right side of the body, and the right hemisphere controls the left side of the body. General differences in cerebral hemispheric function appear to exist in humans. The left hemisphere, which is usually dominant, is involved in language, logic, analytic thinking, and ordering of events and symbols. The right hemisphere has been linked to imagination, creativity in art and music, and spatial and depth perception.

The *corpus striatum* of each cerebral hemisphere consists of a mixture of white and gray matter, giving it a striated appearance. The gray matter of the corpus striatum is represented by a number of nuclear masses called the *basal ganglia.* The white matter of the corpus striatum consists of projection fibers that connect the cerebral cortex with other parts of the central nervous system.

The *rhinencephalon* is more developed in animals than in humans. It is primarily associated with a sense of smell and is sometimes referred to as the olfactory brain.

REVIEW B

1. Another name for the central nervous system is the ________________________ system.
2. The three meningeal membranes are the ____________________, ____________________, and ____________________.
3. The three divisions of the brain are the ____________________, ____________________, and ____________________.
4. Using the following drawing, indicate the area corresponding to the forebrain by stippling and the hindbrain areas by shading. The areas corresponding to the midbrain will remain in white.
5. The ________________________ and ________________________ together are called the forebrain.
6. The outer surface of gray matter in the cerebrum is called the ____________________.
7. The cerebral cortex is made up of four lobes: the ________________, ________________, ________________, and ________________.
8. The left cerebral hemisphere controls the ____________________ side of the body, and the right cerebral hemisphere controls the ____________________ side of the body.
9. The ____________________ of each cerebral hemisphere consists of a mixture of white and gray matter, giving it a striated appearance.
10. The olfactory brain is called the ____________________.

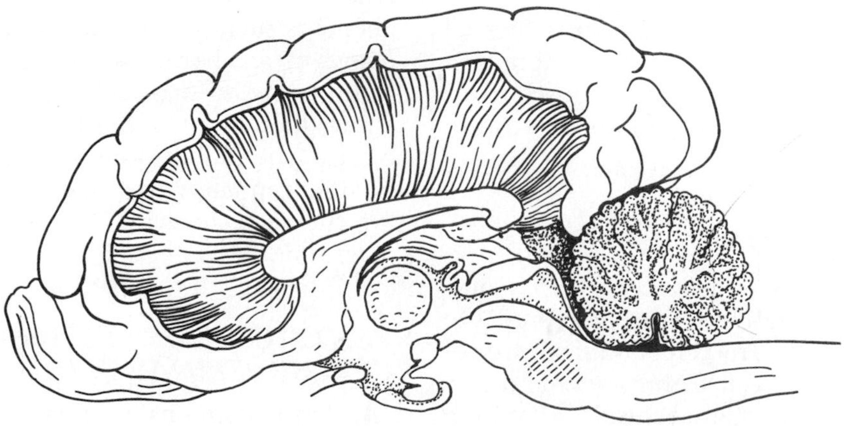

The Diencephalon

The diencephalon is the part of the forebrain that contains the *thalamus,* the *epithalamus,* and the *hypothalamus* (*thalamus* means chamber). The thalamus is a large, gray, oval mass that acts as a center to receive sensory impulses and transmit them to the cerebral cortex. The thalamus has been called the great integrating center of the brain because it plays a role in integrating visual, auditory, tactile, temperature, pain, and taste sensations. The epithalamus contains an olfactory correlation center and the pineal body. The pineal body regulates gonadal hormones and certain *circadian rhythms.* Circadian rhythms are the regular recurrence of biological activities that occur at about the same time each day or night regardless of constant exposure to darkness or light. The hypothalamus is a small but important structure located beneath the thalamus. It plays a role in controlling body temperature, sleep, and the behavior for feeding and drinking. The hypothalamus functions in association with the autonomic nervous and endocrine systems. The *optic chiasm,* part of the visual pathway, is also located in the diencephalon (Fig. 14-6, *B*).

THE MIDBRAIN

The midbrain, or *mesencephalon,* is located between the forebrain and the hindbrain. It contains auditory, visual, and muscle control centers and is involved in body posture and equilibrium.

THE HINDBRAIN

The hindbrain or *rhombencephalon* is composed of the *cerebellum,* the *pons,* and the *medulla oblongata.* The cerebellum consists of a central portion called the *vermis* and two larger sections, one on each side, called the right and left *cerebellar hemispheres.* The cerebellum fine-tunes motor activity and muscle tone, which are essential for precise and complicated voluntary movement and the maintenance of posture. Infection of a pregnant cat with panleukopenia virus (feline distemper) or treatment with certain drugs can cause *cerebellar hypoplasia,* a degeneration and deficiency of cerebellar cells, in the kittens.

The pons, made up of a reticular formation or network and white matter, serves as a bridge connecting the cerebrum, cerebellum, and the medulla oblongata.

The medulla oblongata is the cranial continuation of the spinal cord, from which it is arbitrarily separated at the *foramen magnum.* The foramen magnum is the largest foramen or natural opening in the skull. Reflex centers for controlling respiration and circulation are located in the medulla oblongata. The medulla oblongata is composed of white matter and reticular formation. The reticular formation is a mixture of white and gray matter. The *reticular activating system,* which functions in maintaining alertness and awareness, is located in the reticular formation.

LIMBIC SYSTEM

The *limbic system* appears to be a center for emotional activity and behavior located in deeper structures of the brain. The term *limbus* means border or marginal and refers to the structures surrounding the ventricular cavities and the border of the cerebral cortex. The limbic system involves areas of the diencephalon and the cerebrum including the *cingulate gyrus, hypothalamus, amygdala,* and *hippocampus.*

VENTRICLES OF THE BRAIN AND CEREBROSPINAL FLUID

The brain contains four large, fluid-filled cavities called *ventricles,* which interconnect with each other. The right and left *lateral ventricles* are located in the respective cerebral hemispheres. The third ventricle is located in the diencephalon. The fourth ventricle, located beneath the cerebellum and above the medulla, communicates with the *subarachnoid space.*

The *cerebrospinal fluid* is a thin, transparent, watery fluid within the ventricles of the brain, the central canal of the spinal cord, and the subarachnoid spaces. The cerebrospinal fluid serves as a protective cushion for the brain and spinal cord and provides some nutrients. It is produced by a network of capillaries called the *choroid plexus.* Cerebrospinal fluid drains from the lateral ventricles to the third and fourth ventricles, finally passing into the subarachnoid spaces. Occasionally, some condition interferes with the flow of cerebrospinal fluid. *Hydrocephalus,* or water on the brain, is caused by an abnormal accumulation of cerebrospinal fluid in the ventricular system.

REVIEW C

1. The diencephalon is part of the forebrain that contains the thalamus, the ________________, and the ________________.
2. The ______________________ is located beneath the thalamus and plays a role in controlling body temperature, sleep, and behavior for feeding and drinking.
3. The ______________________ is located between the forebrain and the hindbrain.
4. The hindbrain is also called the ______________________.
5. The hindbrain is composed of the ______________________, ______________________, and ______________________.
6. The ______________________ is responsible for fine-tuning motor activity and muscle tone.
7. The ______________________ is the cranial continuation of the spinal cord.
8. The ______________________ system is a center for emotional activity and behavior and is located deep in the brain.
9. The ______________________ fluid acts to protect and cushion the brain and spinal cord.
10. Cerebrospinal fluid is produced by a network of capillaries called the ________________.

Spinal Cord

The spinal cord is an essential extension of the central processing unit, the brain. Sensations received by the sensory nerves are relayed to the spinal cord, where they are transferred to the brain or to motor nerves. If the sensation is transferred to a motor nerve, it travels out to a muscle or gland and produces an action.

The spinal cord resembles a flattened cylinder, extending from the medulla oblongata to the lower lumbar vertebrae. The spinal cord is enclosed in the vertebral column, which protects it from injury. Like the brain, it has three membranous coverings—the pia mater, arachnoid, and dura mater—and is bathed in cerebrospinal fluid. The spinal cord is made up of an inner core of gray matter and an outer core of white matter. In cross-section, the gray matter of the spinal cord resembles a butterfly with its wings divided into two dorsal and two ventral parts, called *horns*. The outer white matter of the spinal cord contains the tracts (Fig. 14-8).

Both ascending and descending tracts are contained in the spinal cord. The ascending tracts conduct the *afferent* (sensory) nerve impulses to the brain. The descending tracts conduct the *efferent* (motor) nerve impulses from the brain. Centers for connections between the afferent and the efferent nerve impulses are provided by the gray matter.

Through the spinal cord and the pairs of spinal nerves along its sides, the brain maintains intimate association with all organs of the body. Injury of the spinal cord in any segment can imperil any or all of its functions. When the spinal cord is injured, the part above the injury functions normally. There is paralysis of the part below the injury, and the brain receives no impulses from that area.

THE PERIPHERAL NERVOUS SYSTEM

12 pairs cranial nerves

The *peripheral nervous system* provides a means of communication by which stimuli are transmitted from receptor organs to the central nervous system and from the central nervous system to the proper effector organs in the body, muscles, or glands. The peripheral nervous system includes all nerves and ganglia located outside the brain and spinal

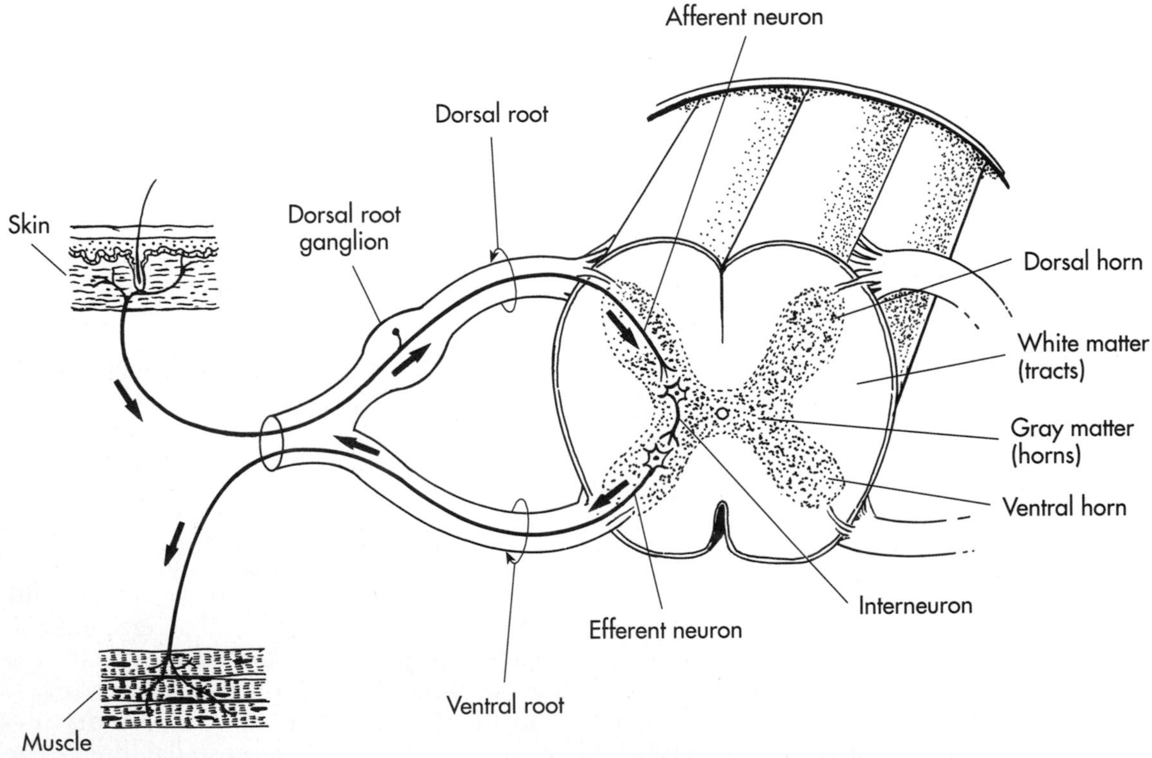
Afferent neuron
Dorsal root
Skin
Dorsal root ganglion
Dorsal horn
White matter (tracts)
Gray matter (horns)
Ventral horn
Interneuron
Efferent neuron
Ventral root
Muscle

FIG. 14-8 Cross-section of the spinal cord showing a reflex arc.

cord, including the cranial nerves, spinal nerves, and autonomic nerves.

Cranial Nerves

The first segment of the peripheral nervous system is the 12 pairs of cranial nerves (Fig. 14-9). Cranial nerves can be identified by name or number. By convention, they are numbered with Roman numerals as they arise from the brain. The trigeminal is the largest of the cranial nerves and the vagus is the longest, having extensive distribution to the body.

Spinal Nerves

The spinal nerves arise from the spinal cord and emerge from the vertebrae. After leaving the spinal cord, the nerves are named after their corresponding vertebrae. A spinal nerve is composed of a dorsal and a ventral root and its branches. The dorsal root enters the dorsal portion of the spinal cord carrying afferent (sensory) impulses from the periphery toward the spinal cord. The nerve cell bodies of the afferent neurons are located in the *dorsal root ganglion,* a swelling on the dorsal root close to the area where the dorsal and ventral roots join to form the spinal nerve. The ventral root emerges from the ventral portion of the spinal cord carrying efferent (motor) impulses from the spinal cord to muscles or organs (Fig. 14-8).

The spinal nerves generally supply sensory and motor fibers to the region of the body in the area where they emerge from the spinal cord. In some areas of the body, they merge to form an interlacing network called a *plexus.* Each forelimb is supplied by nerves that arise from the *brachial plexus.* The *radial* nerve is part of the brachial plexus. Each hind limb is supplied by nerves that arise from the *lumbosacral plexus.* The *sciatic* nerve is part of the lumbosacral plexus and is the largest nerve in the body. The spinal nerves extend beyond the level of the spinal cord in parallel strands. This terminal portion is called the *cauda equina* because it resembles a horse's tail.

CRANIAL NERVES

Number	Name	Function
I	Olfactory	Sense of smell
II	Optic	Vision
III	Oculomotor	Eye movements, focus, pupil changes, accommodation
IV	Trochlear	Eye movements, proprioception
V	Trigeminal	Sensations of head and face, chewing movements
VI	Abducens	Abduction of the eye
VII	Facial	Facial expressions, secretion of saliva, and taste sensation
VIII	Acoustic (auditory)	Hearing (cochlear branch) and maintaining balance and equilibrium (vestibular branch)
IX	Glossopharyngeal	Taste sensations, swallowing, and salivary secretions
X	Vagus	Sensations and movements of organs supplied; slows heart, increases peristalsis
XI	Accessory	Shoulder movements, turning movements of head, movements of viscera
XII	Hypoglossal	Tongue movements

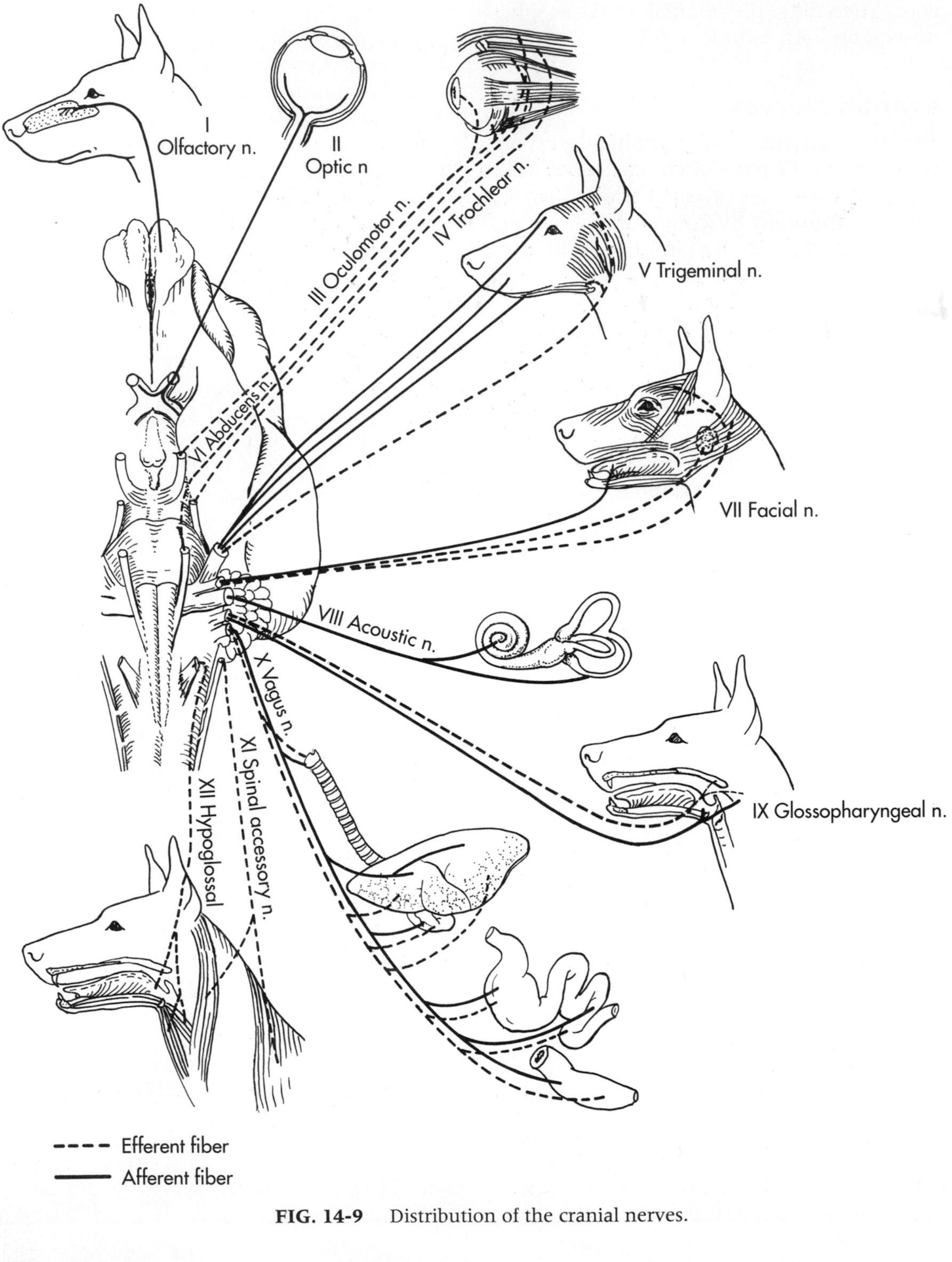
I
Olfactory n.
II
Optic n
III Oculomotor n.
IV Trochlear n.
V Trigeminal n.
VI Abducens n.
VII Facial n.
VIII Acoustic n.
IX Glossopharyngeal n.
X Vagus n.
XI Spinal accessory n.
XII Hypoglossal
Efferent fiber
Afferent fiber

FIG. 14-9 Distribution of the cranial nerves.

REVIEW D

1. The spinal cord has ______________________ membranous coverings.
2. The spinal cord is made up of an inner core of ______________________ matter and an outer core of ______________________ matter.
3. The spinal cord has both ______________________ and ______________________ tracts.
4. The tracts are contained in the ______________________ matter.
5. The peripheral nervous system includes all nerves and ganglia located outside the brain and spinal cord, including the ______________________ nerves, the ______________________ nerves, and the ______________________ nerves.
6. There are ______________________ pairs of cranial nerves.
7. The first cranial nerve, for the sense of smell, is called the ______________________ nerve.
8. The vagus or ______________________ cranial nerve is the longest cranial nerve and has extensive distribution to the thoracic and abdominal viscera.
9. A spinal nerve is composed of a/an ________________ root and a/an ________________ root and its branches.
10. The largest nerve in the body, the ______________________, is a part of the lumbosacral plexus.

AUTONOMIC NERVOUS SYSTEM

Although the autonomic nervous system is an element of the peripheral nervous system, it is an integral part of the entire nervous system. It functions automatically, innervating smooth muscle, cardiac muscle, and glands. The autonomic nervous system is composed of two divisions: the *sympathetic* and the *parasympathetic.* Most organs receive both sympathetic and parasympathetic innervation.

Sympathetic Division

The sympathetic trunk lies close to the vertebrae. It is composed of a series of *ganglia* (nerve cell clusters) on each side, forming a nodular cord resembling a string of beads. The nerve cells of origin for the sympathetic nerves are located in the thoracic and lumbar segments of the spinal cord, so the term for their origin is *thoracolumbar* (Fig. 14-10, *A*).

Parasympathetic Division

The parasympathetic or *craniosacral* division originates in the brain stem and sacral regions. The centers of the brain stem send out impulses through the oculomotor, facial, glossopharyngeal, and vagus cranial nerves. The sacral group sends out impulses through the sacral nerves (Fig. 14-10, *B*).

Functions of the Autonomic System

The sympathetic and parasympathetic divisions generally oppose each other in func-

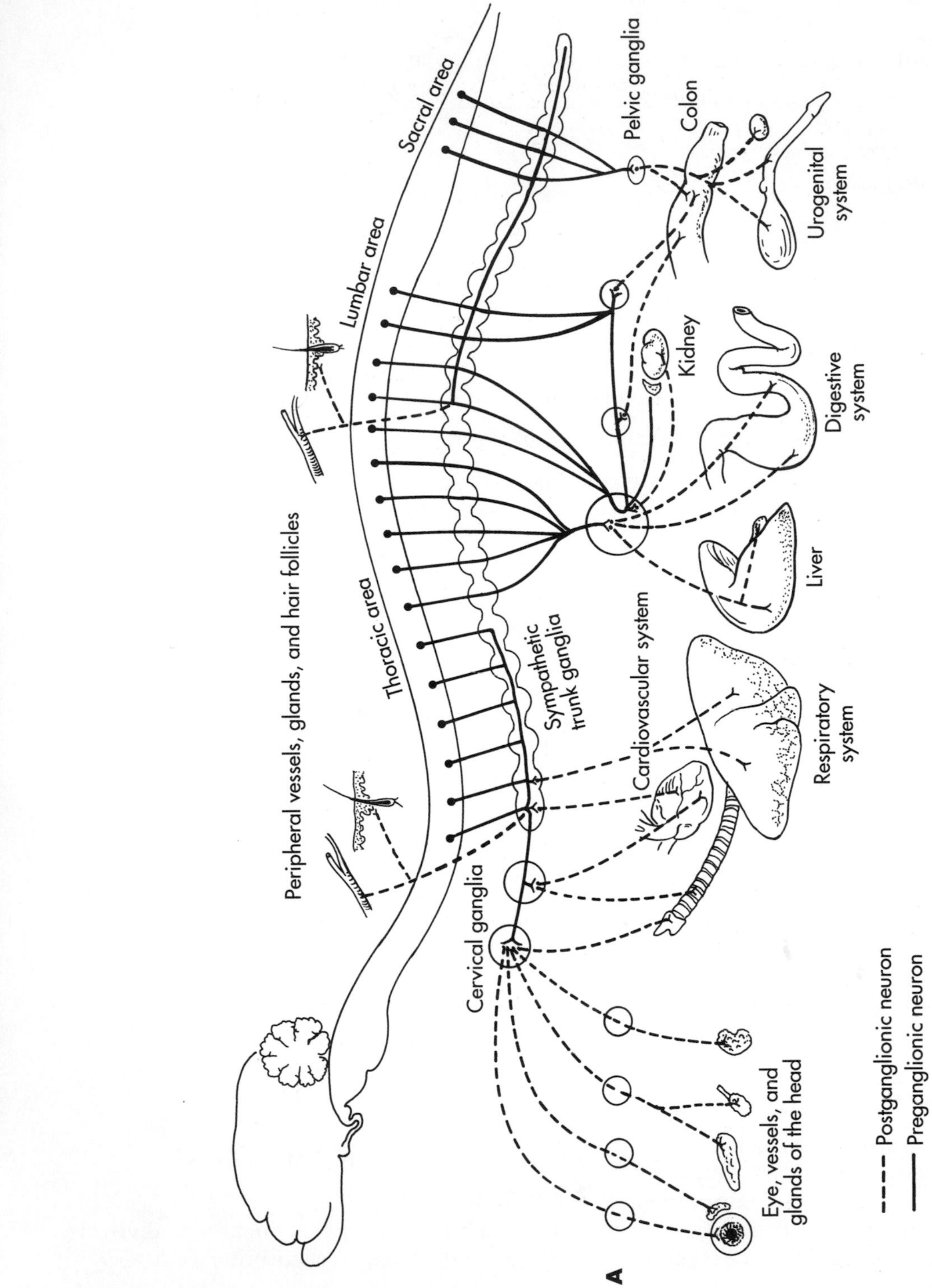
A
Eye, vessels, and glands of the head
Cervical ganglia
Peripheral vessels, glands, and hair follicles
Thoracic area
Sympathetic trunk ganglia
Cardiovascular system
Respiratory system
Liver
Digestive system
Kidney
Lumbar area
Sacral area
Pelvic ganglia
Colon
Urogenital system
Postganglionic neuron
Preganglionic neuron

FIG. 14-10 A, Sympathetic division of the autonomic nervous system.

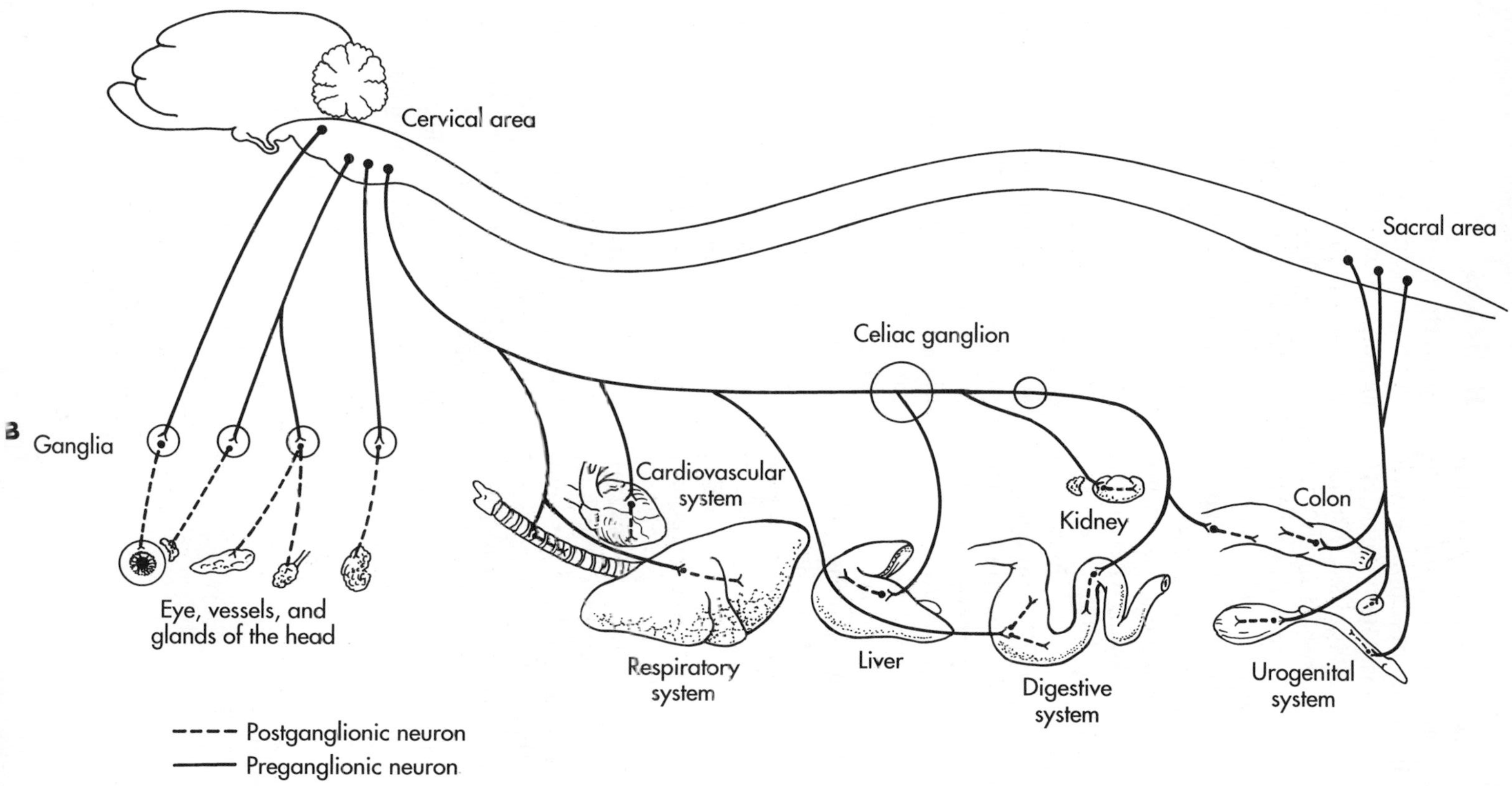
B
Cervical area
Sacral area
Celiac ganglion
Ganglia
Cardiovascular system
Kidney
Colon
Eye, vessels, and glands of the head
Respiratory system
Liver
Digestive system
Urogenital system
Postganglionic neuron
Preganglionic neuron

FIG. 14-10, cont'd **B,** Parasympathetic division of the autonomic nervous system.

tion. The sympathetic nerves are involved in fight-or-flight responses. The parasympathetic nerves are involved in actions associated with restful situations. The sympathetic and parasympathetic divisions, through their antagonistic responses, maintain the delicate balance in body mechanisms.

Some examples of opposition of the divisions are the sympathetic division dilating the pupils and the parasympathetic constricting them. The sympathetic accommodates the eyes to distant vision, whereas the parasympathetic accommodates the eyes to near objects. The sympathetic dilates the bronchial tubes, and the parasympathetic constricts them. The action of the heart is quickened by the sympathetic division, whereas the parasympathetic slows its action. The blood vessels of the skin and viscera are constricted by the sympathetic division so that more blood goes to the muscles where it is needed for fight or flight under stress. The parasympathetic division dilates the blood vessels when the stressful situation has passed. The gastrointestinal tract and bladder are relaxed by the sympathetic system and contracted by the parasympathetic. The sympathetic division causes contractions of the sphincters to prevent leakage from the anus or urethra, and the parasympathetic relaxes these sphincters so that waste matter can be expelled. In a similar fashion, the nerves regulate body temperature, endocrine glands, and salivary and digestive secretions.

Reflexes

A reflex is an autonomic or unconscious response of an effector organ to an appropriate stimulus. When consciousness is involved in an action, it is under the control of the brain. A reflex occurs below the brain level, within the spinal cord, and is not conscious or voluntary.

A reflex involves a chain of at least two neurons, making up a *reflex arc.* A reflex arc has an afferent (sensory or receptor) neuron and an efferent (motor or effector) neuron. Usually, one or more connector neurons called *interneurons* are between the receptor and effector neuron (Fig. 14-8). The *spinal reflex* is the simplest type of reflex. The *knee jerk reflex* is an example of a spinal reflex. The knee jerk reflex can be illustrated by tapping the patellar ligament, causing the leg to extend.

More complicated reflexes are mediated through reflex centers found in the brain. The medulla contains a reflex center for control of heart action, respiration, swallowing, and vomiting. The *pupillary reflex,* in which the size of the pupil of the eye varies with light intensity, is associated with a cranial nerve. The cerebellum contains reflex centers associated with movement and posture. Many of the reflexes are inborn but are subject to modification during learning processes. Think about a newborn foal running after its mother. At first, it is wobbly in its attempts, but after a learning process it becomes very graceful in its movements.

REVIEW E

1. The autonomic nervous system has two divisions: the ____________________ and the ____________________.
2. The sympathetic division is known as the ____________________, noting its origin.
3. The parasympathetic or ____________________ division originates in the brain stem and sacral regions.
4. The sympathetic and parasympathetic divisions generally ____________________ one another in function.
5. The ____________________ nerves are involved in fight-or-flight organ responses.
6. The ____________________ nerves are involved in actions associated with restful situations.
7. An unconscious, involuntary action occurring below the brain level is called a ____________________ action.
8. A reflex involves a chain of at least __2__ neurons.
9. In the ____________________ reflex, the leg extends in response to tapping of the patellar ligament.
10. In the ____________________ reflex, the pupil of the eye contracts in response to exposure of the retina to a bright light.

Chapter 14 Answers

Review A

1. central, peripheral
2. axon, dendrites
3. nuclei
4. ganglia
5. myelin
6. neurilemma
7. blood-brain barrier
8. sensory, motor, connector
9. impulses
10. synapse

Review B

1. cerebrospinal
2. dura mater, arachnoid, pia mater
3. forebrain, midbrain, hindbrain
4. see illustration below

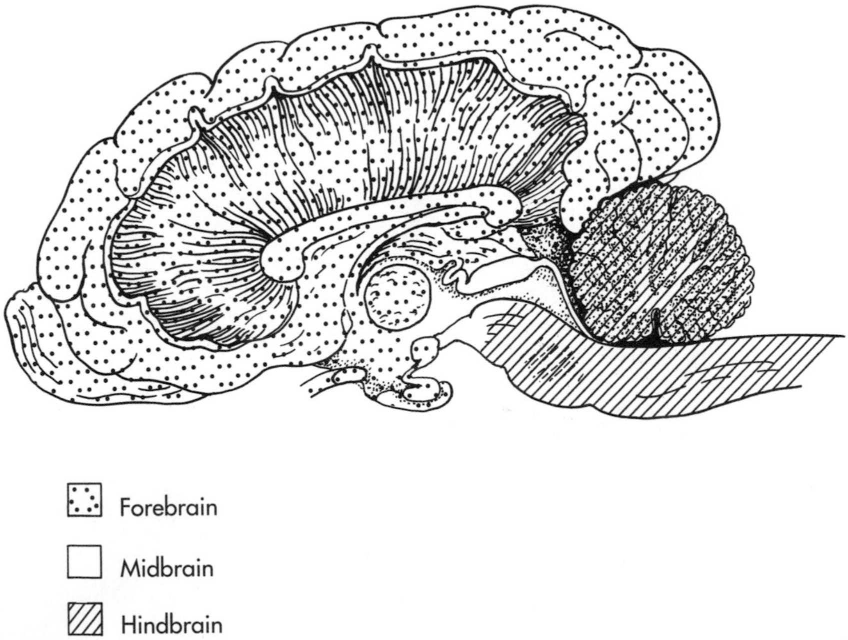
Forebrain
Midbrain
Hindbrain

5. telencephalon, diencephalon
6. cortex
7. frontal, temporal, parietal, occipital
8. right, left
9. corpus striatum
10. rhinencephalon

Review C

1. epithalamus, hypothalamus
2. hypothalamus
3. midbrain
4. rhombencephalon
5. cerebellum, pons, medulla oblongata
6. cerebellum
7. medulla oblongata
8. limbic
9. cerebrospinal
10. choroid plexus

Review D

1. three
2. gray, white
3. ascending, descending
4. white
5. cranial, spinal, autonomic
6. 12
7. olfactory
8. tenth
9. dorsal, ventral
10. sciatic

Review E

1. sympathetic, parasympathetic
2. thoracolumbar
3. craniosacral
4. oppose
5. sympathetic
6. parasympathetic
7. reflex
8. two
9. knee jerk
10. pupillary

Chapter 14 — EXERCISES

THE NERVOUS SYSTEM
THE CENTRAL PROCESSING UNIT

Exercise 1: Complete the following statements.

1. The brain and spinal cord are located in the ____________________ system.
2. The cranial and spinal nerves are located in the ____________________ system.
3. The sympathetic and parasympathetic divisions are part of the ____________________ system.
4. Groups of neuron cell bodies that occur outside the central nervous system are called ____________________ .
5. The membranes that envelop the central nervous system are called ____________________ .
6. The three membranes that envelop the nervous system are called the ____________________ , the ____________________ , and the ____________________ .
7. The cerebral hemispheres are located in the ____________________ , a portion of the forebrain.
8. The part of the forebrain in which the thalamus, epithalamus, and hypothalamus are located is the ____________________ .
9. The thin, transparent, watery fluid found in the ventricles of the brain, the central canal of the spinal cord, and the subarachnoid space is called ____________________ .
10. The passage for the spinal cord through the occipital bone of the cranium is called the ____________________ .

Exercise 2: Using the list of terms below, identify each part in Fig. 14-11 below by writing the name in the corresponding blank.

Rhinencephalon	Occipital lobe	Pineal body
Frontal lobe	Pons	Medulla oblongata
Fourth ventricle	Parietal lobe	Third ventricle
Pituitary (hypophysis)	Cerebellum	Spinal cord
Optic chiasm	Thalamus	Mesencephalon

1. ______________________
2. ______________________
3. ______________________
4. ______________________
5. ______________________
6. ______________________
7. ______________________
8. ______________________
9. ______________________
10. ______________________
11. ______________________
12. ______________________
13. ______________________
14. ______________________
15. ______________________

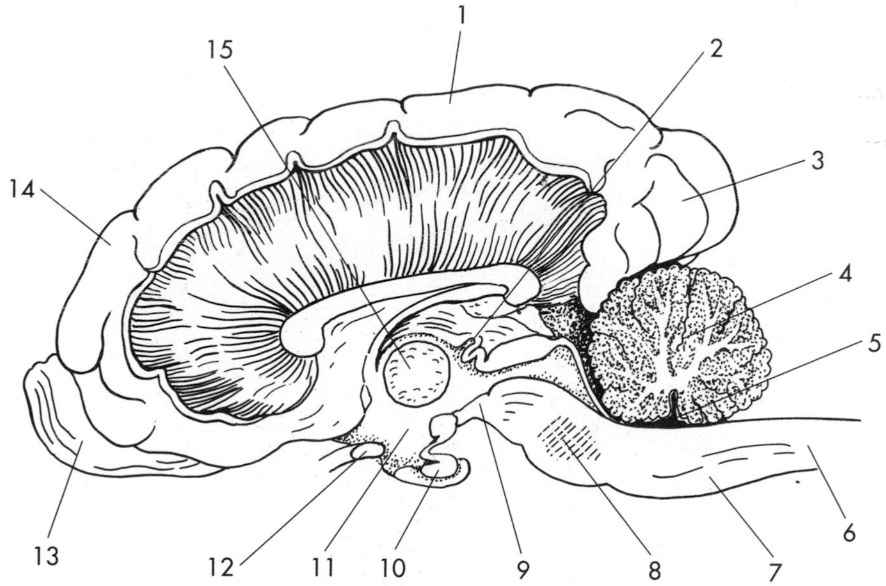
1
2
3
4
5
6
7
8
9
10
11
12
13
14
15

FIG. 14-11

Exercise 3: Match the terms with the correct definitions or statements in the left-hand column and place the corresponding letters in the spaces provided.

H 1. Long nerve cell processes that carry impulses from the cell body

F 2. Numerous short nerve cell processes that conduct nerve impulses toward the cell body

N 3. Neurons concerned with muscle or gland action

K 4. Peripheral neurons that conduct afferent impulses from the sense organs to the spinal cord

D 5. Region of connection between processes of two adjacent neurons for transmission of impulses

G 6. Axon ending

A 7. Space between the pia mater and the arachnoid

I 8. Space between the dura mater and the arachnoid

M 9. Central body of the cerebellum

C 10. A furrow or groove separating folds of the brain

L 11. Second cranial nerve, which innervates the retina of the eye

E 12 Third cranial nerve, which innervates the eye muscles and the sphincter of the pupil and ciliary processes

J 13. Interlacing network of spinal nerves

B 14. Nerve that has extensive distribution to pharynx, thorax, and abdomen

A. Subarachnoid

B. Vagus

C. Sulcus

D. Synapse

E. Oculomotor

F. Dendrites

G. Terminal twig

H. Axons

I. Subdural

J. Plexus

K. Sensory neurons

L. Optic

M. Vermis

N. Motor neurons

Exercise 4: Give the meaning of the components in the following words, and then define the word as a whole.

1. Encephalomyelitis
   encephalo brain
   myel spinal cord
   itis inflammation
   ____

2. Hydrocephalus
   hydro water
   cephalus head
   ____

3. Choriomeningitis
   chorio choroid
   mening meninges
   itis inflammation
   ____

4. Polyradiculoneuritis
   poly many
   radiculo nerve roots
   neur nerves
   itis inflammation
   ____

5. Polioencephalomalacia
   polio gray matter of brain
   encephalo brain
   malacia softening
   ____

6. Craniotomy
   crani skull
   otomy opening
   ____

7. Meningoencephalitis
   meningo meninges
   encephal brain
   itis inflammation
   ____

8. Cephalocele
   cephalo head
   cele protrusion
   ____

CHAPTER 14 PUZZLE

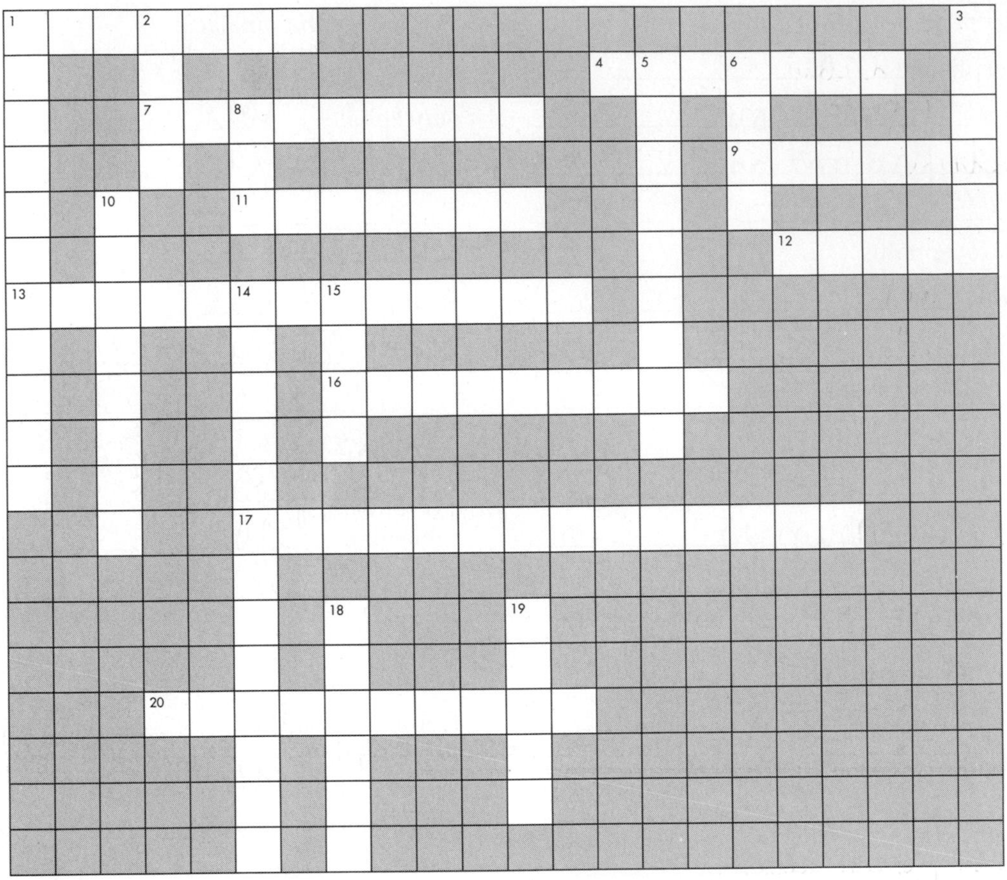

ACROSS CLUES

1. Point at which an impulse is transmitted from axon of one neuron to dendrite of another
4. Nerve cell clusters outside CNS
7. Posterior lobe of cerebral cortex
9. Unconscious response to a stimulus
11. Afferent neurons
12. Tenth cranial nerve
13. Water on the brain
16. Hold and support nerve cells
17. Associated with sense of smell
20. Fifth cranial nerve

DOWN CLUES

1. Fight-or-flight; autonomic nervous system division
2. Neuron process
3. Network of spinal nerves
5. Weblike meninx
6. Cerebral hemisphere convolutions
8. Central nervous system abbreviation
10. Mesencephalon
14. Fluid that protects and bathes brain and spinal cord
15. Part of hindbrain
18. Nerve coating
19. Part of the CNS

Chapter 14 Answers

Exercise 1

1. central nervous
2. peripheral nervous
3. autonomic nervous
4. ganglia
5. meninges
6. dura mater, arachnoid, pia mater
7. telencephalon
8. diencephalon
9. cerebrospinal fluid
10. foramen magnum

Exercise 2

1. parietal lobe
2. pineal body
3. occipital lobe
4. cerebellum
5. fourth ventricle
6. spinal cord
7. medulla oblongata
8. pons
9. mesencephalon
10. pituitary (hypophysis)
11. third ventricle
12. optic chiasm
13. rhinencephalon
14. frontal lobe
15. thalamus

Exercise 3

1. H
2. F
3. N
4. K
5. D
6. G
7. A
8. I
9. M
10. C
11. L
12. E
13. J
14. B

Exercise 4

1. brain; spinal cord; inflammation; inflammation of the brain and spinal cord
2. water; head; accumulation of fluid with enlargement of the head
3. choroid; meninges; inflammation; inflammation of the meninges and choroid plexus
4. many; nerve roots; nerves; inflammation; inflammation of the spinal ganglia, nerve roots, and peripheral nerves
5. gray matter of the brain; brain; softening; softening of the cerebrocortical gray matter
6. skull; opening; surgical procedure for opening the cranium
7. meninges; brain; inflammation; inflammation of the brain and meninges
8. head; protrusion; protrusion of a part of the cranial contents through a defect in the skull

ANSWERS: CHAPTER 14 PUZZLE

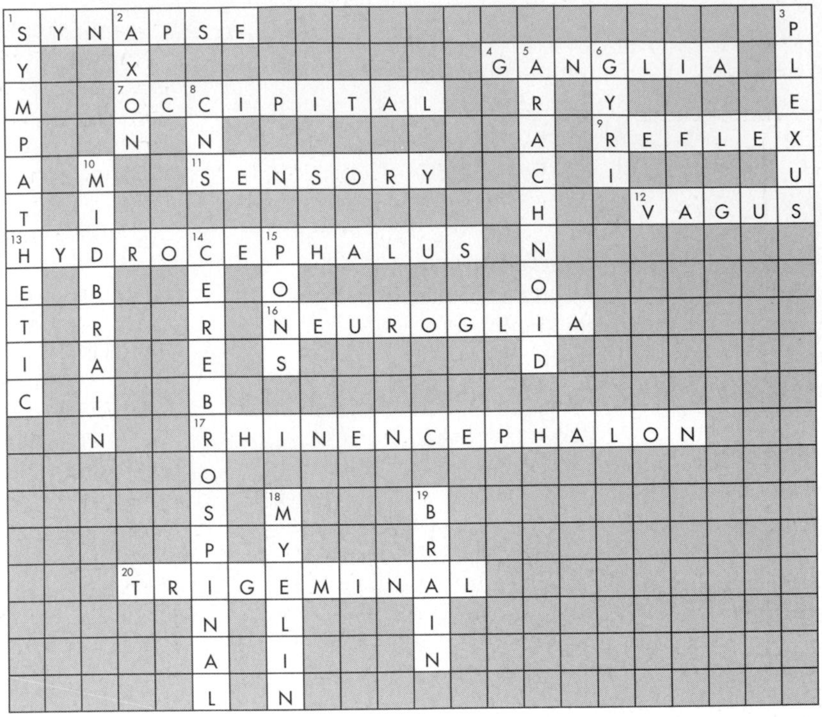
1 SYNAPSE
4 GANGLIA
7 OCCIPITAL
9 REFLEX
11 SENSORY
12 VAGUS
13 HYDROCEPHALUS
16 NEUROGLIA
17 RHINENCEPHALON
20 TRIGEMINAL
1 SYMPATHETIC
2 AXON
3 PLEXUS
5 ARACHNOID
6 GYRI
8 CNS
10 MIDBRAIN
14 CEREBROSPINAL
15 PONS
18 MYELIN
19 BRAIN

GLOSSARY

DIVISIONS OF THE NERVOUS SYSTEM

autonomic: part of peripheral nervous system that functions automatically; activates involuntary, smooth, cardiac muscles and glands serving vital systems and cannot be controlled voluntarily.

central: division of nervous system that includes brain and spinal cord.

cerebrospinal system: the central nervous system; includes the brain and spinal cord.

parasympathetic: one of two divisions of autonomic system, arising from central nervous system by preganglionic neurons, with cell bodies located in brain or in second, third, and fourth sacral segments of spinal cord (also called *craniosacral system*).

peripheral: division of nervous system that consists of nerves and ganglia peripheral to or outside the spinal cord and brain, including cranial and spinal nerves and autonomic nervous system.

sympathetic: one of two divisions of autonomic system, arising from central nervous system by preganglionic neurons, with cell bodies located in thoracic and first three lumbar segments of spinal cord and with ganglia extending from base of skull to coccyx (also called *thoracolumbar*).

BRAIN, SPINAL CORD, AND RELATED TERMS

amygdala: an almond-shaped mass of gray matter located in the anterior portion of the temporal lobe.

analgesia: insensibility to pain.

anesthesia: loss of feeling in part or in body generally.

apathy: indifference to environment.

arachnoid: middle meningeal membrane resembling spider's web (*arachnoid* means spider).

ascending tracts: tracts located in spinal cord, carrying afferent or sensory nerve fibers that conduct nerve impulses to brain.

astrocyte: star-shaped cell of the neuroglia (*astro* means star).

basal ganglia: paired masses of gray matter in each cerebral hemisphere.

blood-brain barrier: an anatomic-physiologic feature that alters the permeability of brain capillaries so that some substances are prevented from entering brain tissue while others are allowed to enter freely.

brain: central part of nerve tissue within cranium, including cerebrum, cerebellum, diencephalon, midbrain, pons, and medulla oblongata.

brain stem: consists of medulla oblongata, pons, and midbrain.

cataplexy: rigidity of muscles, with limbs tending to remain where placed; characterized by trancelike state.

cerebellar hemispheres: the two parts, or hemispheres, that comprise the cerebellum.

cerebellum: second largest division of brain, situated above medulla oblongata and beneath rear portion of cerebrum.

cerebral cortex: outer portion of cerebrum containing gray matter; the cell bodies of neurons.

cerebrospinal fluid: thin, transparent, watery fluid found around spinal cord and in ventricles of brain, central canal of spinal cord, and subarachnoid spaces; supports brain, serving as protective cushion and source of nutrients for brain and spinal cord.

cerebrum: largest part of the brain, occupying most of cranial cavity; divided into two cerebral hemispheres.

choroid plexus: vascular folds of pia mater in third, fourth, and lateral ventricles; secretes cerebrospinal fluid.

cingulate gyrus: one of the divisions of the limbic system of the brain.

circadian rhythm: regular recurrence of biological activity that occurs at about the same time each day or night regardless of exposure to constant darkness or light.

cisterna magna: enlarged subarachnoid space between caudal surface of cerebellum and dorsal surface of medulla oblongata; sample of cerebrospinal fluid may be collected or pressure measured at this site.

convolution: fold in surface of cerebral hemisphere (also called *gyrus*).

corpus striatum: the basal ganglia and the white matter separating them, seen as alternating bands of grey and white matter in each cerebral hemisphere.

corpora striata: plural form of corpus striatum.

descending tracts: tracts located

in spinal cord carrying nerve fibers that conduct efferent or motor impulses from brain.

diencephalon: part of forebrain that contains thalamus, epithalamus, and hypothalamus.

disorientation: situation in which animal appears to suffer loss of bearings or state of mental confusion as to time, place, or identity.

dura mater: outermost membrane of brain and spinal cord.

endorphins: natural, opiate-like substances produced in both brain and pituitary gland that have narcotic action on receptor sites in brain; believed to play role in pain experience.

epithalamus: portion of diencephalon that includes pineal body and olfactory (smell) centers.

fissure: deep groove or furrow of brain on cortical surface of cerebrum.

foramen magnum: passage for spinal cord through occipital bone of cranium.

forebrain: anterior portion of the brain composed of the telencephalon and diencephalon.

fourth ventricle: most posterior ventricle in hindbrain, which produces some cerebrospinal fluid.

frontal lobe: the most anterior lobe of the cerebral cortex, which serves as the center for voluntary movement.

gyri: plural form of gyrus.

gyrus: either lateral half of cerebrum or cerebellum.

hindbrain: also called the rhombencephalon, it is composed of the cerebellum, pons, and medulla oblongata.

hippocampus: part of limbic system often called *gatekeeper for memory.*

horns: projections of gray matter within the spinal cord. In cross sections of the spinal cord there are two horns pointing dorsally and two ventrally.

hyperkinesis: increased motor function or activity.

hypnosis: induced state of altered awareness or trance; immobility state can be produced in various species such as rabbit.

hypothalamus: portion of diencephalon located below and between lobes of thalamus; contains the optic chiasm and part of pituitary gland.

lateral ventricle: cavity in each cerebral hemisphere containing cerebrospinal fluid and communicating with third ventricle.

leptomeninges: pia mater and arachnoid membranes of brain.

limbic system: center for emotional activity and behavior located in deeper structures of brain; involves cingulate gyrus, hypothalamus, amygdala, and hippocampus.

lobes of cerebrum: cerebral cortex is divided into four lobes named for cranial bones above them: occipital, frontal, temporal and parietal.

medulla oblongata: posterior part of brain, continuous with spinal cord.

meninges: three membranes enveloping central nervous system: dura mater, pia mater, and arachnoid.

mesencephalon: one of the three parts of the brainstem, lying just below the cerebrum and just above the pons. Also called the midbrain.

microglia: phagocytic cells of nervous system.

midbrain: located between forebrain and hindbrain; contains auditory, visual, and muscle control center and is involved in body posture and equilibrium.

neuroglia: specialized type of nervous tissue that holds nerve cells and their gossamer filaments together.

neurotransmitters: chemical substances that act at synapse to stimulate or inhibit transmission of impulses; most well known are acetylcholine, norepinephrine (adrenaline), dopamine, and serotonin.

nucleus: mass or cluster of gray matter in brain or spinal cord (see *ganglion* under Nerve Structures).

olfactory brain: also called the rhinencephalon; it is primarily associated with the sense of smell and is more developed in animals than in humans.

oligodendroglia: cells that aid in holding nerve fibers together and forming myelin sheath of nerves.

optic chiasm: crossing of optic nerves on ventral surface of brain (*chiasm* means crossing).

pachymeninges: plural form of *pachymeninx.*

pachymeninx: dura mater.

pia mater: innermost, thin, compact membrane closely adapted to surface of spinal cord and brain.

pons: portion of brain that serves as bridge to connect cerebellum, cerebrum, and medulla oblongata (*pons* means bridge).

reticular activating system: a functional (rather than morphologic) system in the brain essential for wakefulness.

rhinencephalon: the part of the forebrain involved in receiving and integrating olfactory impulses.

Schwann cell: a specialized cell that covers a nerve fiber in the peripheral nervous system, forming the neurilemma.

spinal cord: lowest part of central nervous system, extending from medulla oblongata to coccyx; contains ascending and descending nerve tracts.

stress: biological reactions to any adverse stimulus (physical, mental, emotional, internal, or external) that tends to disturb well-being of animal.

subarachnoid space: space between pia mater and arachnoid.

subdural space: space between dura mater and arachnoid.

sulci: plural form of *sulcus.*

sulcus: furrow or groove separating gyri from each other.

telencephalon: the cerebrum, the corpora striata, and the rhinencephalon.

thalamus: part of diencephalon, known as great integrating center of brain; large, gray, oval mass that acts as center to receive sensory impulses and transmit them on to cerebral cortex.

third ventricle: located in diencephalon; connects to fourth ventricle by way of cerebral aqueduct.

ventricles: four interconnected cavities in the brain filled with cerebrospinal fluid.

vermis: central body of cerebellum, has wormlike shape (*vermis* means worm).

NERVE STRUCTURES AND RELATED TERMS

afferent neurons: neurons that conduct impulses from sense organs to spinal cord and brain.

axon: long nerve cell process carrying impulses from cell body.

collaterals: side branches of axon.

connectors: neurons in which dendrites and axons are connected to other neurons.

dendrites: numerous short nerve cell processes that conduct nerve impulses toward cell body.

dorsal root: part of spinal nerve that enters dorsal portion of spinal cord, carrying afferent impulses from periphery toward spinal cord.

efferent neurons: motor neurons that convey impulses from brain and spinal cord to muscles and glands.

ganglia: plural form of *ganglion.*

ganglion: mass of nerve cells located outside brain and spinal cord that serves as center for nerve impulses.

interneuron neurons: also called connector neurons, a neuron that transmits impulses from sensory to motor neurons or to other interneurons in the central nervous system.

knee jerk reflex: a spinal reflex initiated by tapping the patellar ligament, causing the leg to extend.

motor neurons: neurons serving muscle or glands.

myelinated nerves: nerves covered with sheath of white fatty material called myelin.

myelin sheath: the insulating envelope of myelin that surrounds a nerve fiber and facilitates the transmission of nerve impulses.

nerve: a bundle of nerve fibers.

nerve fibers: the dendrites and axons of a neuron.

nerve trunk: white, glistening, cordlike bundle formed by nerve fibers bound together by connective tissue.

neurilemma: tubelike membrane covering nerve fibers, which may or may not be myelinated (also spelled *neurolemma;* also called *sheath of Schwann*).

neuron: single nerve cell with cell body, axon, and dendrites; structural unit of nervous system.

nociceptive receptor: receptor for pain.

nonmyelinated fibers: nerve fibers that have only a thin coating of myelin surrounding them.

plexus: interlacing network of spinal nerves in several areas of body.

proprioceptive receptors: any sensory nerve endings that give information about movements and position of body.

pupillary reflex: constriction of the pupil of the eye in response to light.

Ranvier's node: interruption or constriction in myelin sheath at regular intervals.

receptors: organs of sensation.

reflex: an involuntary response to a stimulus.

reflex arc: the path of a reflex, involving at least two neurons over which impulses are conducted from a receptor to the brain or spinal cord and then to an effector.

sensory neurons: peripheral nerves that conduct afferent impulses from sense organs to spinal cord.

soma: the body of a cell.

spinal reflex: the simplest type of reflex, one whose arc passes through the spinal cord but not the brain.

synapse: microscopic space between axon of one neuron and dendrites of another, across which impulse is transmitted (*synapse* means connection).

terminal twigs: peripheral nerve endings.

tract: neuronal axons grouped together to form a pathway.

ventral root: part of spinal nerve that emerges from ventral portion of spinal cord, carrying efferent impulses from spinal cord to muscles or organs.

Cranial nerves

abducens: sixth cranial nerve; motor nerve that supplies retractor and lateral rectus muscle of eye.

acoustic: eighth cranial nerve having two sensory division: *cochlear,* which supplies cochlea of ear (hearing), and *vestibular,* which supplies vestibule and semicircular canals of ear (equilibrium); also called the *auditory* nerve.

facial: seventh cranial nerve; sensory and motor nerve, which originates in pons, supplies facial muscles, some taste buds, and salivary glands.

glossopharyngeal: ninth cranial nerve; originates in medulla oblongata and supplies tongue, pharynx, and parotid salivary glands.

hypoglossal: twelfth cranial nerve; motor nerve that originates in medulla oblongata and innervates muscles of tongue.

oculomotor: third cranial nerve, both sensory and motor, which supplies most of eye muscles, pupillary sphincter, and ciliary processes.

olfactory: first cranial nerve; sensory nerve that innervates nasal mucous membrane to supply sense of smell.

optic: second cranial nerve; sensory nerve supplying retina of eye for sight.

spinal accessory: eleventh cranial nerve; motor nerve to muscles of shoulder and neck.

trigeminal: fifth cranial nerve, both sensory and motor; supplies muscles of mastication, eye, and face.

trochlear: fourth cranial nerve; motor nerve that supplies dorsal oblique muscle of eye.

vagus: tenth cranial nerve; both sensory and motor; supplies visceral structures in thorax, abdomen, pharynx, and larynx.

Spinal nerves

The following list includes only a portion of the many spinal nerves. Spinal nerve origins are identified using letters to show their anatomic locations and numbers to indicate positions in the spinal column. *C* refers to cervical, *T* to thoracic, *L* to lumbar, and *S* to sacral, and the number after the letter indicates the corresponding vertebra (for example, *C1* indicates the first cervical vertebra).

brachial plexus: network of nerves derived from last three or four cervical and first one or two thoracic nerves (depending on species); supplies front limbs.

cauda equina: nerves that supply hind limbs, extending below level of spinal cord, deriving their name from arrangement of their strands, which resemble a horse's tail; terminal part of spinal cord, meninges, and nerves.

femoral: key nerve of hind limb; innervates major extensor muscles of stifle; loss of innervation results in inability to bear weight on the hind limb.

lumbosacral plexus: network of nerves derived from last few lumbar and first one, two, or three sacral nerves; supplies hind limbs.

obturator: sensory and motor nerve that supplies muscles of thigh and skin of hip, thigh, and knee joint; paralysis of nerve can occur with parturition, especially in cows.

peroneal: sensory and motor nerve that originates in sciatic nerve and supplies muscles of lower hind limb and skin of foot and toes.

phrenic: sensory and motor nerve that supplies diaphragm, lung, pericardium, and peritoneum.

pudendal: sensory and motor nerve that supplies skin, erectile tissue, and muscle of perineal area.

radial: sensory and motor nerve of brachial plexus that innervates forelimb; provides innervation to major extensors of elbow joint; loss of innervation results in inability to bear weight on forelimb.

sciatic: sensory and motor nerve, largest in body; supplies main extensor muscles of hip and flexor muscle of stifle; paralysis results in profoundly abnormal gait and posture.

suprascapular: supplies muscles of shoulder; paralysis causes atrophy of supraspinatus muscle (called *sweeny* in horses).

PATHOLOGIC CONDITIONS OF THE NERVOUS SYSTEM

ataxia: muscular incoordination.

Aujeszky's disease: disease primarily of pigs caused by a herpes virus; produces neurologic, respiratory, and reproductive signs (also called *pseudorabies* or *mad itch*).

bovine spongiform encephalopathy (BSE): a prion disease of cattle, also known as mad cow disease, characterized by degeneration of brain tissue; thought to be transmissible to humans.

cerebellar hypoplasia: a degeneration and deficiency of cerebellar cells; can be caused by viral agents such as panleukopenia in cats.

cerebral hemorrhage: bleeding into structure of cerebrum, usually caused by rupture of artery or congenital aneurysm; may be followed by destruction of brain tissue, with ensuing paralysis, sensory losses, and cognitive confusion and losses.

cerebrovascular accident (CVA): commonly called a *stroke;* includes rupture or obstruction of artery of brain, producing severe headache, nausea, vomiting, confusion, accompanied by localized and widespread neurologic deterioration.

cervical vertebral malformation: incoordination in dogs and horses associated with caudal cervical vertebral malformation of instability (also called *wobblers*).

chorea: repetitive, rhythmic contractions of group of skeletal muscles; result of encephalitis or myelitis caused by distemper virus in dogs.

choriomeningitis: inflammation of cerebral meninges with infiltration of choroid plexus by lymphocytes.

coma: stuporous condition of depressed responsiveness, with absence of response to strong stimuli.

decerebration: loss of higher mental functions because of brain damage.

discospondylitis: destructive, inflammatory process involving vertebral bodies, seen in dogs and pigs.

encephalitis: inflammation of brain, with variety of types; associated with several viral agents including canine distemper virus.

encephalomalacia: softening of brain tissue caused by reduced blood supply.

encephalomyelitis: inflammation of brain and spinal cord.

encephalopathy: any degenerative disease of brain.

epilepsy: hereditary or idiopathic nervous system disorder, with or without convulsions, which may also result from infection or trauma; characterized by temporary disturbance of brain impulses, with several types: *grand mal* (loss of consciousness with convulsions), *petit mal* (temporary loss of awareness and suspension of activity), and *focal* (seizure affects limited body area).

hemiplegia: paralysis of one side of body.

hydrocephalus: abnormal accumulation of fluid in cerebral ventricles, with thinning of cortex and enlargement of head resulting from separation of cranial bones.

intervertebral disc disease: syndrome of pain and neurologic deficits resulting from displacement of part or all of nucleus of intervertebral disc; seen most often in dogs, particularly in dachshunds and beagles.

listeriosis: infectious disease affecting all species, caused by *Listeria monocytogenes;* typically produces meningoencephalitis and syndrome of circling, facial paralysis, and head pressing.

macrocephaly: excessively large size of head (also called *megacephaly*).

meningioma: benign, encapsulated tumor originating in arachnoid.

meningitis: inflammation of meninges of brain or spinal cord, caused by viral or bacterial infection.

meningoencephalitis: inflammation of brain and meninges; can be caused by feline infectious peritonitis.

meningoencephalomyelitis: inflammation that involves brain, meninges, and spinal cord.

meningomyelitis: inflammation of spinal cord and its membranes.

microcephaly: condition of excessively small head.

myelitis: inflammation of spinal cord (*myel* refers to both spinal cord and bone marrow, and context in which it is used determines which tissue is involved).

myelopathy: any functional disturbance or pathologic change in spinal cord; often used to describe nonspecific lesions.

narcolepsy: uncontrollable urge to sleep or sudden attacks of sleep.

neuralgia: pain in nerve or nerves.

neuritis: inflammation of nerve or nerves, caused by infection, toxicity, or trauma.

neuromyopathy: any disease of muscles and nerves combined.

neuromyositis: neuritis with inflammation of corresponding muscles.

neurotoxin: substance that is poisonous or destructive to nerve tissue.

opisthotonos: tetanic spasm in which head and tail are bent upward and abdomen is bowed downward.

paralysis: loss of muscle function or loss of sensation.

paraplegia: paralysis of posterior part of body and extremities.

paresis: slight or incomplete paralysis.

polioencephalomalacia: softening and necrosis of cerebrocortical gray matter.

polioencephalomyelitis: inflammation of gray matter of brain and spinal cord.

polyneuritis: inflammation of large number of spinal nerves at same time.

polyradiculoneuritis: inflammation of peripheral nerves and spinal nerve roots leading to progressive paralysis with slow recovery; condition follows raccoon bites in some dogs, hence the name *coonhound paralysis.*

rabies: highly fatal infection of nervous system that affects all warm-blooded animal species; transmitted by bite of infected animal or existing wound coming in contact with infected saliva; furious and dumb forms are described.

radiculitis: inflammation of spinal nerve root.

roaring: sonorous respiration caused by air passing through stenosed larynx; most common cause in horses is laryngeal hemiplegia, caused by degeneration of fibers in left recurrent laryngeal nerve (branch of vagus).

scrapie: a chronic, fatal disease of sheep and goats with progressive degeneration of the central nervous system, possibly caused by prion infection. Named for the tendency of infected animals to scrape itching parts of the skin against objects.

seizure: convulsion or attack of epilepsy.

senility: deterioration, both physical and mental, related to aging.

spina bifida: developmental anomaly characterized by defective formation of bony spinal canal through which spinal membranes or cord may protrude.

tetanus: highly fatal disease of all animal species caused by neurotoxin of *Clostridium tetani;* bacterial spores are deposited in tissues, usually by traumatic injury, and under anaerobic conditions vegetate; horses are particularly susceptible to this disease; *lockjaw* is popular synonym and symptom, along with generalized muscle spasms and seizures.

tick paralysis: several species of ticks elaborate neurotoxin that typically causes ascending paralysis in many species, including humans.

tremor: continuous repetitive twitching of skeletal muscle that is usually visible; may be caused by degenerative disease of nervous system or by toxins.

vestibular disease: sudden onset of head tilt, nystagmus, rolling, falling, and circling; seen in older dogs and in cats of all ages.

SURGICAL PROCEDURES

craniotomy: surgical opening of skull.

disk fenestration: removal of intervertebral disk material by perforation and curettage of intervertebral disk space.

laminectomy: procedure in which portion of vertebral arch is removed to relieve signs caused by ruptured intervertebral disk.

neuroanastomosis: anastomosis or connection between nerves.

stereotactic surgery: production of sharply localized lesions in brain after precise localization of target tissue by use of three-dimensional coordinates.

LABORATORY TESTS AND PROCEDURES

brain scan: scanner is used in conjunction with intravenous injection of radioactive substance, which circulates to brain, concentrating in areas of abnormality, to diagnose lesions, tumors, and areas of necrosis.

cerebral angiography: using contrast medium injected into carotid, brachial, subclavian, or femoral arteries, series of X rays is taken to visualize blood vessels of brain.

cerebrospinal fluid tap: examination for presence of abnormal or excessive cell count, protein content, or pressure; obtained via cisterna magna or lumbar puncture.

computed tomography (CT): use of thin beam of X rays to derive cross-sectional images (tomograms) of head, which are put together and analyzed to form picture on computer screen that shows tumors, tissue atrophy, and other anatomic abnormalities; more effective tool for diagnosis than ordinary X ray (also called *computed axial tomography* or *CAT scan*).

electroencephalograph (EEG): a machine used to reveal patterns of electrical activity of brain in form of brain waves; aids in diagnosing epilepsy, tumors, and other abnormalities reflected in electrical activity.

magnetic resonance imaging (MRI): noninvasive method of scanning body using electromagnetic field and radio waves; provides visual images on computer screen and magnetic tape recordings.

myelography: X ray of spinal cord and subarachnoid space, using contrast medium to identify spinal lesions caused by disease or trauma.

vitamin B tests: group of tests done on blood and urine to detect vitamin deficiency, which relates to nervous system problems.

15 The Special Senses

The sources of information

CHAPTER OVERVIEW

In this chapter we discuss the five special senses—smell, taste, vision, hearing, and touch—and their unique structures and sensation mechanisms. Nonmammalian vertebrates have tremendous variations in the kind and location of senses. Even mammals vary widely in the exact nature and site of sensory receptors. This chapter deals mostly with domestic species.

THE SENSE OF SMELL

Smell is one of the most primitive senses. In many animals it is very acute and of paramount importance because it serves to warn the animal of approaching enemies, guides it in its quest for food, and even motivates the sex reflexes.

The peripheral organ for smell is the nose (*naso* and *rhino* refer to the nose), with its external parts and nasal cavities. The organ of smell is the *olfactory epithelium* of the nose, and odor is perceived through stimulation of its cells. The olfactory (*olfact* refers to smell) receptors are situated in the nasal mucosa over a small area just rostral to the cranial cavity. A supplementary olfactory organ, the *vomeronasal organ,* is found in the septum separating the nasal and oral cavities. It consists of two small parallel sacs lined with olfactory epithelium and with openings into the nasal cavity and the mouth. It is important in detecting sexual *pheromones,* hormonal substances that mediate communication between animals. In some species this can be seen in the characteristic behavior of males in the presence of estrous females. When a bull, for example, sniffs the urine or vaginal secretions of a cow in estrus he may extend his head upward while lifting and curling his upper lip, a behavior called *flehmen,* or lip-curl.

The *nostrils (nares)* are the two openings separated from one another by the lower part of the septum (wall between two nasal cavities). The *philtrum* is the groove in the middle of the nose separating the nostrils. It is deep in carnivores and small ruminants and shallow or absent in the pig, cow, and horse.

The nose is formed by the nasal bones and cartilage. The nasal bones are the *turbinates,* upper (dorsal), middle (medial), and lower (ventral) *conchae.* Nasal cartilages are connected to each other and to the bones by fibrous tissue. Just inside the nasal cavities is a lining of skin with a ring of coarse hairs whose function is to trap dust and foreign particles during inspiration.

The mucous membrane lining the nose is continuous with particular connecting areas, and infections of this membrane are easily spread to them. These connecting areas include the nasopharynx; the eustachian tube (auditory canal); the middle ear cavity; the sphenoidal, ethmoidal, frontal, and maxillary sinuses; and the palatine bones and tear ducts.

The stimulation of the olfactory epithelium is initially transmitted to the olfactory bulb and from there continues to the olfactory centers in the brain. In humans, six basic odors have been identified, interacting with each other to produce the variety we experience: flowery, fruity, spicy, resinous, burned, and putrid. The sense of smell is far more sensitive than the sense of taste, and complements it, as is evident when a respiratory infection blocks the sense of smell, causing food to lose its customary flavors. Deficits in the sense of smell are difficult to evaluate in animals.

THE SENSE OF TASTE

The organs of taste are the taste buds, located mainly on the tongue; a few also may be found in the mucous membrane that covers the soft palate, the *fauces* (opening from the mouth to the pharynx), and the epiglottis.

The sense of taste is limited to four primary, or fundamental, tastes: sweet, sour (acid), salt, and bitter. The various other tastes experienced are blends of these. For a substance to arouse a sensation of taste, it must be dissolved either in solution or by the saliva, which accounts for the location of the taste buds on a moist surface. As with smell, deficits in taste are difficult to evaluate in an examination of a domestic animal.

REVIEW A

1. The five special senses are ____________, ____________, ____________, ____________, and ____________.
2. The organ of smell is the ____________ epithelium of the nose.
3. The groove in the middle of the nose, separating the nostrils, is called the ____________.
4. The organs of taste are the ____________, located on the surface of the ____________.
5. The four primary tastes are ____________, ____________, ____________, and ____________.

VISION

The organ of vision is the eye, with its various accessory organs, such as the extrinsic muscle, the eyelids, and the *lacrimal* (tear) apparatus. Strictly speaking, the eye includes only the bulb of the eye (the eyeball) and the optic nerve, which connects it with the brain. This system constitutes the essential part of the organ of vision. The terms *orbit* and *optic* refer to the eye, as do the combining forms *oculo* and *ophthalmo.*

The eyeball occupies the anterior half of the orbital cavity, where it is cushioned in fat and connective tissue (Fig. 15-1). Attached to the eyeball and contained in its orbital cavity are the optic nerve, ocular muscles, and certain other nerves and vessels. The eyes are protected by the eyelids, called *palpebrae* (combining form *blepharo*). In some species, such as the horse, the edges of the eyelids are fringed with eyelashes, or *cilia.* Other species, such as the dog, lack cilia entirely. A soft, transparent mucous membrane called the *conjunctiva* covers the inner surface of the eyelids (the *palpebral conjunctiva*) and the exposed, nontransparent part of the eyeball (the *bulbar conjunctiva*). In many animals a third eyelid, the *nictitating membrane,* is present. It originates at the medial canthus and spreads laterally across the eye when the upper and lower lids close. It is stiffened by a thin piece of cartilage, contains lymphatic and lacrimal tissue, and is covered by conjunctiva. The lacrimal apparatus provides for the production and drainage of tears, which moisten and protect the eye.

Movement of the eyeball is by six slender muscles, attached to each eye, that act together. The eyes are free to move in any direction, upward, downward, and sideways, or the gaze may be fixed and straight ahead.

The eyeball is like a hollow sphere whose wall is made up of three concentric coats and whose cavity is filled with transparent *refracting media* (tissues and fluid that transmit light). The outer fibrous coat *(sclera)* has a white, opaque, posterior portion and a transparent, anterior portion called the *cornea.* The intermediate coat *(choroid)* is vascular and pigmented. The choroid is divided into a posterior portion and a smaller anterior portion, which has three structures: the *ciliary body,* the *suspensory ligament,* and the *iris.* The internal coat *(retina)* is the light-sensitive layer made up of differentiated nervous receptors continuous with the optic nerve. Three transparent refractive media fill the optic cavity: the *vitreous body* (semigelatinous substance contained in a thin, clear membrane), between the retina and the lens, and two *aqueous humor* (watery fluid) chambers anterior to the lens (Fig. 15-1).

The eye is like a camera, with an opening in front, the *pupil,* that lets light in, and a *crystalline lens* behind the pupil focusing the rays of light to form an image on the retina, which contains the vision sense organs, the *rods* and *cones.* The optic nerve carries the impulses from the rods and cones to the visual area.

Structures of the Eye

SCLERA

The sclera is the opaque posterior portion of the fibrous coat of the eye. It is continuous with the cornea, which it meets at the *limbus* (*limbus* means border). The sclera is the white of the eye, and its small superficial blood vessels can be seen through the transparent conjunctiva. The appearance of the sclera varies widely with different disease states, reflecting the condition of the animal. Its inspection is an important part of any physical examination.

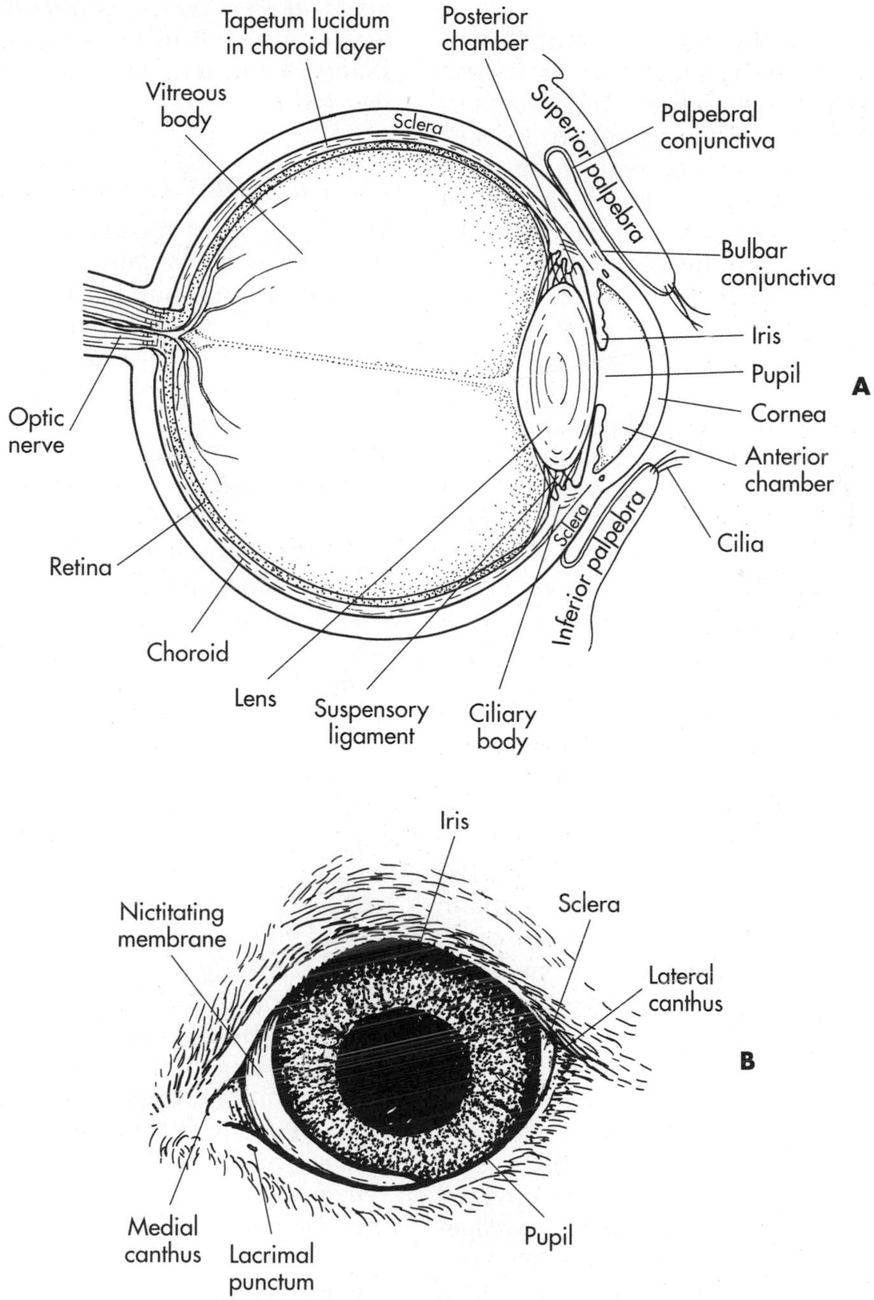
Tapetum lucidum
in choroid layer
Posterior
chamber
Vitreous
body
Sclera
Superior palpebra
Palpebral
conjunctiva
Bulbar
conjunctiva
Iris
Pupil
A
Cornea
Anterior
chamber
Optic
nerve
Cilia
Sclera
Inferior palpebra
Retina
Choroid
Lens
Suspensory
ligament
Ciliary
body
Iris
Nictitating
membrane
Sclera
Lateral
canthus
B
Medial
canthus
Lacrimal
punctum
Pupil

FIG. 15-1 **A,** Cross-section of the eye. **B,** External view of dog's eye.

CORNEA

The cornea is the anterior, transparent portion of the fibrous coat of the eyeball through which light enters the eye. It is nearly circular in shape, and its marked curvature makes it bulge with a domelike protrusion. It is devoid of blood and lymph vessels, except at the extreme periphery. Its avascularity makes the cornea subject to infection after injury.

CHOROID

The choroid is located between the sclera and retina, and its posterior part is a thin membrane with a rich vascular layer. Most animals (swine and humans being exceptions) also have a *tapetum lucidum* as a layer of the choroid. The tapetum is a reflective layer responsible for the shining of most animals' eyes in the dark when light is directed into them.

The cells of the choroid are filled with melanin, a black or dark brown pigment, which gives the choroid a dark brown appearance. Extra light is absorbed by the pigment, which helps to prevent blurring of an image by internally reflected light. The chief function of the choroid is to maintain the nutrition of the retina through its capillary plexus and numerous small arteries and veins.

CILIARY BODY

The ciliary body, an extension of the choroid, is a thickened portion of the vascular layer, which extends from the visual layer to the iris. The ciliary body is a wedge-shaped, flattened ring, with muscles connected to the *suspensory ligament,* which attaches the lens to it, and *processes* (ridges) that secrete the *aqueous humor* (fluid). The ciliary processes consist of a rich vascular plexus embedded in pigmented *stroma* (connective tissue). Focusing on far or near objects, which is called *accommodation,* is accomplished through changing the shape of the lens by action of the *ciliary muscles.*

SUSPENSORY LIGAMENT

The suspensory ligament is the second structure of the anterior extension of the choroid, continuous with the capsule that encloses the lens and attaching it to the ciliary muscles.

IRIS

The iris, the most rostral portion of the vascular layer, continuous with the ciliary body, is doughnut-shaped. Its central opening, the pupil, appears to be black. The iris is composed of rings of muscle fibers, some of which are arranged circularly, contracting to reduce the size of the pupil, with others arranged radially, contracting to increase the size of the pupil, regulating the amount of light admitted to the lens.

The shape of the constricted pupil may not be round (as in cats). In birds the muscles of the iris are skeletal (voluntary), rather than smooth (involuntary). Horses and ruminants have several black masses, the *corpora nigra,* at the upper and lower edges of the iris.

The iris is suspended in the aqueous space between the cornea and lens, dividing it into anterior and posterior chambers. The larger anterior chamber is between the iris and the cornea, and the posterior chamber is between the lens and the iris. These chambers are filled with the lymphlike aqueous humor, which aids in maintaining the shape of the eyeball and empties into the *canal of Schlemm,* an oval channel circling the anterior chamber. The aqueous humor, which is secreted by the ciliary processes, flows through the pupil into the anterior chamber, and the pressure maintained by the balance between secretion and removal of fluid is known as *intraocular pressure.*

The reflection of light scattered by pigment substances in the iris results in different colors, with dark eyes having abundant pigment and blue eyes having less pigment. Some neonates have blue eyes because the pigment does not develop in the *stroma* (connective tissue fibers forming the major part of the iris) until after birth; however, others have brown eyes at birth because the stromal pigment is already developed.

LENS

The transparent crystalline lens is directly behind the iris of the eye, enclosed in an elastic capsule supported by the suspensory ligament, and focuses light rays on the retina. The shape of the lens is altered by the action of the ciliary muscles, which affect the *refraction* (bending) of light rays.

RETINA

The innermost of the three coats of the eyeball, the retina, is a soft, delicate membrane that is in contact with and nourished by the vascular coat. The retina is the nervous tissue layer with special neuroepithelial cells, the *rods* and *cones,* named for their shapes, which serve as the photosensitive receptors of light stimuli. The cones are much less numerous than the rods and are adapted for bright light and color perception as well as fine detail. The rods are much more sensitive for low light vision but are color-blind. Animal classes vary in their ability to discern color. Near the center of the back of the retina in humans is a small yellow area called the *macula lutea,* with a central depression, the *fovea centralis,* the region of clearest vision, in which the cones are most concentrated and no rods are found. The retina also contains numerous sensory and connector neurons and their processes. At a point in the back of the retina, nearer the nose, there is an *optic disk,* where the nerve fibers from the entire eye converge to form the *optic nerve,* producing a blind spot because there are no rods or cones present. At the point where the optic nerve pierces the sclera, it is accompanied by the optic central artery and vein, which come from the choroid.

LACRIMAL APPARATUS

The lacrimal apparatus includes the lacrimal gland proper, a lacrimal gland in the third eyelid, several accessory glands in the eyelids, and a duct system for tear drainage. Tears moisten and clean the surfaces of the eye and contain antibacterial substances such as *lysozyme.* The lacrimal gland is located dorsolaterally under the bony orbit. It secretes tears through several small ducts into the conjunctival *fornix,* the archlike fold where the palpebral conjunctiva curves onto the surface of the globe to become the bulbar conjunctiva. The blinking of the lids spreads the tears medially across the surface of the eye and directs them to a lacrimal lake at the *medial canthus* (nasal corner). The edge of each eyelid has a tiny opening, the *lacrimal punctum* (plural *puncta;* Fig. 15-1B). Tears drain through this opening into the *nasolacrimal* duct. The duct extends from the eyelids along the ventral surface of the nasal cavity, opening just inside the nostril in most species. Failure of drainage can occur in some dog breeds (e.g., miniature poodles) with prominent eyes. The tears then run down the outside of the eyelid, a condition known as *epiphora.*

The Mechanism of Vision

Vision occurs when light rays enter the pupil and are focused on the retina by the lens, cornea, and aqueous and vitreous humors. This process of focusing or *refraction* is accomplished by all four components, any of which may develop defects.

Stimulations of the retinal receptors (rods and cones) are transmitted through the optic nerves to the *optic chiasma*, then to midbrain areas and the visual cortex areas of the occipital lobe. In the optic chiasma, the optic nerve fibers from the inner (or nasal) half of each retina cross over and join those from the outer (or temporal) half of the retina of the other eye before continuing on. For example, the fibers from the right half of the left eye link up with those from the right half of the right eye. The degree to which this happens depends on the species.

Visual acuity varies widely among animals. Predators such as the dog and cat have eyes placed close together. The overlapping of the visual fields of the two eyes gives *binocular* vision. As a result these species have good depth perception and clear focusing of nearby objects. Herbivores such as the horse and cow, on the other hand, have their eyes placed farther back on the sides of their heads. This gives them mostly *monocular* vision because the two visual fields only overlap at a distance. They lose depth perception, but they can see a much wider area around them without moving their heads than can predator species. Blindness *(amaurosis)*, though devastating for wild and range animals, is surprisingly well tolerated by most domestic animals, especially pets. The keenness of their other senses compensates so well that their owners may not even be aware of their blindness.

REVIEW B

1. Two combining forms meaning eye are ____________________ and ____________________ .
2. When referring to the eye, the word *cilia* means ____________________ .
3. The third eyelid is also called the ____________________ .
4. Another word for tear gland is ____________________ gland.
5. The eyeball is made up of three concentric coats. The outer fibrous coat is the __________ . The intermediate coat, vascular and pigmented, is called the ____________________ . The internal light-sensitive layer is the ____________________ .
6. The semigelatinous medium that fills most of the optic cavity is called the ____________ . The fluid anterior to the lens is the ____________________ .
7. The white of the eye is covered by a thin transparent mucous membrane called the ____________________ .
8. Most animals' eyes shine in the dark when light is directed into them. The pigmented layer responsible for this is called the ____________________ .
9. The two solid transparent avascular parts of the eye are the ____________________ and the ____________________ .
10. From the name, you would expect the *corpora nigra* of the horse's iris to be ____________ in color.
11. The inner corner of the eye is properly called the ____________________ .
12. Its name tells you that *macula lutea* means ____________________ spot.

HEARING

We usually think of the ear as the organ of hearing. However, the ear also contains structures responsible for equilibrium. The ear is divided into the *external ear, middle ear,* and *inner ear.* The combining forms *oto* and *auris* refer to the ear; *audi* refers to hearing.

Structures of the Ear

EXTERNAL EAR

The external ear is made up of the *pinna* and the *external auditory meatus* (*meatus* means opening), which is a short, tortuous passage that leads to and penetrates the temporal bone. The external auditory canal is entirely lined by skin and ends blindly at the *tympanic membrane* (eardrum). Sound waves reach the eardrum through this canal and are picked up by the inner bones of the ear and transmitted by the cochlear branch of cranial nerve VIII to the brain (Fig. 15-2).

MIDDLE EAR

This small, air-filled cavity in the skull is lined by a mucous membrane and situated between the internal ear and the tympanic membrane, communicating through the *eustachian tube* with the pharynx. This tube keeps the air pressure equal on both sides of the tympanic membrane, making the air pressure in the middle ear the same as that of the atmosphere. The pharyngeal orifice of the tube normally is closed but opens during swallowing and yawning or when high pressure is created in the nasopharynx, as when a forced expiration is made with the nostrils and mouth closed. Horses have a large ventral diverticulum of each eustachian tube called a *guttural pouch,* located just lateral to the pharynx.

In the middle ear, there are three tiny connected bones called the *auditory ossicles* (*ossicle* means little bone), deriving their names from their shape: the *malleus* (hammer), the *incus* (anvil), and the *stapes* (stirrup). These bones are connected by joints and bridge the middle ear (tympanic cavity) to transmit sound waves by the mechanical action of the ossicles to the inner ear.

INNER EAR

The inner ear (labyrinth) begins at the oval window, against which the stapes presses, and continues in a labyrinthine *cochlea* (which means spiral or snail-shell shape), which contains three canals separated from each other by thin membranes and almost converge at the apex. Two of these canals are bony chambers filled with a *perilymph fluid,* one of which, the bony *vestibular canal,* is connected to the oval window that leads to the middle ear. Another, the *tympanic canal,* is also bony and is connected to the round window opening into the middle ear. The third canal, the *cochlear canal,* is a membranous chamber filled with *endolymph,* situated between the other two canals, containing the *organ of Corti,* a spiral-shaped organ located on the *basilar membrane* of the cochlear canal, made up of cells with projecting hairs that transmit auditory impulses to the cochlear nerve.

Mechanism of Hearing

Sound waves enter the external ear and strike the tympanic membrane, causing vibration, which sets into motion the three ossicles (the malleus, the incus, and the stapes, in that order). The stapes is the last to vibrate, and it strikes against the oval window of the vestibular canal, setting into motion the perilymph fluid in the vestibular and tympanic canals of the cochlea. The vibrating perilymph sets into motion the basilar membrane that separates these two canals, thereby disturbing the endolymph fluid in the membranous area of the cochlea. Hair cells of the organ of Corti, located in this

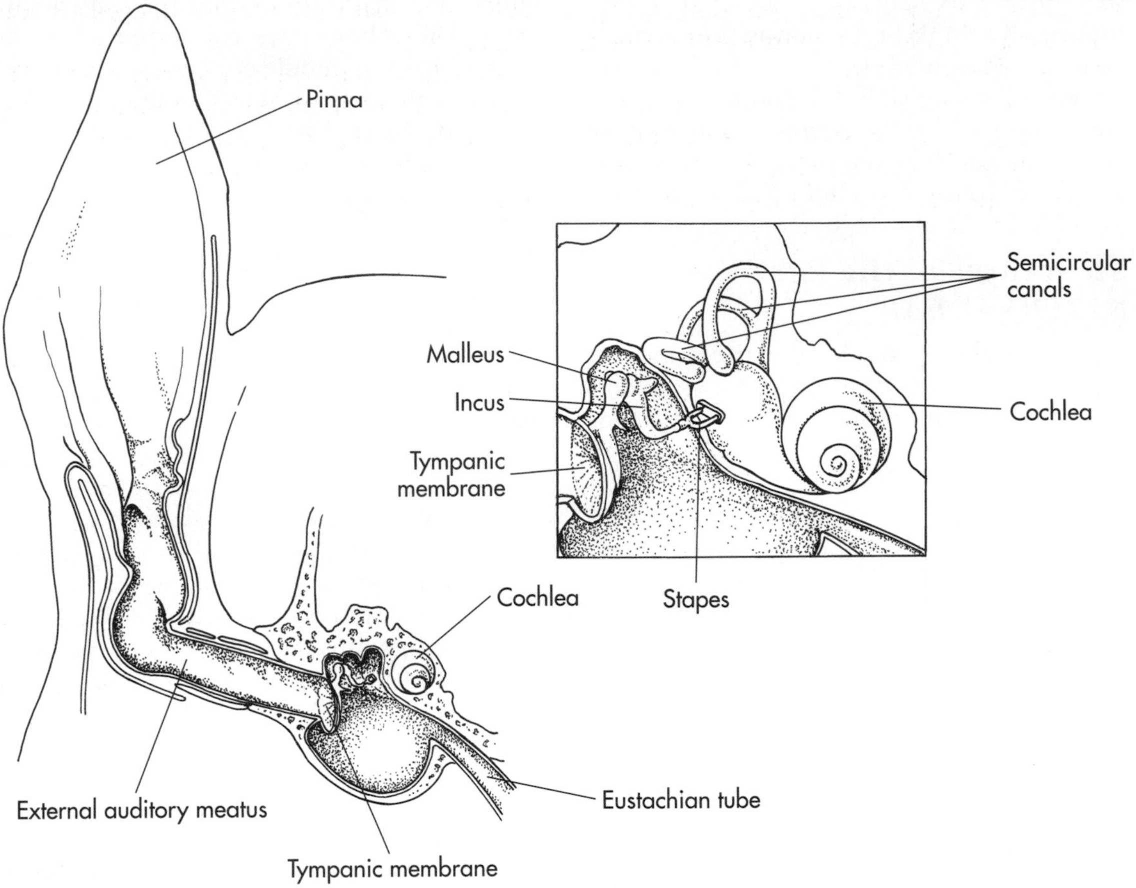
Pinna
Semicircular canals
Malleus
Incus
Tympanic membrane
Cochlea
Cochlea
Stapes
External auditory meatus
Eustachian tube
Tympanic membrane

FIG. 15-2 Cross-section of dog's ear with middle and inner ears enlarged.

area, are stimulated by the movement of the endolymph. By bending against another membrane (the *tectorial*), the hair cells transmit the impulse to the brain by way of the vestibulocochlear nerve. The final interpretation of sound is made by the brain. Some animals, such as dolphins and bats, have mechanisms for amplifying sound waves for echolocation of distant objects.

SENSE OF EQUILIBRIUM

In addition to the structures just described, there are three *semicircular canals* in the labyrinth that lie in planes at right angles to each other, plus a *utricle* and a *saccule* in each inner ear. These are the structures of equilibrium (Fig. 15-2).

The saccule and utricle are small sacs that are lined with sensitive hairs and contain particles, called *otoliths* (*lith* refers to stone), that are made up of calcium carbonate. The otoliths press on the hair cells through the pull of gravity and stimulate the initiation of impulses from the hair cells to the brain through their basal sensory nerve fibers. The utricles and saccules, which together are called the *vestibule,* are responsible for the reactions that result from position change and change of *rectilinear* motion (movement in a straight line).

The semicircular canals, which are liquid-filled, respond to *rotary* or turning movement. They are positioned at right angles to each other, each corresponding to one of the three spatial planes. Turning the head in any direction stimulates at least one of the canals. Inside each canal are hair cell receptors that bend in response to rotary motion, stimulating nerve fibers that carry impulses to the vestibular branch of the vestibulocochlear nerve (cranial nerve VIII) and then to the brain.

TOUCH AND OTHER CUTANEOUS SENSES

The skin is a receptor for the sensations of touch, as well as those of heat, cold, and pain. (Refer to Chapter 8 and Table 15-1.)

Touch (also called light pressure) is experienced as a function of stimulation of *free sensory nerve endings (dendrites)* everywhere in the skin, but especially around hair follicles. Other structures in the corium (layer below the epidermis) called *Meissner's corpuscles* (or *tactile corpuscles*) are believed to mediate light pressure sensations. Heavier pressure stimulates the *Pacinian corpuscles,* which are *lamellated* (layered) bodies of sensory nerve tissue located in the subcutaneous layer.

Thermal sensations of heat and cold appear to be experienced in response to changes of even a few degrees from skin temperature, but the precise mechanisms are not known. Free nerve endings are believed to be the main receptors, along with the *Krause end bulbs* (also called *Krause's corpuscles*) and *Ruffinian corpuscles,* which are

Table 15-1 THE SPECIAL SENSES

Sense	Organ	Receptors	Stimulus
Smell (olfaction)	Mucous membranes of dorsal nasal cavity	Olfactory epithelium hair cells	Chemical gas
Taste (gustation)	Surface of tongue	Taste bud papillae	Dissolved chemicals
Sight (vision)	Retina of eye	Rods Cones	Wavelengths of light
Hearing (audition)	Basilar membrane of cochlea (inner ear)	Hair cells of the organ of Corti	Sound vibrations
Balance (equilibrium)	Utricle, saccule, and semicircular canals of inner ear	Hair cells	Mechanical and fluid pressure
Touch pressure	Layers of skin	Free nerve endings, Meissner's corpuscles, Pacinian corpuscles	Mechanical pressure
Pain	Layers of skin	Nociceptors	Tissue injury
Warmth and cold	Layers of skin	Free nerve endings, Krause end bulbs, Ruffinian corpuscles, skin capillaries	Thermal energy

sensory end structures located in the corium. Also considered as mediators of heat and cold are the capillaries of the skin.

Pain is an unpleasant sensory experience associated with actual or potential tissue damage resulting from intense mechanical, thermal, or chemical stimuli. Specialized receptors called *nociceptors* (*noci* means pain) in the skin and other organs respond to such actual or threatened damage. They connect with *nociceptive* pathways in the central nervous system that can ultimately result in *nociperception,* the perception of pain, in the conscious centers of the brain. Tissue injury can produce a state of *hyperalgesia* (excessive sensitivity to pain) at the site of injury.

The skin areas of the body have varying sensitivities to sensation as a function of the distributions of receptors in the differing areas. The most sensitive areas generally are those that are most involved in obtaining information about oneself and the external world, such as the lips, and fewer receptors are found on dorsal surfaces of the appendages.

Vibrissae (whiskers) are long, tactile hairs that are especially sensitive to touch. Many mammals depend on their vibrissae to give them information about their environment.

REVIEW C

1. The combining forms ________________ and ________________ refer to ear. The combining form for hearing is ________________ .
2. The portion of the ear that is erect in a horse and floppy in a beagle is called the ________________ .
3. The ________________ is the passage that leads from the outside to the eardrum.
4. The structure that keeps the air pressure equal on both sides of the tympanic membrane is the ________________ .
5. The three auditory ossicles are ________________ , ________________ , and ________________ .
6. The word *cochlea* tells you that this structure has a ________________ shape.
7. Hearing impulses are transmitted to the brain by the ________________ nerve.
8. The semicircular canals are responsible for the sense of ________________ .
9. Long tactile hairs that are especially sensitive to touch are the ________________ .
10. The word *lamellated* means ________________ .
11. The skin's main receptors for heat and cold are ________________ .
12. Specialized receptors in the skin that respond to tissue damage are called ________________ .

Chapter 15 Answers

Review A

1. smell, taste, vision, hearing, touch
2. olfactory
3. philtrum
4. taste buds, tongue
5. sweet, sour, salty, bitter

Review B

1. oculo, ophthalmo
2. eyelashes
3. nictitating membrane
4. lacrimal
5. sclera, choroid, retina
6. vitreous body, aqueous humor
7. conjunctiva
8. tapetum lucidum
9. cornea, lens
10. black
11. medial canthus
12. yellow

Review C

1. oto, auris, audi
2. pinna
3. external auditory meatus
4. eustachian tube
5. malleus, incus, stapes
6. spiral or snail-shell
7. vestibulocochlear
8. equilibrium
9. vibrissae
10. layered
11. free nerve endings
12. nociceptors

Chapter 15 — EXERCISES

THE SPECIAL SENSES

Exercise 1: Complete the following statements:

1. The ________________________ separates the external ear from the middle ear.
2. *Ossicle* means ________________________ .
3. Pacinian corpuscles and Meissner's corpuscles are associated with the sense of __________ .
4. The turbinates are the ________________________ bones.
5. The opening from the mouth to the pharynx is the ________________________ .
6. Nociperception is the perception of ________________________ .
7. The lens is attached via the suspensory ligament to the ________________________ .
8. The bending of light rays by the various transparent parts of the eye is called __________ .
9. The retinal cells sensitive to colors are the ________________________ ; the color-blind cells important in low light vision are the ________________________ .
10. The palpebrae are the ________________________ . The combining form for this structure is ________________________ .
11. The border between the cornea and the sclera is the ________________________ .
12. The tiny opening in each eyelid is called the ________________________ . It leads into the ________________________ duct.
13. *Amaurosis* means ________________________ .
14. The guttural pouch in the horse is a large diverticulum of the ________________________ .
15. A state of excessive sensitivity to pain at the site of an injury is called ________________________ .
16. The light-sensitive layer of the eye is the ________________________ . It receives its blood supply from the layer just outside it, the ________________________ .

Exercise 2: Using the following list of terms, identify each part in Figure 15-3 by writing the name in the corresponding blank.

Vitreous body	1. ________________________
Bulbar conjunctiva	2. ________________________
Lens	3. ________________________
Retina	4. ________________________
Iris	5. ________________________

Sclera
Anterior chamber
Optic nerve
Cornea
Ciliary body
Choroid
Pupil
Suspensory ligament
Cilia
Posterior chamber
Inferior palpebra
Superior palpebra
Palpebral conjunctiva

6. ______________________
7. ______________________
8. ______________________
9. ______________________
10. ______________________
11. ______________________
12. ______________________
13. ______________________
14. ______________________
15. ______________________
16. ______________________
17. ______________________
18. ______________________

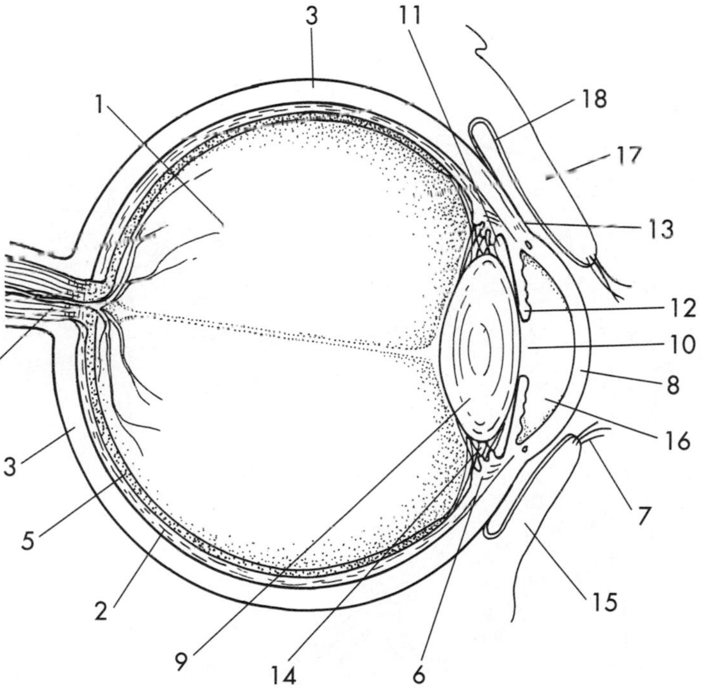
3
11
18
1
17
13
12
10
4
8
16
3
7
5
15
2
9
14
6

FIG. 15-3

Exercise 3: Using the following list of terms, identify each part in Figure 15-4 by writing the name in the corresponding blank.

Pinna	1. ____________
Cochlea	2. ____________
Incus	3. ____________
Eustachian tube	4. ____________
Tympanic membrane	5. ____________
External auditory meatus or canal	6. ____________
Malleus	7. ____________
Stapes	8. ____________
Semicircular canals	9. ____________

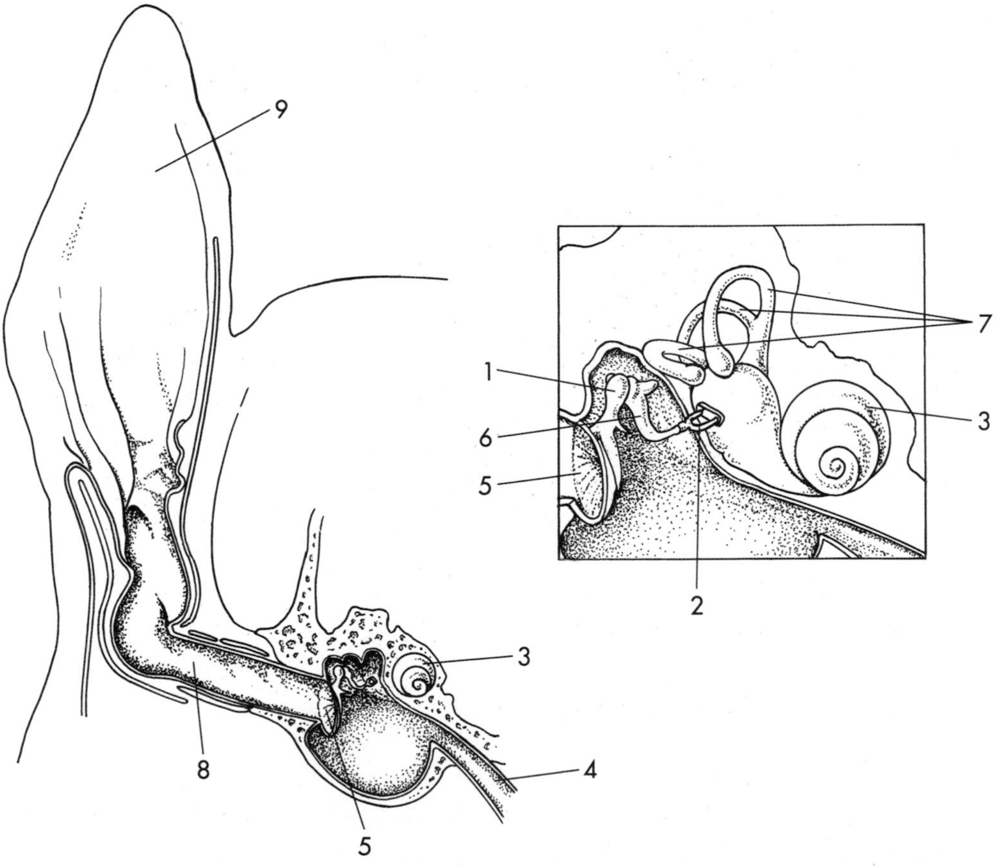
9
8
5
3
4
7
1
6
5
3
2

FIG. 15-4

Exercise 4: Match the terms in the right column with the definitions in the left column by placing the appropriate letter in the blank space provided.

_____	1. The depressed area in the center of the back of the retina; the area of clearest vision.	A. Eustachian tube
_____	2. Angles at the ends of the slits between the eyelids.	B. Canthi
_____	3. Specialized outer ends of the visual cells in the retina that are adapted to bright light, acute vision, and color perception.	C. Rods
_____	4. Special cylindrical neuroepithelial cells in the retina, highly sensitive to low light.	D. Semicircular canals
_____	5. The partition separating the nares.	E. Cones
_____	6. Special organ of hearing located on the basilar membrane of the cochlea.	F. Tympanic membrane
_____	7. The projecting part of the ear that lies outside the head.	G. Septum
_____	8. Structures for equilibrium in the labyrinth.	H. Fovea
_____	9. Structure leading from the ear to the throat.	I. Pinna
_____	10. Structure that separates the middle ear from the external ear.	J. Organ of Corti

Exercise 5: Give the meaning of the components of the following words and then define the word as a whole. Check the glossary if necessary.

1. Blepharitis

   blephar ______________________

   itis ______________________

   ____

2. Conjunctivitis

   conjunctiv ______________________

   itis ______________________

   ____

3. Iritis

   ir ______________________

   itis ______________________

   ____

4. Keratoconjunctivitis sicca

   kerato ______________________

   conjunctiv ______________________

   itis ______________________

   sicca ______________________

   ____

5. Trichiasis

   trich ______________________

iasis ______________________

____

6. Achromatopsia

a ______________________

chromat ______________________

opsia ______________________

____

7. Panophthalmitis

pan ______________________

ophthalm ______________________

itis ______________________

____

8. Otitis media

ot ______________________

itis ______________________

media ______________________

____

9. Anisocoria

an ______________________

iso ______________________

cor ______________________

ia ______________________

____

10. Aural hematoma

aural ______________________

hemat ______________________

oma ______________________

____

11. Blepharoplasty

blepharo ______________________

plasty ______________________

____

12. Xerophthalmia

xer ______________________

ophthalm ______________________

ia ______________________

____

CHAPTER 15 PUZZLE

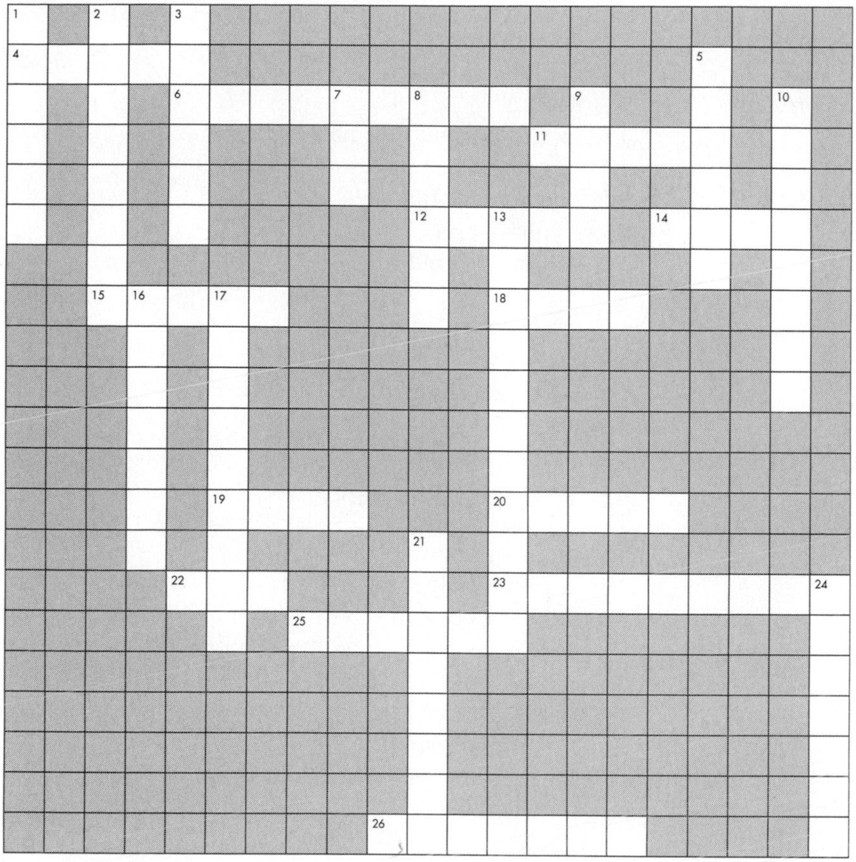

ACROSS CLUES

4. One of special senses
6. Eyelids
11. Visual receptors for color
12. Anvil (auditory ossicle)
14. Number of primary tastes
15. One of special senses
18. Organ of smell
19. Colored portion of eye
20. One of special senses
22. Combining form meaning ear
23. Utricles and saccules together
25. Transparent portion of eyeball
26. One of special senses

DOWN CLUES

1. Stirrup (auditory ossicle)
2. Little bones
3. Wall between nasal cavities
5. One of special senses
7. Organ of vision
8. Light-sensitive layer of eye
9. Visual sense receptors
10. Glands forming tears
13. Membrane covering exposed eyeball
16. Hammer (auditory ossicle)
17. Inner ear
21. Free sensory nerve endings
24. Tympanic membrane

Chapter 15 Answers

Exercise 1

1. tympanic membrane
2. small bone
3. touch (light pressure)
4. nasal
5. fauces
6. pain
7. ciliary body
8. refraction
9. cones, rods
10. eyelids, blepharo
11. limbus
12. lacrimal punctum, nasolacrimal
13. blindness
14. eustachian tube
15. hyperalgesia
16. retina, choroid

Exercise 2

1. vitreous body
2. choroid
3. sclera
4. optic nerve
5. retina
6. ciliary body
7. cilia
8. cornea
9. lens
10. pupil
11. posterior chamber
12. iris
13. bulbar conjunctiva
14. suspensory ligament
15. inferior palpebra
16. anterior chamber
17. superior palpebra
18. palpebral conjunctiva

Exercise 3

1. malleus
2. stapes
3. cochlea
4. eustachian tube
5. tympanic membrane
6. incus
7. semicircular canals
8. external auditory meatus or canal
9. pinna

Exercise 4

1. H
2. B
3. E
4. C
5. G
6. J
7. I
8. D
9. A
10. F

Exercise 5

1. eyelid; inflammation; inflammation of the eyelids
2. conjunctiva; inflammation; inflammation of the conjunctiva
3. iris; inflammation; inflammation of the iris
4. cornea; conjunctiva; inflammation; dry; inflammation of the cornea and conjunctiva with dryness (caused by lack of tears)
5. hair; condition; irritation of the eye from abnormal hairs that impinge on the corneal surface
6. without; color; vision; lack of color vision

7. entire; eye; inflammation; inflammation of entire eye
8. ear; inflammation; middle; inflammation of the middle ear
9. not; equal; pupil; condition; unequally sized pupils
10. ear (pinna); blood; tumor (swelling); collection of blood in the pinna
11. eyelid; changing; surgical change to eyelid
12. dry; eye; condition; dryness of eye (caused by lack of tears)

ANSWERS: CHAPTER 15 PUZZLE

1 S		2 O		3 S																
4 T	A	S	T	E													5 V			
A		S		6 P	A	L	P	7 E	B	8 R	A	E		9 R			I		10 L	
P		I		T				Y		E			11 C	O	N	E	S		A	
E		C		U				E		T				D			I		C	
S		L		M						12 I	N	13 C	U	S		14 F	O	U	R	
		E								N		O					N		I	
		15 S	16 M	E	17 L	L				A		18 N	O	S	E				M	
			A		A							J							A	
			L		B							U							L	
			L		Y							N								
			E		R							C								
			U		19 I	R	I	S				20 T	O	U	C	H				
			S		N					21 D		I								
				22 O	T	O				E		23 V	E	S	T	I	B	U	L	24 E
					H		25 C	O	R	N	E	A								A
										D										R
										R										D
										I										R
										T										U
									26 H	E	A	R	I	N	G					M

GLOSSARY

SENSE OF SMELL AND TASTE

ageusia (ah-gu'ze-ah): lack or impairment of sense of taste (also called *ageustia; geusia* refers to taste).

anosmia: absence of sense of smell.

concha (kong'kah): shell-shaped turbinate bones of nose.

fauces (fô'sēz): opening from mouth to pharynx.

flehmen: a sexually related behavior in which a male animal sniffs the urine or vaginal secretions of a female, then extends his head upward while lifting and curling his upper lip (also called lip-curl).

nares (nair'eez): the openings of the nasal cavity; nostrils (singular *naris*).

olfactory center: center for smell located in brain.

olfactory epithelium: organ of odor reception located in small area in nasal mucosa.

pheromone (fear'ah-moan): a hormonal substance secreted by an animal that elicits a particular response from another individual of the same species.

vomeronasal organ: a supplementary olfactory organ located at the base of the nasal cavity, with openings into the nasal cavity and mouth.

SENSE OF VISION

Vision-related anatomic and other terms

anterior chamber: space between iris and cornea that contains aqueous humor.

aqueous humor: clear, colorless fluid that fills anterior and posterior chambers of the eye.

binocular vision: the use of both eyes simultaneously so that a single image is seen, permitting stereoscopic perception (compare with *diplopia*).

blepharon: eyelid (also called *palpebra*).

canal of Schlemm: exit duct for aqueous humor, located in anterior cavity, which keeps intraocular pressure constant under normal conditions.

canthi: plural form of *canthus.*

canthus (kan'thus): angle at either end of slit between eyelids, lateral canthus, and medial canthus.

chiasma (key-as'mah): the crossing of two lines or tracts, as at the optic chiasma (also spelled *chiasm*).

choroid (ko'roid): coat, located between the sclera and the retina, with cells filled with melanin, whose posterior part is thin membrane with rich vascular layer.

cilia: eyelashes.

ciliary body (sil'e-er"e): thickened extension of choroid from visual layer to iris, consisting of ciliary processes and muscles, assisting in accommodation and secreting aqueous humor.

cones: specialized neuroepithelial cells of retina, which serve as color and fine-detail receptors of vision.

conjunctiva (kon"junk-ti'vah): mucous membrane lining the inner surfaces of the eyelids and the anterior part of the sclera.

cornea (kor'ne-ah): transparent structure that forms anterior part of external tunic of eye.

corpora nigra: black masses at edge of iris in horses and ruminants.

extrinsic muscles: six slender muscles attaching outside of eyeball to bones of orbit, acting together to move eyeballs.

fornix: an archlike structure or space, such as the conjunctival fornix, where the palpebral conjunctiva curves onto the surface of the eye to become the bulbar conjunctiva.

fovea (fo've-ah): depressed area in center of macula of retina, with no rods and greatest concentration of cones, producing area of clearest vision.

iris: most anterior portion of vascular layer of eye, a doughnut-shaped, pigmented ring of muscles that regulates size of pupil.

lacrimal glands: organs of secretion of tears, which cleanse and lubricate conjunctiva.

lens: transparent part of eye, directly behind iris, that focuses light rays on retina (also called *crystalline lens*).

levator palpebrae muscles: muscles that raise upper lid.

limbus: corneoscleral junction.

lysozyme (lye'so-zime): an enzyme with antibacterial properties; found in saliva, tears, sweat, and other body fluids.

macula: yellow spot near center of back of retina with central depression, the fovea (also called *macula lutea*).

meibomian glands: sebaceous glands on margins of each eyelid.

monocular vision: the situation in animals whose eyes are placed on the sides of their heads; the visual fields of the eyes do not overlap sufficiently to give good depth perception.

nasolacrimal duct: the tubular structure that drains tears from the lacrimal puncta of the eyelids to the nasal cavity.

nictitating membrane (nictitans): third eyelid, complete in birds, incomplete in many mammals; originates at medial canthus and contains cartilage, lacrimal tissue, and lymphatic tissue.

optic: term referring to eye.

orb: eyeball.

orbit: bony socket that contains eye.

palpebra: eyelid (plural, *palpebrae*).

posterior chamber: space between iris and lens that contains aqueous humor.

pupil: an opening in the iris that changes in size to regulate the amount of light entering the eye; its shape varies between species.

refracting media: transparent tissues and fluids in eye through which light passes and by which it is refracted and brought to focus.

retina: innermost, nervous tissue or sensory layer of three coats of eyeball; contains rods and cones.

rods: highly specialized, cylindric, neuroepithelial cells of retina; react to light but not color and are most sensitive to low light intensity.

sclera (skle'rah): tough, white, supporting tunic of eyeball.

tapetum lucidum: reflective layer of choroid in most animals.

uvea: term used to include iris, ciliary body, and choroid.

vitreous body: semigelatinous transparent substance that fills membrane-enclosed space between lens and retina.

Pathologic conditions relating to the eye

INFLAMMATIONS AND INFECTIONS OF THE EYE

acute contagious conjunctivitis: purulent infection of conjunctiva (also called *pinkeye*).

blepharitis: inflammation of eyelid.

chorioretinitis (ko″re-o-ret″ĭ-ni'tis): inflammation of choroid and retina (also called *retinochoroiditis*).

choroiditis: inflammation of choroid.

conjunctivitis: inflammation of conjunctiva.

dacryoadenitis (dak″re-o-ad″ĕ-ni'tis): inflammation of lacrimal gland (also called *dacryadenitis*).

dacryocystitis: inflammation of lacrimal sac.

iritis: inflammation of iris.

keratitis: inflammation of cornea.

keratoconjunctivitis (ker″ah-to-kon-junk″tĭ-vi'tis) *sicca:* inflammation of cornea and conjunctiva because of a deficiency in tear production (also called *dry eye*).

ophthalmitis: inflammation of deeper structures of eye (also called *ophthalmia*).

optic neuritis: inflammation of optic nerve.

panophthalmitis: inflammation of all structures of eye.

retinitis: inflammation of retina.

scleritis: inflammation of sclera.

uveitis: inflammation of uvea, which includes iris, ciliary body, and choroid.

HEREDITARY, CONGENITAL, AND DEVELOPMENTAL DISORDERS OF THE EYE

achromatopsia: absence of color vision from degeneration of the retinal cones; a hereditary disease of humans and malamute dogs.

albinism: absence of pigment in eye.

anophthalmos (an″of-thal'mos): absence of or rudimentary development of one or both eyes (also called *anophthalmia*).

cherry eye: prolapse of gland of third eyelid in dogs.

congenital cataract: opacity of lens originating before birth.

ectopia of lens: misplacement of lens.

ectropion: rolling outward of eyelid, common in St. Bernards.

entropion: rolling inward of eyelid, common in chow chows and shar-peis.

epiphora: excessive tearing, common in poodles.

microphthalmos: abnormally small eyes.

OTHER ABNORMAL CONDITIONS OF THE EYE

adhesions of iris: fibrous bands or strictures present in iris or adhering iris to other eye structures.

altered pupillary reflexes: hyper- (over) or hypo- (under) contraction of pupil on exposure to light.

amaurosis: blindness.

anisocoria: uneven size of pupils.

aphakia (ah-fa'ke-ah): absence of lens, usually used to describe absence of lens after cataract surgery, but it may also be congenital anomaly.

astigmatism: defective curvature of refractive surfaces of eye, causing light rays to spread over a more or less diffuse area and not sharply focus on retina (*stigma* means point).

blepharospasm: spasm of eyelid or excessive winking of eyes.

blindness: lack or loss of sight, with variety of causes and a number of types.

cataract: opacity of crystalline lens or its capsule, with a number of types and varying causes.

corneal opacity: opacity of cornea.

corneal ulcer: lesion of cornea.

diabetic retinopathy (ret″ĭ-nop′ah-the): noninflammatory degeneration of retina, characterized by retinal ischemia, hemorrhages, and exudation.

diplopia: double vision (*diplo* means double).

glaucoma (glaw-ko′mah): disease characterized by excessive intraocular pressure, with hardness of eye, atrophy of retina, and possible progression to blindness.

hypertensive retinopathy: retinal degeneration caused by hypertension.

hypopyon (hi-po′pe-on): accumulation of pus in anterior chamber of eye.

lenticular opacity: opacity in lens.

myopia: nearsightedness, caused by refraction error, which focuses parallel rays in front of retina.

nuclear sclerosis: drying out of lens with age.

nystagmus (nis-tag′mus): involuntary, rapid, horizontal, vertical, rotary, or mixed movements of eyeball (*nys* means nod).

ophthalmoplegia: paralysis of eye muscles.

pannus: abnormal membrane-like corneal vascularization (*pannus* means cloth).

proptosis: displacement of eye out of its orbit.

ptosis: dropping or falling of eyelid.

retinal detachment: separation of retina from choroid that causes loss of vision; caused by abscesses or hemorrhages in vitreous body, trauma, complications of intraocular surgery, inflammation or tumors of choroid, and passage of vitreous or aqueous humor through hole in retina.

strabismus (strah-biz′mus): deviation of eye, with various forms called *tropias* (meaning turning), including *esotropia* (turning inward; also called *convergent strabismus* or crossed eyes and seen in some Siamese cats); *exotropia* (turning outward; also called *wall-eye*), *hypertropia* (upward deviation of one eye); and *hypotropia* (downward deviation of one eye).

synechia (sĭ-nek′e-ah): adhesion of one part of eye to another, especially iris to cornea or lens (*synechia* means continuity).

trichiasis: irritation of the cornea caused by abnormal hairs growing from the palpebral margins and impinging on the corneal surface.

xerophthalmia: a condition of dry corneas and conjunctivae.

SURGICAL AND OTHER PROCEDURES OF THE EYE

blepharoplasty (blef′ah-ro-plas″te): plastic repair of eyelid.

blepharorrhaphy: suturing together of eyelid margins (also called *tarsorrhaphy*).

blepharotomy: incision of eyelid (also called *tarsotomy*).

canthoplasty (kan′tho-plas″te): plastic surgery of palpebral fissure, especially section of canthus to lengthen fissure and surgical restoration of defective canthus (also called *cantholysis*).

canthotomy: incision of canthus.

capsulectomy: excision of capsule of crystalline lens.

capsulotomy: incision of capsule of crystalline lens.

cataract implant: procedure for implantation of permanent artificial lens after cataract removal.

conjunctivoplasty: plastic repair of conjunctiva.

cyclodialysis (si″klo-di-al′i-sis): procedure for glaucoma, to form communication between anterior chamber of eye and suprachoroidal space.

dacryoadenectomy (dak″re-o-ad″ĕ-nek′to-me): excision of tear gland.

dacryocystectomy: excision of lacrimal (tear) sac.

dacryocystotomy: incision of lacrimal gland or duct (also called *lacrimotomy*).

enucleation: excision of eyeball.

iridectomy: excision of part of iris.

iridencleisis (ir″ĭ-den-kli′sis): procedure used to reduce intraocular pressure, forming permanent drain for aqueous humor by strangulation of slip of iris in corneal incision.

keratectomy: excision of portion of the cornea.

keratocentesis: puncture of cornea for aspiration of aqueous humor.

keratoplasty: corneal transplant or repair of cornea.

keratotomy: incision of cornea.

laser surgery: use of instrument that concentrates light energy into narrow beam so that treatment of tissue can be done so quickly that surrounding areas are not affected; use within eyeball to repair the retina.

VISUAL TESTS AND DIAGNOSTIC INSTRUMENTS

electroretinogram (ERG): measures functioning of retina.

fluorescent eye stain: test to detect abnormalities or injuries in cornea.

goniometry: measures drainage angle of eye.

menace reflex: indication of vision in animals.

ophthalmoscope (of-thal″mo-skōp): instrument that examines interior of eye using light source, perforated mirror, and system of lenses.

Schirmer tear test: measures tear production.

sonogram: use of ultrasound to detect diseases of eye.

tonometry: measures intraocular pressure.

SENSE OF HEARING

Ear and related anatomic terms

auricle: external projecting part of ear (also called *pinna*).

auris: term that refers to ear.

cerumen: earwax.

cochlea (kok′le-ah): snail-shaped canal in inner ear.

endolymph: fluid that fills semicircular canals and membranous labyrinth of ear.

eustachian tube (u-sta′ke-an): tube that leads from ear to throat (also called *auditory tube*).

guttural pouch: ventral diverticulum of eustachian tube in equine.

incus: anvil-shaped bone in middle ear (also called *anvil*).

labyrinth (lab-ĭ-rinth): inner ear, consisting of numerous canals and membranes and organ of hearing, the organ of Corti.

malleus: hammer-shaped bone in middle ear (also called *hammer*).

meatus: opening to ear; both internal and external.

organ of Corti: spiral organ of hearing located on basilar membrane of cochlear membrane.

ossicles: little bones of middle ear.

otolith: stone in utricle and saccule of inner ear (*lith* means stone).

perilymph: fluid that fills some chambers of inner ear.

pinna: see *auricle.*

saccule: small, hair-lined sac of inner ear, which together with utricle and semicircular canals is organ for equilibrium.

semicircular canals: three membranous canals (lateral, superior, and posterior) contained within bony semicircular structures of labyrinth, involved with equilibrium.

stapes (sta′pēz): stirrup-shaped bone in middle ear (also called *stirrup*).

tympanic membrane: membrane *(eardrum)* that separates middle ear from external ear and transmits vibrations to ossicles.

utricle (u′tre-k′l): small hair-lined sac of inner ear that is concerned with equilibrium.

vestibulocochlear nerve: cranial nerve VIII; has branches for transmitting sound and equilibrium to brain.

Pathologic conditions of the ear

INFLAMMATIONS AND INFECTIONS OF THE EAR

eustachitis (u″sta-ki′tis): inflammation of eustachian tube.

labyrinthitis: inflammation of inner ear or labyrinth.

myringitis: inflammation of eardrum.

otitis media, externa, and interna: inflammation of middle ear (also called *tympanitis*), external ear, and inner ear, respectively.

panotitis: inflammation of all parts of ear.

vestibulitis: inflammation of vestibular system.

OTHER ABNORMAL CONDITIONS AND DESCRIPTIVE TERMS OF THE EAR

deafness: complete or partial loss of sense of hearing; cause in white cats with blue eyes is perinatal degeneration of cochlea; similar condition also occurs in dalmations and other dogs.

hematoma (aural): blood-filled swelling of ear pinna.

mites (ear): ear infection with *otodectes spp.*

otalgia: earache.

otorrhea (o″to-re′ah): discharge from ear.

vertigo: dizziness.

Oncology

Other tumors occur in the structures of the ear, as they do in other parts of the body, but only one peculiar to the ear is given here.

ceruminous gland adenocarcinoma: malignant tumor of wax-producing cells in ear canal.

Surgical procedures of the ear

ablation: removal of ear canal.

Zepp and Lacroix operations: procedures to bypass narrowed portions of ear canal.

SENSE OF TOUCH AND OTHER CUTANEOUS SENSES

free nerve ending: sensory dendritic nerve endings located close to surface of skin and around hair follicles.

hyperalgesia: a state of excessive sensitivity to pain at the site of an injury.

Krause end bulb: globular nerve structure deep in skin, believed to be receptor for heat and cold, along with free nerve endings and capillary responses (also called *Krause's corpuscle*).

Meissner's (tactile) corpuscle: small, oval body in corium (layer of skin below epidermis) with interlaced sensory fibrils and epithelioid cells believed to be receptors for light touch, along with free nerve endings.

nociception: the peripheral and central nervous system processing of information about the internal or external environment related to tissue damage, including the quality, intensity, location, and duration of stimuli.

nociceptors: specialized peripheral receptors that signal actual or potential tissue damage by mechanical, thermal, or chemical stimuli.

nociperception: the conscious interpretation of sensory information as unpleasant; the perception of pain.

Pacinian corpuscle: oval sensory body located deep in subcutaneous layer; appears to be receptor for heavy pressure (also called *lamellated corpuscle*).

pain: an unpleasant sensory or emotional experience associated with actual or potential tissue damage.

Ruffini corpuscle: oval sensory end structure in corium believed to be receptor for warmth; also seems to be function of free nerve endings and capillary responses.

vibrissae: large tactile hairs found on the faces of many animals, commonly called whiskers.

16 The Immune System

The defenders of the body

CHAPTER OVERVIEW

The Latin term *immunis,* meaning exempt, is the source of the English word *immunity.* The immune system consists of cells and chemicals that protect the body against invasion by foreign substances and maintain its general health. Weak immune system responses can result in failure to combat infections or malignancies. Excessively strong immune system responses can result in *hypersensitivities* or *autoimmune disease.*

There are many mechanisms in the various systems of the body that are involved in preventing infection and disease (Fig. 16-1) Some systems, such as the cardiovascular and lymphatic, function directly to destroy invading organisms. Other systems have more indirect roles in protecting the body. This chapter describes the immune system and its component parts and mechanisms.

NONSPECIFIC IMMUNE MECHANISMS

Nonspecific immune defenses protect against foreign cells or matter without having to recognize their specific identities. These defenses recognize a general property that marks the invader as foreign. The nonspecific immune defenses include defenses at the body surfaces, the response to injury known as *inflammation,* and a family of antiviral proteins called *interferons.*

The integumentary system poses both a physical and a chemical barrier to invading organisms. Sweat, sebum (from the sebaceous glands), and cerumen (from the ceruminous glands) all help to maintain the skin environment. The respiratory system provides mechanical and chemical barriers to infection. Ciliated mucous membranes of the respiratory system filter the incoming air of impurities. Mucus, which coats the walls of the upper respiratory tract, entraps foreign material and has antiseptic properties. Products of the gastrointestinal tract, such as saliva and hydrochloric acid, prevent many pathogens from multiplying. Other mechanisms include tears from the eyes and urine from the genitourinary tract. Tears and urine can wash foreign substances out of the body, limit the growth of bacteria, or even kill certain organisms.

Other substances are involved in protecting the body from disease. Natural body chemicals such as *histamines* and *prostaglandins* produce vasodilation and inflammation. Histamines and prostaglandins increase the local vascular permeability, bringing more leukocytes and phagocytes to the area to combat the infection. Chemicals called *pyrogens* (*pyr-* means fire or heat) are released by invading bacteria and by the defending leukocytes. Pyrogens cause the body temperature to increase, producing a fever. This activates the phagocytic action of the immune system. *Phagocytosis* is a process whereby particulate matter is engulfed and destroyed.

A large group of plasma proteins known as *complement* provides another means for killing microbes. Complement proteins are

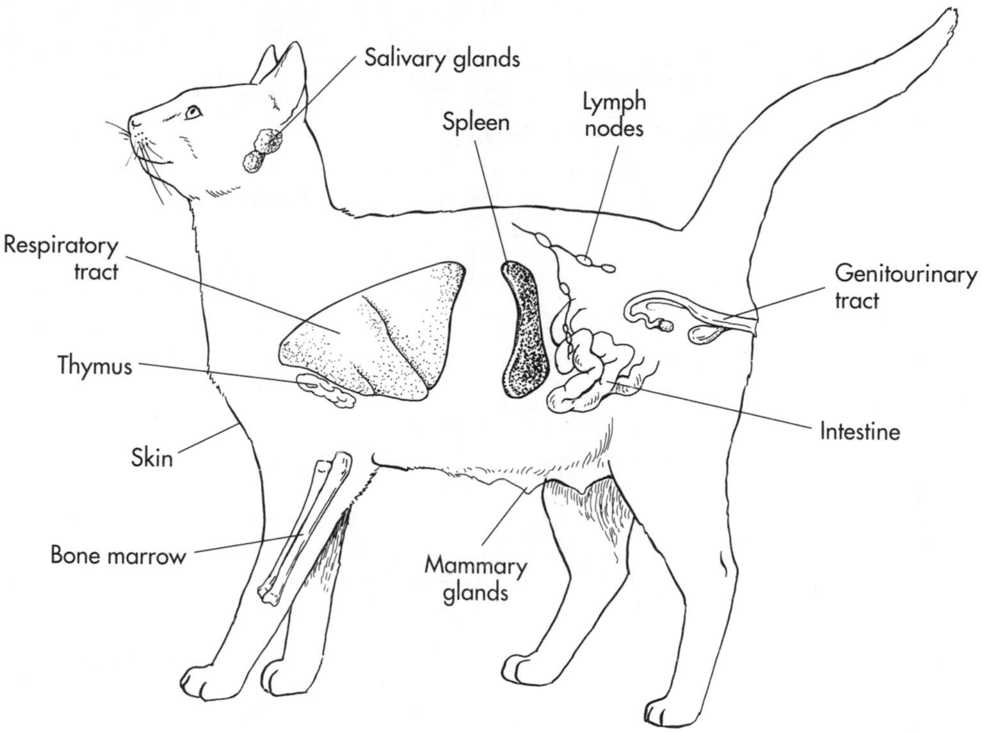
Salivary glands
Spleen
Lymph nodes
Respiratory tract
Genitourinary tract
Thymus
Skin
Intestine
Bone marrow
Mammary glands

FIG. 16-1 Major body defense mechanisms.

activated by invading organisms in a specific sequence to produce phagocytosis and inflammation. The cells of the immune system release protein messengers called *cytokines* that regulate host cell growth and function in immune defense. *Interferons* are a family of cytokines that are synthesized by body cells stimulated by the invasion of viruses. Interferon nonspecifically inhibits viral replication inside host cells and promotes antitumor activities.

SPECIFIC IMMUNE MECHANISMS

Specific immunity is the response of the defenses of the body to specific substances that are recognized as harmful. Substances that are capable of producing such immune system reactions are called *antigens*. Antigens can be foreign to the body, such as bacteria, viruses, and parasites, or can be part of the body's immune mechanisms.

White blood cells called *lymphocytes* are the essential cells in specific immune defense. There are three main types of *lymphocytes: B cells, T cells,* and *null cells.* B cells are formed and mature in the bone marrow. They are involved in producing *humoral immunity* (Fig. 16-2). The term *humoral* denotes communication by way of soluble chemical messengers, in this case antibodies in the blood. B cells produce proteins called *antibodies* or *immunoglobulins* that respond to antigens in the blood. There are five main classes of antibodies: IgG, IgM, IgE, IgA, and IgD. IgG, commonly called *gamma globulin,* is the most abundant immunoglobulin in the

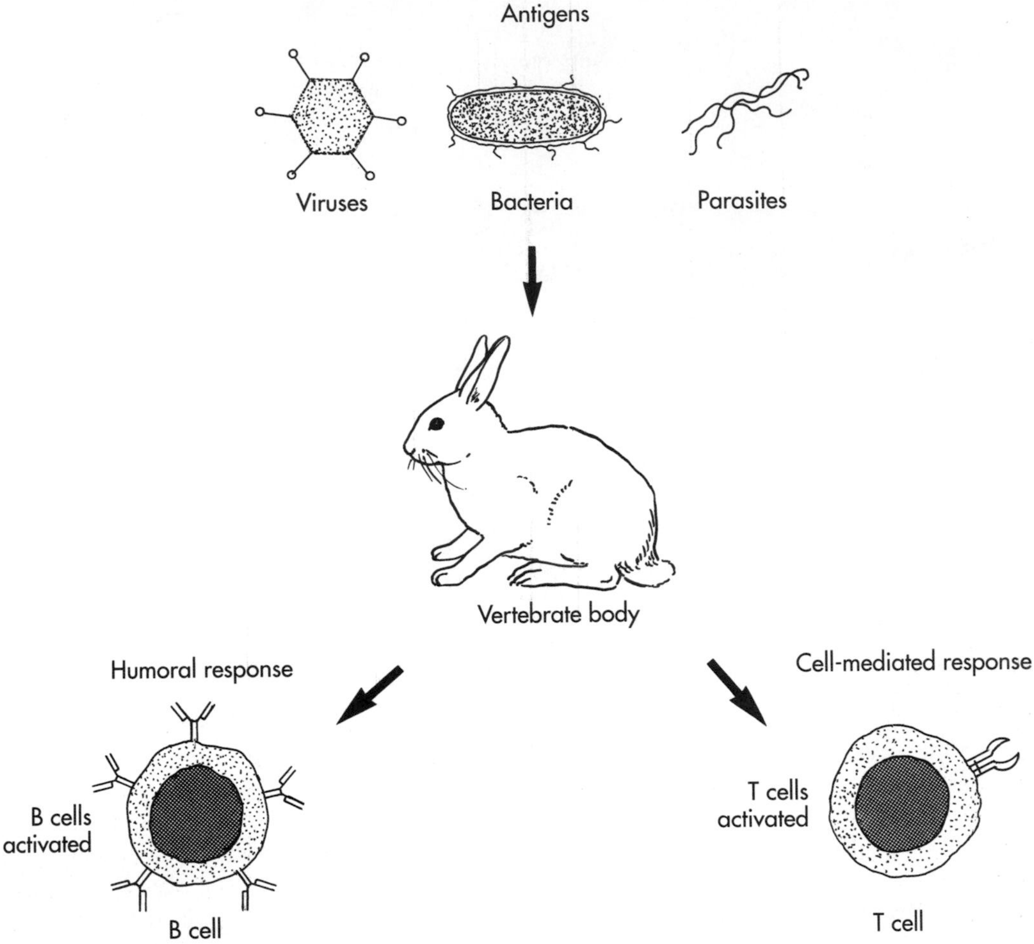
Antigens
Viruses
Bacteria
Parasites
Vertebrate body
Humoral response
Cell-mediated response
B cells activated
B cell
T cells activated
T cell

FIG. 16-2 Immune response to antigen.

body. IgM is the first immunoglobulin produced when antigens invade. IgE is associated with allergic reactions. IgA is found in saliva, tears, and milk and in the mucous membrane lining the intestines and bronchi. The function of IgD is still unclear.

Antibodies work by binding to the antigens, preventing them from functioning and accelerating their destruction or elimination. The binding of antigen to antibodies on a B cell's surface stimulates it to differentiate, forming two types of cells: *plasma cells* and *memory cells*. Plasma cells are responsible for the initial antibody response, called the *primary response*. The primary response takes some time to produce sufficient antibodies to be effective, and usually some disease develops. The *secondary* or *memory response* is facilitated by the ability of B cells to develop into memory cells. Memory cells do not secrete antibodies initially. When memory cells recognize a previously encountered antigen, they develop into plasma cells to rapidly produce large amounts of specific antibodies in response. This effect causes the animal to have a high antibody

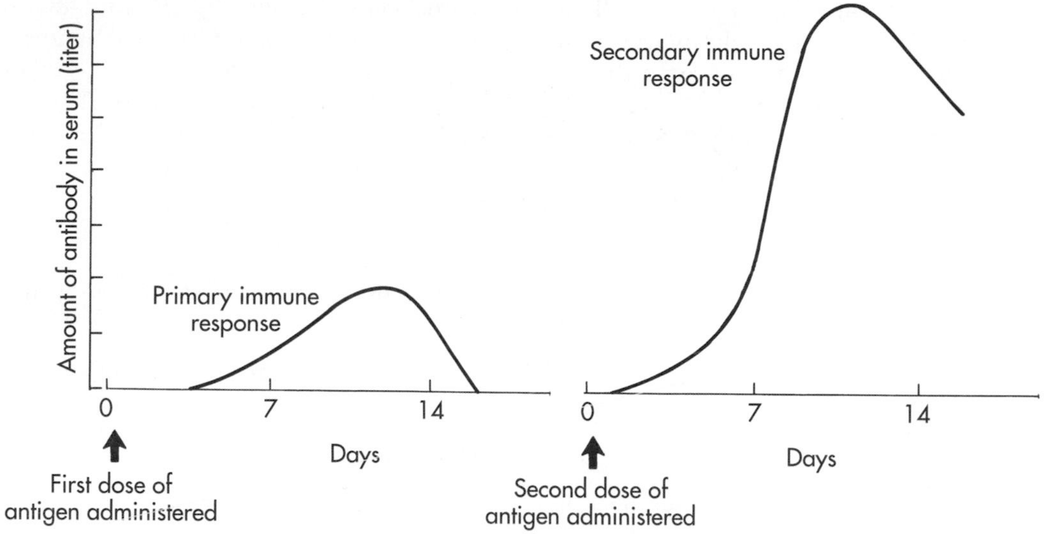
Amount of antibody in serum (titer)
Primary immune response
Secondary immune response
0
7
14
0
7
14
Days
Days
First dose of antigen administered
Second dose of antigen administered

FIG. 16-3 Humoral immune response.

level or high *titer* (Fig. 16-3). The antibodies attack the antigens, preventing development of that specific disease. Long-term immunity is produced to the specific invading microorganism.

T cells also arise in the bone marrow, but they derive their name from their site of maturation, the thymus. T cells are involved in *cellular or cell-mediated immunity* (Fig. 16-2). There are two major types of T cells: *cytotoxic T cells* and *helper T cells.* Cytotoxic T cells are also called *CD8+ cells* because they have the protein CD8 in their plasma membranes. Cytotoxic T cells are attack cells. They have a vital function in monitoring the cells of the body. They can destroy virus-infected cells, cancer cells, and cells of a transplanted foreign tissue. Like the B cells, cytotoxic T cells also can become memory cells. They respond rapidly and vigorously to the presence of previously encountered antigens, producing long-term immunity. Helper T cells are also called *CD4+ cells* because they have the protein CD4 in their plasma membranes. Helper T cells secrete *cytokines.* Cytokines, host cell growth factors, play an important role in stimulating the immune response of T cells and B cells.

T cells can bind antigen only when the antigen appears on the plasma membrane of a host cell complexed with the cell's *major histocompatibility complex (MHC)* proteins. The major histocompatibility complex is a tightly linked cluster of genes whose products, the MHC proteins, are associated with intercellular recognition and self/nonself discrimination. There are two classes of MHC proteins: I and II. *Class I MHC proteins* are found on the surface of all cells of an animal's body except red blood cells. Cytotoxic T cells need antigen to be associated with class I MHC proteins. *Class II MHC proteins* are found on the surfaces of macrophages and B cells. Helper T cells need antigen to be associated with class II MHC proteins.

The third type of lymphocytes, null cells, do not have the surface molecules that characterize B cells and T cells. Null cells cannot develop into memory cells. A type of null cell called a *natural killer (NK) cell* plays an important role in the body's defense against tumor cells. Natural killer cells can kill tumor cells and viral infected cells by *lysis*. Lysis is a process in which a specific antibody causes destruction of a cell.

Once an attack of the antigen is successfully completed, the great majority of B cells, plasma cells, helper T cells, and cytotoxic T cells that participated in it die by *apoptosis*. Apoptosis is a type of programmed cell death in which the cell self-destructs. The timely death of these cells prevents the immune defense from becoming excessive.

REVIEW A

1. ____________ immune defenses protect against foreign substances without having to recognize their specific identity.
2. ____________ immune defenses depend on specific recognition of the foreign substance.
3. Substances capable of producing an immune response are called ____________.
4. There are three main types of lymphocytes: ____________, ____________, and ____________.
5. B cells are formed and mature in the ____________.
6. B cells are involved in a specific type of immunity called ____________.
7. B cells produce proteins called antibodies or ____________ that respond to antigens in the blood.
8. B cells differentiate into two types of cells: ____________ and ____________.
9. ____________ are responsible for the initial antibody response called the primary response.
10. T cells mature in the ____________.
11. T cells are involved in a specific type of immunity called ____________.
12. There are two type of T cells: ____________ and ____________.
13. A natural killer cell is type of ____________ cell.
14. ____________ is a process in which a specific antibody causes destruction of a cell.

PROTECTIVE IMMUNITY

Immunity can develop passively or actively. *Passive immunity* develops when antibodies are transferred from a mother to her fetus or are injected into an individual animal. Antibodies can be transferred from a mother to her fetus through the placenta. Some animals such as ruminants, horses, and pigs receive low levels of antibodies from the mother before birth. These animals receive most of their antibodies from the *colostrum,* or first milk. If an animal does not receive colostrum or is unable to absorb the antibodies, *failure of passive transfer (FPT)* occurs. Failure of passive transfer predisposes a young animal to infection. Passive immunity provides the animal with short-term immunity.

Active immunity is acquired by *vaccination* or by natural infection with a microorganism. Vaccination is the administration of an *antigen* (vaccine) to stimulate a protective immune response against an infectious agent. In active immunity, the immune system plays an active role to provide the animal with long-term immunity.

IMMUNE SYSTEM PROBLEMS

There are two major types of immune system problems: a weakness or deficiency in the effectiveness of the system or an excessively strong reaction by the system.

Immune System Weakness or Deficiency

Problems that produce deficiencies in the immune system can arise from congenital factors in which blood cells are insufficient or ineffective. Animals with *agammaglobulinemia* have no gamma globulins (antibodies) circulating in their blood. These animals are highly susceptible to fatal infections. *Severe combined immunodeficiency disease (SCID)* results from defects in both humoral and cell-mediated immunity. Severe combined immunodeficiency occurs in Arabian foals. A special strain of mice called SCID mice are used in immunology research. These mice, like their human counterparts, fail to develop mature T and B cells. SCID mice can be kept alive by housing them in a sterile environment. *Cyclic hematopoiesis* is an inherited condition occurring in collies that have a silver-gray coat. These dogs have cyclic fluctuations in their numbers of white blood cells and are more susceptible to infections.

Immunosuppression can be induced by viruses, bacteria, and parasites. Viruses such as *feline immunodeficiency virus (FIV), feline leukemia virus (FeLV),* and *bovine viral diarrhea virus (BVD)* suppress the immune system. Examples of bacterial disease that cause immunosuppression are tuberculosis and Johne's disease in cattle. Animals that are affected by malignancies often exhibit immunosuppression. This occurs in animals that have *lymphoma* (cancer of the lymphatic tissue) and *multiple myeloma* (cancer of the plasma cells). An immunosuppressed debilitated animal is susceptible to *opportunistic* infections. In opportunistic infections, disease is produced by microorganisms that normally would not produce disease.

Immunomodulator or *immunostimulant drugs* sometimes are used in veterinary medicine. Drugs such as levamisole are thought to stimulate the immune system. These drugs are used to treat cancer and immune-mediated diseases.

Excessively Strong Immune System Reaction

In some situations the immune system response to an antigen produces excessive inflammatory reactions and other complications. Various foods and parasites, such as fleas, can produce allergic reactions, which are a type of hypersensitivity reaction. Some animals have a genetic tendency to develop *atopy,* a hypersensitivity reaction that usually involves the skin. Animals that are stung by bees or have a severe reaction to a vaccination can develop *anaphylaxis,* a severe response to a foreign substance. Symptoms such as swelling, airway blockage, and tachycardia can develop acutely and can be life-threatening. Perhaps the greatest problem of overreaction is *autoimmune disease.* The immune system cannot adequately distinguish between foreign antigens and those of its own cells. In autoimmune disease, the body attacks its own cells and tissues. Diseases of this sort include *rheumatoid arthritis* (in which joint tissue is attacked), *myasthenia gravis* (in which the action of the neurotransmitter acetylcholine is affected), and *hemolytic anemia* (in which the red blood cells are destroyed). *Systemic lupus erythematosus* is a multisystem autoimmune disease in which skin, blood vessels, joints, and kidneys are attacked.

Antiinflammatory and *immunosuppressant drugs* are used therapeutically to treat various conditions in animals. Antiinflammatory drugs such as corticosteroids, aspirin, and ibuprofen act by suppressing inflammation. Immunosuppressant drugs such as cyclophosphamide and cyclosporin are used in organ or bone marrow transplants. These drugs suppress the immune system to reduce the potential for organ rejection.

REVIEW B

1. ______________________ immunity develops when antibodies are transferred from a mother to her fetus.
2. ______________________ immunity is acquired by vaccination or by natural infection with a microorganism.
3. The term ______________________ means no gamma globulins circulating in the blood.
4. The acronym SCID stands for ______________________________________.
5. Lymphoma is cancer of the ______________________ tissue.
6. Multiple myeloma is cancer of the ______________________ cells.
7. ______________________ is a hypersensitivity reaction that usually involves the skin, as in food allergies.
8. ______________________ is a severe, often life-threatening response to a foreign substance.
9. Rheumatoid arthritis and systemic lupus erythematosus are examples of ______________________ diseases.
10. Aspirin and ibuprofen are examples of ______________________ drugs.

Chapter 16 Answers

Review A

1. nonspecific
2. specific
3. antigens
4. B cells, T cells, null cells
5. bone marrow
6. humoral
7. immunoglobulin
8. plasma, memory
9. plasma cells
10. thymus
11. cellular (cell-mediated)
12. helper, cytotoxic
13. null
14. lysis

Review B

1. passive
2. active
3. agammaglobulinemia
4. severe combined immunodeficiency disease
5. lymphatic
6. plasma
7. atopy
8. anaphylaxis
9. autoimmune
10. antiinflammatory

Chapter 16 EXERCISES

THE IMMUNE SYSTEM

Exercise 1: Match the term in the right column with the correct definition or statement in the left column by placing the appropriate letter in the blank space provided.

_____ 1. Serum proteins that act in a specific sequence to produce phagocytosis and inflammation	A. Apoptosis
_____ 2. Helper T cells secrete these growth factors	B. FPT
_____ 3. Natural body chemical that increases vascular permeability to bring more white blood cells to area	C. Titer
_____ 4. Condition that occurs if an animal does not receive colostrum	D. Complement
_____ 5. Result of defects in both humoral and cellular immunity	E. IgG
_____ 6. Administration of an antigen to stimulate a protective immune response against an infectious agent	F. Opportunistic
_____ 7. Antibody associated with primary response	G. Pyrogen
_____ 8. Type of disease caused by debilitation when disease normally would not be present	H. MHC
_____ 9. Protein associated with intercellular recognition and self/nonself discrimination	I. SCID
_____ 10. Programmed cell death	J. Histamine
_____ 11. Type of disease that occurs when immune system cannot adequately distinguish between foreign antigen and its own	K. Vaccination
_____ 12. Most abundant antibody in the body	L. IgM
_____ 13. Antibody level measure	M. Cytokines
_____ 14. Cytotoxic T cell	N. CD8+
_____ 15. Chemical that causes the body temperature to increase and activate the immune system	O. Autoimmune disease

CHAPTER 16 PUZZLE

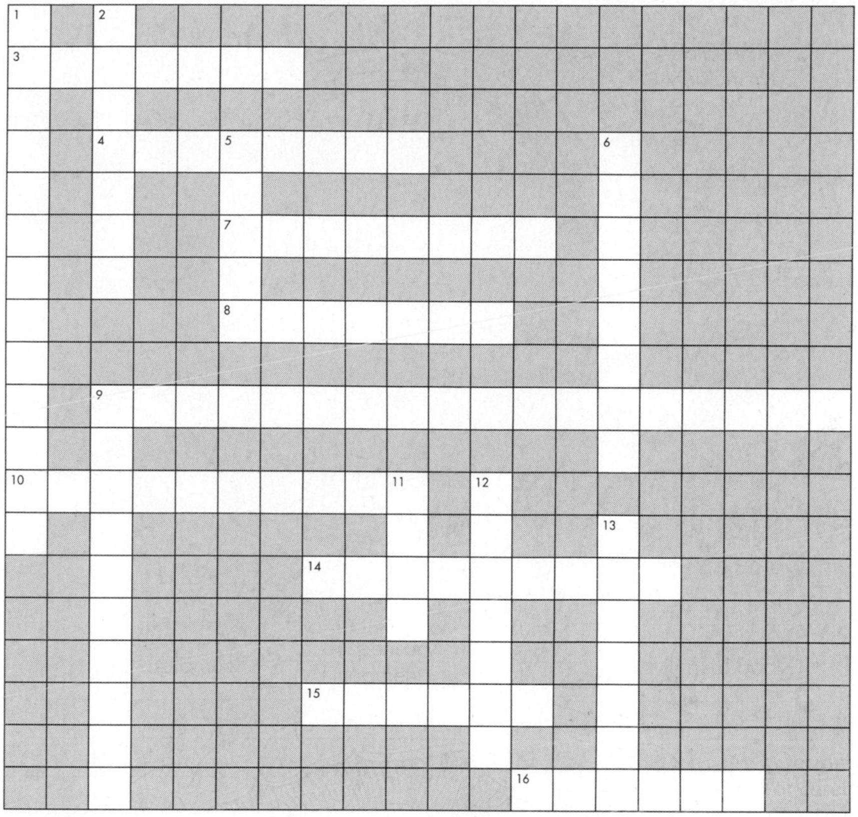
1
2
3
4
5
6
7
8
9
10
11
12
13
14
15
16

ACROSS CLUES

3. Cancer of plasma cells
4. Cancer of lymphatic system
7. Antigen
8. Substance capable of producing an immune response
9. No gamma globulins circulating in blood
10. Protein that protects body against infection and some types of cancer
14. Milk high in antibodies
15. Vaccination gives this type of immunity
16. Type of T cell

DOWN CLUES

1. Antibody
2. Immune response mediated by T cell
5. Type of B cell associated with primary immunity
6. CD8+ cell
9. Rheumatoid arthritis and systemic lupus are this type of disease
11. Type of lymphocyte with no B or T cell surface marker
12. Type of immunity involved when antibodies are transferred from a mother to her fetus
13. B cell involved in this type of immunity

Chapter 16 Answers

Exercise 1

1. D
2. M
3. J
4. B
5. I
6. K
7. L
8. F
9. H
10. A
11. O
12. E
13. C
14. N
15. G

ANSWERS: CHAPTER 16 PUZZLE

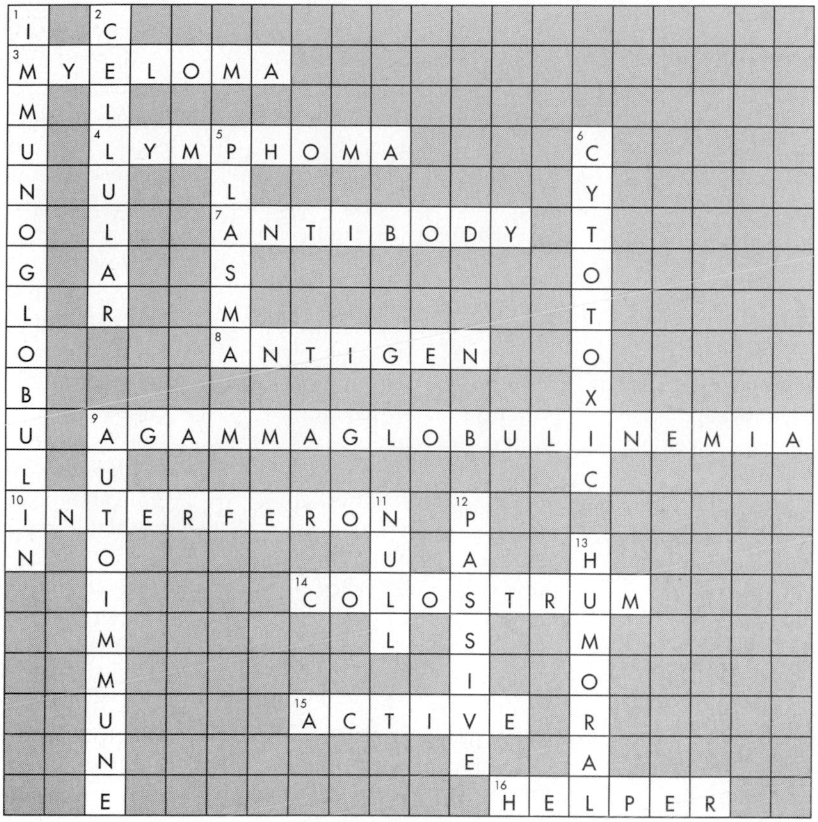
1 IMMUNOGLOBULIN
2 CELLULAR
3 MYELOMA
4 LYMPHOMA
5 PLASMA
6 CYTOTOXIC
7 ANTIBODY
8 ANTIGEN
9 AGAMMAGLOBULINEMIA
9 AUTOIMMUNE
10 INTERFERON
11 NULL
12 PASSIVE
13 HUMORAL
14 COLOSTRUM
15 ACTIVE
16 HELPER

GLOSSARY

active immunity: immunity that follows exposure to antigen; exposure can be natural or by vaccination.

agammaglobulinemia: condition in which animal has no circulating gamma globulins (antibodies) in its blood, causing it to be highly susceptible to infection.

anaphylaxis: severe response to a foreign substance; acute life-threatening symptoms such as swelling, airway blockage, and tachycardia may develop.

antibody (immunoglobulin): specialized serum proteins produced by B lymphocytes in response to particular foreign antigen; facilitates removal or clearance of antigen.

antigen: foreign substance that binds specifically to antibody or T cells and elicits immune response.

antiinflammatory drug: drug such as aspirin or ibuprofen that counteracts or suppresses inflammation.

apoptosis: programmed cell death in which the cell self-destructs.

atopy: clinical syndrome involving hypersensitivity or allergy with hereditary predisposition, often seasonal and characterized by pruritus.

autoimmune disease: disease caused by immune attack against animal's own tissues.

B cells: lymphocytes that mature in bone marrow and are precursors of antibody-secreting plasma cells.

bovine virus diarrhea (BVD): infectious viral disease of cattle causing diarrhea, stomatitis, and rhinitis in young animals.

cell-mediated immunity (cellular immunity): immune response mediated by T cells that play a role in protection against various bacteria, viruses, and cancer.

colostrum: thick, yellow secretion present in mammary gland after parturition; first milk is very rich in maternal antibodies and plays important part in providing passive immunity to neonate.

complement: group of serum proteins that participates in sequence of reactions, resulting in cell lysis.

cyclic hematopoiesis: inherited condition occurring in collies that have silver-gray coat; these dogs have cyclic fluctuations in their number of white blood cells, causing them to be more susceptible to infections.

cytokines: protein messengers released by cells of immune system that regulate host cell growth and function in immune defense.

failure of passive transfer (FPT): occurs when neonate does not receive colostrum or is unable to absorb antibodies, predisposing animal to infection.

feline immunodeficiency virus (FIV): lentivirus that infects cats and gradually destroys selected populations of T lymphocytes, resulting in immunodeficient state.

feline leukemia virus (FeLV): oncovirus that produces variety of conditions in cats including neoplasia, anemia, and reproductive failure; immunosuppression predisposes animal to wide spectrum of secondary diseases.

gamma globulin: immunoglobulin G, most abundant immunoglobulin circulating in body.

hemolytic anemia: can occur as result of disorder of immune system in which antibodies fail to recognize body's own red blood cells and destroy them.

histamine: naturally occurring chemical found in body tissues; involved in hypersensitivity reactions, causing capillary dilation and smooth muscle contraction.

humoral immunity: immunity that can be transferred by antibodies present in plasma, lymph, and tissue fluids.

hypersensitivity: exaggerated immune response causing damage to animal.

immunomodulator (immunostimulant): drugs, such as levamisole, that modulate or stimulate immune system.

immunosuppression: suppression of immune response.

immunosuppressive drugs: drugs, such as cyclophosphamide and cyclosporin, that suppress immune system.

interferon: natural protein produced by variety of cell types that induces antiviral state in cells and helps to regulate immune response.

lymphoma: any cancer of lymphatic tissue.

lysis: destruction of cells or other antigens by specific antibody; *lyse* is the verb form.

major histocompatibility complex (MHC): tightly linked cluster of genes whose product, the MHC proteins, are associated with intercellular recognition and self/nonself discrimination.

memory cell: clonally expanded progeny of T cells and B cells formed after primary antigen response; responsible for speed and higher level of secondary immune response.

multiple myeloma: malignant neoplasm in which plasma cells proliferate and invade bone marrow, causing bone destruction.

myasthenia gravis: action of neurotransmitter acetylcholine is affected, producing syndrome of episodic muscle weakness, which is aggravated by activity; may be acquired as autoimmune disease.

natural killer cell (NK): type of null cell that has cytotoxic ability.

null cells: small group of lymphocytes that fail to express surface molecules characteristic of B cells and T cells.

opportunistic: type of disease caused by immunosuppression or debilitation when disease normally would not occur.

passive immunity: transient immunity; protection of one individual conferred by administration of antibody produced in another individual.

phagocytosis: condition whereby matter is engulfed and destroyed.

plasma cells: antibody-producing cells derived from activated B cells.

primary immune response: initial humoral and cellular immune response to antigen.

prostaglandins: naturally occurring chemicals that cause vascular permeability and help to control inflammation.

pyrogens: agents released by invading bacteria and by defending leukocytes, causing body temperature to increase and immune system to be activated.

rheumatoid arthritis: chronic autoimmune disease that causes erosion and destruction of joints, producing swelling and lameness.

secondary immune response (memory response): more rapid and heightened immune response that occurs after second exposure to antigen.

severe combined immunodeficiency disease (SCID): congenital immune system deficiency disease in which animal must be kept in sterile environment to prevent illness or death from infections.

systemic lupus erythematosis (SLE): chronic disease of autoimmune origin involving many organ systems, characterized by joint, renal, skin, and hematologic disorders.

T cells: lymphocytes that depend on thymus for their differentiation; involved in cellular immunity.

T cytotoxic cells: T lymphocytes that are attack cells; also called *CD8+* cells.

T helper cells: T lymphocytes that, when activated, release growth and differentiation factors to enhance both cell-mediated and humoral immune responses; also called *CD4+* cells.

titer: amount of one substance needed to correspond with a given amount of another substance; used to denote antibody or antigen levels.

vaccination: administration of antigen (vaccine) to stimulate protective immune response against infectious agent.

vaccine: suspension of living or inactivated organisms used as antigen to confer immunity.

LABORATORY PROCEDURES

electrophoresis: technique using electric current to separate proteins; used to identify gross deficiencies or excesses of types of immunoglobulins.

enzyme-linked immunosorbent assay (ELISA): assay in which antibody or antigen can be quantitated by using enzyme-linked antibody and colored substrate to measure activity of bound enzyme.

immunofluorescence assay (IFA): immunologic test using antibodies chemically conjugated with fluorescent dye.

titration: measurement of level of specific antibodies in serum by testing increasing dilutions of serum for antibody activity.

virus isolation: use of special culturing techniques to isolate virus from blood or body fluids.

Western blot: detection of protein antigens that have been electrophoretically separated and transferred to filter by labeling antigenic bands with radioactive or enzyme-conjugated antibodies.

IV

TERMINOLOGY OF THE ANIMAL INDUSTRY

The animal industry encompasses all aspects of animal use in our society. Section IV of *Learning Veterinary Terminology* consists of seven chapters that introduce you to the main branches of the animal industry. Each segment is based on a single species or group, each with its own needs and peculiarities. Species terminology reflects the way in which animals are used by humans. Therefore it is very different from the veterinary medical terminology in earlier sections. It is based on ordinary language rather than Greek and Latin, and it varies regionally. It is the language used daily by farmers, breeders, trainers, fanciers, pet owners, and any others whose lives most closely intersect with those of animals. This section's purpose is to enable you to communicate knowledgeably with these animal owners.

Chapter 17 gives an overview of dogs and cats, the species with which most readers are likely to be familiar. Chapter 18, "Equine Industry," describes the many ways in which horses are used and the basic vocabulary that results. Chapter 19, "Cattle Industry," explains why these animals are kept and describes the basic management procedures on which that industry's terminology is based. Chapter 20 deals with swine and the terminology unique to that species. Small ruminants, including sheep, goats, and llamas, are covered in Chapter 21. An overview of rodents, rabbits, and laboratory animal science is given in Chapter 22. Chapter 23 is an introduction to the widely variable subject of exotic animals and deals mostly with reptiles and birds. In every case it can be seen that the terminology used results not only from the specific characteristics of the species involved but also from the ways in which the species is used or managed for the benefit of human beings.

17 Dogs and Cats

CHAPTER OVERVIEW

Dogs, cats, and people are three species whose natural history has been linked for millennia. Living and working together has created a relationship between the three that can be viewed as a kind of coevolution. Originally domesticated for their help in the economic life of early communities, dogs and cats are now increasingly kept for social and psychologic reasons as pets and companions. The more recent and future development of these domesticated animals cannot be separated from that of *Homo sapiens.* Our species has altered the natural world. Both consciously and unconsciously we exert selective forces on the rest of the planet's living things. That selection is largely responsible for the animals we know today as dogs and cats.

DOGS

Canis familiaris has lived with humans for at least 12,000 years. Dogs are extremely social animals. They evolved living in groups, and their original social organization probably was much like that of their close cousins, wolves. Intimate and long association with humans permits dogs to include their owners in their *pack,* or family group. Therefore dogs may assume a *dominant* or *submissive* role with their owners, in contrast to cats, who maintain a strong sense of independence. A dominant animal will not easily accept discipline and direction from its owner. A submissive one accepts a nondominant role in the family.

Most dogs today in developed countries are kept as companions or pets. Some still work at traditional jobs such as hunting, guarding, retrieving, and herding. In the United States, dogs are also used as guide dogs for people with disabilities; as guard dogs and sled dogs; and in customs inspections, bomb squads, rescue missions, police patrols, biomedical research, and pet-facilitated therapy. Many compete in shows and are used for breeding. Other uses for dogs are racing, notably by greyhounds, and fighting, although this is *inhumane* and illegal.

Dog shows and performance trials bring pleasure and often profit to dog owners. The most famous organization involved with showing is the American Kennel Club (AKC), but many other groups exist, some devoted to specific breeds. Many of these organizations run shows of various types. When dogs compete at shows, they are not compared with each other but with the ideal specimen of their breed. *Unbenched* shows are now the most common. When the dogs are not being exhibited in the ring, they are with their owners, not assigned to any specific place. During dog shows run by licensed or member dog clubs, championship points are awarded. A *bench show,* now very rare, required dogs to be leashed or caged on a platform when not being exhibited. A *match* show is one in which no championship points are awarded; it is mostly a practice event for dogs and their exhibitors. *Field trials* are competitions for hounds and sporting breeds in which the animals are judged on ability and style in hunting, tracking, and retrieving. Some dogs excel at *obedience trials* demonstrating their ability to interpret and carry out commands.

CATS

Over the centuries the cat, *Felis catus,* has been both worshiped by the ancient Egyptians and persecuted for witchcraft in the Dark Ages. The association of cat and humans probably began about 6000 or 7000 years ago as society was able to produce agricultural surpluses of grains and other foods. The cat was needed to protect these storage sites from rodents.

Only in very recent times has the relationship between *Felis catus* and *Homo sapiens* expanded. Cats now number more than 60 million and are the most popular pet in the United States. Because of its small size, low maintenance, and independent personality, the cat fits into our increasingly busy urban and suburban life. This popularity is reflected by the growing national veterinary organizations devoted to cats and the exclusively *feline* practitioners and hospitals. Cats are also used in biomedical research and pet-facilitated therapy, shown in competitions, bred for profit, and still used for rodent control.

Organizations of owners and breeders of felines, such as the Cat Fanciers Association, sponsor shows in which cats are judged on their *conformation,* their external physical appearance.

BREEDING

Breeding dogs and cats has become a major business. A purebred dog or cat has a known *sire* (male parent) and *dam* (female parent). *Registration papers* are the documents that show the animal's pedigree and indicate that it is registered with the American Kennel Club or breed association.

BREEDS

Dogs often are classed as *purebreds* or *mixed breeds.* A purebred dog is a member of a recognized breed eligible for registration. A mixed breed dog is a combination of different breeds. The original dog was a medium-sized animal resembling its wolflike ancestor. All purebred domestic dogs are derived from this type canine by selective breeding over millennia. Size ranges from a toy breed, such as a Chihuahua weighing 3 pounds, to a giant breed of more than 100 pounds, such as a Russian wolfhound.

Breeds that have some behavioral, physical, or historical similarity to one another often are organized into groups. A common classification system categorizes dogs as working, sporting, terriers, nonsporting, hounds, and toys. Examples of breeds in each group are given in the box on the following page.

Some mixed breed dogs resemble purebreds and may have names such as *poodle mixes* or *shepherd mixes.* Some are called simply mixed breed dogs. *Mongrel* and *mutt* are terms generally not used for mixed breed dogs in a veterinary hospital setting.

Many cat breeds exist. The most common cat is the *domestic short hair (DSH).* These are *not* mixed breed cats. Also common are domestic long hairs, Siamese, Persian, Himalayan, Abyssinian, Burmese, Manx, and Maine coon cats. Other breeds include Scottish folds, ragdolls, Somalis, rex, Birman, sphinx, and ocicats.

Cat markings and colors are important in identification. *Calicos* and *tortoiseshells* have two X-chromosome–linked colors, black and orange (also called red, yellow, or ginger). Calicos have discrete patches of the two colors on white, whereas tortoiseshells have the black and orange interspersed. They are all female unless genetically abnormal. Other genetic factors produce deafness in white cats with blue eyes.

Tabbies have black stripes or spots over a brown or gray undercoat. They may have white fur, too. Other common colors are black, black and white, orange, gray, gray and white, and white.

Siamese and *Himalayans* are described by the hair color of their *points* (Fig. 17-1). Points are the face (mask), ears, feet or legs, and tail. The rest of the body generally is a lighter color. The cat may be a seal point, chocolate point, flame point, lilac point, or blue point, among others.

DOG BREEDS

Working breeds

German shepherd
Doberman pinscher
Great Dane
rottweiler
Old English sheepdog
St. Bernard

Sporting breeds

golden retriever
Labrador retriever
weimaraner
Irish setter
cocker spaniel

Terriers

cairn terrier
fox terrier
Scottish terrier
West Highland white terrier

Nonsporting breeds

Boston terrier
bulldog
poodle
dalmatian
Lhasa apso

Hounds

basset hound
Afghan hound
greyhound
Russian wolfhound
beagle
dachshund

Toys

Chihuahua
Maltese
Pekingese
toy poodle
shih tzu
Yorkshire terrier

REVIEW A

1. The scientific name for the domestic dog is ______________________________.
2. The scientific name for the domestic cat is ______________________________.
3. The name for the male parent is ______________________________.
4. The scientific name for human beings is ______________________________.
5. The species adjective for the domestic cat is ______________________________.
6. The term for the female parent is ______________________________.
7. Deaf cats often have ______________________ coats and ______________________ eyes.

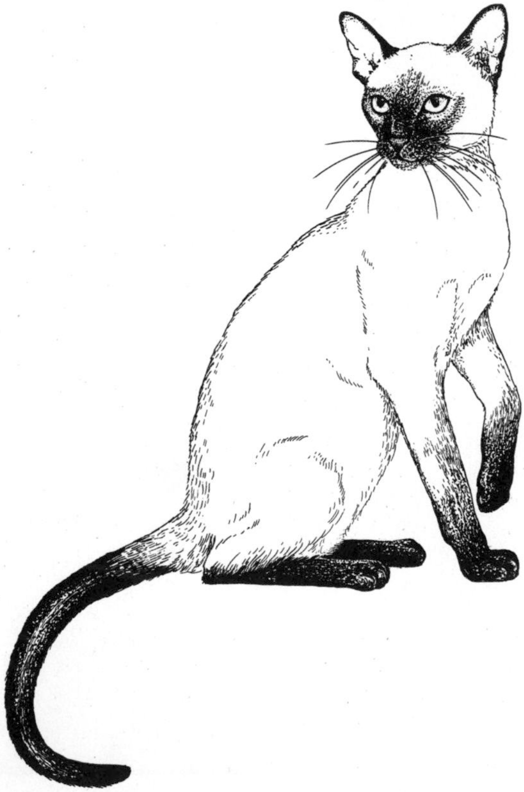

FIG. 17-1 Siamese cat points.

REPRODUCTION

Dogs reach *puberty* somewhere between 8 months and 2 years, with smaller dogs maturing earlier than large ones. Puberty is the time at which an animal reaches sexual maturity and can reproduce. The female comes into *estrus* or heat about once every 7 months (basenji and wolf-crosses once a year).

Ovulation is the release of an egg from the ovary. It is spontaneous in dogs and occurs approximately 12 to 14 days after the onset of vaginal bleeding. Serum *progesterone* rises after ovulation. Progesterone is a hormone associated with the maintenance of pregnancy. In mating dogs, a portion of the penis becomes especially enlarged, and the penis is held in the bitch's vagina by muscular contractions. This is called the *tie* (Fig. 17-2). When so attached, the animals may rotate their bodies and face away from each other while still mating. The tie is not a common behavior among animals other than dogs. It may last up to 1 hour but is not essential for *ejaculation* or *fertilization*.

Duration of pregnancy is 63 days, and the female dog or *bitch* often gives birth to litters of up to 12 or more. *Whelping* is the process of canine *parturition*, or giving birth. Most dogs whelp normally, but some experience difficulty giving birth. This is called *dystocia* and is more common in very small dogs such as Chihuahuas. Puppies can be separated from their mothers after 8 weeks. *Weaning* or withdrawal from mother's milk may be done earlier than 8 weeks. Early contact with humans helps puppies and kittens have good relationships with owners because the process of *socialization* occurs during the first two or three months of life.

False pregnancy is also called *pseudocyesis*. It is common in dogs and may mimic the signs of pregnancy. The mammary glands enlarge and may even produce milk. The animal may exhibit "mothering" behavior, such as nest building. *Spaying* or *ovariohysterectomy* is the cure. Ovariohysterectomy is the removal of ovaries and uterus. *Castration* is the removal of the testes. *Orchiectomy* is the correct term for castration.

Feline reproduction is somewhat different from that of other domestic species. Females, called *queens*, are *induced* ovulators, like ferrets, rabbits, and mink. They ovulate only if sexual activity occurs. They are seasonally *polyestrous*, meaning that they undergo heat cycles several times a year; the frequency is determined by the season.

Gestation or duration of pregnancy is approximately 63 days. One to 10 or more fe-

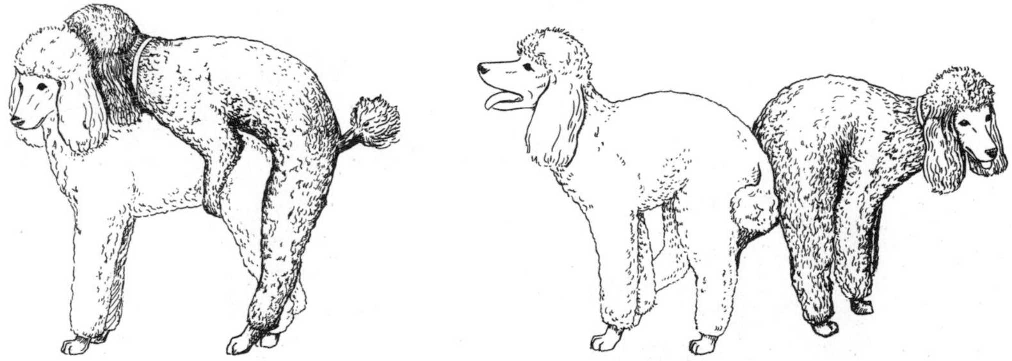

FIG. 17-2 Canine mating: the tie.

tuses may be present, possibly sired by more than one male. Giving birth is called *queening* in cats. It is almost always trouble-free. Kittens are born with their eyes and ears sealed, and they are unable to walk. *Lactation,* or milk production, is also usually problem-free. Kittens should remain with their mother until about 8 weeks of age. Young cats reach puberty around 6 to 9 months of age and should be spayed or castrated at around 6 months. Neutering as early as a few weeks of age is increasingly common, especially in humane organizations.

BEHAVIOR

Dogs are *social* animals and usually adapt well to being cooperative members of a human family. However, the occasional dog shows signs of *aggression* or other behavioral abnormality. *Behavior modification* methods have been useful in treating these animals. These techniques seek to change actions rather than deal with motivations or emotions. Most current opinion favors training dogs by *positive reinforcement* of desirable behavior with rewards and praise rather than punishment.

Some normal dog behavior may be disturbing, irritating, or embarrassing to people, but it should not be judged as "bad" behavior to be punished. Dogs engage in barking, chewing, licking, sniffing, and other actions that would not be appropriate for people. In fact, *anthropomorphism,* or attributing human emotions to animals, is a common error in training and disciplining animals. *Ethology* is the science of studying animal behavior.

Feline behavior, including social behavior, probably has changed little since the cat was domesticated. However, the asocial image of the cat may not be entirely accurate. The domestic cat may be primarily solitary but exhibits long-term group associations, complete with complex social structures. The focus of both socialized and *feral* feline social groups is the female and her kittens. Feral domestic cats have reverted to a wild, untamed state.

A cat in heat shows characteristic and often disturbing behaviors. She rubs her face on objects, rolls around, and assumes a position of *lordosis,* with her lumbar spine curved downward and her tail pulled over to one side (Fig. 17-3). While loudly vocalizing or *calling,* she may knead, especially with her hind feet. Some females urinate outside the litter pan when in heat. Others come into heat very frequently, especially during spring and summer.

Intact *toms* (male cats) at maturity begin to *spray* their urine around the house. In-

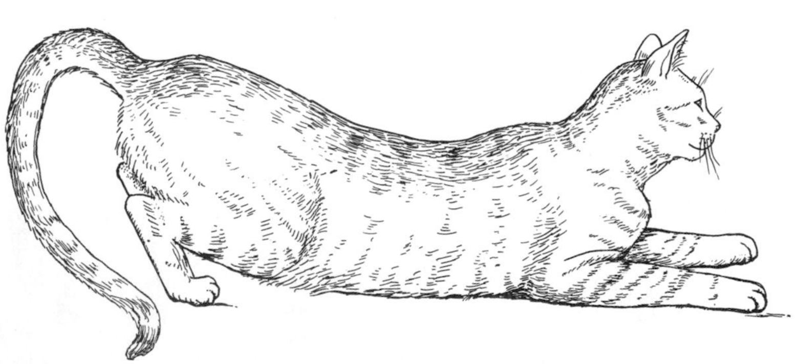

FIG. 17-3 The queen exhibiting lordosis.

stead of squatting, they usually back up toward a vertical surface and spray urine. Their urine becomes extremely pungent and difficult to deodorize. Cats spray to mark their territory, alerting other toms to their presence. These and other secretions contain *pheromones,* biochemicals that convey messages to other animals.

Cats need to claw or scratch on something. Regular nail trimming, providing a *scratching post* (a structure of wood or carpeted material), covering the nail with a commercial plastic cap, and *declawing* or *onychectomy* are methods used to prevent furniture damage. Onychectomy is the surgical removal of most of the bone that contains the growing nail. Some humane groups and veterinarians consider this surgery inhumane.

Some cats may begin urinating or defecating outside the litter box. These are called *elimination problems.* Once physical causes are ruled out, a behavioral diagnosis may be considered.

REVIEW B

1. The age at which an animal can first reproduce is called ______________________.
2. The process of giving birth is called ______________________. In dogs, the particular name is ______________________. In cats, it is ______________________.
3. The hormone most closely associated with maintenance of pregnancy is ______________________ ______________________.
4. Difficulty giving birth is called ______________________.
5. Another word for false pregnancy is ______________________.
6. Attributing human traits to animals is called ______________________.
7. The release of eggs from the ovary is called ______________________.
8. *Spay* is the common word for the surgical procedure ______________________.
9. The cyclic period of sexual and nonsexual activity is called the ______________________ cycle.
10. The surgical removal of the testes is called ______________________.
11. A female cat is called a(n) ______________________.
12. A female dog is called a(n) ______________________.
13. A male cat is called a(n) ______________________.
14. A domestic cat that lives in a wild state is called ______________________.

NUTRITIONAL CONSIDERATIONS

Although dogs are *carnivores,* an all-meat diet is unbalanced and unhealthy. Cats are much stricter carnivores and need more protein than do most other domestic species. Because of the availability of good commercial pet foods, nutritional problems are not as common as in the past.

The *magnesium* content of food has been associated with *feline lower urinary tract disease (FLUTD).* For cats who have had FLUTD, special low-magnesium, urine-acidifying diets have been formulated and are commercially available.

COMMON DOG AND CAT DISEASES

Among the tasks of the veterinary profession is to diagnose and treat animal disease, alleviate pain and suffering, prevent disease where possible, and protect public health.

An animal presented to a veterinary clinic or hospital with a health problem is given a *physical examination.* This process includes inspection, *palpation, percussion, auscultation,* and smell to determine the animal's health. Palpation is a technique in which the examiner uses his or her hands to feel the texture, size, and consistency of various parts of an animal's body. Percussion is the tapping of a part of the animal's body with the fingertips to evaluate the size and consistency of its internal organs. It can also be used to detect the presence of fluid or gas in a body cavity and evaluate its quantity. Auscultation is listening for sounds in an animal's body, using a stethoscope. An *otoscope* and *ophthalmoscope* are used to examine the ears and eyes, respectively. The examiner should know the animal's *history,* a systematic account of its life and factors that may have a bearing on its present condition. *Signs* and *symptoms* are important to the examiner. In human medicine, signs are objective findings, as perceived by the examiner, whereas symptoms are the subjective perceptions of the patient. The two terms generally are used interchangeably in veterinary medicine. If blood tests are needed, *venipuncture* (insertion of a needle into a vein) is performed to collect a sample. *Radiography* (use of X rays) and other tests may be used if indicated. An *indication* is a symptom or circumstance that calls for a certain treatment or test to be done. Its opposite, a *contraindication,* means that a certain treatment should *not* be used. The physical examination, history, and laboratory tests constitute the data base on which a *diagnosis,* the identification of the disease, is made and on which a plan of treatment is developed. The diagnosis may make possible a *prognosis,* a prediction of the probable outcome of the disease based on the condition of the animal and the usual course of the disease.

Information is recorded into the animal's permanent record, often a type of *problem-oriented veterinary medical record.* In such systems, use of a *master problem list* makes assessing a patient's medical problems much easier.

If an animal is treated and sent home, it is called an *outpatient.* If it is hospitalized, it is an *inpatient.* For example, a dog with *kennel cough* or a cat with an *upper respiratory infection (URI)* often is treated at home as an outpatient. These conditions resemble colds and flu in people and occur with or without *anorexia,* or loss of appetite. However, a dog with a *pyometra* or pus-filled uterus usually is treated surgically as an inpatient. For inpatients, the medical record can be *SOAPed,* an acronym that stands for *subjective, objective, assessment,* and *plan or procedure.* SOAPing ensures the orderly recording of data about the patient, an early assessment or diagnosis (tentative or definitive), and a treatment or diagnostic plan.

Other problems the veterinary clinic may treat range from a *high rise* cat or dog who has jumped or fallen from a height to *ringworm,* a *zoonotic* fungal infection of the skin. A zoonotic disease, or zoonosis, is transmissible between humans and animals. Other common problems encountered are fleas, ticks, ear mites, and *mange.* Mange is a skin condition caused by tiny arthropod parasites called mites. Some mange mites are also zoonotic.

PREVENTIVE MEDICINE

Routine preventive care includes vaccinations. *Vaccination* is the inoculation of the patient with a substance to produce immunity against disease. Dogs are routinely vaccinated against *infectious canine distemper, infectious canine hepatitis* (or canine adenovirus 1 and 2), canine *parvovirus,* canine *parainfluenza, leptospirosis,* and *rabies.*

A standard cat vaccine is often called *FVRCP.* This includes such viral diseases as feline viral rhinotracheitis, feline calicivirus, and feline panleukopenia (feline distemper). Rabies is also an important vaccine. Newly acquired cats generally are tested for the presence of the *feline leukemia virus (FeLV)* and sometimes *feline immunodeficiency virus (FIV).* Cats at risk are also vaccinated against FeLV.

Preventive care also means checking the animals for a variety of intestinal parasites, most commonly *roundworms, hookworms, whipworms,* and *tapeworms.* In most parts of the United States, dogs are tested for *heartworm,* a large worm that causes heart and lung disease. Older animals may have *periodontal disease,* in which the soft tissues holding the tooth in its socket are destroyed. *Dental prophylaxis,* or preventive removal of *plaque,* may avoid tooth loss.

Orchiectomy in dogs and cats is more complicated if the animal is a *cryptorchid.* Cryptorchids have one or both testicles retained in the abdomen or groin.

Polydactyly can make onychectomy more difficult. A polydactyl cat has extra toes. In dogs and cats, the first (most medial) digit is called the *dewclaw.* Both dogs and cats normally have front dewclaws, but cats and most breeds of dogs lack rear dewclaws.

Veterinarians and veterinary technicians care for animals as a team. Although only a veterinarian can diagnose and prescribe treatment, veterinary technicians perform many diagnostic tests and treatment regimens and are a critical part of the health care team.

REVIEW C

1. The instrument used to examine the eyes is called a(n) ______________________.
2. Insertion of a needle into a vein is called ______________________.
3. Diseases that are transmissible from animals to humans are called ______________________.
4. Onychectomy is also known as ______________________.
5. An animal that eats both animal and vegetable foods is called a(n) ______________________.
6. An animal with one or both testicles not in the scrotum is called ______________________.
7. A pus-filled uterus is called ______________________.
8. The presence of extra toes is called ______________________.
9. Preventive cleaning of plaque from the teeth is called ______________________.
10. The most medial digit on the front leg of dogs is called a(n) ______________________.

Chapter 17 Answers

Review A

1. *Canis familiaris*
2. *Felis catus*
3. sire
4. *Homo sapiens*
5. feline
6. dam
7. white, blue

Review B

1. puberty
2. parturition, whelping, queening
3. progesterone
4. dystocia
5. pseudocyesis
6. anthropomorphism
7. ovulation
8. ovariohysterectomy
9. estrous
10. orchiectomy
11. queen
12. bitch
13. tom
14. feral

Review C

1. ophthalmoscope
2. venipuncture
3. zoonotic
4. declaw operation
5. omnivore
6. cryptorchid
7. pyometra
8. polydactyly
9. dental prophylaxis
10. dewclaw

Chapter 17 EXERCISES

DOGS AND CATS

Exercise 1: Match the definition in the right column with the word in the left column by placing its letter in the blank provided.

____ 1. *Felis catus*	A. Removal of ovaries and uterus
____ 2. Dominant	B. Study of animal behavior
____ 3. Himalayan	C. Declaw
____ 4. Calico	D. Intestinal parasite
____ 5. Queen	E. Viral disease of dogs
____ 6. Ovariohysterectomy	F. Reproductive behavior of canines
____ 7. Orchiectomy	G. Controlling, leading
____ 8. Onychectomy	H. Genus and species name of cat
____ 9. Ethology	I. Cat breed with points
____ 10. Tie	J. Black/orange/white cat
____ 11. Infectious canine distemper	K. Removal of testes
____ 12. Hookworms	L. Female cat

Exercise 2: Complete the following statements.

1. The most common type of dog show for judging conformation is called a(n) ____________ ____________ show. Competitions in hunting, tracking, or retrieving ability are called ____________ .
2. The acronym *SOAP* stands for ____________ , ____________ , ____________ , ____________ .
3. The most common cat breed is the ____________ .
4. Calico cats have the colors ____________ , ____________ , and ____________ . Tortoise shell cats have the colors ____________ , and ____________ .
5. Where are a Siamese cat's points? ____________ , ____________ , ____________ , and ____________ .
6. The process of withdrawing a puppy from its mother's milk and switching it to solid food is called ____________ .

7. FIV is the acronym for ______________________.
8. A queen in estrus may assume a characteristic posture called ______________________.
9. The science of animal behavior is called ______________________.
10. Biochemicals that convey messages from one animal to another are called ______________________ ______________________.
11. Another name for declawing is ______________________.
12. X-ray pictures are properly called ______________________.
13. The term used to describe loss of appetite is ______________________.
14. A member of a recognized breed eligible for registration is called a(n) ______________________.
15. *Orchiectomy* is another term for ______________________.
16. FLUTD, or ______________________, has been associated with a high ______________________ content of food.

CHAPTER 17 PUZZLE

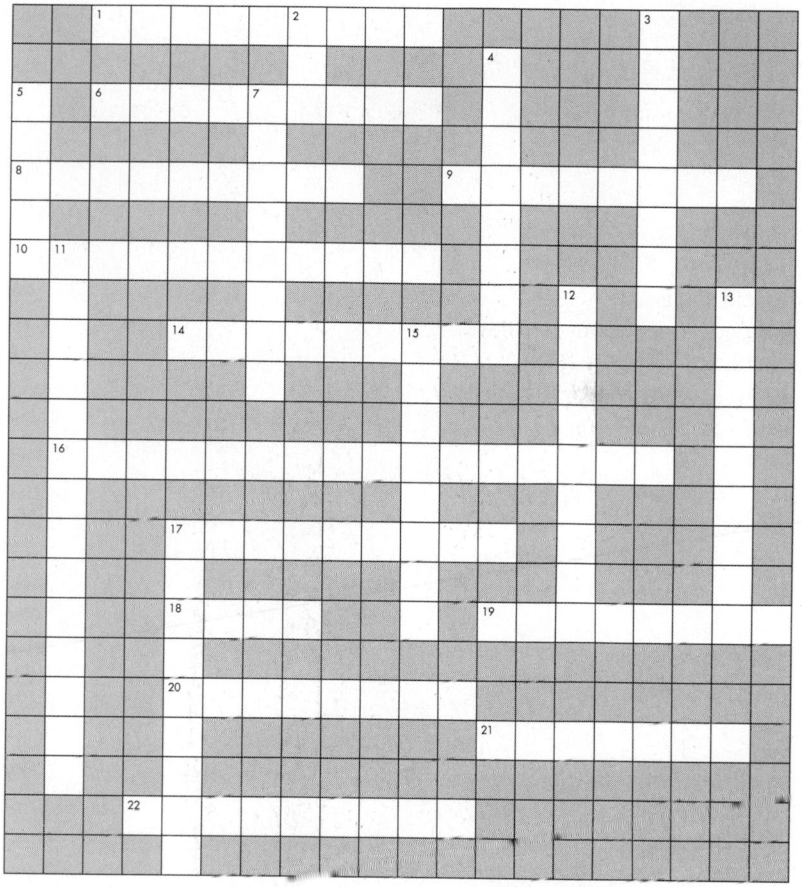

ACROSS CLUES

1. Milk production
6. Chemical transmitting information to another animal
8. Intestinal parasite
9. Fungal infection of the skin
10. Having extra toes
14. Hospitalized animal
16. Attributing human feelings to animals
17. Worm causing heart and lung disease
18. Impolite word for mixed breed dog
19. Giving birth to puppies
20. Position assumed by queen in heat
21. Vocalization by a queen in heat
22. Mineral important in feline urinary tract disease

DOWN CLUES

2. Male cat
3. Transmissible from animal to human
4. Controlling, in charge
5. Common initials for cat vaccination
7. Instrument to examine ears
11. Instrument to examine eyes
12. Meat eater
13. Period of development of the fetus
15. Study of animal behavior
17. Cat breed with points

Chapter 17 Answers

Exercise 1

1. H	7. K
2. G	8. C
3. I	9. B
4. J	10. F
5. L	11. E
6. A	12. D

Exercise 2

1. unbenched; field trials
2. subjective, objective, assessment, plan
3. domestic short hair
4. black, orange, white; black, orange
5. face, ears, feet, tail
6. weaning
7. feline immunodeficiency virus
8. lordosis
9. ethology
10. pheromones
11. onychectomy
12. radiographs
13. anorexia
14. purebred
15. castration
16. feline lower urinary tract disease, magnesium

ANSWERS: CHAPTER 17 PUZZLE

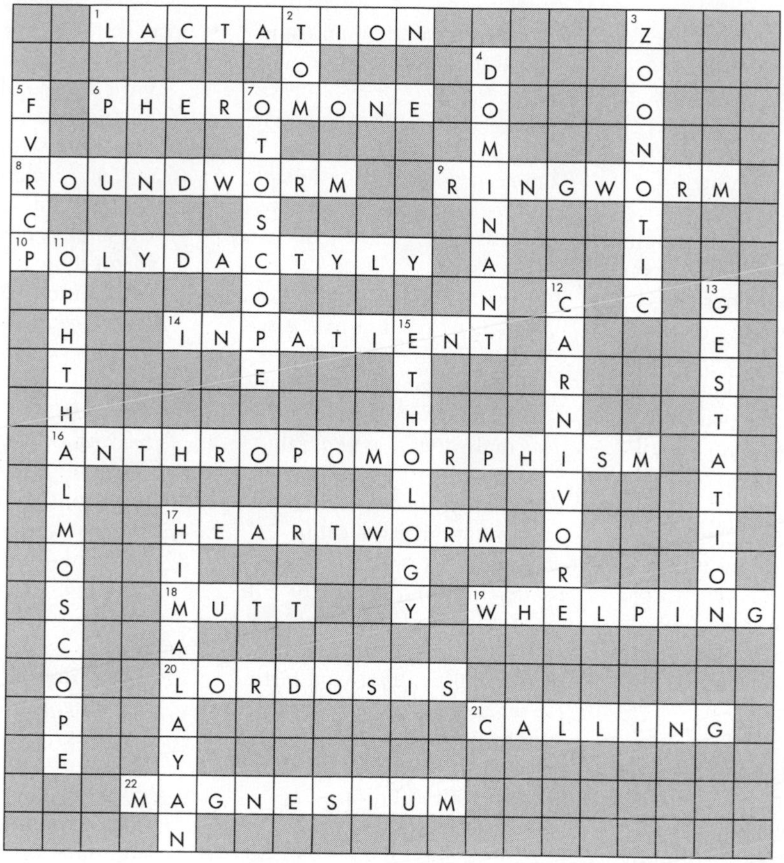
1 LACTATION
2 TOO
3 ZOONOTIC
4 DOMINANT
5 FVRC
6 PHEROMONE
7 OTOSCOPE
8 ROUNDWORM
9 RINGWORM
10 POLYDACTYLY
11 OPHTHALMOSCOPE
12 CARNIVOR
13 GESTATION
14 INPATIENT
15 ETHOLOGY
16 ANTHROPOMORPHISM
17 HEARTWORM
18 MUTT
19 WHELPING
20 LORDOSIS
21 CALLING
22 MAGNESIUM
HIMALAYAN

GLOSSARY

anorexia: lack of appetite.
anthropomorphism: attributing human qualities to nonhuman organisms.
auscultation: the act of listening for sounds in an animal's body, using a stethoscope.
behavioral modification: technique that attempts to change actions without emphasizing motivations or inner conflicts.
bench show: competition during which animals are kept leashed at specific place on platform while not being exhibited in ring.
bitch: female dog.
calico: cat having patches of black and orange on white.
canine distemper (infectious canine distemper): viral disease of dogs, associated with respiratory, digestive, or neurologic symptoms.
canine parainfluenza: viral disease of dogs causing coldlike or flulike symptoms.
canine parvovirus: viral disease of dogs causing severe vomiting and diarrhea.
Canis familiaris: genus and species name of dogs.
carnivore: member of order *Carnivora;* meat eater.
castration: removal of testes; orchiectomy.
catheterization: passage of tube into body for evacuating or injecting fluids.
cryptorchid: individual with one or both testes not descended into scrotum.
cystitis: inflammation of urinary bladder.
dam: mother.
declawing: removal of part or all of bone containing claw; onychectomy.
dental prophylaxis: preventive treatment of teeth and supporting structures by removal of plaque.
dewclaw: first (most medial) digit; both dogs and cats normally have front dewclaws, and cats and most breeds of dogs lack rear dewclaws.
diagnosis: the identification of a disease or condition by a scientific evaluation of physical signs, symptoms, history, and laboratory tests.
dog: male dog; also general name for canine species.
domestic short hair (DSH): most common breed of cat in United States.
dominant: commanding or controlling of others.
DSH: domestic short hair cat.
dystocia: difficulty giving birth.
ear mites: arthropod ectoparasites of ear canal.
ejaculation: ejection of semen from male urethra.
elimination problems: behavioral abnormality of dogs and cats that urinate or defecate in inappropriate places.
estrus: phase of estrous cycle during which female accepts male and ovulation occurs.
estrous cycle: cyclic period of sexual activity in nonhuman female mammals.
ethology: study of behavior of animals.
false pregnancy (pseudocyesis): condition common in dogs that mimics pregnancy.
feline: adjective describing anything pertaining to cats.
feline calicivirus: viral cause of upper respiratory infections in cats.
feline distemper: viral disease of cats; feline panleukopenia.
feline immunodeficiency virus (FIV): viral disease of cats.
feline leukemia virus (FeLV): fatal viral disease of cats.
feline lower urinary tract disease (FLUTD): most common cause of cystitis in cats; formerly feline urological syndrome (FUS).
feline panleukopenia (feline distemper): viral disease of cats causing severe vomiting and diarrhea.
feline viral rhinotracheitis: viral cause of upper respiratory infections in cats.
Felis catus: genus and species name of domestic cat.
fertilization: union of egg and sperm.
field trial: competition during which dogs are judged on tracking, retrieving, and hunting.
fleas: arthropod ectoparasites of dogs and cats.
FVRCP: common cat vaccine combination consisting of feline viral rhinotracheitis, feline calicivirus, and feline panleukopenia.
gestation: length of time from conception to birth.
heartworm: *Dirofilaria immitis,* a helminth infecting the heart of dogs and other species.
high rise syndrome: group of clinical signs related to jumping from height.
history: a systematic account of a patient's life and of factors that may have a bearing on its present condition.
Homo sapiens: genus and species name of humans.

hookworm: parasitic worm that may infest small intestine.
immunosuppression: decrease of body's ability to resist disease.
indication: sign or circumstance that indicates treatment of disease or certain course of action.
induced ovulator: animal that ovulates only as result of sexual activity, such as cat, mink, ferret, rabbit, or llama.
infectious canine hepatitis: contagious viral disease of dogs.
inhumane: cruel; lacking in compassion.
inpatient: one who has been admitted into hospital for treatment.
intact: unneutered; capable of reproduction.
intestinal parasite: organism in gastrointestinal tract that lives at expense of another organism.
kennel cough: upper respiratory infection in dogs caused by several microorganisms.
lactation: milk production.
leptospirosis: bacterial zoonotic disease of dogs.
leukemia: cancer of white blood cells.
lordosis: position of female cat in heat; her vertebral column assumes downward curvature.
magnesium: mineral important for body function.
mange: skin disease caused by mites.
master problem list: part of medical record concisely listing animal's medical history.
match show: sanctioned event mostly for practice; dogs are not awarded championship points or credits toward obedience awards.
mixed breed: combination of two or more breeds.
mongrel: a dog ineligible for registry in any recognized breed, especially a dog whose appearance gives little or no clue to its ancestry.
mutt: same as mongrel, but a more derogatory term.
neutering: removal of gonads (ovaries or testes).
obedience trial: competition during which dogs are judged on their response to commands.
obesity: abnormal amounts of fat on body; 20% to 30% over normal weight.
omnivore: animal that eats both meat and vegetables.
onychectomy: declaw operation.
ophthalmoscope: instrument to examine eyes.
orchiectomy: removal of testes; castration.
otoscope: instrument to examine ears.
outpatient: animal treated without being admitted to hospital.
ovariohysterectomy: removal of ovaries and uterus.
ovulation: discharge of egg from ovary.
palpation: a technique of physical examination in which the examiner uses his hands to feel the texture, size, consistency, and location of various parts of an animal's body.
papers: documents showing animal's pedigree as eligible for registration in a specific breed.
parturition: giving birth.
percussion: a technique in physical examination of tapping an animal's body with the fingertips to evaluate the size, borders, and consistency of some internal organs and to discover the presence and evaluate the amount of fluid or gas in a body cavity.
periodontal disease: disease of supporting structures of teeth including alveolar bone to which teeth are anchored.
pheromone: chemical secreted by animal that influences specific patterns of behavior by other members of same species.
physical examination: an investigation of an animal to determine its health using inspection, palpation, percussion, auscultation, and smell.
plaque: gummy mass of microorganisms that grows on crowns and spreads along roots of teeth.
points: areas of hair differently colored than on rest of body in Siamese, Himalayan, and similar cats; usually found on face (mask), ears, feet, tail.
polydactyly: more than normal number of toes on any foot.
positive reinforcement: influencing behavior by rewarding desired actions.
POVMR: problem-oriented veterinary medical record; system of recordkeeping that is organized around animal's medical history and current status.
progesterone: hormone important in pregnancy.
prognosis: a prediction of the probable outcome of a disease based on the condition of the animal and the usual course of the disease as observed in similar situations.
pseudocyesis: false pregnancy; common in dogs.
puberty: period at which animal becomes capable of reproduction.

purebred: an animal that is eligible for registration by a recognized breed association.
pyometra: pus in the uterus.
queen: female cat.
queening: cat giving birth.
rabies: viral disease fatally affecting central nervous system of mammals.
radiograph: X-ray.
ringworm: fungal infection of skin.
roundworms: large intestinal parasites sometimes visible in animal's feces.
seasonally polyestrous: animals in which frequency of their estrous cycle correlates with season of year.
Siamese: breed of cat with points.
sign: an objective finding as perceived by an examiner.
sire: father.
SOAP: acronym for *subjective, objective, assessment, plan;* method of organizing information on inpatient records.
socialization: process of adapting individual to fit into its society.
spay: ovariohysterectomy.
spraying: act of male cat discharging urine to mark territory.
stethoscope: instrument to listen to sounds from within body cavity.
submissive: docile, yielding.
symptom: a subjective indication of a disease as perceived by a patient (usually used as synonymous with *sign* in veterinary medicine).
tabby: cat having stripes or spots.
tapeworm: flat, segmented intestinal parasite.
tie: mating behavior of dogs during which male's swollen penis is kept within vagina by muscular spasms.
tom: male cat.
tortoiseshell: cat having black and orange hairs intermingled with each other.
unbenched show: majority of dog shows, where dogs are kept with their owners in place of their choosing when not being exhibited in ring.
upper respiratory infection: viral or bacterial infection of upper airway.
vaccination: to inoculate with substance to produce immunity against disease.
venipuncture: blood collection from vein.
weaning: gradual withdrawal of mother's milk, substituting puppy or kitten food.
whelping: giving birth to puppies.
whipworm: intestinal parasite.
zoonosis (zoonotic): disease transmissible between animals and humans.

18 Equine Industry

CHAPTER OVERVIEW

This chapter discusses terminology important to an understanding of the horse and the equine industry. In today's world, the horse serves humanity for transportation, recreation, and work purposes. As a result of people's interest in the horse and the horse's multiple uses, the equine industry is financially strong and growing. Horses have been used for thousands of years for transportation and as beasts of burden. Horses are well suited temperamentally and behaviorally to serve our needs. The horse is also appealing for its beauty, speed, and grace.

Two conventions are used to describe the horse. All horses are considered to turn 1 year older each January 1, regardless of the date of birth. This is because of the racing industry's need for a consistent way to separate groups of young racehorses (for example, 2-year-olds versus 3-year-olds). The next constant refers to a means of measuring the height of the animal. Horses are measured using a system of *hands*. The hand equals 4 inches and is used to measure from the ground to the top of the *withers* (base of the neck). The number to the right of the decimal or hyphen is a number of inches, not a percentage. For example, a horse that stands 15.3 hands would be 63 inches tall. This system of measuring height is one of the ways used to distinguish different groups of adult equines.

GROUPS OF BREEDS

There are two distinct ways to classify groups of horse breeds. Sometimes horses are divided into groups by height, using measurement in hands (Table 18-1). Horses may also be grouped based on physiologic differences. Variation exists within breeds in each of the following groups:

Miniature breeds (for example, American miniature horse) are adults less than 8.2 hands.

Pony breeds (e.g., Shetland, Welsh) are those between 10 and 14.2 hands.

Table 18-1 GROUPS OF HORSES BASED ON HEIGHT OF ADULT

Breed	Height (hands)	Height (inches)	Weight (lb)	Weight (kg)
Miniature	<8.2	<34	200	90
Pony	10.0-14.2	40-58	300-600	136-273
Light	14.2-17.2	58-70	800-1200	364-545
Draft	17.0-19.2	68-78	>1300	>591

Light breeds (e.g., Arabian, quarter horse, thoroughbred) are those generally between 14.2 and 17.2 hands.

Draft breeds (e.g., Belgian, Clydesdale, Percheron) are usually between 17 and 19.2 hands.

Another way to classify horses relates to physiology. Horses may be considered *cold blooded* or *hot blooded.* Basal body temperature may be the same. However, cold-blooded horses such as the draft breeds have lower heart and respiratory rates and lower normal blood parameters. Hot-blooded horses include most of the light horse breeds (e.g., thoroughbreds, Arabians, quarter horses). Hot bloods are quicker to react to stimuli and have higher physiological parameters than the cold bloods. A number of breeds are crosses of these characteristics and are considered *warmbloods* (e.g., Hanoverian, Trakehners).

CORRECT TITLES FOR HORSES

As mentioned previously, all horses turn 1 year older each January 1. Horse owners typically use a combination of age-related terms in combination with a sex-determined term (refer to Appendix E) when referring to a horse. Most horses less than 5 years old are described using two terms together. For example, a *yearling filly* is a female horse that is 1 year old. Most horses are considered mature by 4 or 5 years of age, and then age references are not used as often. See Table 18-2 for age-related terms and Table 18-3 for common combination terms.

Table 18-2 AGE-RELATED TERMS FOR HORSES

Suckling	A foal that is still nursing or suckling from the mare.
Weanling	A foal that has been weaned or separated from the mare. Usually foals are weaned at 3 to 6 months of age.
Yearling	One-year-old horse.
Two-year-old	Self-explanatory.
Three-year-old	Self-explanatory.
Four-year-old	Self-explanatory.
Aged	After 4 or 5 years of age, especially in horse shows, the mature horse is referred to as aged.

Table 18-3 ROUTINE COMBINATIONS FOR HORSE NAMES

Suckling colt	A young male horse still nursing from the mare.
Suckling filly	A young female horse still nursing from the mare.
Weanling colt	A young male horse that has been weaned.
Weanling filly	A young female horse that has been weaned.
Yearling gelding	A 1-year-old horse that has been castrated.
Two-year-old filly or mare	A 2-year-old female horse. From about 2 or 3 years of age, the female is called a mare.
Three-year-old stallion	A 3-year-old male horse. From about 2 or 3 years of age, the male is called a stallion.
Aged gelding	A castrated male horse 4 years of age or older.

REVIEW A

1. Hands used to measure horses equal ______________ inches each.
2. All horses are considered 1 year older on ______________ each year.
3. Pony breeds are equines that are usually less than ______________ hands.
4. The largest horses belong to the ______________ breed group.
5. Horses that have highest physiological parameters are considered to be ______________ .
6. The correct term for a 1-year-old horse is ______________ .
7. The correct two-word term for a seven-month-old male horse just separated from his dam or the mare is ______________ .
8. The correct two-word term for a newborn female foal is ______________ .

PURPOSE

Different types of horses are used for various purposes. Many horses serve multiple purposes or uses. Horses can be ridden for pleasure during the week and then compete in horse shows on weekends. Some people use horses as meat-producing animals. A great number of terms are associated with the different purposes for which people use horses. Some common terms are introduced in the following pages (Fig. 18-1).

Pleasure

Many horses are kept as pets or companion animals. Some are ridden, and some are used to pull buggies, wagons, or sleighs for our enjoyment. Horses that pull are considered *driving horses.* Two general types of riding (both for pleasure and competition) are *Western* and *English.* The type is determined by what type of *tack* (equipment and saddlery) is used and what type of apparel the rider may wear. Western riding usually is done with a heavy *stock* saddle, and the rider may wear Western clothing. English riding usually is done with a lighter saddle, and the rider may wear English apparel (Fig. 18-2).

A form of English riding that may be done for pleasure or competition is *dressage.* Dressage is a classic form of training in which the horse is trained to perform movements in a balanced, supple, and obedient manner.

Competition

Horse owners often compete for awards or prize money in various events. Competitive events often began as an extension of work or racing activities. Many horses are entered into competition against each other in *halter* (conformation) classes. *Equestrian* competitive events include *performance* riding or driving classes, *equitation* (rider's ability), dressage, jumping, *3-day eventing, polo, rodeo, gymkhana* (games), and others.

Work

Horses are used for all types of work and as basic transportation for some people. Breeds such as the quarter horse are still used to work on ranches and to traverse areas that automobiles cannot. Ponies may be used for children's rides. Horses are used for police work, as circus performers, as pack animals

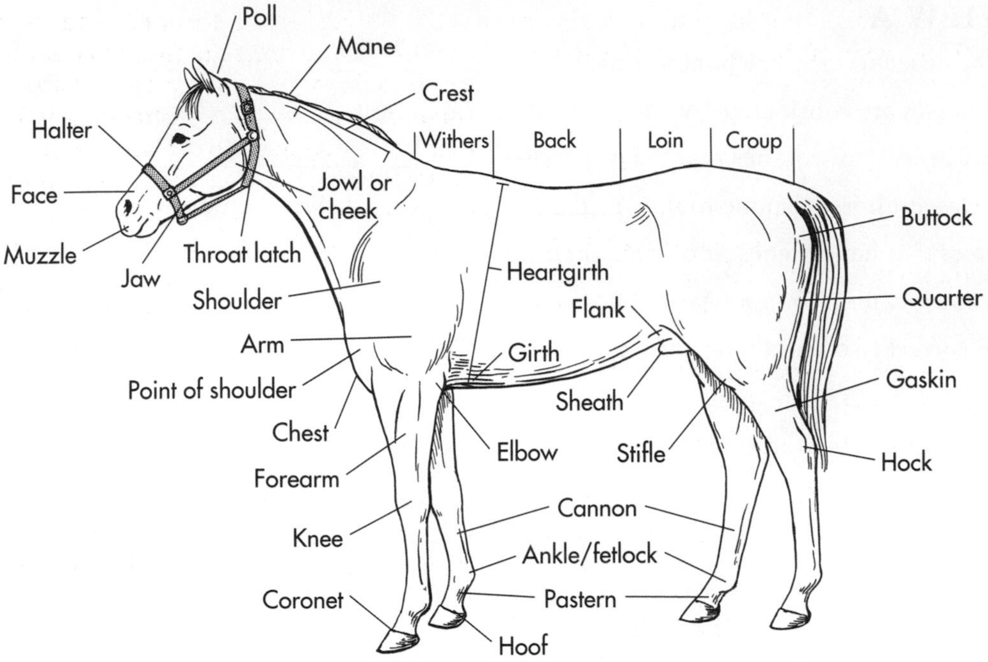
Poll
Mane
Crest
Withers
Back
Loin
Croup
Halter
Face
Muzzle
Jaw
Jowl or cheek
Throat latch
Shoulder
Arm
Point of shoulder
Chest
Forearm
Knee
Coronet
Heartgirth
Flank
Girth
Sheath
Elbow
Stifle
Cannon
Ankle/fetlock
Pastern
Hoof
Buttock
Quarter
Gaskin
Hock

FIG. 18-1 External anatomy of the horse.

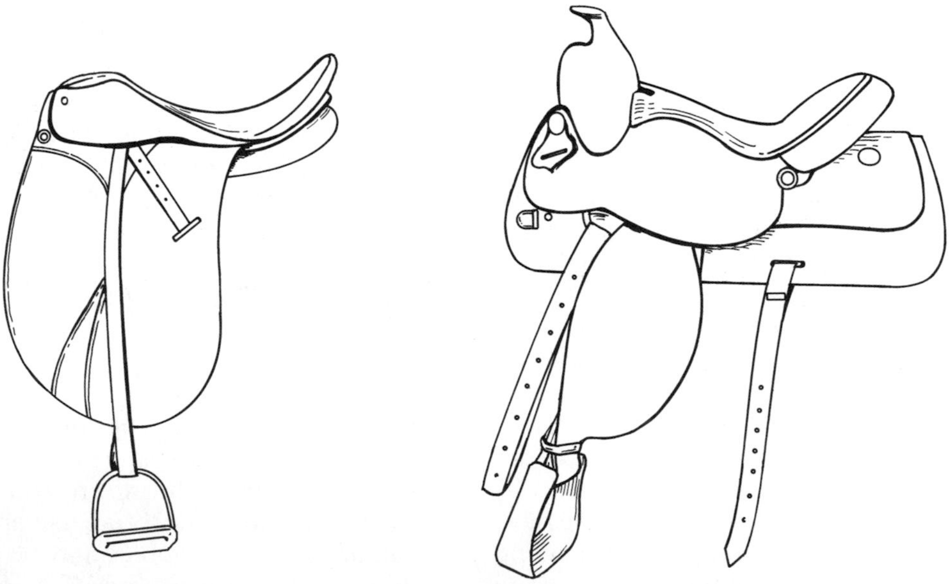

FIG. 18-2 *Left,* English-type saddle. *Right,* Western-type saddle.

in remote locations, and for pulling wagons or sleighs. Some draft breeds are still used to pull farm equipment.

Racing

Horses are used for numerous types of racing activities. Many breeds are ridden in *flat* races. The most popular breed used for flat racing is the thoroughbred. The best-known flat racing event in North America is the Kentucky Derby. Flat races, in which the horse *gallops,* may be run on a soil or *turf* (grass) track. Betting on races is done with a *parimutuel* system. In parimutuel betting, the total amount bet (less taxes) is divided between the winners in proportion to the size of their bets. Another type of parimutuel racing is *harness* racing. In this form of racing, the horse pulls a small cart called a *sulky* or *bike* (Fig. 18-3). The horse performs at either the *trot* or *pace.* Horses are disqualified if they break their gait.

Steeplechasing is a form of distance racing in which the horses are jumped over a series of obstacles while racing against the rest of the horses in the *field* (participants). Steeplechasing originated in Ireland, where originally the racers took the most expeditious cross-country route to a distant point, which was often a church steeple. Other forms of distance racing include *endurance racing* and *competitive riding.* Endurance races are those in which the horse competes against other racers over distances of 50 to 100 miles. The race is won by the fastest competitor. Strict rules apply to protect the well-being of the horse. Checkpoints during the race are managed by veterinarians. Strict criteria are used at the checkpoints to allow only the racer whose health is not compromised to continue. Competitive riding is an event in which a horse's fitness or condition is evaluated (usually by veterinarians) before, during, and after a specified distance. The distance must be covered in a specific

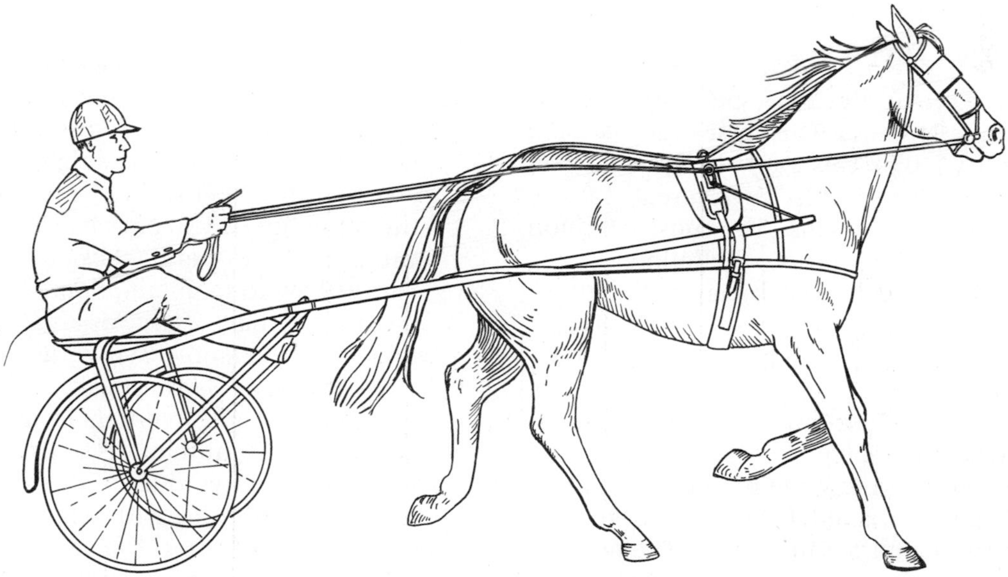

FIG. 18-3 Pacer pulling a sulky.

predetermined ride time. The winner in this event is the horse who has evidence of the best physical conditioning and who maintains the condition throughout the ride.

Horses differ from other domestic species because of their sweat production. A horse working hard or racing can lose more than 2 gallons of sweat per hour. Sweat losses can lead to dehydration and *electrolyte* imbalances. Depending on the condition of the horse and the electrolyte composition of the sweat, we may see an accumulation of sweat that is thick and frothy. We would say that this horse is *lathered.* In hot or humid weather, the intense muscle activity associated with work or racing can lead to dangerous levels of *hyperthermia.* After significant work or racing, horses must be *cooled out* to allow evaporation of the sweat and a slow decrease in core body temperature.

REVIEW B

1. A system of betting on horse races in which the winnings are divided among bettors in proportion to the size of their bet is called a ______________________ system.
2. A form of racing in which horses compete against other racers over a long distance and the horses are examined at veterinary checkpoints is called ______________________ racing.
3. Horses that pull buggies, wagons, or sleighs are considered ______________________ horses.
4. A horse that is covered with thick, frothy sweat is considered to be ______________________ .
5. A classic form of training in which the horse is trained to perform movements in a balanced and obedient manner is called ______________________ .

GAITS OF THE HORSE

Horses have survived as a species by outrunning their enemies. The horse is a *quadruped* (four legs) that can vary the sequence in which it moves its legs. Therefore, the horse has several basic gaits. The most common gaits of the horse include the following:

Walk—a four-*beat* (step) gait with equal intervals between the beats; this is the slowest gait of the horse and the one it uses most often.

Trot—a medium-fast two-beat gait in which the diagonal feet strike the ground at the same time (for example, right front and left rear feet strike the ground at the same time). The period of time when none of the feet are in contact with the ground is called the moment of *suspension.*

Pace—a medium-fast two-beat gait in which the legs on the same side of the body strike the ground simultaneously (for example, the right fore and right rear feet strike the ground at the same time). The pace is a faster gait than the trot and takes more athletic energy to maintain. Some horse breeds may have a pace as a natural gait (for example, standardbreds).

Gallop—the horse's fastest gait, a four-beat gait. The gallop differs from the other gaits in that it is not symmetric on the two sides of the horse. The front leg with which the horse would start the gallop is called the *lead* (for example, starting the gait with the left front leg is the left lead).

Many breeds have natural or trained variations of these four basic gaits. Gaits such as the *jog, canter,* and *running walk* are variations of the basic four gaits.

UNUSUAL EQUINES

Horses *(Equus caballus),* donkeys *(Equus asinus),* and zebras *(Equus zebra)* are all considered equines descended from an ancestor known as *Hyracotherium* or *Eohippus.* The domestic horse has 32 pairs of chromosomes, whereas the donkey and zebra have 31 pairs. Successful mating between these species does exist. Usually, species hybridization results in a sterile *foal.* A *jack,* a male donkey, when mated to a mare, produces a *mule.* A *jenny,* a female donkey, when mated to a stallion, produces a *hinny.* Usually a mule is larger than a hinny. Most mules are sterile. Different breeds of donkeys and horses have been used to produce various mule types including draft-type mules (crosses with draft horses). Mules and donkeys are used for work, competition, and pleasure purposes.

BREEDING

The breeding of horses is a large component of the equine industry. A valuable stallion may be bred to as many as 100 mares in a breeding season using artificial insemination. Successful breeding stallions or mares whose *get* (progeny) are successful racehorses or show horses may be worth millions of dollars.

The breeding of horses and sales of their get are a very large and active component of the horse business. Stallions that are used primarily for breeding purposes are considered to *stand at stud.* The number of mares financially consigned to be bred to a stallion in 1 year is called the stallion's *book* for that year.

A mare used primarily for breeding purposes is called a *broodmare.* To identify which broodmare is in estrus, the mare is *teased.* Usually this is done by walking the broodmare past a *teaser.* A teaser may be a stallion, a pony stallion, or even a gelding that has been treated with hormones. The teaser attempts to breed the mare and thereby identifies which mare is ready to be bred. Once identified as in estrus, the broodmare is bred with the stallion by *natural cover* (normal mating) or by artificial insemination. Some breed registries do not allow artificial insemination (for example, thoroughbreds).

Horses are *seasonally polyestrous,* with heat cycles every 21 days during the spring and summer (in the Northern Hemisphere). When a broodmare is determined to be pregnant, she is considered to be *settled,* or in foal. After an 11-month gestation, foaling (parturition) usually occurs in the spring or summer. Before parturition, a broodmare's mammary glands or udder may fill with milk. The mare is said to be *bagging up.* Immediately before parturition, some mares get an accumulation of colostrum on their nipples. The colostrum on the nipples is called wax; the mare is said to be *waxing.* After parturition, mares usually come back into estrus in 7 to 12 days. This first postfoaling heat is called *foal heat.* The next estrus occurs approximately 21 days after foal heat. This second heat is called the *30-day heat* (approximately 9 + 21 days).

A term that has two meanings for the horse is *maiden.* When applied to breeding, a maiden mare is a mare that has not had a foal. When applied to race horses, maiden can mean a horse of either sex that has never won a race.

HOUSING

Horses are housed or stabled in a variety of ways. In many areas, horses may be kept in a pasture all the time. A *corral* or a *paddock* is a smaller outdoor confinement. When housed, horses usually are considered to be kept in a barn. Horses housed at the racetrack are said to be in a *shedrow.* In barns, we typically find two different types of individual stalls for horses. The *box stall* is a large enough enclosure to allow the horse to move and lie down. In contrast, the *tie, slip,* or *standing stall* creates greater confinement, and usually the horse is not able to move very much. While in the tie, slip, or standing stall, most horses are tied to the front of the stall. Horses often are ridden in a confined area called an *arena.* Arenas may be indoor or outdoor. Exhibitions of horses usually are held in a *coliseum, pavilion,* or arena.

REVIEW C

1. A medium-fast two-beat gait in which the legs on the same side of the body strike the ground simultaneously is called the ______________________ .
2. A hybrid equine that is a cross between a jack and a mare is called a(n) ________________ .
3. A female horse used primarily for breeding is called a(n) ______________________ .
4. Foal heat occurs ______________________ days after parturition.
5. When colostrum accumulates on the nipples before parturition, the mare is said to be ______________________ .

FEEDING

The horse is a monogastric herbivore (see Fig. 11-2). It evolved from a dog-sized plant browser. Fiber or cellulose is digested in the *hindgut* (large intestine). The equine teeth have evolved to allow grinding of rough grasses. The teeth are considered to be *hypsodont.* Hypsodont teeth are long-crowned, progressively erupting teeth. The horses' teeth erupt for approximately 20 years. The maxilla of the horse is 30% wider than the mandible. Because of the jaw width and the slowly erupting teeth, horses may get points on the *buccal* surface of the upper teeth and the *lingual* surface of the lower teeth. These points can interfere with proper mastication and cause pain. The points may need to be filed smooth in a procedure called *floating.*

The first upper premolar of the horse usually is small or absent and serves no purpose. This tooth is called the *wolf tooth* and is situated in the mouth immediately behind the place where the bit would go into the mouth for riding or driving. The wolf tooth can interfere with the bit and cause the horse discomfort. Wolf teeth, when present, often are extracted for this reason.

Horses can survive nutritionally on good-quality pasture or hay. Horses that are performing in racing, competition, work, breeding, or other activities usually need additional feed to supplement the hay or pasture. Various cereal grains such as corn, oats, and barley can be successfully fed to horses. Vitamin and mineral supplementation depends on the quality of the feedstuffs used, the geographic locale, and the activity of the horse. Horses always need access to clean water. A normal 1000-pound (440-kg) horse consumes 5 to 10 gallons (20 to 40 liters) of water per day for maintenance.

RESTRAINT

Understanding the behavior of the horse is paramount to restraint. Horses have survived as a species by a behavior of "fear and flight" from predators. When frightened, horses may kick with the hind limbs, strike forward with the forelimbs, or run from enemies. The major defense of the species is speed. Horses evolved a hoofed digit on elongated legs to outrun enemies. The pupil of the eye is elongated horizontally to allow tremendous peripheral vision (up to 350 degrees). Horses prefer to remain in groups or herds. When given the opportunity, horses eat small amounts almost continually throughout the day. Horses can be kind, affectionate, giving animals when handled regularly. The species does not have the intelligence to reason but has an excellent memory, which is beneficial for training. If we remember these basic behavioral traits, our ability to work with and benefit from the horse improves.

Always approach a horse slowly toward its head or from the side. Speak softly to the horse. Using food expedites catching the horse. Avoid startling the animal. The basic instrument of restraint is the *halter.* Some horses may have a halter on at all times. A lead rope or *lead shank* usually is attached to the halter with a snap of some sort. The lead rope or shank provides a longer means of attachment for control purposes. Horses are accustomed to being handled or led from the *near side* (left). The horse may balk when led or handled from the *far side* (right). Additional restraint in horses is commonly provided by the use of a *twitch.* A twitch is a handle that has a loop of rope or chain on one end. The loop is tightened over the upper lip or muzzle to facilitate restraint. The mechanism of action of the twitch is the release of *endorphins* (the body's natural analgesics). Other forms of physical or chemical restraint may be needed for uncooperative horses.

The horse is ridden or driven with a *bridle.* The bridle is used to replace the halter as the primary means of restraint on the head for these activities. In many situations, the bridle has an attached piece of metal called the *bit* in the horse's mouth for controlling the riding or driving activity. A *harness* is the device that attaches a horse or *team* of horses to a wagon, sulky, cart, or sleigh to allow for pulling or towing.

HOOF CARE

A horse's hooves grow approximately ¼ inch per month. Excess hoof must be removed to allow the foot to retain its normal shape and function. Horses do not need to be shod unless they are being ridden on a hard surface regularly or have a specific need for a shoe. Horseshoes can be made of different metals or even rubber. Shoes can come in many different types or styles depending on the activity of the horse and the terrain on which the horse is ridden or driven. Horseshoes usually are attached to the insensitive portion of the hoof with horseshoe nails. People trained in proper hoof care and shoeing are called *farriers.*

Cleaning of the debris that accumulates in the hooves is an important part of routine husbandry. A bacterial infection of the *frog* (soft portion of the palmar hoof) is called *thrush.*

PREVENTIVE HEALTH CARE

Routine preventive care is important to the health of the horse. Parasite control and immunization for preventable infectious diseases are important. The most serious parasites that can cause disease and debilitation in the horse are the *Strongyles* (bloodworms). The most common infectious diseases of the horse include *tetanus, Eastern* or *Western encephalomyelitis, rhinopneumonitis, influenza, rabies, Potomac horse fever,* and *equine viral arteritis.* Geographic location affects the incidence of these diseases and the need for immunization.

Horses may also need to be tested for *equine infectious anemia* (*EIA* or *swamp fever*). This viral disease can cause acute hemolytic anemia leading to death. Horses can survive the viremia and become chronic inapparent carriers. The carriers can be a significant risk to other horses because the disease is spread by the transfer of blood. The virus usually is spread by biting insects or contaminated needles. Most states and countries require that horses being transported be tested for this disease. The test for EIA is the *Coggins test.* Positive carriers must be quarantined or euthanatized. No vaccination is available for EIA at this time.

COMMON DISEASES

In addition to the infectious diseases mentioned in the previous section, the horse also can be affected by colic, heaves, laminitis, and lameness.

Colic simply means abdominal pain. Colic can have many causes: the peculiar gastrointestinal anatomy of the horse, its variable tolerance of pain, parasites, and management errors. Colic can be a simple gastrointestinal disturbance such as a gas accumulation, or it can be a life-threatening displacement or twist of the intestines. An affected horse may exhibit anorexia, sweating, anxiety, rolling, stretching to urinate, or even violently throwing itself on the ground in pain. If in a stall, the horse may become trapped up against the wall and unable to move. A horse so trapped is *cast.* Horses also can become cast in a stall because of rolling that is not necessarily a result of colic pain. Thorough examination of the horse to determine the severity and the cause of the colic is an important aspect of equine veterinary practice.

Heaves is the common name used for a disease that is known as *chronic obstructive pulmonary disease (COPD).* Heaves is a chronic, asthmalike disease that usually is a result of allergies. Horses exhibit this disease by chronic cough, some nasal discharge, and forced or labored expiration. Expiratory effort can be so great that some horses acquire an increased abdominal wall musculature called a *heave line.* Because of the chronic nature of this disease, treatment is directed at environmental changes and various therapies to aid breathing.

Laminitis is an acute inflammation of the sensitive structures of the foot. *Laminae* are the fingers of tissues that hold the hoof wall to the underlying supportive tissues of the foot. Laminitis has many causes and inciting factors. Horses with laminitis may have systemic hypertension. The shunting of blood directly from arterioles to venules bypassing the capillary beds of the laminae results in hypoperfusion of the laminae. Most of the changes that occur in the hoof are caused by this lack of blood supply to the laminae. Untreated laminitis can lead to permanent damage and interruption in normal hoof growth. This chronic condition is exhibited by varying degrees of lameness and abnormal hoof growth. Chronic lameness associated with laminitis may render the horse unsuitable (unsound) for riding or driving uses. The common term used to describe the hoof changes seen in chronic laminitis is *founder.*

Horses can exhibit numerous types of lameness depending on the inciting cause, anatomic location, and severity of the condition. Some lameness can be minor, and other types can lead to chronic pain and debilitation. Because horses are used for so many competitive and work-related activities, proper diagnosis and treatment for lameness are important. Lameness diagnosis, as well as caring for other aspects of the equine industry, often is the responsibility of veterinarians who restrict their practice to horses. These veterinarians are called *equine practitioners.*

REVIEW D

1. The process of filing the sharp points on the teeth of a horse is called ________________ .
2. Horses usually are handled or led from the left or ________________ side.
3. A bacterial infection of the frog of the hoof is called ________________ .
4. The blood test for equine infectious anemia is called the ________________ test.
5. The term used for abdominal pain in a horse is ________________ .

Chapter 18 Answers

Review A

1. 4
2. January 1
3. 14.2
4. draft
5. hot blooded
6. yearling
7. weanling colt
8. suckling filly

Review B

1. parimutuel
2. endurance
3. driving
4. lathered
5. dressage

Review C

1. pace
2. mule
3. broodmare
4. 7 to 12 days
5. waxing

Review D

1. floating
2. near
3. thrush
4. Coggins
5. colic

Chapter 18 — EXERCISES

EQUINE INDUSTRY

Exercise 1: Complete the following sentences.

1. Horses are measured in hands. One hand equals ______________________ inches.
2. The birthday for all horses is ______________________ .
3. Pony breeds are considered to be breeds less than ______________________ hands.
4. Harness race horses pull a small cart called a ______________________ .
5. A form of racing in which the fitness of the horse is evaluated before, during, and after the timed and specific distance event is called ______________________ .
6. A form of English riding in which the horse is trained to perform movements in a balanced, supple, and obedient manner is called ______________________ .
7. The name used for the equine that is the result of the mating of a jack and a mare is ______________________ .
8. A number of breeds are crosses of cold-blooded and hot-blooded horses. These crosses often have characteristics of each and are considered to be ______________________ .

Exercise 2: Match the definition in the right column with the gait in the left column. Place the appropriate letter in the blank space provided:

_____	1. Walk	A. Medium-fast, two-beat diagonal gait
_____	2. Trot	B. Medium-fast, two-beat gait in which the legs on the same side of the body strike the ground simultaneously
_____	3. Pace	C. Fastest four-beat gait
_____	4. Gallop	D. Four-beat slow gait
_____	5. Lead	E. The front leg with which the horse would start the gallop

Exercise 3: Multiple choice.

1. Where is fiber or cellulose digested in the horse?
   a. Stomach
   b. Small intestine
   c. Large intestine
   d. Cecum only

2. The first upper premolar tooth of the horse is called a(n)
   a. Canine tooth
   b. Wolf tooth
   c. Incisor tooth
   d. Hypsodont tooth
3. The procedure of filing the points off the premolar and molar teeth of a horse is called
   a. Floating
   b. Crowning
   c. Wolfing
   d. Enameling
4. The most basic instrument of restraint placed on the horse's head is a
   a. Bridle
   b. Harness
   c. Bit
   d. Halter
5. The instrument of restraint commonly applied to the lip or muzzle of a horse is the
   a. Lead shank
   b. Halter
   c. Twitch
   d. Bridle
6. A bacterial infection of the soft portion of the hoof is called
   a. Farrier
   b. Thrush
   c. Pododermatitis
   d. Laminitis
7. Horses can be routinely immunized for all of the following diseases *except*
   a. Equine infectious anemia
   b. Rhinopneumonitis
   c. Tetanus
   d. Rabies

8. An equine disease in which there are asymptomatic carriers is
   a. Laminitis
   b. Colic
   c. Equine infectious anemia
   d. Chronic obstructive pulmonary disease
9. *Founder* is the common term used to describe the chronic changes of the hoof in horses suffering from
   a. Heaves
   b. Laminitis
   c. Colic
   d. Coggins
10. Positive carriers of equine infectious anemia must be
    a. Vaccinated
    b. Transported
    c. Treated
    d. Quarantined

Exercise 4: Complete the following sentences.

1. The blood test for equine infectious anemia is called the ________________________ test.
2. Horses usually are handled or led by the halter from the ________________________ side.
3. A horse caught in recumbency and unable to rise is said to be ________________________ .
4. The term for abdominal pain is ________________________ .
5. A mare used primarily for reproductive purposes is a ________________________ .
6. The first heat or estrus cycle seen after foaling occurs ________________ days after parturition.
7. A female donkey is called a ________________________ .
8. A horse that is used to determine which mares are in estrus is called a ________________________ .
9. The prominent bulge at the base of the neck dorsally is called the ________________________ .

Exercise 5: Match the definition of the equine activity with the appropriate name in the left column. Place the appropriate letter in the space provided.

_____ 1. Rodeo	A. Distance riding in which horses are jumped over a series of obstacles
_____ 2. Gymkhana	B. Exhibition of conformation
_____ 3. Dressage	C. Dressage, cross-country, and jumping completed in 1 to 3 days
_____ 4. English	D. Exhibition of cowboy skills
_____ 5. Halter class	E. Form of riding using a stock saddle
_____ 6. 3-day eventing	F. Games emphasizing speed, action, activity
_____ 7. Steeplechasing	G. Form of riding using a light saddle
_____ 8. Western	H. Racing over distances usually greater than 40 miles
_____ 9. Endurance racing	I. Classic form of horse training

CHAPTER 18 PUZZLE

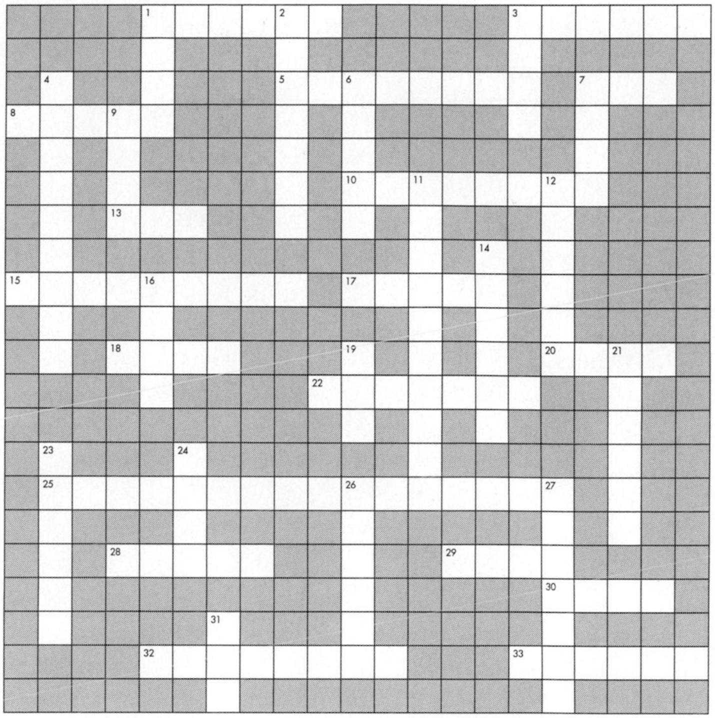
1
2
3
4
5
6
7
8
9
10
11
12
13
14
15
16
17
18
19
20
21
22
23
24
25
26
27
28
29
30
31
32
33

ACROSS CLUES

1. Bacterial infection of frog
3. Another term for paddock
5. Ancestral horse
7. Placed in horse's mouth
8. Large types of horses
10. Classic form of training
13. Offspring
15. Inflammation of foot structure
17. Enclosed area for exhibition
18. Male donkey
20. 2-beat lateral gait
22. Horseshoer
25. Herpes-caused respiratory disease
28. Abdominal pain
29. Speed and sequence of moving feet
30. Riding equipment
32. Filing teeth
33. Asthmalike disease

DOWN CLUES

1. Two-beat diagonal gait
2. Racetrack barn
3. Trapped; unable to rise
4. Female horse used primarily for breeding
6. Unit of measuring horse's height
7. Sulky
9. Soft part of hoof bottom
11. Horse rider
12. Fastest four-beat gait
14. Headgear for restraint
16. Left side of horse
19. Right side of horse
21. Slower 3-beat gait
23. Tack put on head for riding
24. Newborn horse
26. Mare who never foaled
27. Term meaning pregnant
31. Slow trot

Chapter 18 Answers

Exercise 1

1. 4
2. January 1
3. 14.2 or 14½
4. bike or sulky
5. competitive riding
6. dressage
7. mule
8. warm bloods

Exercise 2

1. D
2. A
3. B
4. C
5. E

Exercise 3

1. C
2. B
3. A
4. D
5. C
6. B
7. A
8. C
9. B
10. D

Exercise 4

1. Coggins
2. left or near
3. cast
4. colic
5. broodmare
6. 7 to 12 days
7. jenny
8. teaser
9. withers

Exercise 5

1. D
2. F
3. I
4. G
5. B
6. C
7. A
8. E
9. H

ANSWERS: CHAPTER 18 PUZZLE

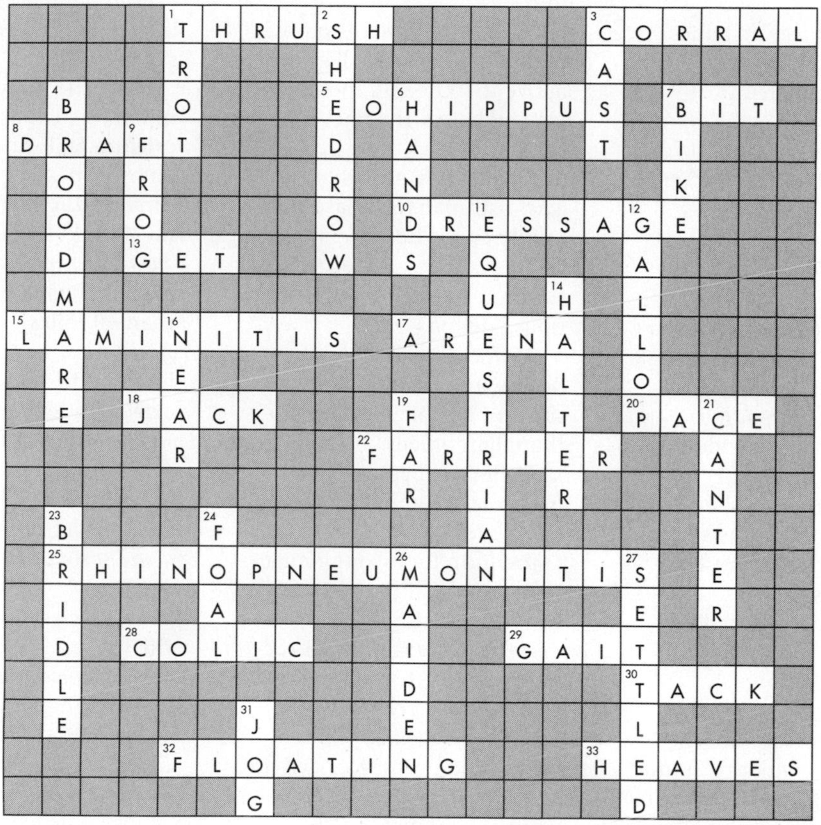
1 THRUSH
3 CORRAL
5 EOHIPPUS
7 BIT
8 DRAFT
10 DRESSAGE
13 GET
15 LAMINITIS
17 ARENA
18 JACK
20 PACE
22 FARRIER
25 RHINOPNEUMONITIS
28 COLIC
29 GAIT
30 TACK
32 FLOATING
33 HEAVES
1 TROT
2 SHEDROW
3 CAST
4 BROODMARE
6 HANDS
7 BIKE
9 FROG
11 EQUESTRIAN
12 GALLOP
14 HALTER
16 NEAR
19 FAR
21 CANTER
23 BRIDLE
24 FOAL
26 MAIDEN
27 SETTLED
31 JOG

GLOSSARY

3-day eventing: three activities (dressage, cross-country, jumping) completed in 1 to 3 days.

30-day heat: estrus that occurs approximately 30 days after foaling.

aged: a mature horse of either sex, usually after 4 or 5 years of age.

arena: large enclosed area used for exhibitions or exercise (indoor or outdoor).

bagging up: swelling of the mammary glands or udder before foaling.

beat: step, as in a gait; the frequency at which one or two feet strike the ground simultaneously.

bike: sulky or cart, typically pulled by harness racing horses (standardbreds).

bit: the part of the bridle that goes in the horse's mouth.

blemish: scar, irregularity, or unsightly defect that does not interfere with serviceability.

book: number of mares listed or signed for a breeding season to a particular stallion.

box stall: enclosure in a stable or barn where the horse can move freely without being tied in one place.

bridle: the part of the horse's tack that is placed on its head for riding or driving.

broodmare: mare used primarily for reproductive purposes.

buccal: cheek side of the teeth (opposite of lingual).

canter: a three-beat gait similar to but restrained and slower than the gallop.

cast: trapped or caught in a recumbent position and unable to rise.

chestnut: horny growths on the medial aspect of the leg, above the knee on the front leg and below the hock on the rear.

chronic obstructive pulmonary disease: asthmalike disease commonly called heaves.

Coggins test: federally recognized serum test for equine infectious anemia.

cold blooded: large breeds of horses that usually have slower physiological functions than light breeds.

colic: abdominal pain.

coliseum: large arena used for exhibition.

colt: the term for a young male horse; sometimes used for a newborn of either sex.

competitive riding: a form of racing in which the horses must complete a specified distance in a specified time.

competition: a purpose or activity accomplished for award, prizes, or money.

cooling out: the act of walking to cool down an exercised horse.

corral: area used for holding, exercising, or enclosing horses (paddock).

dam: the mare or mother animal of a young horse.

draft: large breed usually over 17 hands, also a body type such as draft pony or draft mule.

dressage: classic form of horse training.

driving: controlling a horse or horses that are harnessed to various carts, wagons, or carriages.

Eastern or Western encephalomyelitis: life-threatening, virus-caused brain and spinal cord infection often called sleeping sickness.

electrolyte: the body's salts or minerals such as sodium, calcium, chlorine, and potassium.

endorphin: the body's own natural chemical analgesics.

endurance racing: racing over distances usually greater than 40 miles.

English: a form of riding using a light saddle and apparel with origins in England.

Eohippus: ancestral horse more accurately called *Hyracotherium.*

equestrian: a horse rider.

equestrian event: horse-related activity.

equine: species name for the horse.

equine infectious anemia: life-threatening viral anemia, sometimes called swamp fever.

equine practitioners: veterinarians whose practice is limited primarily to the horse.

equine viral arteritis: virus-caused vascular inflammation with multisystemic clinical signs.

equitation: equine competitive events that are judged primarily on the rider's abilities.

Equus asinus: genus and species of donkeys.

Equus caballus: genus and species of horses.

Equus zebra: genus and species of zebras.

ergot: small, horny mass on the palmar or plantar surface of the fetlock.

farrier: a person who has been

trained to trim hooves and make horseshoes, commonly called a blacksmith, smithy, or horseshoer.

far side: right side of the horse, the side not usually used for leading the horse or mounting into the saddle.

field: participants in a racing or competitive event.

filly: a young female horse.

flat race: race in which the horse is ridden by a jockey over a specified distance.

floating: filing or removing the points on the teeth.

foal: newborn horse of either sex.

foal heat: first estrus after foaling, usually in 7 to 12 days after foaling.

foaling: the act of parturition or giving birth for horses.

founder: common term for chronic laminitis.

frog: soft portion of the underside of the hoof.

gait: the speed and sequence of moving the feet.

gallop: the fastest of the three basic gaits, a four-beat gait.

gelding: a castrated horse.

get: progeny, offspring.

gymkhana: equestrian events emphasizing speed, action, and activity; games on horseback.

halter: the basic headgear used for restraint, also used in confirmation competition classes.

hands: a means of measuring height of horses; one hand equals 4 inches.

harness: equipment used to attach a horse or horses to carts, wagons, sulkies, or sleighs.

heave line: increased abdominal musculature associated with the extra effort of expiration in horses with heaves or COPD.

heaves: common name for chronic obstructive pulmonary disease (COPD), an asthmalike, chronic respiratory condition.

hindgut: collective term for the cecum and small and large colon.

hinny: sterile hybrid offspring of a female donkey (jenny) and a male horse (stallion).

hot blooded: group of horses with faster physiological functions than others.

hyperthermia: elevated body temperature.

hypsodont: tooth type characterized by long crowns and progressive eruption.

Hyracotherium: ancestral horse (formerly called *Eohippus*).

influenza: common virus-caused respiratory disease.

jack: a male donkey.

jenny: a female donkey.

jog: a slow trot.

lameness: alteration in gait or stride or inability to bear weight on a limb.

lamina: singular of *laminae.*

laminae: fingers of tissue that attach the hoof to the underlying structures of the foot.

laminitis: inflammation of the laminae in the foot.

lather: an accumulation of sweat on the horse's body.

lead: the starting or leading foot in the three- or four-beat gaits (canter or gallop).

lead shank: a strap, rope, or chain attached to the halter and used to lead the horse.

light: breeds of horses intermediate in size and stature, usually more than 14.2 hands.

lingual: tongue side of the teeth (opposite of buccal).

maiden: a mare that has not had a foal, or a race horse of either sex that has not won a race.

mare: a mature female horse.

miniature: breeds of horses; small breeds usually less than 8.2 hands.

mule: hybrid cross between a male donkey (jack) and female horse (mare).

natural cover: normal mating, as opposed to artificial insemination.

near side: left side of the horse, usually the side from which the horse is led or mounted.

pace: medium-fast, two-beat lateral gait.

paddock: area used for holding, exercising, or enclosing horses (corral).

parimutuel: betting system in which the total amount bet (less taxes) is divided between winners proportionally to the size of their bets.

pavilion: large arena used for exhibition.

performance: indicator of success in competitions, as in riding or driving.

pleasure: riding or driving of horses for enjoyment.

polo: an equestrian sport that originated in Persia, probably the most ancient goal game.

pony: small breeds of horses usually between 8.2 and 14.2 hands, a horse for a child.

Potomac horse fever: fever and diarrheal disease with bacterial origin.

progeny: offspring, get.

proud flesh: excessive or exuberant scar tissue that sometimes forms, especially on limbs.

quadruped: an animal that walks on four legs.

rabies: fatal virus-caused neurologic disease.

rhinopneumonitis: herpesvirus–caused respiratory disease or abortion.

rodeo: exhibition of cowboy skills.

running walk: a faster variation of the four-beat gait exhibited by some breeds.

seasonally polyestrous: having many heat cycles during a certain season of the year.

settled: pregnant or in foal.

shedrow: barn or groups of barns where horses are stabled at the racetrack.

sire: the stallion or father of a young horse.

slip stall: a stall in which the horse is tied in place and cannot move about (standing or tie stall).

stallion: a mature male horse; sometimes called a stud, especially when used for breeding.

stand at stud: a stallion being used primarily for breeding is said to stand at stud.

standing stall: a stall in which the horse is tied in place and cannot move about (slip or tie stall).

steeplechasing: a form of distance racing in which horses are jumped over a series of obstacles.

stock saddle: type of saddle with a high front (pommel) and high rear (cantle) that is used for riding (Western style).

strike: movement quickly and cranially with a front leg of the horse as a means of defense or aggression.

Strongyles (bloodworms): the most health-threatening family of internal parasites of the horse.

suckling: a foal of either sex that is still nursing or sucking milk from its dam.

sulky: cart or bike, typically pulled by harness racing horses (standardbreds).

suspension: period of time when none of the feet are in contact with the ground.

tack: equipment used in riding or driving horses.

teaser: horse used to determine which mares are in estrus (heat).

teasing: act of determining which mares are in estrus (heat).

tetanus: bacteria-caused neurologic disease leading to muscle rigidity; often called lockjaw.

thrush: bacterial infection of the frog in the hoof.

tie stall: a stall in which the horse is tied in place and cannot move about (standing or slip stall).

trot: medium-fast, two-beat diagonal gait.

turf: grass or sod used for flat racing.

twitch: means of restraint in horses, often by using a device twisted on the upper lip or muzzle.

unsoundness: defects or lameness causing a horse to be unserviceable or unsuitable.

warm blooded: group of horses exhibiting some characteristics of both cold and hot blooded horses.

waxing: accumulation of colostrum on the nipples of a mare, usually before foaling.

weanling: a young horse of either sex that has been weaned or separated from its dam.

Western: a form of riding using a stock saddle and apparel with origins in the western United States.

withers: base of the neck.

wolf tooth: first upper premolar tooth.

yearling: a young horse of either sex that is 1 year old or officially 1 year old after January 1.

19 Cattle Industry

CHAPTER OVERVIEW

This chapter discusses terminology important to an understanding of dairy and beef cattle and the cattle industry. Cattle are second only to dogs in terms of their long association with humans and may be the most important of our domestic animals. They were probably first domesticated in Asia and Europe in or around the New Stone Age. Cattle are used as draft animals and provide humans with meat, milk, hides, and many byproducts.

Although there have been many changes in cattle since they were first domesticated, all modern-day cattle possess the blood of one or both of two ancestors. Cattle belonging to *Bos taurus* originated in and are adapted to temperate zones and are of European descent. Most cattle found in the United States are of this particular descent. *Bos indicus* are cattle that originated in Asia and are of Indian descent. The humped cattle of today have their origin in the zebu or Brahman cattle. These humped cattle have a characteristic fleshy hump dorsal to the withers; large, drooping ears; and an extremely large, fleshy dewlap. Cattle belonging to *Bos indicus* appear to be more heat tolerant and can survive on less water because of the hump (similar to that of the camel). They also seem to be more disease and ectoparasite resistant than their *Bos taurus* relatives. Crossbreeding *Bos taurus* to *Bos indicus* results in progeny that are considered *hybrids* and possess *hybrid vigor.* This type of cross has occurred with several breeds of beef cattle currently found in the United States.

BREEDS OF CATTLE

Modern-day cattle have been bred for two primary purposes: milk and meat production. Some breeds are considered *dual-purpose,* having desirable traits of both dairy and beef cattle. Dairy cattle have been selected and bred so that the dietary foodstuffs they consume are converted into milk. Beef cattle have been selected and bred so that the dietary foodstuffs they consume are converted into flesh.

If we examine the body type of a typical dairy cow (Fig. 19-1), we note that she has a very angular (almost triangular) body, with many of her skeletal structures exposed through her hide. This anatomic feature indicates that she is converting her feed into milk and not into flesh. Her legs are long, lacking excessive flesh, making it easier to place a milking machine under her. Her neck is long and slender, thus indicating a greater ability to produce milk. Her *body capacity* is characterized by the circumference of her *heart girth* and *barrel.* A large heart girth indicates great heart and lung capacity or the ability to pump more blood and oxygen through her udder to manufacture milk. A large barrel indicates a large abdominal region, which is indicative of large feed capacity or the ability to consume more feed. The consumption of increased amounts of feed will result in more nutrients being pumped through the udder and thus more milk being produced. The *udder* of the dairy cow is large, attached high and wide, with four teats equally placed and of uniform length and diameter, which makes milking easy.

If we examine the typical body style and type of beef animals (Fig. 19-2), we note that they are extremely rectangular in stature and appear fleshy, with very few skeletal anatomic structures revealed. Beef animals have shorter legs because they are not milked, and the flesh from these areas is of lower quality. Their necks are shorter and fleshy, with an udder conducive in size to just suckling a calf. They should also have a large heart girth for the purpose of pumping more nutrient-containing blood through the body to produce a better quality *carcass.* The barrel should be large and well sprung, indicative of great feed capacity. Dual-purpose breeds of cattle (for example, Brown Swiss) have qualities conducive to both dairy and beef production.

Dairy Breeds

Today five major breeds of dairy cattle are recognized in the United States: Ayrshire, Brown Swiss, Guernsey, Holstein-Friesian, and Jersey. As a result of almost exclusive use of *artificial insemination* in dairy cattle, bull calves are used for *veal* or dairy beef production. However, the calves of Jerseys and Guernseys normally are not used for veal or beef production because of a high carotene content that makes their fat yellow and undesirable to the consumer. The Holstein-Friesian accounts for approximately 90% of the dairy cattle in the United States. Holstein bull calves are used almost exclusively for veal and some dairy beef production. Table 19-1 indicates color, size, milk production ranking, and milkfat ranking of each.

Breeds of Beef Cattle

Beef cattle breeds are divided into four major categories: European breeds, Indian breeds, U.S.-developed breeds, and new and exotic breeds. Although there are 60 to 70 recognized breeds of beef cattle in the United

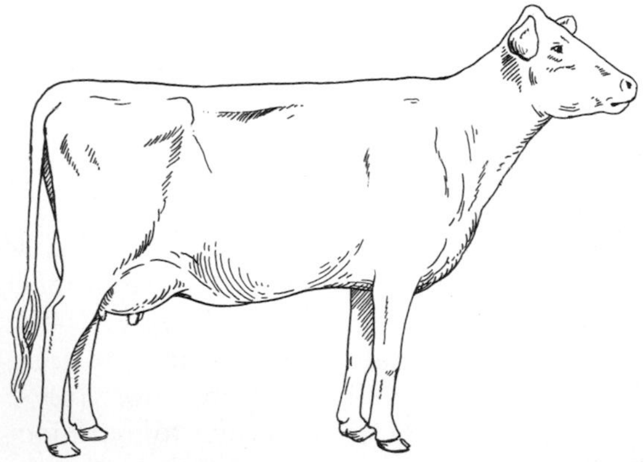

FIG. 19-1 Typical body type of a dairy cow.

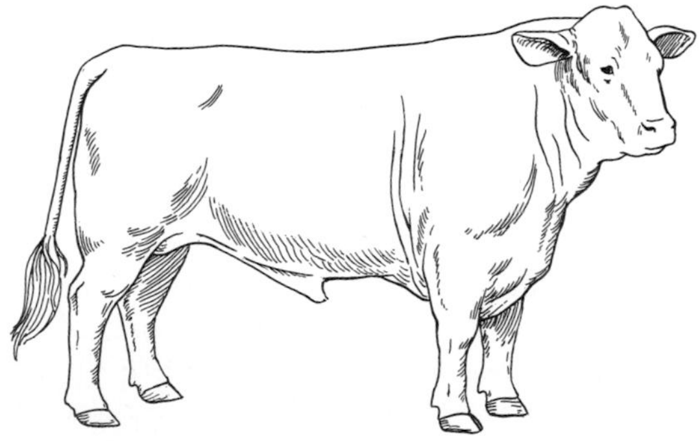

FIG. 19-2 Typical body type of a beef animal.

States, the Angus, polled Hereford, and Hereford remain the three most popular breeds. These three breeds account for approximately 90% of total beef cattle numbers. Table 19-2 indicates color, distinguishing characteristics, and classification of the most popular breeds of beef cattle.

Table 19-1 BREEDS OF DAIRY CATTLE AND DISTINGUISHING CHARACTERISTICS

Breed	Size (lb)	Color	Milk production ranking*	Milkfat ranking*
Ayrshire	1200	distinct red or mahogany and white	3	4
Brown Swiss	1400	solid brown ranging from light to dark	2	3
Guernsey	1100	any shade of fawn with distinct white markings	4	2
Holstein-Friesian	1500	distinct black-and-white markings, some red and white	1	5
Jersey	1000	any shade of fawn with or without white markings	5	1

*Number 1 is the highest, and number 5 is the lowest.

Table 19-2 BREEDS OF BEEF CATTLE AND DISTINGUISHING CHARACTERISTICS

Breed	Color	Distinguishing characteristics	Classification
Angus	black	polled, small, calf-limited dystocia, high weaning weight, good muscle-to-bone ratio	European breed
Brahman	varying shades of gray	humped, heat tolerant, disease and insect resistant, drooping ears, loose skin on neck, loose excessive dewlap	Indian breed
Brangus	black	polled, hybrid vigor resulting from cross of Brahman and Angus	U.S.-developed breed
Charolais	white	heavily muscled, polled or horned, noted for lean meat, heat and cold tolerant, high dressing percentage, good mothering ability	Exotic breed
Hereford	red body with white face, underline, and switch	horned, hardy, good grazing ability, thick muscling, reproductively efficient, good temperament	European breed
Polled Hereford	same as Hereford	same as Hereford except polled	U.S.-developed breed

REVIEW A

1. The genus and species of cattle of European descent is ______________________; that of cattle originating in Asia is ____.
2. Brahman cattle are also called ______________________ cattle.
3. The cow's mammary glands are collectively called the ______________________________.
4. The most common breed of dairy cow in the United States is the ______________________.
5. The three most common breeds of beef cattle in the United States are ____________________, ______________________, and ______________________.

DAIRY CATTLE REARING AND HOUSING SYSTEMS

There are several different types of housing systems for dairy cattle. The three most popular types of housing systems used are *free-stall, loose* or *pen,* and *stanchion* barns. Today all systems of rearing are highly mechanized to reduce labor intensity.

Stanchion barns effectively restrain each animal in a confined area by means of a stanchion. A stanchion has a wood-lined metal yoke, which is fastened at the top and bottom by a bolt and chain. The yoke is allowed to pivot from side to side so the animal can eat and drink water. Water cups normally are automatic so the animal can drink *ad libitum.* The yoke is adjustable for varying neck thicknesses. The stall to which the stanchion is attached must be long enough for the cow to lie down comfortably. It must be wide enough to allow the animal to get up without injuring its udder and teats. Bedding composed of straw, sawdust, or wood chips is used in stanchion housing to prevent abrasions and injury. Rubber mats are also commonly used. Stanchion-type housing does allow for more individual attention than other systems because it is easier to keep a visual watch over individual animals. It also facilitates handling and treatment.

A free-stall system uses loose housing with pens provided for the animals. The animals are not confined or restrained and may enter and leave the stalls at will. The barn usually is divided into a feeding area and a resting area. The stalls are situated in the resting area. This system allows more effective use of automatic feeding systems. The animals seem to stay cleaner than in stanchion housing; however, more bedding is needed. There are fewer injuries to teats and udders. Free-stall housing works well with the use of a milking parlor.

The most efficient use of housing is loose or pen-type housing. With loose housing, all animals are housed in one large, open pen or building. The floor is slotted, with a manure pit under the building.

Most dairy farms today use automatic milking machines and *milking parlors,* in which the cows come to you to be milked. A milking parlor is composed of a weigh jar for collecting milk, a milking machine, and a vacuum system to move milk from the weigh jar to the bulk refrigerated milk tank. Various types of milking parlors are available, and the type selected depends on the number of animals being milked. The use of the milking parlor has reduced time and labor involved with the milking process. Cows are milked twice a day all year. Individual cows are milked for approximately a 305-day *lactation* period. Cows are "dried off" for 60 days, which corresponds to the last 60 days of their gestation period. The use of the milking parlor has improved sanitation involved with the milking process.

BEEF CATTLE REARING AND HOUSING SYSTEMS

There are several rearing systems for beef cattle. Confinement rearing of beef cattle seems to be the least practical and is not recommended because it is costly and very labor intensive. Most beef cow and calf operations have very simple housing facilities. Cows normally calve on open pasture with little difficulty. Animals can be kept out during the winter if there is some shelter from the elements. This shelter can be a simple wind block using natural tree lines.

Other systems of rearing beef cattle include feedlot, pasture, and open range. Feedlots are confined rearing, and all food is brought to the animals. Pasture rearing allows the animals to graze on land that has been improved by planting various types of forages. More animals can be kept in a given area than when reared on open range. Open range has the animals hunt for food on unimproved land. Each animal needs a lot of land to completely balance its diet.

Animals kept on feedlot normally are separated by size and age. Pasture and open range are considered the least expensive systems of rearing, but feedlot operations are needed for *finishing* cattle. With the exception of pasture and open range rearing, feed must be brought to the animals. Cleaning up after the animals is also unnecessary with open range and pasture rearing. Animals reared on open range effectively convert coarse forage into flesh. Open range is land that cannot sustain a crop for direct human consumption and therefore is considered unproductive land. Cattle, as *ruminant* animals, can convert this forage into a marketable product. They also keep this unproductive land clear of overgrowth while fertilizing it with their manure.

No matter which system of beef cattle rearing is used, effective cattle handling facilities are essential to the proper operation of a beef enterprise. These handling facilities can be either permanent or temporary. (See section on restraint of cattle.)

REVIEW B

1. A wood-lined metal yoke placed behind the head to restrain cattle is called a ______________ ______________________________.
2. The most efficient type of housing for dairy cattle is ______________.
3. Cows generally are milked ______________ times a day for a lactation period of ______________ days and allowed a dry period of ______________ days.
4. The process of finishing beef cattle usually is done in a ______________, rather than on the range.

FEEDING CATTLE

Cattle are *ruminant* herbivores possessing a stomach that has four functional compartments. The compartments of the ruminant stomach are the rumen, reticulum, omasum, and abomasum, or "true stomach" (see Fig. 11-2). A calf is born as a monogastric and gradually with age develops into a true ruminant.

Cattle do not have upper incisors; instead, they have a dental pad. It appears that they do not need upper incisors because they are able to graze efficiently without them. Cattle prehend food with their tongues. When cattle graze, they form a *bolus* of food and swallow it almost immediately, with little chewing. They consume all the food they desire, lie down in the pasture, and ruminate, or "chew their cud." This process of *rumination* includes regurgitating the previously swallowed food back into the mouth for reinsalivation, remastication, and redeglutition. After this bolus of food is swallowed, another bolus is regurgitated. This process of rumination continues until all fibrous roughage is broken down.

The first and largest compartment of the ruminant stomach is called the *rumen* or fermentation vat. Here saliva, bacteria, and protozoans soften and break down carbohydrates and proteins of coarse forage. Fermentation also takes place in the *reticulum,* whose surface looks like a honeycomb. The reticulum also traps foreign objects such as screws, wire, nails, and stones and is sometimes called the "hardware compartment." Many cattle are fed rumen magnets to prevent a disease condition called *traumatic gastritis* or *hardware disease.* Smaller food particles move on to the *omasum* or "manyplies," which has the appearance of large leaves. Movement through this organ mixes the food and grinds it. It is in the omasum that large quantities of water are absorbed. Ingesta then moves on to the *abomasum,* or true stomach. Here the ingesta is mixed with gastric juices, and digestion takes place. Digestion in the abomasum is the same as in monogastric animals.

Both beef and dairy cattle consume large quantities of *roughage,* which they obtain by grazing on pasture or being fed hay or *silage.* Most beef cattle eat only what they graze, with an occasional protein supplement during the winter. A beef calf runs with its dam until it is *weaned* at about 6 months of age. From 6 months to approximately 12 to 15 months, beef animals graze on pasture or open range with no additional supplements. At about 15 months of age, the animals are removed from pasture, placed in a feedlot, and put on a high-protein complete ration, which increases both the yield and quality of the carcass at slaughter. This is the most economic way of rearing beef cattle. A constant supply of water must be available to help soften and digest the coarse forage consumed.

Dairy animals normally are fed according to the amount of milk they produce. Some dairy farmers do *challenge feeding.* They keep increasing the amount of feed the cow receives just as long as she keeps increasing the amount of milk produced. Most dairy cattle graze on roughage about 6 to 9 months per year. They are then given a protein, mineral, and vitamin supplement and hay to complete their ration. Free access to fresh water must be available. An average dairy cow in production consumes about 30 to 50 gallons of water per day. In confinement rearing, dairy cattle are fed a complete pelleted ration. Both dairy and beef cattle should be given mineral blocks *ad libitum.*

REVIEW C

1. The four compartments of the ruminant stomach are the ______________________________ , ______________________________ , ______________________________ , and ______________________________ .
2. Cattle have ____________________ upper incisors.
3. *Rumination* means ____________________ .
4. "Hardware disease" is properly called ____________________ . The part of the stomach it usually affects is the ____________________ .
5. The "true stomach" of ruminants is the ____________________ .
6. An average dairy cow in full production consumes about ____________________ gallons of water per day.

RESTRAINT OF CATTLE

Cattle do not show the variable individual differences that horses do, but they also do not respond to commands and reasoning as do horses. Because dairy cattle are handled regularly, they seem to be a little easier to handle than are beef cattle, which respond to the natural fight-or-flight instinct. When handling bulls, whether they be dairy or beef, the animal should never be trusted. Because of their size and unpredictable nature, they can cause severe injury to their handlers. Bulls normally have a ring that is placed through the septum of their nose. A staff usually is attached to the ring so that the handler can handle the bull from a distance. Another effective means of restraining a bull is to drive him into a *squeeze chute* equipped with a head gate (Fig. 19-3). The bull can be effectively restrained so that the handler is not kicked, head butted, or thrown. Because cattle are herd oriented, they will crowd and bunch up when driven. They sometimes create a domino effect by climbing the back of the animal in front of them. Herding cattle too quickly should be avoided to prevent bruising and other injuries.

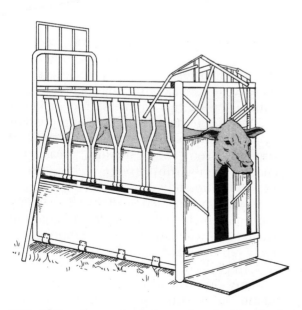

FIG. 19-3 A squeeze chute equipped with a head gate is used to restrain cattle.

Beef cattle normally are handled by the use of mechanical devices such as corrals, working chutes, dodge gates, and head gates. They include a series of corrals containing sorting pens, holding pens, blocking gates, loading chutes, squeeze chutes, head gates, and working chutes (Fig. 19-4).

Corrals are fenced areas that enclose and

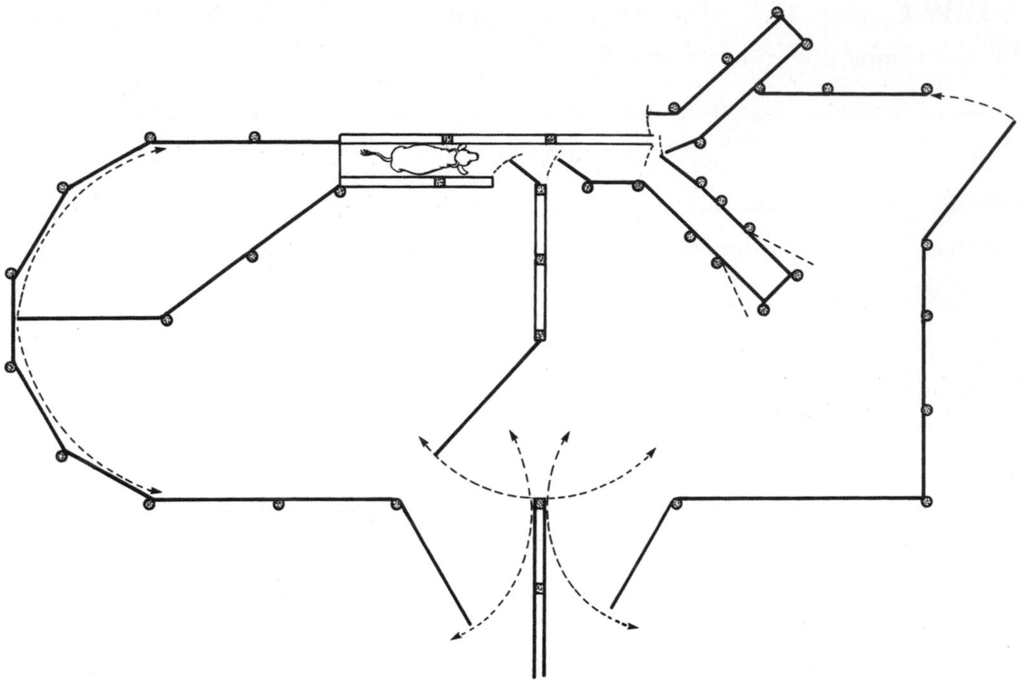

FIG. 19-4 A typical beef cattle handling system with corrals, gates, and chutes.

facilitate the restraint of cattle. Various types of chutes are available for animal restraint. There are portable chutes, built-in chutes, and custom chutes designed for various procedures. Each type of chute has various attachments to hold the head in a certain position. These head gates effectively restrain the head and prevent injury to the handler and the animal. Other components of a chute allow easy access to other parts of the animal's body. Chutes normally have a squeeze apparatus that squeezes the body of the animal to effectively restrain it.

These handling facilities make it easier to handle beef cattle. Because beef cattle are not handled as dairy cattle are, they are not as docile to work with and are stressed more easily if handled inappropriately. The corral system reduces the amount of labor and time needed to handle beef cattle, reduces injury by effectively restraining them, reduces weight loss resulting from stress and overexertion, makes the handling of beef cattle safer for the handlers, and makes it much easier to diagnose, treat, and prevent injury and disease. Animals are worked and funneled from large holding areas into smaller corrals, run through a chute single file, and ultimately restrained in a squeeze chute with an attached head gate. By moving and funneling beef cattle from larger to smaller restricted areas, they are more effectively immobilized so procedures may be performed.

Many other means of restraint are used on individual cattle. Dairy cattle can be rope haltered and led manually by the handler using a rope or nylon halter. Nose leads or nose tongs are used to restrain the head of an animal. The fingers of the handler can be used if nose leads are not available. When handlers work around the caudal aspect of cattle, they may find the constant tail movements annoying, particularly when the *switch* flicks across the handler's eyes. A tail tie can be used to immobilize the tail by securing it to a front leg. Hobbles or antikickers may be used to prevent the animal from kicking the handler while he or she is milking or working on the ventral portion. Hobbles are placed above the animal's hocks. Lifting the legs of cattle for hoof trimming is much more difficult than with horses. Ropes, pulleys, and leverage can be used, but the animal often kicks constantly, making it almost impossible to perform the trimming. The most effective restraint method for hoof trimming is the use of the tilt table. It offers the most control and comfort to the animal and the handler. If an animal needs to be placed in a lateral recumbent position, the handler can use ropes to cast the animal. A calf may be restrained by flanking it and bringing it to the ground. This restraint method is effective for dehorning and castration.

REVIEW D

1. The end of a cow's tail is called the ______________________________.
2. Devices used to prevent cattle from kicking are called ______________________________.
3. The restraint technique of placing a calf in lateral recumbency is called ______________________________.
4. Nose rings normally are used only to restrain ______________________________.

COMMON TECHNIQUES AND PROCEDURES

Many procedures are performed on both dairy and beef cattle. The following is a brief discussion of the most common procedures and the instruments and tools used.

Identification

The permanent identification of all animals is important so that accurate records can be maintained on each animal. Beef cattle normally are branded on their rump. This procedure is performed by using either hot irons or chemicals. Both metal and plastic ear tags are also used. These are less permanent because they can be torn out. Dairy cattle normally are identified by the use of ear tags, ear tattoos, and neck chains with plastic identification tags affixed to them.

Dehorning

Almost all dairy animals in the United States are dehorned for the safety of both the animal and the handler. Dehorning should be performed as early as possible in the animal's life (usually at less than 2 months of age) to minimize animal stress and setbacks resulting from infections. The ideal time of year to dehorn is in the early spring and late fall, before and after the time that flies appear. Electric (hot) dehorners and chemical dehorners can be used throughout the year. Chemical dehorning using caustic paste burns the *corium,* which surrounds the horn button. Electric dehorning uses heat to burn the corium around the horn button to prevent horn growth. Electric dehorning is considered the most humane. The Roberts tube dehorner actually cuts around and scoops out the horn button. The Barnes dehorner is designed to dehorn animals that are between 4 and 12 months of age. This tool lifts (scoops) the horn out by the roots and crushes the blood vessels. Keystone dehorners contain a set of guillotinelike blades and are used for dehorning in older cattle with full-grown horns. Another method of removing mature horn is a manual or electric saw.

Castration

Castration is the removal of the testicles either surgically or nonsurgically. Bulls can be castrated at any time during their lives, but it is usually done when the bulls are less than 3 months of age to minimize stress. Calves usually are castrated from birth up to 2 weeks of age. Castration is performed to remove the source of testosterone, the male sex hormone.

Surgical castration includes the use of a knife or scalpel to remove the lower third of the scrotum. After the testicles are exposed an *emasculator* is applied to the spermatic cord. The emasculator is an instrument that crushes and cuts.

Two nonsurgical and bloodless methods of castration are the use of the *Burdizzo emasculatome* and the elastrator. The emasculatome crushes the spermatic cord and blood vessels while leaving the scrotum intact. The *elastrator* has a small elastic band that is placed over the scrotum as close to the body as possible without incorporating the rudimentary teats. The elastic band is released, eliminating nerve and blood supply to the scrotum and testicles. The scrotum and testicles atrophy and slough off in 3 to 4 weeks.

Medication

Pills can be administered to cattle by means of a *balling gun.* The *bolus* (pill) is placed in the balling gun, and the gun is inserted over the lingual torus to the rear of the animal's mouth. The plunger is engaged, and the bolus is inserted into the rear of the oral cavity. Liquid medication can be administered by using a drencher, dose syringe, or stomach tube. If using a stomach tube, a Frick speculum must be placed into the oral cavity first to prevent the animal from biting down on the actual tube.

Removal of Supernumerary Teats

Many dairy calves are born with more than the usual four teats. These *supernumerary* (extra) teats can develop and grow just like a normal teat. These teats can be the source of infection, especially *mastitis,* and can interfere with the placement of the milking machine on the functional teats. Supernumerary teats should be removed surgically from heifers.

REVIEW E

1. Permanent identification of range beef cattle normally is done by ______________________.
   Methods for permanent identification of dairy cattle are ______________________, ______________________, and ______________________.
2. Surgical removal of the testicles is called ______________________ and is done to remove the source of ______________________. The instrument used is the ______________________.
3. Two instruments used for nonsurgical (bloodless) removal of the testicles are the ______________________ and the ______________________.
4. The device used to administer pills to cattle is called a(n) ______________________.
5. If dairy heifers are born with more than four teats, the extra ones are called ______________________ teats.
6. The most humane method for dehorning young calves is by using a(n) ______________________.
7. When passing a bovine stomach tube, a(n) ______________________ must be placed in the animal's mouth to prevent it from chewing the tube.

REPRODUCTION, PREGNANCY, AND MANAGEMENT OF THE NEWBORN CALF

The breeding of cattle is a large component of the cattle industry. Dairy cattle are bred so that they drop a calf approximately every 12 months. This is called the *calving interval.* The purpose of having a calf once a year is so that the cow comes back into full milk. A cow does not reach her full milk potential until her fourth *lactation,* at which time she is 6 years old. Heifer calves serve as replacement stock for the herd. Almost all bull calves, with the exception of Jersey and Guernsey bull calves, are used for veal production. Beef heifer calves are used as replacement animals and are also reared for meat, as are beef bull calves that are castrated and reared as steers.

Cattle are polyestrous animals with estrus occurring every 21 days. Heifers normally are bred at about 15 months of age, even though puberty is reached much earlier. It is thought that the heifer should reach anatomic as well as sexual maturity before breeding. Heifers should drop their first calf by 24 months of age. The *gestation* period for cattle is about 280 days, or 9 months. Gestation varies among breeds. The estrus period of the bovine lasts approximately 18 hours. The female bovine is the only animal that does not ovulate until about 12 hours after the completion of *estrus* (heat). All other farm animals ovulate during estrus.

Beef cattle traditionally are bred by using natural servicing by the bull. The bull runs with the heifers and the cows, breeding them naturally. Dairy cattle, on the other hand, are almost exclusively bred by means of *artificial insemination (AI).* One of the major problems with AI breeding is the detection of estrus and proper timing of insemination. Because cattle do not ovulate until after the completion of estrus, it is the responsibility of the manager to be observant about when a cow or heifer is in heat. When a female is noticed riding another female and the female on the bottom remains to be mounted, she is said to be in *standing heat.* If standing heat is noticed in the morning, the female should be bred that evening. Standing heat lasts about 18 hours.

Because the life span of the egg is very short in comparison with the life of the sperm, viable sperm must be available to impregnate the ovum, no matter when it is ovulated. Once the female is bred, she should be checked for pregnancy about 30 to 45 days after breeding, by rectal palpation. A cow that is not pregnant is said to be *open.* If heat periods are missed and conception does not take place, the calving interval is increased, resulting in longer *dry* periods and fewer overall profits because of decreased milk production. A pregnant cow is milked for approximately 305 days after her last calving and dried off for the last 60 days of gestation so she can build her body reserves of nutrients. This dry period is important so that she does not exhibit any nutritional deficiencies when she *freshens* and comes into full milk. About 2 to 3 weeks before parturition, the diet of the heifer or cow should be altered and calcium intake lowered. This reduces the chances of the cow coming down with *milk fever (parturient paresis)* immediately after calving. After a cow calves, she is bred again approximately 60 days later.

After the calf is born, it should be rubbed vigorously with a burlap bag or towel to get its circulatory system functioning. Normal birth position is forelegs and head first in a diving position, head between legs. A piece of hay or straw can be inserted into the calf's nostril to cause it to sneeze and force fluids out of the respiratory system. The calf's umbilical cord must be dipped in 7% iodine to prevent the invasion of organisms and a condition called *navel ill (omphalitis)*. The iodine also helps to dry the wet cord. The calf should be forced to consume about 8% of its body weight in *colostrum* within the first 12 hours after birth. It is critical that the calf gets 2 quarts of colostrum by 6 hours after its birth. Colostrum contains antibodies that protect the calf from anything that the dam was protected against. This is called *passive immunity*. Colostrum is beneficial not only because of the passive immunity it provides but also because it contains about 10 times more vitamin A and 3 to 4 times more protein than milk. Colostrum may also increase intestinal motility, thus preventing bacterial colonization of the small intestine and assisting in the prevention of *scours*, or diarrhea. The ability of the calf's intestines to absorb antibodies from the colostrum lasts only the first 36 hours of life. After 36 hours, postpartum intestinal absorption is zero. After the dairy calf has received sufficient amounts of colostrum, it should be removed from its dam and placed in a pen or calf-hutch. A dairy calf should not remain with its dam for more than 24 hours. The cow or first calf heifer should be returned to the milking herd for production purposes. The calf is fed via a pail with bottled milk or milk replacer.

REVIEW F

1. At 30 to 45 days after breeding, a cow may be checked for pregnancy by ____________________.

   If she is not pregnant she is said to be ____________________.
2. During the time when a dairy cow is not milking she is said to be ____________________.

   When she calves she is said to ____________________.
3. *Parturient paresis* is the correct name for ____________________ in cows.
4. Navel ill is an infection of the ____________________ and is also called ____________________.
5. The cow's first milk is called ____________________.
6. *Scours* is a common name for ____________________ in calves.
7. Because cows continue to cycle regularly every 21 days (unless bred), they are said to be

   ____________________.

MILK PRODUCTION

The primary purpose of the dairy cow is to produce milk. A cow is milked for 305 days per year, two times per day. A cow's udder is made up of four mammary glands, which are called quarters. Specific quarters are identified as left rear, left fore, right rear, and right fore. The basic milk producing structures of the udder are the alveoli. (See Chapter 12, Fig. 12-8.) Blood traveling through the alveoli contributes the raw materials for milk manufacturing. Within the alveoli are epithelium-lined milk cavities that produce the milk. There are thousands of these alveoli throughout the udder tissue. Small tubes lead from each individual alveolus to small milk ducts, which in turn lead to larger milk ducts. These large milk ducts direct the milk into a *gland cistern* (collecting basin). Each gland cistern can hold about a pint (16 ounces) of milk. Milk then passes from the gland cistern into the teat cistern and through the *streak canal,* which is located at the ventral end of the teat. A sphincter muscle at the terminal ventral end of the teat prevents the milk from leaking out before milking. Milk is then expressed to the exterior into the milking machine or calf's mouth.

Because most cows are milked twice a day, the milk produced between milkings is stored in the alveoli milk cavities, tubules, and small ducts. Milk letdown is stimulated by the washing action of the udder before milking. This conditioned reflex stimulates the pituitary gland to release a hormone called *oxytocin.* Oxytocin enters the circulatory system and travels to the udder, stimulating muscle fibers to contract and forcing the milk out of the alveoli and milk ducts. Milk then empties into larger ducts and into the cisterns and is eventually expressed through the sphincter of the teat to the exterior.

After the cow's udder is washed, each teat is tested by stripping a few squirts of milk into a *strip cup. Stripping* is the removal of a few squirts of milk from the teat before placing the milking machine on the cow. A strip cup lets the milker do a gross examination of the milk to inspect for flakes, sloughed cells, and blood. If any of this debris is present, the cow probably has a condition called *mastitis.*

After the cow is stripped, the milking machine is placed on the animal, and the animal is milked for approximately 5 minutes. During milking, the cow's udder can be massaged to assist in milk letdown. The cow must be watched to make sure that she is not overmilked. Overmilking can cause trauma to milk-producing tissue and is a predisposing cause of mastitis. After milking is completed and the machine is removed, each of the cow's teats is dipped in antibacterial solution *(teat-dip).* Any cow being treated with antibiotics should be milked last; that way, antibiotic milk will not mix with regular milk. If this occurs, it could be extremely dangerous to humans who are allergic to antibiotics. The animal is then released and returned to the barn or pasture to begin the process all over. Recently, dairy animals have been injected with bovine somatotropic hormones (growth hormones) to increase the overall amount of milk they produce.

PREVENTIVE HEALTH CARE

Routine preventive care is important to the health of cattle. Parasite control and immunization for preventable infectious diseases is important. Testing for nonpreventable diseases must be done to remove the carriers and eventually eliminate the disease. Simple management procedures can be used to prevent disease. An example is the use of a 5% copper sulfate footbath to prevent foot rot in dairy cattle.

Several endoparasites can cause disease and debilitate both dairy and beef cattle, thus reducing profits by reducing milk production and carcass yield and quality. They include liver flukes, tapeworms, gastrointestinal roundworms, lungworms, and coccidiosis. Both gastrointestinal roundworms and coccidiosis are a common problem.

It is important to use approved deworming compounds and adhere to milk withdrawal times and preslaughter times. Withdrawal times are important for preventing contamination of milk and meat that are to be consumed by humans.

Ectoparasites cause tremendous losses in the cattle industry by lowering milk production, increasing feed costs, decreasing carcass quality, reducing weight gains, and in extreme cases causing loss of animals. The ectoparasites that affect cattle and cause severe problems include flies, lice, mosquitoes, ticks, and mites. They can be controlled by spraying, dusting, fogging, dipping, cattle tube oilers, dust bags, and feed additives. Feed additives are used to control the larvae found in the feces from becoming adults.

Federal and state governments require that dairy cattle be tested for tuberculosis and brucellosis. *Tuberculosis* is an infectious disease characterized by a chronic debilitated state despite good nutrition. Brucellosis is a highly contagious disease characterized by abortion. The control method for these diseases is the test-and-slaughter method. When infected animals are found, they are removed for slaughter. The herd is quarantined and retested until it is free of the disease.

Mastitis testing is necessary to prevent tremendous monetary losses in the dairy industry. The disease causes an inflammation of the mammary glands, usually involving the alveoli, secretory cells, and connective tissue. With severe cases of mastitis, the secretory tissue is replaced with scar tissue, thus reducing the amount of functional milk-producing tissue. Mastitis changes not only the quantity but also the quality of the milk. If mastitis is suspected, a test called the *California mastitis test (CMT)* is performed. If the animal tests positive for mastitis, the cow is given intramammary infusions of broad-spectrum antibiotics.

Cattle usually are vaccinated on the basis of age. Cattle may be immunized against one or more or all of the following diseases depending on their geographic location: *brucellosis, bovine rhinotracheitis, bovine viral diarrhea, campylobacteriosis, leptospirosis, rotavirus,* and *corona virus, E. coli, pasteurellosis, parainfluenza,* and *Clostridium*. Male cattle should never be vaccinated for brucellosis.

COMMON DISEASES OF CATTLE

In addition to the infectious diseases mentioned in the previous section, cattle also can be affected by the following diseases and conditions: *abomasal displacement, abomasal ulcers, traumatic reticulitis (hardware disease), bloat, ketosis, pink eye, ringworm, warts, white muscle disease,* and *lymphosarcomas.*

REVIEW G

1. The udder of a cow is made up of ______________ separate mammary glands, each called a(n) ______________ .
2. The basic milk-producing structures of the mammary gland are called ______________ .
3. The passage from the teat cistern to the outside is the ______________ .
4. Milk letdown results from release of the hormone ______________ .
5. Inflammation of the udder is called ______________ .
6. A 5% copper sulfate foot bath is used to prevent ______________ in cattle.
7. Two cattle diseases that are controlled by the test-and-slaughter method are ______________ and ______________ .
8. CMT stands for ______________ .

Chapter 19 Answers

Review A

1. *Bos taurus, Bos indicus*
2. zebu
3. udder
4. Holstein-Friesian
5. Angus, polled Hereford, Hereford

Review B

1. stanchion
2. loose (pen-type)
3. two, 305, 60
4. feedlot

Review C

1. rumen, reticulum, omasum, abomasum
2. no
3. chewing the cud
4. traumatic gastritis (or traumatic reticulitis), reticulum
5. abomasum
6. 30 to 50

Review D

1. switch
2. hobbles (antikickers)
3. flanking
4. bulls

Review E

1. branding, ear tags, ear tattoos, neck chains
2. castration, testosterone, emasculator
3. emasculator, elastrator
4. balling gun
5. supernumerary
6. electric dehorner
7. Frick speculum

Review F

1. rectal palpation, open
2. dry, freshen
3. milk fever
4. umbilicus, omphalitis
5. colostrum
6. diarrhea
7. polyestrous

Review G

1. four, quarter
2. alveoli
3. streak canal
4. oxytocin
5. mastitis
6. foot rot
7. tuberculosis, brucellosis
8. California mastitis test

Chapter 19 EXERCISES

CATTLE INDUSTRY

Exercise 1: Match the term in the right column with the correct definition or statement in the left column by placing the appropriate letter in the blank space provided.

_____ 1. At pleasure, free choice

_____ 2. Loss of hair

_____ 3. Device used to pill large animals

_____ 4. Castrated male bovine

_____ 5. Test for inflammation of the bovine udder and mammary glands

_____ 6. First milk produced immediately after parturition

_____ 7. Naturally or genetically hornless

_____ 8. Difficult or labored parturition

_____ 9. Bred for both dairy and beef

_____ 10. Phase of the female reproductive cycle, in standing heat

A. Steer
B. Balling gun
C. Colostrum
D. California mastitis test
E. *Ad libitum*
F. Polled
G. Dystocia
H. Estrus
I. Dual-purpose
J. Alopecia

Exercise 2: Define the following terms.

1. Freshen
2. Hybrid vigor
3. Milk fever
4. Marbling
5. Range
6. Ruminant
7. Squeeze chute
8. Supernumerary teats
9. Traumatic reticulitis
10. Veal

CHAPTER 19 PUZZLE

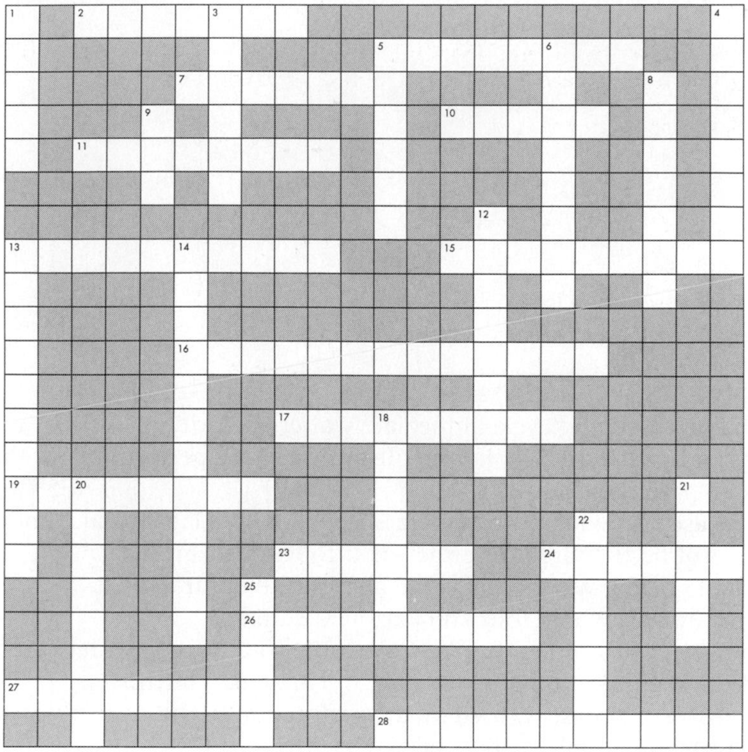

ACROSS CLUES

2. To begin lactation cycle
5. Difficult or labored parturition
7. Caused by *Moraxella bovis*
10. Caudal region of bovine neck
11. Loss of hair
13. Substance used to fight bacterial diseases
15. Period of time cow is milking
16. Flies, lice, and ticks
17. Feeding beef cows to increase carcass quality and yield
19. A cud-chewing animal
23. Mating of two different species
24. Device used to prevent kicking
26. First milk after parturition
27. Feed high in TDN
28. Having more than one estrous cycle per year

DOWN CLUES

1. Accumulation of gas in rumen
3. Female bovine not yet calved
4. Hormone that causes milk letdown
5. Loose skin over brisket
6. Remove testicles
8. Of long duration
9. Mature female bovine
12. Infectious disease of mammary gland
13. Placental membranes that surround fetus, expelled at birth
14. Mechanical means of impregnating cows
18. Presence of bile pigments; jaundice
20. Streaks or lines of fat in lean meat
21. Ball of food or large pill
22. Also called pododermatitis
25. Underdeveloped horns not attached to skull

Chapter 19 Answers

Exercise 1

1. E
2. J
3. B
4. A
5. D
6. C
7. F
8. G
9. I
10. H

Exercise 2

1. The beginning of a lactating cycle immediately after parturition.
2. The effect of producing a hybrid; hybrid offspring usually perform better than either of their individual parents.
3. A paralytic disease following parturition associated with a lack of calcium in the blood.
4. Streaks or lines of fat that are interdispersed throughout lean meat.
5. An open area of grazing where beef cattle harvest the natural feed.
6. A cud-chewing animal with a four-compartment stomach.
7. A restraint device used to effectively restrain cattle so that procedures can be performed.
8. An excess of the regular number of four teats; removed at birth.
9. Also called hardware disease; caused by the perforation of the recticulum wall by a sharp foreign object such as a nail, a screw, or baling wire.
10. Generally a young dairy bull calf, under 12 weeks of age, kept in the dark and fed only milk or milk replacer; used to produce a pale, soft, and tender carcass.

ANSWERS: CHAPTER 19 PUZZLE

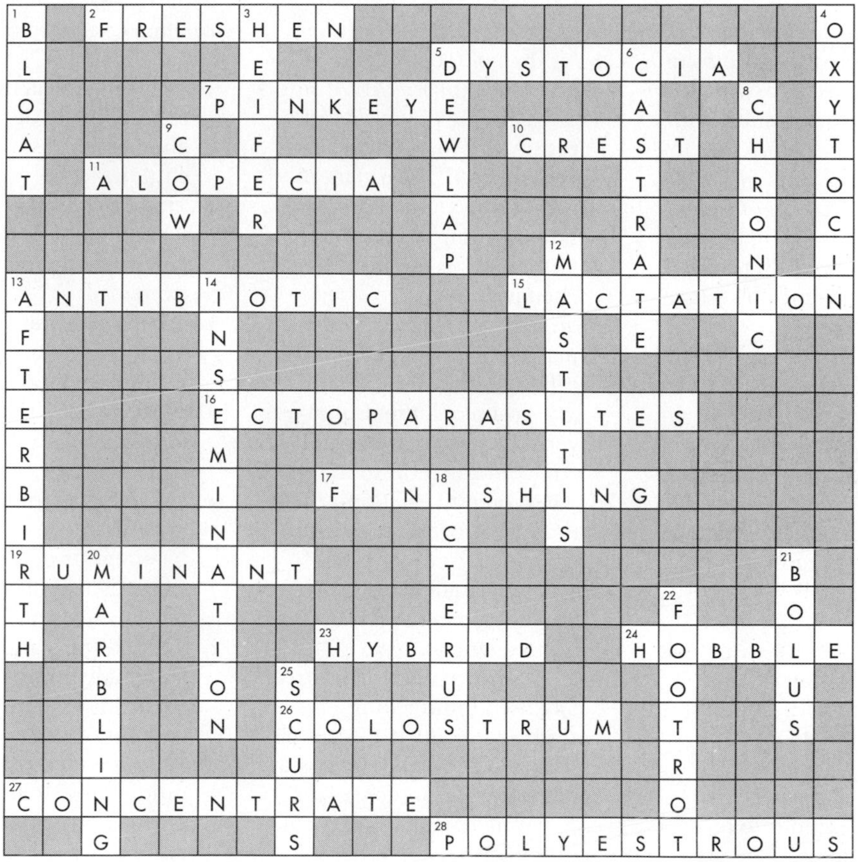
1 BLOAT
2 FRESHEN
3 HEIFER
4 OXYTOCIN
5 DYSTOCIA
5 DEWLAP
6 CASTRATE
7 PINKEYE
8 CHRONIC
9 COW
10 CREST
11 ALOPECIA
12 MASTITIS
13 ANTIBIOTIC
13 AFTERBIRTH
14 INSEMINATION
15 LACTATION
16 ECTOPARASITES
17 FINISHING
18 ICTERUS
19 RUMINANT
20 MARBLING
21 BOLUS
22 FOOTROT
23 HYBRID
24 HOBBLE
25 SCOURS
26 COLOSTRUM
27 CONCENTRATE
28 POLYESTROUS

GLOSSARY

abomasal displacement (right): disease of newly calved cows in which abomasum assumes abnormal position resulting in abdominal distension and loss of appetite.

abomasopexy: fixation of the abomasum by suturing to ventral abdominal wall; used to prevent recurrence of abomasal displacement.

abortion: termination and expulsion of fetus before completion of normal gestation.

ad libitum: at pleasure: used to indicate feeding or supplying water on a free-choice basis.

afterbirth: placental membranes that surround fetus during gestation; usually expelled from uterus directly after parturition.

alopecia: loss of hair.

antibiotic: substance that kills bacteria or prevents their growth.

artificial insemination: act of introducing semen into female's genital tract by use of mechanical methods.

bacterin: preparation administered to develop immunity against bacterial diseases.

balling gun: mechanical device, either metal or plastic, used to pill large animals.

barrel: circumference of abdominal region; used as indication of feed capacity.

bloat: accumulation of gas in rumen of cattle; excess gas is removed by stomach tubing or puncturing abdomen and rumen with trocar and cannula.

body capacity: heart girth and barrel; large heart girth means larger heart and lung and greater feed capacity.

bolus: ball of food or large pill.

bovine viral diarrhea (BVD): infectious disease of young cattle causing profuse diarrhea.

brand: method of permanently identifying animal by scarring skin on rump; usually performed using hot irons or chemicals.

bred: animal that has been mated and is pregnant; also called "with calf."

breed: group of animals that are genetically similar in color and conformation so that when bred to each other will produce progeny with same characteristics.

brucellosis: contagious disease of bovine causing abortion late in pregnancy.

bull: mature male bovine, usually used for breeding.

butterfat: fat content of whole milk; rises to top of milk that has not been homogenized.

calf: young bovine, either male or female, usually under 1 year of age.

California mastitis test: test for bovine mastitis; measures number of somatic cells and leukocytes.

campylobacteriosis: bacterial disease of cattle causing abortion and infertility; also called vibriosis.

carcass: after slaughter, dressed (head, blood, hide, and offal removed) body of beef animal.

casein: milk protein often used in purified diets.

castrate: to remove testicles from male animal.

cattle: two or more members of genus *Bos,* regardless of sex or age.

chronic: condition of long duration.

chute: mechanical device used to restrain cattle or make handling easier (as in *squeeze* chute).

cistern: collecting basin in udder where milk is secreted before entering teat and being expressed.

close breeding: practice of breeding son to dam, sire to daughter (inbreeding).

Clostridium: genus of spore-forming, anaerobic bacteria; can cause tetanus, blackleg, and enterotoxemia in cattle.

cod: remnants of scrotum of steer; usually filled with fat.

colostrum: first thick, yellowish milklike substance produced by female immediately after parturition; high in protein and antibodies.

concentrate: feed that is high in total digestible nutrients (TDN) and low in fiber and moisture content.

conformation: overall shape and body type (form) of bovine.

copulation: act of mating.

corium: specialized cells that form horns of cattle.

cow: mature female bovine that has given birth and is lactating.

cow hocked: animal whose hocks turn in and rub together, reducing udder capacity.

creep feed: high-energy feed given to calves by means of special feeding panels that allow access to calves but not to adult animals.

crest: caudal region of neck; most prominent on mature male bovine.

crossbred: offspring resulting from mating of two different breeds within same species.

cud: bolus of regurgitated food from stomach (rumen) of bovine.

cull: animal that is usually removed from herd because it does not meet standards of overall herd; unproductive animal.

dam: female bovine who is mother of calf.

dehorn: mechanical removal of horn buttons or horns of bovine.

dewlap: loose skin that covers brisket and portion of neck; more prominent on dairy and certain beef cattle.

DHIA: Dairy Herd Improvement Association.

dressing percentage: percentage dressed weight of animal is to live weight.

dry: cow that is not lactating; usually last 60 days of gestation in dairy cows.

dual-purpose: dairy and beef cattle that are bred and used for both milk and meat production.

dystocia: difficult or labored parturition.

ear tagging: placement of tag in ear for identification purposes.

ectoparasites: parasites that inhabit external body surfaces.

E. coli: normal inhabitant of intestinal flora; pathogenic form causes epidemic diarrhea in newborn calves.

elastrator: bloodless castration device using small bands.

emasculatome: bloodless castration device that crushes spermatic cord without breaking skin (also called a Burdizzo).

emasculator: surgical castration instrument that both crushes and cuts spermatic cord.

estrous cycle: recurrent set of physiologic and behavioral changes that take place in female animal from one estrus period to next.

estrus: stage of estrous cycle in which female is receptive to male (heat).

feeder: beef cattle old and heavy enough to be placed in feed lot to improve carcass quality and yield.

fertile: able to reproduce at regular intervals.

finishing: feeding beef cattle high-quality feed before slaughter to increase carcass quality and yield.

foot rot: bacterial disease characterized by inflammation of interdigital tissue and heel of hoof; also called *pododermatitis.*

freemartin: heifer calf born twin to bull; usually sterile.

free-stall: open stall system of rearing beef cattle.

freshen: beginning of lactating cycle immediately after parturition.

gestation: period between conception and parturition.

globule: fat particles that make up butterfat component of milk.

heart girth: circumference around thoracic cavity; measurement of heart and lung capacity; also used as indicator of animal's weight.

heat (estrus): period of sexual acceptance; female usually stands for service.

heifer: female bovine that is old enough to breed but has not yet calved.

hobble: device placed on caudal aspect of hocks to restrain hind legs of cow and prevent her from kicking while being milked.

hormones: substances produced by ductless glands that have physiologic effect on animal.

hybrid: progeny resulting from mating two different species.

hybrid vigor: increase in vitality resulting from mating of unrelated animals; hybrid offspring usually perform better than either parent.

icterus: presence of bile pigments; jaundice.

impaction: overfilling and plugging of stomach with feed that is exceptionally dry.

inbreeding: mating together of closely related animals.

infectious bovine rhinotracheitis (IBR): highly contagious respiratory disease of cattle; more prevalent in cattle that are crowded together in feedlots.

ingest: to eat or take in through mouth.

ketosis: disease characterized by accumulation of ketones in blood and tissue; cow has sweet-smelling breath and urine; also called *acetonemia.*

lactation: period of time cow is producing milk.

leptospirosis: acute infectious disease that causes abortion storms and subacute febrile illness.

lymphosarcoma: most common malignant lymphoid tumor found in cattle; also called *bovine leukosis.*

mammary (milk) veins: found on ventral underline of cow; carry blood away from udder.

marbling: streaks or lines of fat that are interdispersed throughout lean meat; makes meat tender and juicy.

mastitis: infectious and contagious inflammation of mammary gland (udder).

milk fever: paralytic disease following parturition associated with lack of calcium in blood.

milk solids: components of milk after all water is removed.

milk well: depression of female bovine's ventral underline where milk veins enter body.

monogastric: having a simple stomach.

nurse cow: cow whose purpose is to nurse multiple calves in addition to its own.

nutrient: substance that nourishes body.

offal: visceral organs and associated tissues removed from carcass of slaughtered animal.

open: not pregnant.

oxytocin: hormone produced by pituitary gland; responsible for milk letdown and uterine contractions.

palatability: relative acceptance of feeds by animals.

palpation: using sense of touch to examine animal; *see rectal palpation.*

parturition: process of calving.

passive immunity: transfer of antibodies produced by one animal and given to another; immunity produced is passive and temporary.

pasteurize: process of heating milk to kill pathogenic organisms.

pedigree: written record of animal's ancestral background.

pinkeye: contagious disease of cattle caused by *Moraxella bovis;* characterized by conjunctivitis, lacrimation, and corneal ulceration and opacity.

poll: top of head between ears.

polled: genetically or naturally hornless.

polyestrous: having more than one estrous cycle per year.

prolopsed vagina: protrusion of vagina resulting from pressure of developing fetus or other cause.

proved: refers to an animal whose ability to transmit traits is known and predictable.

puberty: age at which reproductive organs become functional.

purebred: offspring of two purebred parents; can be registered by breed association.

quarter: term used to specify a particular gland of cow's udder, such as left front quarter or left hind quarter.

range: open area of grazing land where beef cattle harvest natural feed.

ration: amount of food animal eats in 24-hour period.

rectal palpation: method of pregnancy determination in cattle; using rubber or plastic sleeve, hand is inserted into rectum to feel fetus or its associated structures.

replacement: animals that are raised from birth for addition to herd: superior animals are selected and retained for breeding purposes.

ringworm: fungal infection of skin and hair; characterized by thick, round, gray crusted patches over skin surface; hair that is in infected areas falls out or breaks off.

rotavirus and corona virus: viruses that cause diarrhea in young calves.

roughage: feedstuffs that are high in fiber and low in total digestible nutrients (TDN); examples include hay and silage.

rumen: first or large compartment of stomach of ruminant animals; also called fermentation vat.

rumenotomy: surgical incision into the rumen, most often done to remove hardware (nails, wire, etc.) from the reticulum.

ruminant: cud-chewing animal with four-compartment stomach.

rumination: process of regurgitating food (bolus) from rumen for remastication.

scours: profuse diarrhea, most commonly seen in young calves.

scrub: inferior animal.

scurs: underdeveloped horns that are not attached to skull surface.

service: process of breeding cattle.

silage: cattle feed (roughage) produced by fermenting chopped whole corn plants or mixed pasture grasses.

sire: male bovine that is capable of breeding and producing offspring; paternal parent of animal.

skim milk: whole milk that has had butterfat removed.

spotter bull: vasectomized bull used to seek out and mark females that are in estrus.

springing: anatomic changes

that indicate that parturition is near.

squeeze chute: restraint device used to effectively restrain cattle so that procedures can be performed.

stag: male bovine castrated after sexual maturity.

stanchion: restraint device that secures cattle around neck.

standing heat: cow or heifer in estrus that will stand to be mounted by bull or another female.

steer: male bovine castrated at young age.

strip cup: metal cup with a black or screened lid; used for detecting mastitis.

supernumerary teats: those in excess of regular number of four teats.

supplement: use of additional high-protein feeds to help improve and balance poorer ration, such as pasture.

switch: distal part of bovine tail, consisting of long, coarse hairs.

tattoo: permanent means of identification of cattle; indelible ink is injected under skin using system of numbers or letters.

teaser: male bovine that is used to seek out females that are in estrus; male is usually vasectomized.

traumatic reticulitis: caused by perforation of reticulum wall by sharp foreign object such as a nail, screw, or baling wire; also called *hardware disease.*

trocar and cannula: instrument used to puncture abdomen and rumen to relieve bloat.

udder: organ of milk production of cow; made up of two mammary glands and four teats.

vaccine: preparation administered to develop immunity against viral diseases.

vasectomized: rendered sterile by removal of portion of vas deferens (in male); vasectomized animal still exhibits libido.

veal: young dairy calf, under 12 weeks of age, kept in dark and fed only milk or milk replacer; used to produce pale, soft, and tender carcass.

warts: caused by viruses, multiple papillomas are located usually on head, neck, shoulders, and back; also called *papillomatosis.*

wean: removal of calf from cow so it can no longer nurse.

white muscle disease: disease of young calves caused by selenium and vitamin E deficiency; usually result of selenium-deficient diet fed to cow or heifer during or before gestation.

whole milk: milk as it is secreted from udder of cow, without anything removed.

yearling: animal that is approximately 1 year old.

20 Swine Industry

CHAPTER OVERVIEW

Pigs are useful in many ways. Pigskin can be tanned to produce soft, durable leather for clothing and equipment. Pigs are especially helpful as biomedical research tools because their physiology is comparable to that of humans. Vietnamese potbelly pigs enjoy life as pets. However, this chapter focuses on swine as a food source, which is the most common use. To accommodate the demands of the market, swine production has become more efficient and economical. In addition, an intermediate body type was developed to meet the demand for a leaner meat product, replacing the earlier trend of short, fat pigs for lard and the long, rangy type for pork.

HISTORY

Animal agriculture has evolved from a family enterprise to a big business. Modern swine production has also been revolutionized. Traditionally, pig production was secondary income to the farmer who raised another major crop, usually grains. The Midwest family raised litters from several sows in low-cost, low-density style. Today, pig production is intensified and specialized. In the last 20 years, massive *farrow-to-finish* operations with 100 to 1000 sows, marketing 18 pigs per sow annually, are common means of production. Improved labor efficiency is the driving force in the current swine industry. Traditional farm help has been replaced by automatic systems. Mechanical devices feed, water, ventilate, regulate environmental parameters, and provide manure disposal. This sophisticated equipment increases the necessary capital investment, which must be offset by expanding the individual operation.

A growing concern for animal welfare is gaining support. Intensively reared pigs are exposed to more stress than extensively raised animals. There is a direct relationship between herd size and disease, injury, piglet morbidity, and mortality. Production methods that consider the physical and mental well-being of swine may be on the horizon.

BREEDS

The genus and species name for the pig is *Sus scrofa.* The common breeds are listed in Table 20-1.

The Landrace and Yorkshire breeds are prolific, are good mothers, and produce abundant milk. The female animals of these breeds are commonly used for maternal lines. The Duroc, Hampshire, and spotted breeds yield a lean carcass with efficient feed conversion and so are often used as sires. By *crossbreeding* or mating a female of one breed with a male of another breed, pig producers capitalize on the parental traits of both breeds and gain hybrid vigor in the offspring.

Table 20-1 COMMON SWINE BREEDS

Breed	Place of origin	Color	Physical features	Qualities
Yorkshire	England	White	Erect ears; dished face	Excellent reproduction; efficient feed conversion
Landrace	Denmark	White	Long, drooping ears; long body	Excellent reproduction
Duroc	New York and New Jersey	Red	Drooping ears	Efficient feed conversion; fast rate of gain
Hampshire	Kentucky	Black with white belt	Erect ears	Efficient feed conversion; low back fat
Spotted	Indiana	White with black spots	Drooping ears	Fast rate of gain
Poland China	Ohio	Black with white spots	Drooping ears	Fast rate of gain

BEHAVIOR

Swine have many positive characteristics that can be used to make their management easier. Pigs are intelligent and are easily trained with some patience to use *farrowing* crates and automatic feed and water systems and to move to designated areas.

Swine are clean animals and have an innate *dunging pattern,* soiling in one area of their pen. They prefer to urinate and defecate in damp areas, usually near the water source. Therefore food should be offered at the opposite end of the pen to promote a clean environment.

Swine can see, hear, and smell very well. Swine are social and need visual and preferably physical contact with others. Their sociability lends to positive contact with human caretakers.

Swine are industrious and curious creatures. They spend hours rooting about with their snouts to explore their surroundings and search for snacks. Unfortunately, rooting destroys pasture and increases intestinal parasitism. *Ringing* is a procedure that discourages rooting behavior. Wire rings are inserted between the pig's nostrils or at the rim of the nose. One ring suffices for young pigs. Sows may need two or three rings spaced about ½ inch apart. Boars may not have rings if they interfere with the male's nuzzling behavior during mating. Hogs raised indoors do not need rings.

Swine are strong and have a low center of gravity. They are adept at rooting under a fence and using their power to escape. Fencing must be *hog-tight,* or sturdy enough to hold hogs.

REVIEW A

1. The genus and species name for the pig is ______________________ .
2. The mating of a female of one breed with a male of a different breed is called ____________ .
3. The Poland China breed of swine originated in ______________________ .
4. Swine prefer to urinate and defecate on one part of their pen, leaving the remainder free of their wastes. This behavior is called ______________________ .
5. Ringing swine is done to prevent them from ______________________ .
6. Fencing that is good enough to prevent swine from escaping is called ________________ .

PHYSIOLOGY

Swine are omnivores with a monogastric stomach. Pigs must consume a balanced diet.

Hogs have four toes on each foot. Only two toes of the four are functional and bear weight. The two toes that do not have ground contact are called *dewclaws.*

Pigs are *homeotherms,* with a body temperature of 102° ±1° F or 38.9° C. Pig hair is coarse, sparse, and bristly and does not provide the protection from the elements that occurs in most other mammals. Swine are well insulated with a layer of body fat. Piglets are an exception. They do not have ample body fat and need an external heat source. Pigs will shiver and pile up in a corner when they are cold. Swine have few sweat glands, so protection from the sun and extreme heat is essential. The following devices can be used to provide a cooler environment for swine:

Shades—trees are a natural source for shade if swine rooting behavior does not destroy the trees: artificially created shade, constructed of four poles with a reflective roof, either portable or stationary, can also be used.

Wallows—pigs construct natural wallows in the form of mud holes; manufactured wallows are shallow, water-tight wading pools made of concrete, metal, or treated lumber; wallows should be equipped with a drain plug and a ramp for easy access.

Spray cooling—simple hosing with water or more sophisticated systems of releasing a mist regularly promotes the comfort of swine.

Air cooling—swine that are housed in confinement can be cooled by common air conditioning, ventilation fans, *evaporative coolers* (pads moistened with cold water; fanned air is then pulled from the outside and directed through the pad, which produces a cooling effect), and *zone cooling* (high-velocity air around the head of the animal as it stands in a crate or small pen, promoting heat loss and thereby cooling the body).

BREEDING

Mature and immature male hogs are called *boars.* A castrated male is a *barrow.* Mature females are known as *sows,* whereas immature females are *gilts.* Newborns of either sex are called *pigs.*

Swine are polyestrous, with heat cycles occurring every 21 days throughout the year. Estrus lasts for 2 to 3 days. The sow ovulates 8 to 12 hours before the end of standing heat. Sixteen to 18 eggs are ovulated, and 10 to 12 piglets are born. Sows have a postpartum estrus but do not ovulate at this time. The sow resumes estrus 4 to 10 days after weaning her litter.

Puberty is attained at 5 to 8 months of age or at 150 to 200 pounds. Moving gilts to fenceline contact with boars stimulates onset of estrus. Gilts usually are not bred on their first heat because ovulation rates increase in the second and third heats. The reproductive life for sows includes mating, gestation, farrowing, lactating, weaning, and interval to remating.

Mating or breeding is performed by pen mating, hand mating, or artificial insemination. In *pen mating,* the boar is housed with a group of females at all times and breeds them as they come into heat. For *hand mating,* boars and sows are housed separately. The sow in heat is taken to the boar, which is allowed to service the sow under controlled conditions. The exact breeding date and expected delivery date can be recorded. *Artificial insemination* requires special equipment and training. A semen sample is collected from the boar, processed, and inseminated into selected sows.

Once mated, the sow's gestation period ranges from 112 to 116 days, with an average of 114 days (easily remembered as 3 months, 3 weeks, and 3 days). The act of birthing is called *farrowing.* Sows are taken to a farrowing crate or pen to limit mobility. This helps prevent the sow from lying on or injuring her newborns.

Farrowing crates usually are 5 feet by 7 feet (Fig. 20-1). Freshly washed sows enter the disinfected crate 3 to 4 days before parturition to adjust to the crate. The sow is confined to the center 2-foot by 7-foot area, with access to food and water. The sow can lie down or move a couple of steps but cannot turn around. Newborn pigs can sleep and feed in the adjacent *creep* area without being crushed by the sow. *Farrowing pens* are larger, with guardrails along the wall and floor junctures. This area provides escape for the pigs.

A sow will build a nest if given material and opportunity. Otherwise she will paw at the ground attempting to nest build. The

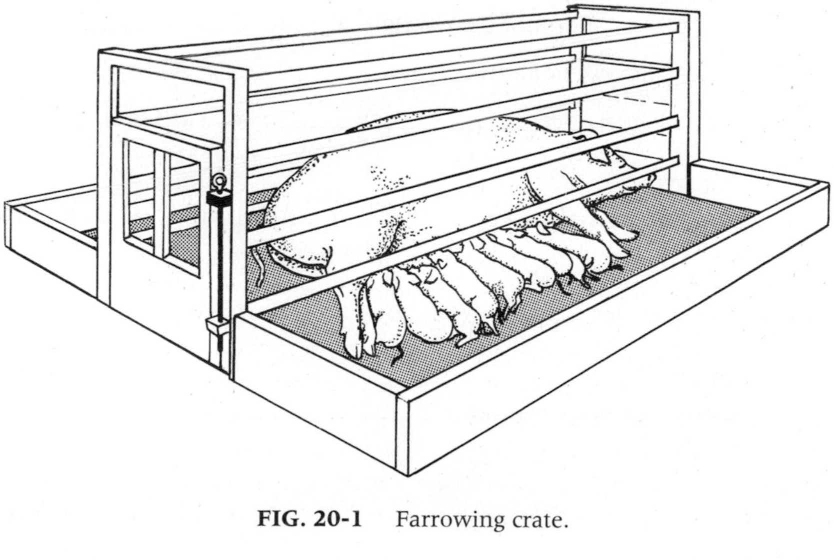

FIG. 20-1 Farrowing crate.

sow prefers ambient temperatures of 15° C, whereas newborns need 21° to 27° C. Therefore space heaters or heat lamps are provided in the creep for pig comfort. Many pig losses occur in the first 72 hours after birth, so attention to farrowing management is important.

Technological advances have produced sophisticated equipment such as the *blow away unit* to reduce pig mortality. The blow away unit houses the sow in a farrowing crate. When she stands, the sow interrupts an infrared beam, which triggers a blower to force cold air under the sow. The piglets find this uncomfortable and move to the creep for warmth. Meanwhile the sow can eat and drink without injuring her pigs. When the sow lies down she does not interfere with the light beam, enabling the pigs to nurse comfortably and safely.

Pigs weigh about 3 pounds each at birth. They are born head or feet first at 20-minute intervals. Farrowing should be complete in about 4 hours, after which the afterbirth is expelled. Newborns cough, start breathing, and are up on their feet immediately. Their eyes are open, but they use their nose to locate a teat for their first meal of *colostrum.* The sow remains still and does not lick newborns but grunts softly to communicate to her litter. By 3 days of age, each piglet has selected a teat, which it nurses exclusively until weaning. After the sow has nursed the litter, she should be encouraged to rise, eat, and drink. Sows are excellent mothers with protective instincts.

Weaning occurs between 3 and 8 weeks of age or at 10 to 12 pounds. Pigs go to market at 5 to 6 months of age when they weigh 200 pounds.

Reproductive failures represent potentially significant losses for pig producers. Only proven breeding sows—those who conceive readily, wean 18 pigs annually, and exhibit a short *interval to remating* period—should remain in the herd. Sows and boars remain productive for 5 to 6 years. Unproductive hogs are culled.

REVIEW B

1. Swine are omnivores with a ______________________ stomach.
2. The two toes on each foot that do not bear weight are called ______________________ .
3. The purpose of a hog wallow is to allow ______________________ .
4. A male hog is called a(n) ______________________ ; if castrated, he is called a(n) ______________________ .
5. The name for an immature female pig is ______________________ ; when mature she is called a(n) ______________________ .
6. Because their estrous cycles occur throughout the year, swine are described as being ______________________ .
7. The act of birthing in swine is called ______________________ .

HOUSING

Commercial swine are sold for two main purposes: slaughter or breeding. Hog producers raise pigs as farrow to finish, farrow to wean, feeder to finish, breeder, or SPF operations.

Farrow-to-finish operations are full-spectrum units. They often use crossbred pigs and market stock at 200 pounds of body weight.

Farrow-to-wean settings serve as nurseries. Pigs are sold as weanlings at 6 to 8 weeks of age to commercial feeder farms.

Feeder-to-finish farms obtain weanlings at 30 to 50 pounds and grow them to market weight of 200 pounds. When feeders reach 100 pounds, the temperature of their environment is lowered from 21° C to 15.5° C to maximize their growth rate. Feeder herds are often *open herds.* They permit animals from several other swine farms to enter their premises and mingle.

Breeders raise purebred gilts and boars to sell to other purebred breeders or commercial farrowing farms. Performance testing programs that measure or estimate carcass yields are done routinely. Breeders can thus provide genetically superior stock.

Specific pathogen free (SPF) herds are designed to eradicate certain diseases. SPF animals originate from cesarean section or hysterectomy of a pregnant sow. The litter is raised in laboratory isolation until weaning. The SPF weanlings serve as breeding stock in closed herds. A *closed herd* is one that forbids outside pigs to enter the herd. New genes are brought into the herd by artificial insemination. Caretakers pay strict adherence to sanitation regulations. SPF herds are costly and generally do not remain SPF for more than a few years.

Management systems are *extensive* (outdoors) or *intensive* (indoors). In extensive management, swine are pastured in groups and are usually pen mated. Sheds or huts are provided for shelter. Benefits of pasturing hogs include less need for specialized equipment, smaller equipment, reduced building investment, and flexible expansion or reduction ability. Intensive or confinement housing enables rearing of large numbers in a small area. The potential problems include high economic investment, manure handling and disposal, and serious concentration of disease outbreaks. Advantages are disease control from wild animals, operator comfort and convenience, closer supervision of stock, potential for automation, and high-volume production.

The flooring used in confinement housing has received much attention. Concrete floors are used because they are durable and easy to sanitize. Other flooring materials include plastic, expanded metal, steel, aluminum, and wood. The floor in the nursery ought to be smooth, to limit knee abrasions of neonates, but not slippery. Slotted or partially slotted floors are popular because there is no need for daily cleaning or bedding. Manure drops through the grids into a pit beneath slatted flooring. The floor and pit are flushed regularly. The waste is then moved to a holding lagoon until it can be spread on fields. With minimal labor, the pens and pigs stay clean.

Whatever the purpose, type of operation, or management system, housing swine is motivated by providing conditions that yield rapid growth. No single production system works best. All have merits and pitfalls. Parameters to consider are suitable environment for animals, minimal routine labor requirements, and convenience for caretakers.

FEEDING

Feed expenses constitute 60% to 80% of the total bill to market swine. Feeding must be done with economic efficiency, which means maximizing feed intake while minimizing feed costs.

Clean, fresh water is an essential nutrient that should be provided *ad libitum (ad lib).* Automatic watering systems often are used.

Energy is provided in most swine rations as carbohydrates and fats. Common sources of energy are corn, wheat, oats, barley, tallow, and vegetable oil. Protein is needed to build muscle. Protein is added to swine diets in the form of soybean meal, cottonseed meal, and fishmeal. Minerals are provided in two ways. Minerals that are needed in large amounts are *macrominerals.* Calcium, phosphorus, sodium, and chlorine are macrominerals. *Microminerals* are iron, zinc, manganese, copper, iodine, and selenium; they are mixed in smaller quantities. Vitamins A, D, E, K, riboflavin, niacin, pantothenic acid, choline, and B_{12} are also added. Commercially prepared diets are complete feeds that reflect the nutritional demands for the stage of production. Feed is also mixed on the farm. This involves producing, grinding, measuring, mixing, and storing food ingredients. Regular analysis is needed to ascertain correct nutrient levels in farm-mixed feed.

The five phases of production are gestation, lactation, starter, grower, and finisher. Dietary changes are noteworthy. During gestation it is important to restrict the sow's diet, or she can become overweight. Gestation diets are low in protein, about 12%. Lactation diets are higher in protein (14%) and minerals to meet the increasing energy needs of the sow. Starter diets are the most complex and fortified. Milk products and antibiotics are added to increase growth rate. The protein in starter diets ranges from 18% to 20%. Protein levels in grower and finisher diets are 16% and 14%, respectively.

Swine are fed using methods designed to meet differing management styles. To keep food clean, pigs that are fed *ad lib* are offered food in a hopper. When the pig is ready to eat, it flips up a cover to access the food. Food is mixed with water and placed in a trough to eliminate dust and reduce waste. This is known as *liquid feeding. Interval feeding* reduces labor because pigs are fed for several hours every other day.

REVIEW C

1. Commercial swine are sold for two main purposes: ________________ and ________________ .
2. SPF stands for ____________________ . Only SPF animals are used to stock ____________________ herds, which forbid entry to other swine.
3. ____________________ is an abbreviation for *ad libitum,* which means ____________________ .
4. Needed in large amounts, calcium, phosphorus, sodium, chlorine, and potassium are called ________________________ ; iron, zinc, manganese, and others needed in smaller quantities are the ________________________ .
5. The five phases of swine production are gestation, ________________ , ________________ , ________________ , and ________________ .

RESTRAINT

Restraint methods should always be used in a safe and effective manner for the animal and handler.

Hog hurdles are portable partitions used to maneuver swine, usually into a corner (Fig. 20-2). They are constructed from plywood about 2 feet long by 3 feet wide, with a handle cut out in the middle along the top of the board. Hogs will move away from the hurdle, which is held between the handler and the animal. Before other restraint methods are used, pigs are confined to a small pen by the use of a hurdle.

A *hog snare* is a device that secures the pig's head (Fig. 20-3). It is used on large or older swine. A loop made from rope, cable, or wire is attached to a long handle. The loop material is passed through the handle and out the opposite end. To apply the snare, place the loop into the pig's mouth around the upper snout. With a quick push-pull action, tighten the loop around the pig's snout. Pigs can inflict severe bites, so control of the head is paramount. Snares can be handheld or tied to a sturdy post.

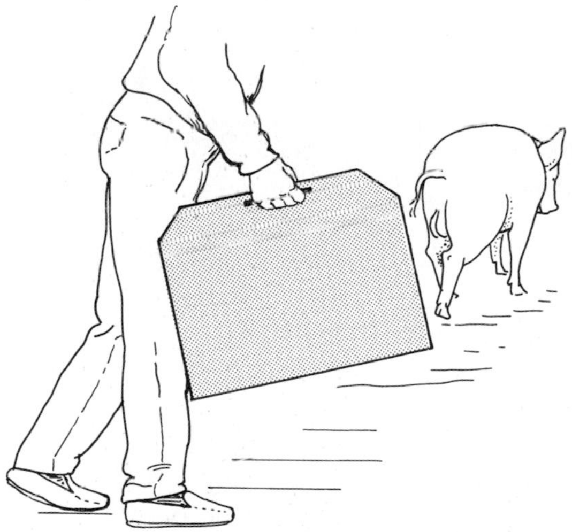

FIG. 20-2 Hog hurdle.

Casting means laying an animal down on its side for restraint purposes. A bowline knot is tied first about the neck in front of the shoulders. A half hitch is tied around the heartgirth, behind the front legs. A second half hitch is tied in front of the rear legs. The half hitches are tied on the same side of the animal and off center along the topline. The handler stands behind the hog and pulls steadily on the rope. The pressure exerted by the half hitches causes the animal to buckle and lie down on the side opposite the half hitches. For greater control, a hog snare is used simultaneously.

A *headgate* is a mechanical instrument at the end of a chute that locks the pig's head on both sides of the neck between the jaws and shoulders. One handler drives the pig into the chute. Another handler closes the headgate quickly when the pig's head is into position.

A *sling* is a swine restraint device commonly used in research (Fig. 20-4). The sling is a canvas hammock with four leg holes. A fifth hole is present to facilitate blood collection from the vena cava. The pig is driven to the sling, positioned over the leg holes, and hoisted up off the ground. The pig is comfortable and well supported.

Young or small pigs, weighing less than 75 pounds, can be handheld. A pig can be held upright, upside down, or on its side. The handler grasps a hind leg first to catch the pig and then holds either hind legs or forelegs. The pig faces away from the handler. The restrainer supports the pig's backbone by squeezing it with her or his legs. If the pig is laid down on the ground, the handler gently rests her or his knee on the pig's side for extra control. When releasing a pig from restraint, observe it for proper recovery.

Pigs are easily moved from one place to another through use of a narrow alley or along a fence line. Hurdles and canes or

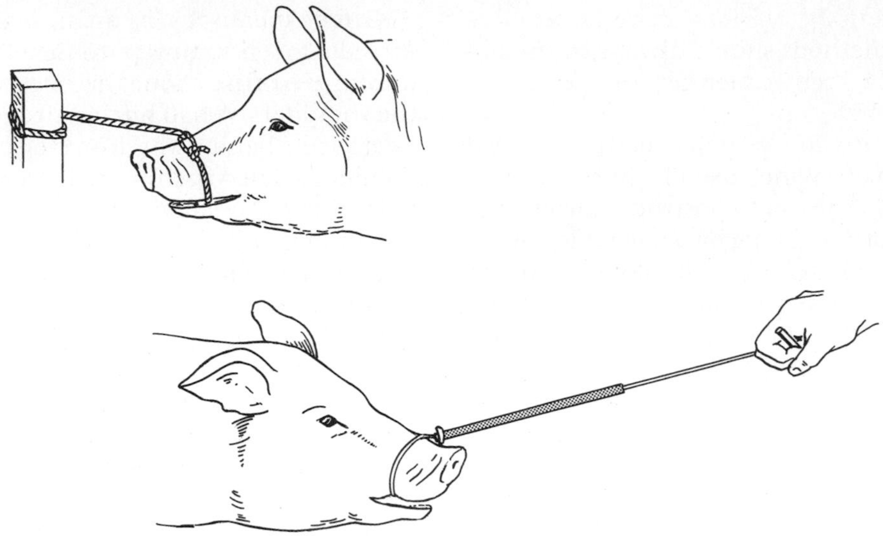

FIG. 20-3 Hog snares.

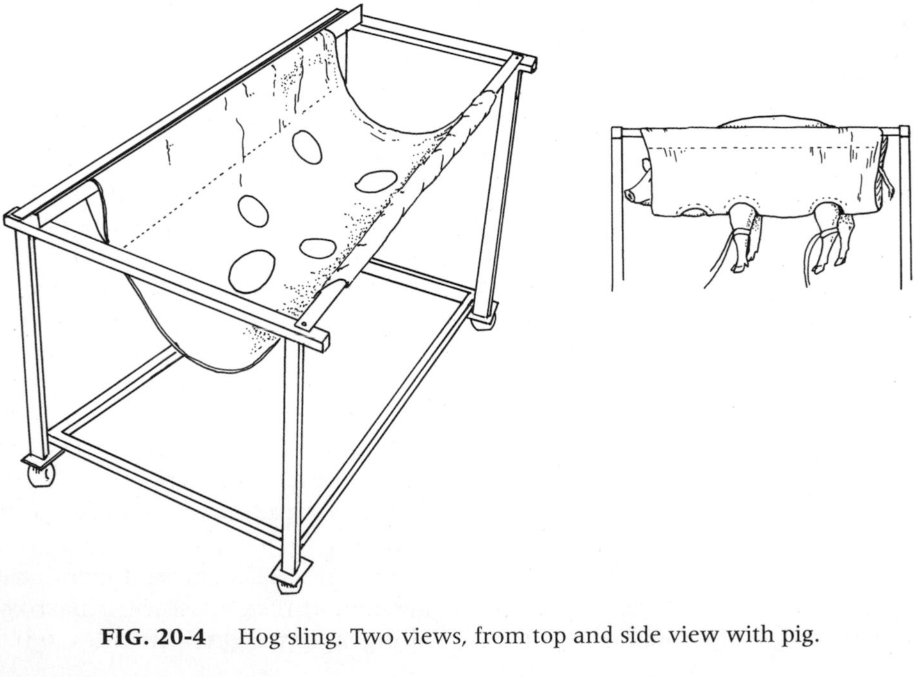

FIG. 20-4 Hog sling. Two views, from top and side view with pig.

whips encourage swine to move along. Handlers should refrain from exciting or hurrying hogs. A little patience goes a long way when working with swine.

HERD HEALTH

In modern pig production, swine often receive medical care as a whole herd rather than as individuals. Preventive medicine is a critical factor in maintaining a productive and economic herd.

Newborn pigs are processed within 12 to 24 hours after birth. This involves caring for navel cords, clipping needle teeth, docking tails, administering iron, identifying each, and castrating males. While performing these tasks, it is best to remove the pigs from the sows. The pigs will squeal, which will in turn upset the sows, who may attack.

Soon after pigs are born, the umbilical cord may be tied off with a square knot or cut off about one inch from the body. The cord is then dipped, swabbed, or sprayed with tincture of iodine. Iodine disinfects the navel opening and helps dry the cord.

Pigs are born with eight teeth called *needle teeth.* The teeth are one incisor and one canine tooth on all four sides of the jaws. Needle teeth are the pig's only means of defense. Pigs can inflict severe bites on each other and on the dam when fighting for a nursing spot. Needle teeth are cut off within 1 to 2 days after birth. Using a disinfected pig teeth nipper, each tooth is clipped off at the gumline. Teeth are still soft soon after birth and do not splinter as readily as 2-day-old teeth.

Cannibalism of penmates' tails is a common problem for confined swine. To control tail biting, the tail is docked within 24 hours after birth. There are several reasons to dock tails at this time: There is less tail hemorrhage and less interest by siblings to investigate healing tails. The pig is easy to restrain. The farrowing pen is clean, and the pigs have received antibody protection from the sow's colostrum. Disinfected pig teeth nippers can be used to cut tails one-half inch from the body. A blunt cutting instrument results in less bleeding than a very sharp tool. Hogs that are pasture raised do not routinely need tail docking.

Iron-deficiency anemia of piglets can be a serious problem in intensively raised swine for several reasons. Sow colostrum and milk are low in iron, and nursing pigs cannot store iron efficiently. The pigs are growing rapidly and have no contact with iron in the soil. The problem is prevented by an intramuscular injection of iron dextran shortly after birth.

Identification methods for swine include ear notching, ear tagging, tattooing, and branding. Ear notching often is used on baby pigs. Ear notching systems match a V-notch in the ear with a number value. Purebred swine associations require a litter number to be placed in the pig's right ear and the individual number notched in the left ear. A disinfected ear notcher is used to make ear cuts. Care is taken to notch firmly and distinctly. Blood stop powder can be applied to the ear if slight bleeding occurs.

Ear tags are plastic or metal tags with a number imprinted on both sides. Ear tags have the advantage of being easily read from a distance. Often breeding animals are notched at birth and later tagged to facilitate quick identification. The pig is restrained using a chute, head gate, or hog snare. The tag is inserted into the ear tag applicator. The ear is disinfected and the tag punched through the ear. Pigs may lose tags and need retagging.

There are two methods of tattooing swine. Ears are tattooed using a pliers-type device that holds numbers and letters, which are imprinted into the skin. Indelible ink is smeared into the tattoo puncture sites to facilitate reading the tattoo. The ear tattoo is a positive identification marker that lasts for life but still requires physical restraint of the pig to read. Ear notches or tags can be used simultaneously for improved visibility. Hog carcasses are tattooed in the shoulder or ham. Numbers or letters are inserted into the *tattoo marker,* a flat mallet that is swung to impregnate the tattoo into the skin. The tattoo is brushed with tattoo paste or ink for permanent marking.

Paint branding is a temporary method of identification. Quick-drying enamel paint is poured into a pan. The brand is pressed into the paint and then applied to the back of the hog, rotating back and forth to improve visibility. Aerosolized spray paints can also be used. Do not overcrowd animals during branding or brands are apt to smear before they have dried.

Only superior males should remain intact for breeding purposes. Males are castrated if they are to be slaughtered because cooking the meat from boars produces an offensive odor. Pigs can be castrated between 1 and 21 days of age. There is less bleeding with younger animals. The pig is held by the hind legs. Another person uses a castration knife, scalpel, or razor blade to make two incisions directly over the testicles. Each testicle is pulled out through its incision, twisted, and cut with a scraping motion. Antiseptic powder or spray may be applied to the incision sites.

Breeding boars grow elongated canine teeth called *tusks.* Tusk development is a result of testosterone stimulation. Tusks may grow to be 5 inches long, with a diameter of ½ inch. To avoid injury to others, tusks are cut with a hacksaw every 4 to 6 months.

From birth to weaning, the piglet is dependent on its dam's colostrum and milk for passive intestinal immunity. At weaning, pigs are vaccinated to stimulate their own antibody production.

Intensive housing has eliminated soil-borne infectious diseases of swine. Pneumonia and enteritis are still troublesome. Growth promotants and antimicrobial agents are fed to herds at therapeutic and prophylactic levels to control gastroenteritis and pneumonia. Antibiotics are withdrawn from feed when swine reach 120 pounds. Caretakers should pay attention to drug withdrawal times. When the herd is faced with epidemics, vaccination against the causative agent is indicated.

Insecticides and anthelmintics are used when necessary. Routine treatment of adult animals minimizes parasitic outbreaks. Weanlings often are treated for external and internal parasites when they are vaccinated. Farrowing swine on slatted floors also reduces the internal parasite load.

During the growing through finishing stages, the caretaker should observe animals daily and treat signs of disease quickly and deliberately. Reduction in disease outbreaks is a result of good management practices. High-quality ventilation, low population density, minimal stress factors, genetic selection for natural disease resistance, adequate vaccination programs, regular sanitation of crates and pens, batch farrowing, and closed-herd status are some techniques to improve herd health.

REVIEW D

1. What is a hog hurdle? ____

2. A swine restraint device consisting of a handle with a cable loop that passes over the animal's snout is called a ______________________ .

3. The use of ropes to lay an animal down on its side for restraint purposes is called ______________________ .

4. The swine restraint device consisting of a canvas hammock with four leg holes is a(n) ______________________ .

5. The needle teeth in newborn pigs are ______________________ in number and consist of two types of teeth, ______________________ and ______________________ .

6. Intramuscular injections of iron dextran are given to newborn piglets to prevent ______________________ .

7. The elongated canine teeth of mature boars are called ______________________ .

Chapter 20 Answers

Review A

1. *Sus scrofa*
2. crossbreeding
3. Ohio
4. dunging pattern
5. rooting
6. hog-tight

Review B

1. monogastric (simple)
2. dewclaws
3. cooling
4. boar, barrow
5. gilt, sow
6. polyestrous
7. farrowing

Review C

1. slaughter, breeding
2. specific pathogen free, closed
3. *ad lib,* free choice
4. macrominerals, microminerals
5. lactation, starter, grower, finisher

Review D

1. a portable partition used to maneuver swine
2. hog snare
3. casting
4. sling
5. eight, incisors and canines
6. iron deficiency anemia
7. tusks

Chapter 20 EXERCISES

SWINE INDUSTRY

Exercise 1: Match the terms in the right column with the definitions in the left column by placing the appropriate letter in the space provided.

_____ 1. A castrated male hog

_____ 2. The innate tendency to eliminate waste products in a certain area

_____ 3. Temporary teeth of pigs that are clipped soon after birth

_____ 4. Management system that pastures stock

_____ 5. Processed pig fat that is soft and white

_____ 6. Identification system that relies on cutting slits in the ears of swine

_____ 7. The swine production unit that serves as the nursery

_____ 8. A breeding system that mates animals of different breeds

_____ 9. The overgrown canine teeth of the boars

_____ 10. Hosing down a hog

A. Lard
B. Extensive management
C. Farrow to wean
D. Spray cooling
E. Tusks
F. Needle teeth
G. Barrow
H. Ear notching
I. Dunging pattern
J. Crossbreeding

Exercise 2: Complete the following statements.

1. The most common use for swine today is for ____________________ .
2. Because swine are social animals, it is important that they have visual and ____________________ contact with others.
3. Swine are polyestrous, with heat cycles every ________ days throughout the year.
4. Of the three mating systems, the one that provides the least accurate date of conception is ____________________ .
5. To pig producers, good farrowing management practices are important because ____________________ .
6. The feeding system that reduces dust and waste is ____________________ .
7. Commercial swine are sold for two reasons: ____________________ and ____________________ .
8. The restraint method using ropes that are strategically tied is known as ____________________ .

9. Processing newborn pigs involves ______________________________,
______________________________,
______________________________,
______________________________,
______________________________, and
______________________________.

10. Two infectious diseases that can cause significant losses for pig producers are
______________ and ______________.

CHAPTER 20 PUZZLE

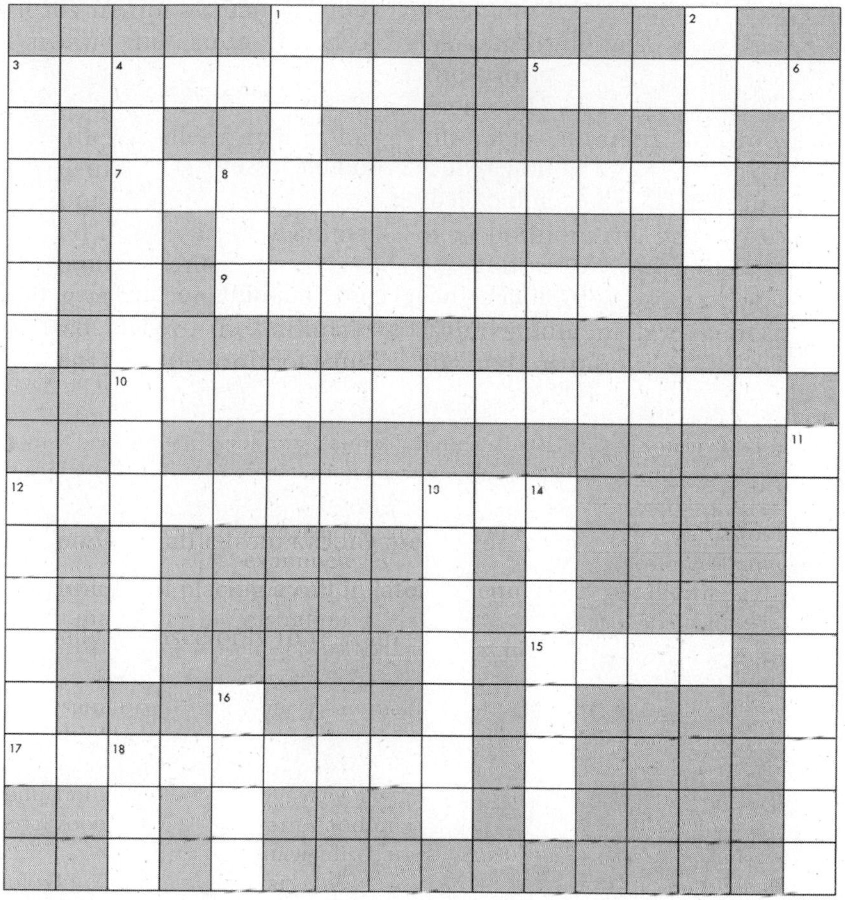
1
2
3
4
5
6
7
8
9
10
11
12
13
14
15
16
17
18

ACROSS CLUES

3. Method of identification
5. Act of giving birth
7. Male hormone
9. Young animal not relying on milk nourishment
10. Minerals added to feed in small amounts
12. Simple stomach
15. Canine tooth
17. Pregnancy

DOWN CLUES

1. Immature female pig
2. Area that offers feed and escape for smaller animals
3. Castrated male hog
4. Agent that destroys or expels worms
6. Mudhole or wading pool
8. Female hog
11. First milk
12. Breeding
13. Discourages rooting behavior
14. Method of restraint
16. Rendered pig fat
18. Specific pathogen free

Chapter 20 Answers

Exercise 1

1. G
2. I
3. F
4. B
5. A
6. H
7. C
8. J
9. E
10. D

Exercise 2

1. food
2. physical
3. 21
4. pen mating
5. they reduce economic losses
6. liquid feeding
7. breeding, slaughtering
8. casting
9. dipping navel cords, clipping needle teeth, docking tails, administering iron, identifying piglets, castrating males
10. gastroenteritis, pneumonia

ANSWERS: CHAPTER 20 PUZZLE

					[1] G								[2] C		
[3] B	R	[4] A	N	D	I	N	G			[5] F	A	R	R	O	[6] W
A		N			L								E		A
R		[7] T	E	[8] S	T	O	S	T	E	R	O	N	E		L
R		H		O									P		L
O		E		[9] W	E	A	N	L	I	N	G				O
W		L													W
		[10] M	I	C	R	O	M	I	N	E	R	A	L	S	
		I													[11] C
[12] M	O	N	O	G	A	S	T	[13] R	I	[14] C					O
A		T						I		A					L
T		I						N		S					O
I		C						G		[15] T	U	S	K		S
N				[16] L				I		I					T
[17] G	E	[18] S	T	A	T	I	O	N		N					R
		P		R				G		G					U
		F		D											M

GLOSSARY

artificial insemination: breeding method in which processed fresh or frozen semen is deposited into female reproductive tract.

barrow: castrated male hog.

boar: male hog.

blow away unit: mechanical device that promotes safety for nursing pigs; when sow stands up, she interrupts infrared beam, which forces cold air to blow beneath her and cold air is uncomfortable to nursing young; when sow lies down, there is no interruption to light beam, enabling pigs to nurse safely.

carcass: dressed body, without organs, of meat animal.

casting: method of restraining livestock that uses ropes to place animal on its side.

closed herd: herd that prevents new animals from entering.

colostrum: thick first milk produced by pregnant dam; rich in antibodies, thus conferring passive immunity to neonates.

creep: area that limits access to certain animals.

creep feed: system of feeding that enables smaller-sized animals to consume extra foodstuff that larger animals cannot access.

crossbreeding: breeding system that mates animals of same species but different breeds.

dunging pattern: tendency for animals to deposit wastes in particular location.

ear notching: making slits in pigs' ears for identification purposes.

evaporative cooling: system of cooling that draws fanned air in through cold water–moistened pads.

extensive management: management system that houses animals outdoors in free-range style.

farrowing: birthing process of pigs.

farrowing crate: small crate that limits mobility of sow during delivery of her young.

farrowing pen: small pen used for sow parturition and designed with guardrails to protect newborns.

farrow-to-finish: a full-service swine operation that houses breeders, newborns, weanlings, and feeder stock.

farrow-to-wean: swine production unit that houses breeding sows and offspring until weaning age or weight.

feeder-to-finish: swine farm that raises weanling pigs to market weight.

gilt: immature female hog.

hand mating: breeding method in which sow is brought to boar for controlled service.

hog-tight: sturdy fencing that prevents animals from escaping.

intensive management: management system that houses large numbers of animals under confinement conditions.

lard: soft, white fat that results from rendering fatty tissue of pigs.

needle teeth: eight temporary incisor and canine teeth of piglets (also called *wolf teeth*).

open herd: herd that permits animals from other herds to join existing herd.

pen mating: breeding system in which male is housed with females and breeds them as they come into heat.

ringing: procedure that implants wire ring through pig's nose to discourage rooting behavior.

shade: natural or artificially constructed shelter from sun and heat.

sling: a swine restraint device resembling a hammock, with four leg holes and a fifth hole under the neck for blood collection from the vena cava.

sow: female hog.

specific pathogen free (SPF): management system that is costly but used to eradicate certain diseases; animals originate from cesarean section or hysterectomy and are raised in isolation; great attention to sanitation and contamination prevention are primary concerns.

spray cooling: cooling system in which swine are manually or automatically misted.

tusk: overgrown canine tooth of boars.

wallow: natural or artificially constructed wading pool to cool swine.

zone cooling: cooling system that uses high-velocity air directed towards hog's head to create heat loss and cool animal.

21 Small Ruminants

CHAPTER OVERVIEW

This chapter introduces various aspects of the small ruminants: sheep, goats, and llamas. *Ruminants* are animals having a multichambered stomach. Sheep and goats have four chambers, and llamas have three. They also have other common characteristics including split hooves, a *lingual torus* (ridge on tongue), a maxillary dental pad rather than upper incisors, and horizontally positioned oval pupils in the eyes. This chapter reviews small ruminant management and health care practices, which vary based on the function of the animal. The topics discussed include purposes, breeds, breeding, neonatal care, housing, feeding, restraint, routine health care, and common diseases.

PURPOSES AND BREEDS

Sheep are compact animals possessing scent glands in the face and hind feet. They are used for meat, wool, milk, and hide and as research models for a variety of diseases and conditions. Sheep often are shown in competitions to determine the best representative of their breed and type. There are about 300 domesticated breeds. Originally, sheep *flocks* were raised for meat or wool production (Fig. 21-1). Today's genetics emphasize the dual and even triple-purpose nature of sheep, producing wool, meat, and milk. Sheep's wool is called *fleece* and is shorn once a year in the spring. It is sorted, washed, dyed, and spun into yarn for the textile industry. *Lanolin,* natural oil secreted by sebaceous glands, is recovered during the washing process, purified, and sold in the cosmetics industry. Studies are being done to improve the method for harvesting wool. Scientists inject sheep with an animal protein called *epidermal growth factor (EGF)*. After about 6 weeks, EGF causes the fleece to fall off the animal in a single sheet. The average fleece weighs about 8 pounds. Meat from young sheep is known as *lamb.* Stronger-tasting and stringier meat from older sheep is *mutton.* Common dual-purpose breeds of sheep include Suffolk and Cheviot for meat and medium wool. Merino and Rambouillet are examples of fine wool breeds.

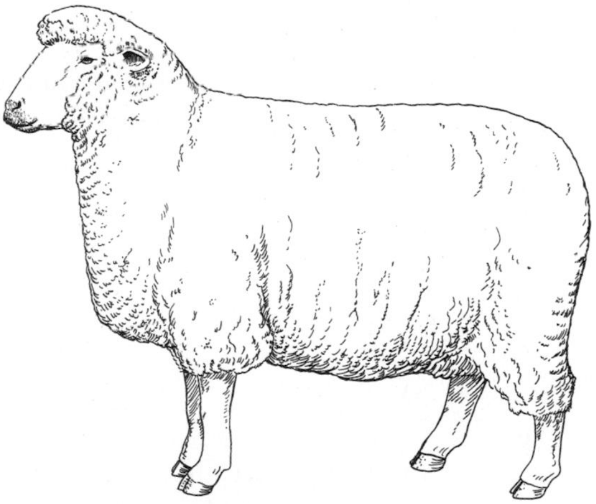

FIG. 21-1 A wool-type sheep.

Goats are used for dairy, meat, hide, and fiber, as research models, and as companions for other animals, for brush and weed control, as pack animals, and as pets (Fig. 21-2). Goats are regularly exhibited for conformation and milk production assessment. Common dairy goat breeds are French Alpine, Saanen, Toggenburg, Oberhasli, Nubian, and LaMancha. The first four breeds listed have erect ears. Nubians have pendulous ears and a Roman nose. The LaMancha breed has very short elf or gopher ears. The South African Boer goat is a popular meat breed. Goat meat is called *chevon*. Angora goats produce mohair, being shorn two or three times each year. Cashmere goats are raised for their cashmere fleeces and are shorn once annually in the spring. The pygmy and Nigerian dwarf are pet breeds selected for their diminutive stature.

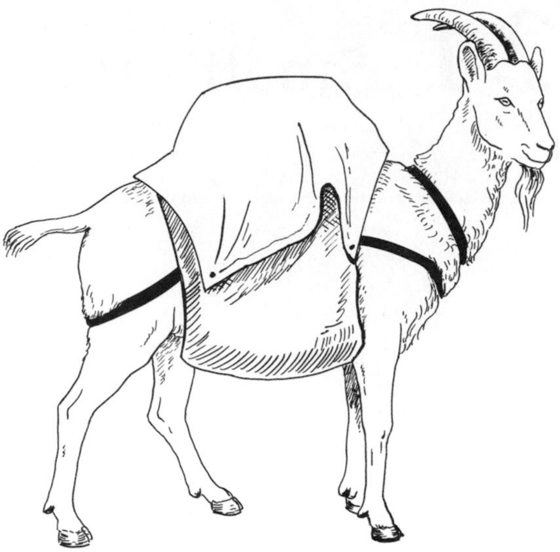

FIG. 21-2 French Alpine goat ready for packing.

Llamas are increasing in popularity in the United States. They are used as companions, or pack animals, for fiber and meat, and as protectors of other livestock, including sheep and goats. Llamas normally are not sheared. Their hair coat takes approximately 2 years to grow back after shearing. The llama pen is easily cleaned because llamas use a *communal dung pile* for waste excretion.

REVIEW A

1. Ruminants such as sheep and goats have _________ stomach chambers. Llamas and other camelids have _________ chambers.
2. The pattern that llamas use for excretion of their wastes is called a _____________________ .
3. A group of sheep is called a _____________________ .
4. Toggenburg dairy goats have _____________________ ears.
5. _____________________ is a natural oil secreted by sebaceous glands in sheep.
6. Goat meat is called _____________________ .

BREEDING

Sheep and goats are seasonally polyestrous breeders because their estrous cycles do not usually continue throughout the year. However, in tropical climates estrus may be observed year round. Cooler nights and shorter periods of daylight initiate the breeding season. Regular estrous or heat cycles occur on average every 18 to 21 days during breeding season, from late summer through late winter. Estrus lasts for 1 to 3 days, with *spontaneous ovulation* occurring about 12 hours after standing heat. *Standing heat* occurs when the female accepts the male's mounting behavior. Ewes are bred to *lamb* at 2 years of age. Does are bred to *kid* between 1 and 2 years of age. Gestation for ewes and does is about 5 months. Before giving birth, the dam's hair or wool is clipped from the udder and perianal areas. This *crotching out* of ewes maintains sanitation and helps lambs find teats to nurse. Many sheep and goat producers synchronize breeding to *freshen* females at times when they can be supervised. Synchronization of estrus can be achieved by hormonal injection or naturally. Because males and females usually are housed apart, the sudden introduction of a male can stimulate breeding activity of females. Females should display signs of estrus 16 to 24 days after exposure to males. This phenomenon, called the *ram effect* in sheep and the *buck effect* in goats, is a natural way to synchronize estrous cycles. Ewes and does remain in the group as long as they are giving birth to and weaning healthy offspring. Some of the reasons for *culling* are unsound feet or legs, injury, or infection of the mammary system or reproductive failure.

Identifiable parentage may not be necessary in commercial flocks. Such sheep normally are *pasture* or *pen bred,* with rams breeding ewes repeatedly during estrus for a period of two estrous cycles. It is common to use ewes of wool-type breeds mated with rams of meat-type breeds to yield crossbred lambs. Crossbred flocks have the advantage of *hybrid vigor (heterosis),* with good rate of gain, high carcass quality, and fine wool.

When the offspring's sire and dam must be known, as in the case of purebred herds, the parents are *hand mated.* Bucks have a distinct odor emanating from scent glands near the base of the horns. To attract does during breeding season, bucks spray urine on their front legs, heads, and beards, in addition to constant rubbing of their scent glands. A doe in heat will vocalize to the male, mount other does and be mounted by penmates, wag her tail, and exhibit a swollen pink vulva. The doe is taken to the buck, which mates readily if the doe is in standing heat. Birth of twins or triplets is common. Dairy goats milk for 10 months after kidding. They are bred in the fall and *dried off* or stopped from milking 2 months before kidding again.

Llamas commonly are hand mated or pasture bred year round. When the female is receptive to the male, she lies calmly in sternal recumbency *(cush),* enabling him to mount. Ejaculation takes place over a period from 15 to 20 minutes during which the male makes a guttural sound *(orgling). Induced ovulation* occurs about 26 hours after mating. Pregnant females may be unreceptive and will run from or *spit* (expell regurgitated stomach fluid) at a male. Gestation is about 11½ months. *Dystocia* (difficult birth) is rare, but malpresentation, such as the head turned back, is seen. The long neck makes turning the head forward to pass through the birth canal a challenge. Single births are usual. Planning for spring or fall births avoids potential *hypothermia* or *hyperthermia* complications for the newborn. Hypothermia results from an abnormally low body temperature, whereas hyperthermia occurs from an abnormally high body temperature. Llama females do not lick newborns, nor do they eat the placenta. A llama female needs only a 15-day period of rest before her next pregnancy.

Pregnancy diagnosis can be determined by hormonal assays that use milk, serum, or urine. Ultrasound and radiology techniques involve specialized equipment. *Ballottement,* bouncing the fetus against the abdominal wall, can be used by an experienced caretaker. For maximum productivity females are not permitted to remain *open* (not bred).

Desired traits are preserved through selective breeding. *Artificial insemination, embryo transfer,* and *cloning* are all technical reproductive processes that have been performed on goats, llamas, and sheep. Each method involves freezing and transplanting semen, ova, and cells, respectively, to maintain genetic lines.

There is confusion about the nomenclature of members of the family Camelidae. For Old World camelids, which include camels, most people use *cow* for female, *bull* for male, and *calf* for young animals. Llamas belong to the South American camelids. Some people use bovine terms, whereas others use equine terms. Because llamas are neither, perhaps it is more appropriate to use *female* and *male* for adults. A castrated male is called a gelding. An infant from birth to weaning is a baby or *cria*. *Juvenile* is used for animals between weaning and adulthood.

NEONATAL CARE

A ewe or doe in labor is separated from its penmates into a lambing or kidding pen. In cold weather an additional heat source, usually a heat lamp, is indicated. After delivery, the mother licks her newborns to clear the respiratory openings, stimulate breathing, and bond with her offspring. A small amount of milk can be drawn from teat orifices to make sure they are patent. The newborns nurse within a few hours of birth. The first milk, *colostrum,* provides maternal antibodies, nourishment, and a laxative for the baby. Weak offspring may need stomach tubing if they cannot nurse. A 7% iodine solution is applied to the umbilical cord to prevent infection *(navel ill, omphalitis)*. The *afterbirth,* placental membranes that are expelled after delivery, is collected and discarded. The lambing or kidding pen is kept clean and the family allowed to bond for a few days before reintroduction to the group.

Very often in goat dairies, kids are taken away from their dams at birth and raised using bottle feeding. Orphaned lambs are also commonly raised this way without difficulty. Llamas react differently. *Berserk male syndrome* is seen when male crias are bottle fed. Because they lose an instinctive fear of humans, the hand-raised males view caretakers as other male llamas. At first, the male may spit at the human without provocation. It may also butt the person with its chest. Llamas can rear up, strike with their front feet, and bite the opponent. To prevent berserk male syndrome, male crias should not be bottle fed and should be castrated between 1 and 6 months of age.

Within a few weeks after birth, lambs' tails are *docked,* and ram lambs are castrated. The *dock* is the part of the tail that remains on the body. The tail is docked 1 inch from the body by severing between the vertebrae surgically or using an emasculator, elastrator, sharp pocket knife, or emasculatome. One reason to dock the tail is to improve sanitation. Long woolen tails that are soaked with urine, blood, or feces are prone to *fly strike.* Long tails may also interfere with breeding and lambing. Docked sheep are more desirable in *conformation* shows and exhibitions.

Some sheep and goats are naturally hornless, or *polled.* Goats raised extensively or used for packing are allowed to grow their horns as a means of defense against predators. However, it is dangerous to house horned goats under intensive management. Kids are *disbudded* between 3 and 14 days of age depending on breed, sex, and size. Disbudding is achieved by burning the horn buds with an electrical hot iron or applying a caustic paste. Surgical amputation of the horn *(dehorning)* may be performed at any age with appropriate anesthesia. The scent glands of buck kids are burned during disbudding to reduce the pungent odor from mature glands. *Wattles* can also be removed easily at this time. They are skin appendages that hang from the ventral surface of the neck and have no known function. The time for castration of buck kids varies with the function of the animal. If they are to be slaughtered before 2 months of age, buck kids are left intact. If they will not be slaughtered before 2 months of age, *bucklings* are castrated between 4 and 14 days of age. The incidence of urinary calculi can be reduced if pet wethers are not castrated until 6 to 8 weeks of age. Castration of lambs and kids is done surgically or by using an emasculator, emasculatome, or elastrator. These procedures are performed in a clean environment, paying attention to fly control, *aseptic technique,* and a tetanus vaccination program.

HOUSING

Small ruminants need minimal housing, such as a *run-in shed.* Shade or shelter from the sun is advisable in the summer. A *windbreak* is adequate for all except the very young during cooler weather. Warm, dry, and draft-free lambing pens are needed in colder climates for better survival of lambs. Lambs are born wet and often weak, which predisposes them to hypothermia.

It is more convenient to house dairy goats in a barn designed with a milking parlor. The free-stall housing system works well for goats. Goats are curious and clever. They escape from inadequate fencing and gates with minimal effort. If goats are housed in low roofed buildings, shelters must not be adjacent to fences. Goats may escape by climbing on the shelter and jumping to the other side of the fence.

Llamas should be watched closely in times of extreme heat or cold. Their hair is very thick, and it may be necessary to use electric fans to prevent hyperthermia during periods of high heat. They should have shelter from winds during periods of extreme cold to prevent hypothermia.

REVIEW B

1. A lamb born without shelter during cold weather may be prone to ____________________.
2. Llamas may suffer ____________________ if not given an adequate cooling system in very hot climates.
3. Two surgical procedures commonly performed on ram lambs are ____________________ and ____________________.
4. The breeding cycles of sheep and goats are described as being ____________________ because females are receptive to the male only during a certain time of year.
5. Male goats have a strong odor resulting from ____________________ glands on the head and their practice of ____________________ on their front legs, heads, and beards.
6. When a female llama is ready to mate she lies in sternal recumbency, a position known as ____________________.
7. Bouncing the fetus against the abdominal wall is a method of pregnancy diagnosis called ____________________.

FEEDING

Sheep and goats are true ruminants with four stomach compartments: rumen, reticulum, omasum, and abomasum. The llama has three compartments: C-1, C-2, and C-3. The esophagus empties into C-1, the largest component. C-1 and C-2 are used for fermentation. Bicarbonate is also secreted, resulting in a pH between 6.4 and 7.0. The function of C-3, the true stomach, is to produce digestive juices, yielding a pH of 3.0. Like the rat and horse, the llama lacks a gallbladder.

Nutrition of all ruminants is similar but varies with management systems and functions of animals. All animals should have a supply of fresh clean water. Small ruminants *browse* (feed on shrubs and bushes) and *graze* (feed on grasses and other plants close to the ground) depending on the forage quality available. Sheep are mostly *grazers*. They are generally managed extensively as range flocks or intensively as farm flocks. In the Western states, range sheep consume primarily brush, shrubs, and grass and are sold for intensive feeding or directly for slaughter if grazing conditions were lush. Farm flocks are seen more commonly in the Corn Belt and in Eastern states where grains are plentiful. Lambs are *creep-fed* so there are rapid gains at an earlier age, producing a finished lamb for slaughter, usually in 3 to 6 months. Farm flocks are pastured from 4 to 8 months a year. They receive hay and grain while housed the remainder of the year in *drylot*. Shepherds use the practice of *flushing* for reproductive gains in their flocks. Flushing involves feeding an increased amount of concentrates to breeding stock during the last few weeks before breeding. Flushing

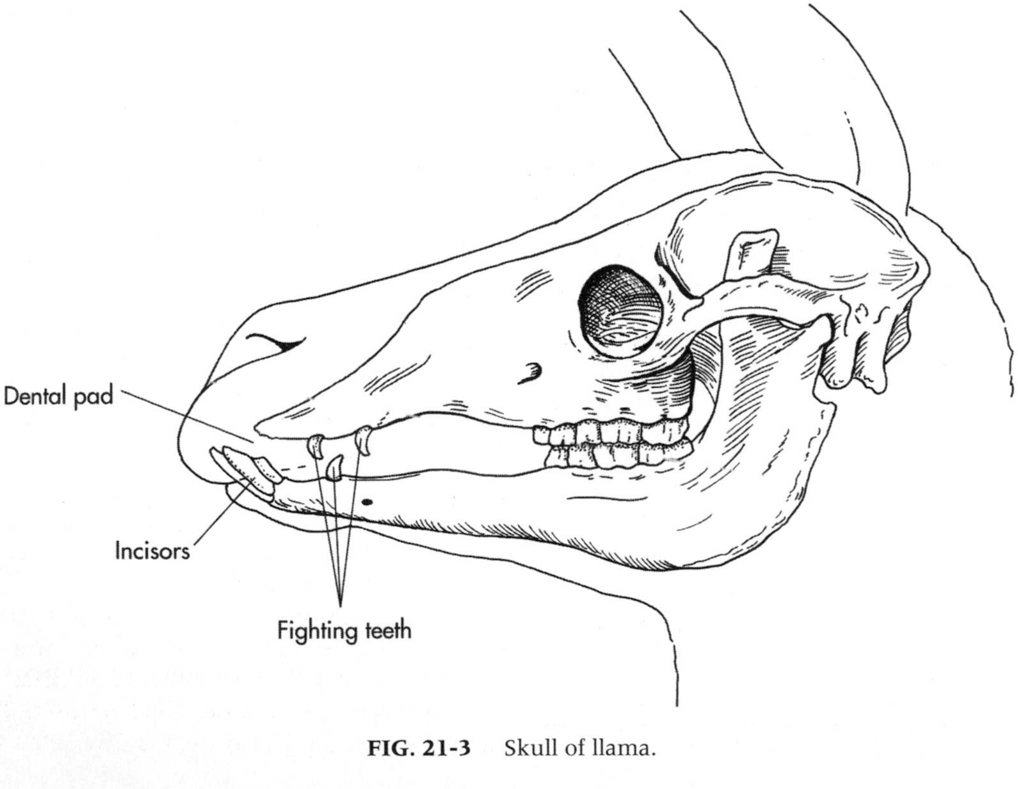
Dental pad
Incisors
Fighting teeth

FIG. 21-3 Skull of llama.

improves semen quality, ovulations, and conception rates, resulting in greater multiple births. While pregnant, ewes and does consume a maintenance diet until the last 4 to 6 weeks before lambing or kidding. Additional grain is fed at the end of gestation to provide extra energy for the fast-growing fetuses and to prevent metabolic diseases, such as *ketosis.*

Llamas normally spend one third of daylight hours grazing and browsing. The llamas' split upper lips permit close grazing without damage to the root of the plant. The upper and lower canines and the single upper incisor* develop into fighting teeth in llamas (Fig. 21-3). Fighting teeth stop growing in geldings and usually do not need to be cut in females. However, males can inflict serious injury by biting at the throat, legs, and genitals of aggressors. Teeth are cut at the gum line with obstetric wire every 2 to 4 years after 3 years of age.

Goats prefer to browse rather than graze. Animals under intensive management should have good-quality hay in ray racks available *ad lib.* Alfalfa hay improves milk production of dairy goats but is too rich for llamas and male sheep and goats. Grain supplementation is suggested for animals that are used for breeding, packing, meat, and milk production. Concentrates are available as ground grains rolled into a *pellet.* Another grain type, *sweet feed,* combines whole, rolled, or cracked grains with molasses for increased palatability. Grain rations are fed in clean buckets or troughs. Often grain is medicated with drugs, such as *coccidiastats,* growth promotants, urinary acidifiers, and antibiotics. *Drug withdrawal times* must be observed when animals are intended for human consumption. The drug must be excreted from the animal's body before slaughter or use of milk.

*An incisor by origin but not by function.

RESTRAINT

The most difficult part of restraining sheep is catching them. A trained herding dog facilitates moving and separating sheep. Sheep are extremely *herd bound,* and startling one member can cause a stampede. It is usually best to drive the entire flock into a holding pen and then single out the desired animal by using a gate or board. A shepherd's crook easily snares the hind leg above the stifle. Lambs are grasped directly by a hind leg. When close to the desired sheep, grip under its chin and tip its head upward. Whenever restraining a sheep, keep in mind not to grab the animal by the wool. Doing so breaks the wool fibers and lessens the value of the fleece. The actual restraint of the animal is done with the animal in standing or sitting position. To restrain in the standing position, place one hand under the animal's chin and the other hand around its dock. Restraining the sheep in the sitting position is known as *rumping* (Fig. 21-4). The animal is lifted into the sitting pose, rests on its rump, and leans backward into the restrainer's legs. Once sheep are immobilized, they usually accept restraint without further struggle.

Goats are more independent and less herd bound than sheep. Goats may be caught and restrained in the standing fashion, as mentioned for sheep. Goats are easily backed into a corner or tied to a fence or post with a rope and collar. When restraining a goat with horns, grasp only at the base of the horns to avoid breaking them. Bearded goats can be held and led by the beard. Because dairy goats are handled frequently and usually wear neck collars, catching a dairy goat poses no problem. Dairy goats are commonly restrained in a *stanchion* (Fig. 21-5) for milking or other procedures.

The immature llama may be restrained with one arm around the chest and the other around the hindquarters. Llamas can be cornered with a long rope because they will not usually jump over a 3½-foot-high

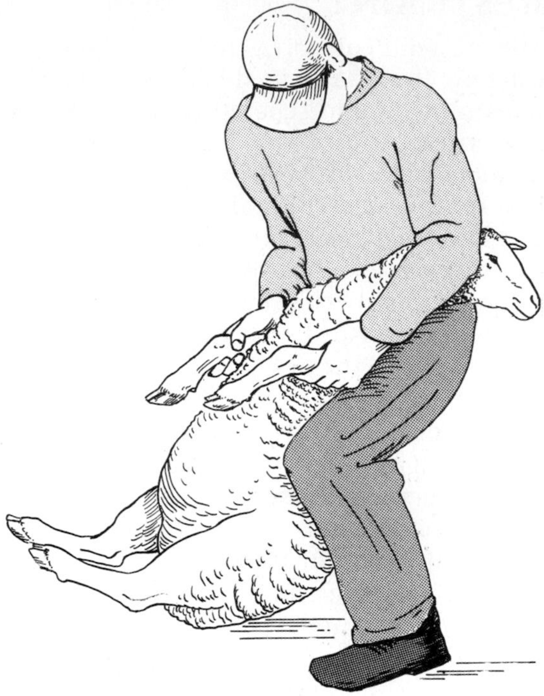

FIG. 21-4 Rumping is a useful restraint method for sheep.

rope. Mature llamas may be restrained by tying to a fence or post using a lead rope and *halter* (Fig. 21-6) or placed in a chute. A halter is a harness of leather, nylon, or rope that extends behind the ears and encircles the nose. The lead rope is attached under the chin to the ring on the halter with a metal snap. Llamas can also be restrained in a squeeze chute. A bar is placed over the shoulders to prevent the animal from rearing up. Keep in mind that any member of the camelid family will spit if provoked, so a second handler may be needed to restrain the head. A feisty llama can be muzzled or a sack placed over its head.

REVIEW C

1. The largest compartment of the llama stomach is ______________________ .
2. The name of the true stomach of the llama is ______________________ .
3. Why should sheep never be caught by grasping their wool?

   ____ .
4. The type of forage eaten determines whether an animal is a ______________________ (feeding on shrubs and bushes) or a ______________________ (feeding mostly on grasses).
5. What is drug withdrawal time? ______________________ .
6. The type of teeth that develop into fighting teeth in male llamas are ______________________ and ______________________ .

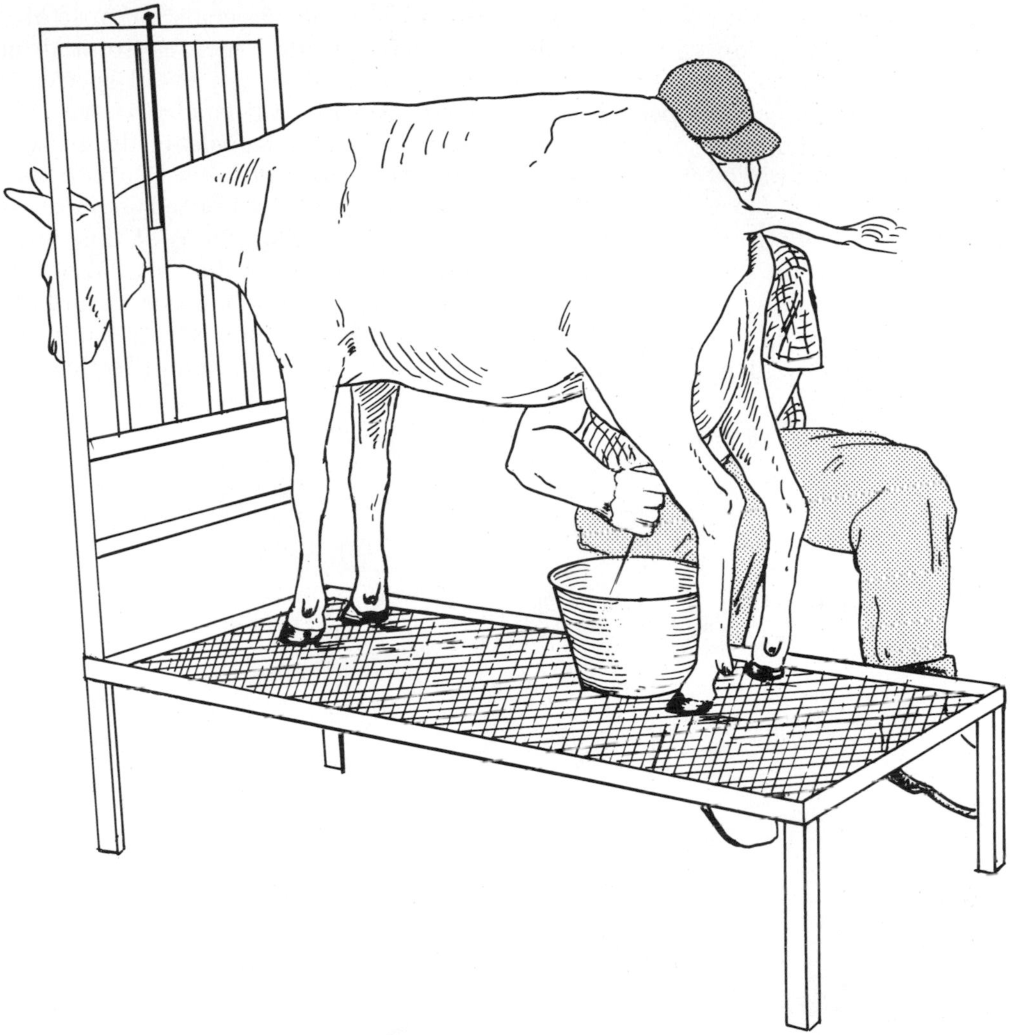

FIG. 21-5 Dairy goat being milked while restrained in a stanchion.

ROUTINE HEALTH CARE

Routine preventive health care is important to the well-being of the animals and to the market value of the meat, milk, and fiber they produce. Common vaccines given to ruminants include *tetanus, Clostridium perfringens* types C & D, and *rabies*. If dams are vaccinated during the last 6 to 8 weeks of pregnancy, their offspring receive maternal antibodies through colostrum. Vaccination boosters should be administered to the adults and neonates at appropriate intervals, following manufacturer's recommendations. Sheep, llamas, and to a lesser extent goats are affected by *white muscle disease*. Periodic administration of selenium and vitamin E is recommended to reduce this muscular affliction.

The thick wool that covers the sheep's body can harbor external parasites, such as lice, keds, and mites. Ivermectin-based injectables or oral medication can eliminate these parasites without contaminating the wool. However, spraying and *dipping* sometimes are still used. In dipping, the animal's entire body is plunged briefly into a tank of insecticide solution.

Llamas are affected by the ectoparasite *Sarcoptes scabiei.* It is the causative agent of *mange,* which is zoonotic. Ivermectin has documented success in treating mange. However, ivermectin is not approved for use in sheep, llamas, or goats. Because of excessive drug-testing expenses, some drugs are not approved for use in all species. Some drugs are used off-label or have *extralabel drug use* status. Extralabel drug use status permits use without species approval.

Young animals housed intensively are prone to *coccidiosis.* Signs of this endoparasitic infestation are diarrhea, loss of condition, frailness, dry hair coat, and failure to thrive. Young animals can be housed in small groups by age, rotated to clean ground

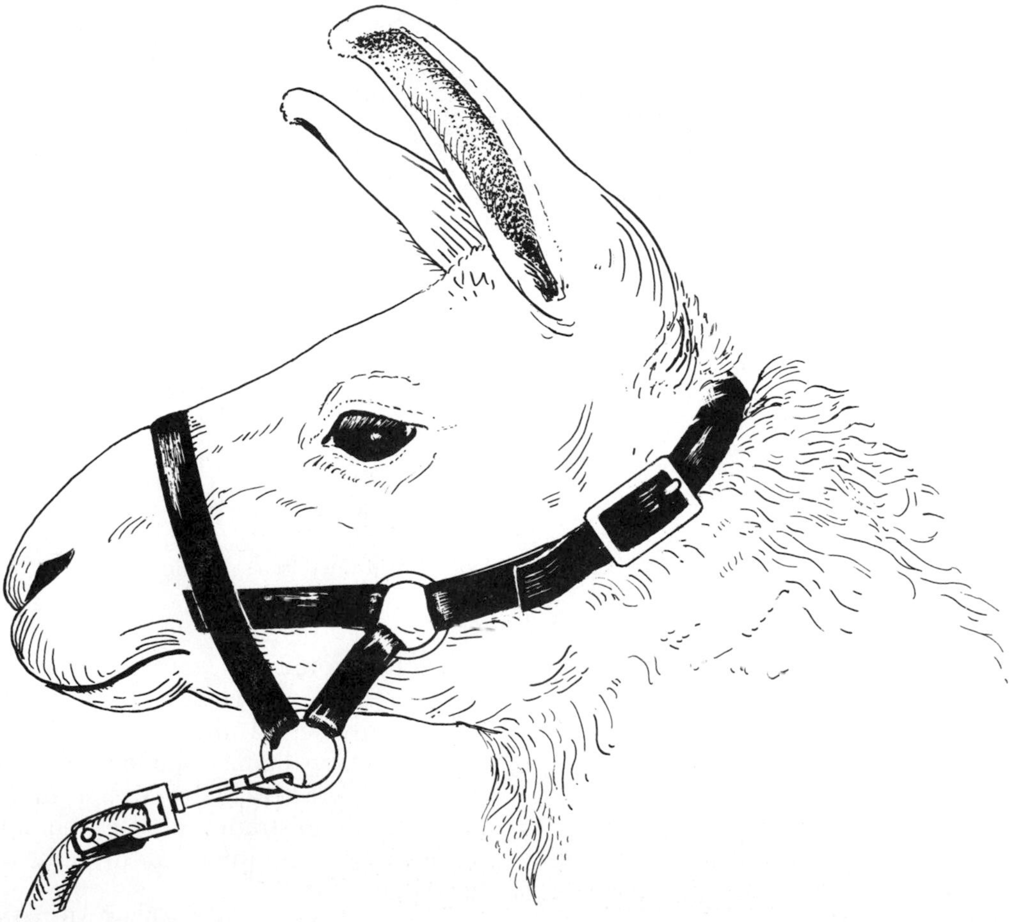

FIG. 21-6 A useful restraint device for llamas is a halter with lead rope.

regularly, medicated with coccidiostats in food and water, fed grain and water in clean buckets, and offered hay in suspended hayracks to control the condition.

Helminthiasis is more commonly observed in extensively reared animals than intensively reared stock. Gastrointestinal parasites, liver flukes, and lungworms infect ruminants of all ages. Clinical signs include weight loss, poor growth, anemia, diarrhea, rough hair coat, persistent coughing (for lungworms), and intermandibular edema (for liver flukes and gastrointestinal parasites). Routine fecal analysis and egg counts with appropriate anthelmintic treatment can effectively manage internal parasitism.

Proper foot care reduces the chances of hoof rot, teat injuries, abnormal gait, and sore feet. All these conditions can contribute to decreased food intake, which negatively influences the function and health of the animal. Small ruminants are encouraged to regularly walk through medicated footbaths or are vaccinated against hoof rot. Hoof trimming varies with exercise, nutrition, climate, and management systems. Llama toenails are trimmed flush to the footpad about every 3 months. These toenails do not bear weight, nor are they worn down by terrain (Fig. 21-7). Sheep and goat hooves, which are worn down by rocky terrain, are trimmed at least 3 times a year.

COMMON DISEASES

Clostridium perfringens types C and D are causative agents of *enterotoxemia,* or overeating disease. It is more common to observe this disease in young confined animals, which are fed heavily for maximum growth. Signs of overeating disease are diarrhea, weakness, anorexia, incoordination, cir-

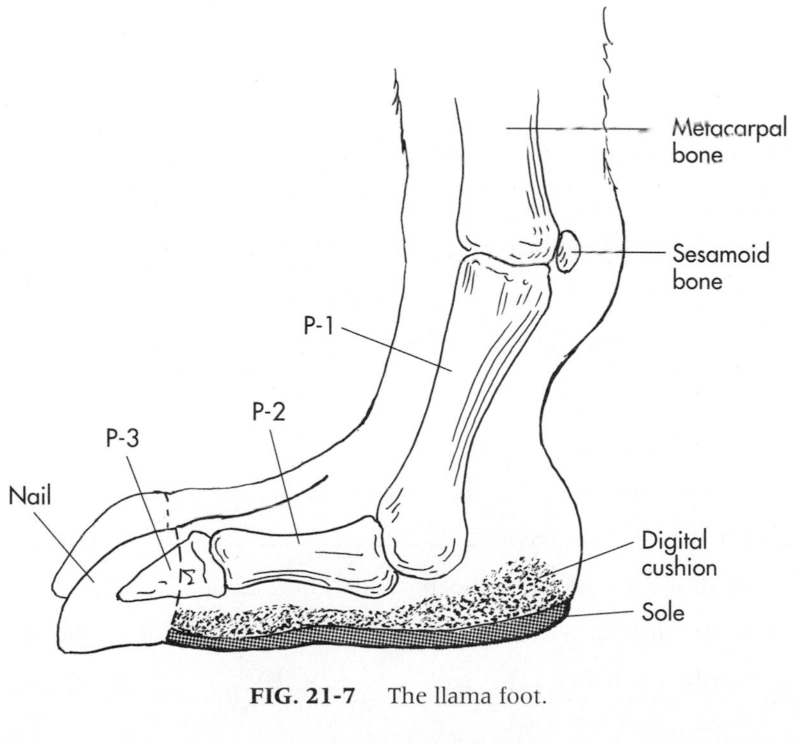
Metacarpal bone
Sesamoid bone
P-1
P-2
P-3
Nail
Digital cushion
Sole

FIG. 21-7 The llama foot.

cling, convulsions, and sudden death. Small ruminants do not respond well to treatment, but vaccination is effective. The causative agent of *tetanus,* or lockjaw, is *Clostridium tetani.* Signs of tetanus include poor coordination, anorexia, stiff limbs, prolapsed third eyelid, bloat, and usually death. Prevention using a tetanus toxoid booster annually is the best control method.

Contagious ecthyma, sore mouth or *orf,* is a highly contagious viral disease that is zoonotic. When an outbreak occurs, small ruminants have swollen lips, mouth, nose, and feet, and the udder swells if affected animals are nursing. There is no cure for sore mouth. However, supportive nursing care, such as antibiotics for secondary bacterial infections and forced feeding, may be necessary until the virus runs its course. Because the virus is hardy, vaccination is suggested once the herd or flock is infected.

Bacteria and viruses can cause *pneumonia.* Very often, stresses such as shipping, changes in weather, a barn that is too warm, or harassment by dogs hasten pneumonia. Signs of pneumonia are fever, lethargy, dyspnea, and coughing. Treatment includes segregation in a warm, dry, and draft-free barn, broad-spectrum antibiotics, forced feeding, expectorants, steaming, and exercise.

Llamas are afflicted with *acute abdomen,* a digestive disorder similar to colic in equines. Signs include anorexia, depression, stomach atony, decreased fecal output, normal to subnormal rectal temperature, and increased pulse and respiration, especially if pain is present. *Bloat* occurs in sheep and goats when they are overfed concentrates or lush legumes. Indigestion results because gas builds up and the animal is unable to belch. Bloated animals experience abdominal pain, stamp their hindfeet, lie down, grunt, and have a firm swelling in the left paralumbar fossa. Treatment involves medical management or surgical intervention. Refer to Chapter 19 for information on mastitis, brucellosis, and tuberculosis, which may affect goats, llamas, and sheep.

REVIEW D

1. Small ruminants are routinely vaccinated against three diseases: ________________, ________________, and ________________.
2. Zoonotic diseases spread by contact with small ruminants include ________________ and ________________.
3. Intensively reared animals are pushed to consume food for maximum growth and production. Two diseases that may result from this type of management are ________________ and ________________.
4. What is extralabel drug use? ________________________________.
5. Contagious ecthyma is also known as ________________ and ________________.
6. Selenium and vitamin E are given to sheep to prevent ________________ disease.
7. *Sarcoptes scabiei* is the cause of ________________. Because it can be spread to humans, the disease is described as being ________________.

Chapter 21 Answers

Review A

1. four, three
2. communal dung pile
3. flock
4. erect
5. lanolin
6. chevon

Review B

1. hypothermia
2. hyperthermia
3. castration, tail docking
4. seasonally polyestrous
5. scent, urinating
6. cush
7. ballottement

Review C

1. C-1
2. C-3
3. Grasping the wool can damage the wool fibers and reduce fleece value.
4. browser, grazer
5. Drug withdrawal time is the period after cessation of drug administration necessary to ensure that drug residues do not contaminate products for human consumption.
6. canines, incisors

Review D

1. tetanus, enterotoxemia, rabies
2. mange, contagious ecthyma
3. enterotoxemia, bloat
4. Extralabel drug use is the practice of permitting drugs to be administered to species that lack approval for such use by the Food and Drug Administration.
5. orf, sore mouth
6. white muscle
7. mange, zoonotic

Chapter 21 EXERCISES

SMALL RUMINANTS

Exercise 1: Fill in the blanks.

1. Skin appendages found along the ventral surface of the necks of goats have no known function and are called ______________________ .
2. To say that a ewe is open means ______________________ .
3. A castrated male llama is called a(n) ______________________ .
4. Omphalitis is inflammation of the ______________________ .
5. In addition to wool and meat, sheep are raised for ______________________ and ______________________ and ______________________ .
6. In the estrous cycle of the goat estrus occurs every ______________________ days.
7. Breeding two sheep of different breeds is called ______________________ . The increased vigor of the resulting offspring is called ______________________ .
8. Sheep are pasture bred when the identification of parents is not critical. When the identity of sire and dam must be known with certainty, the method of choice is ______________________ .
9. A baby llama is called a(n) ______________________ .
10. The method of pregnancy diagnosis in which the fetus is pushed and then felt bouncing back against the abdominal wall is called ______________________ . Other methods that can be used are ______________________ , ______________________ , and ______________________ .
11. Bottle feeding of baby llamas is not recommended because of the danger of causing ______________________ .
12. Mature llamas are led and restrained by using ______________________ .
13. Dipping is a method for treating ______________________ .
14. The meat from mature sheep is called ______________________ .
15. *Clostridium tetani* is the cause of ______________________ in several species.
16. Natural synchronization of estrus in a group of does can be achieved by using the ______________________ effect. The same phenomenon in sheep is called the ______________________ effect.

17. Induced ovulation occurs in llamas as a result of ________________________ . A different situation occurs in ewes, which are considered ________________________ ovulators.

Exercise 2: Match the terms in the right column with the statements in the left column by placing the appropriate letter in the space provided.

_____ 1. Goat meat

_____ 2. Used in cosmetics industry

_____ 3. Ovulation for which no male need be present

_____ 4. Producer of mohair

_____ 5. Preparturient sanitation practice

_____ 6. Prevents white muscle disease

_____ 7. A group of goats

_____ 8. Used to treat protozoan parasites

_____ 9. Method of pregnancy diagnosis

_____ 10. Restrains milking goats

_____ 11. Used to treat external parasites

_____ 12. Device used for castration

_____ 13. Naturally hornless

_____ 14. Practice of increasing food

_____ 15. A group of sheep

A. Angora goat
B. Polled
C. Ultrasound
D. Chevon
E. Lanolin
F. Stanchion
G. Emasculator
H. Spontaneous
I. Vitamin E
J. Herd
K. Crotching out
L. Flushing
M. Flock
N. Coccidiastats
O. Ivermectin

CHAPTER 21 PUZZLE

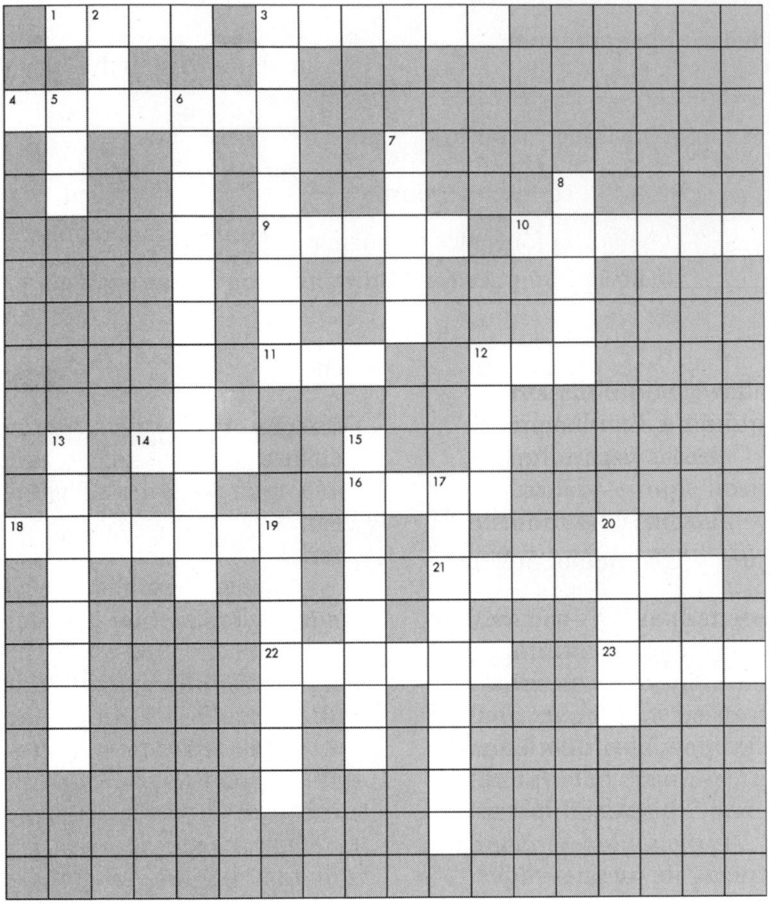

ACROSS CLUES

1. Group of goats
3. Castrated goat
4. First flush of lactation
9. Fermenting vat of ruminant
10. Consume leafy shrubs and bushes
11. Baby goat
12. Female goat
14. Contagious ecthyma
16. Male goat
18. Ruminating
21. Oil found in sheep wool
22. Dehorn
23. Baby llama

DOWN CLUES

2. Female sheep
3. Three-sided shelter
5. Male sheep
6. Increased body temperature
7. cut wool off sheep
8. eat plants close to the ground
12. cut off
13. increase feed before breeding
15. true stomach of ruminant
17. fibrous material inedible for nonruminant
19. neutered male llama
20. group of sheep

Chapter 21 Answers

Exercise 1

1. wattles
2. she is not pregnant
3. gelding
4. umbilicus
5. milk, hide, as research animals
6. 18 to 21
7. crossbreeding, heterosis (hybrid vigor)
8. hand mating
9. cria
10. ballottement, hormonal assays, ultrasound, radiology
11. berserk male syndrome
12. halters
13. ectoparasites
14. mutton
15. tetanus
16. buck, ram
17. mating, spontaneous

Exercise 2

1. D
2. E
3. H
4. A
5. K
6. I
7. J
8. N
9. C
10. F
11. O
12. G
13. B
14. L
15. M

ANSWERS: CHAPTER 21 PUZZLE

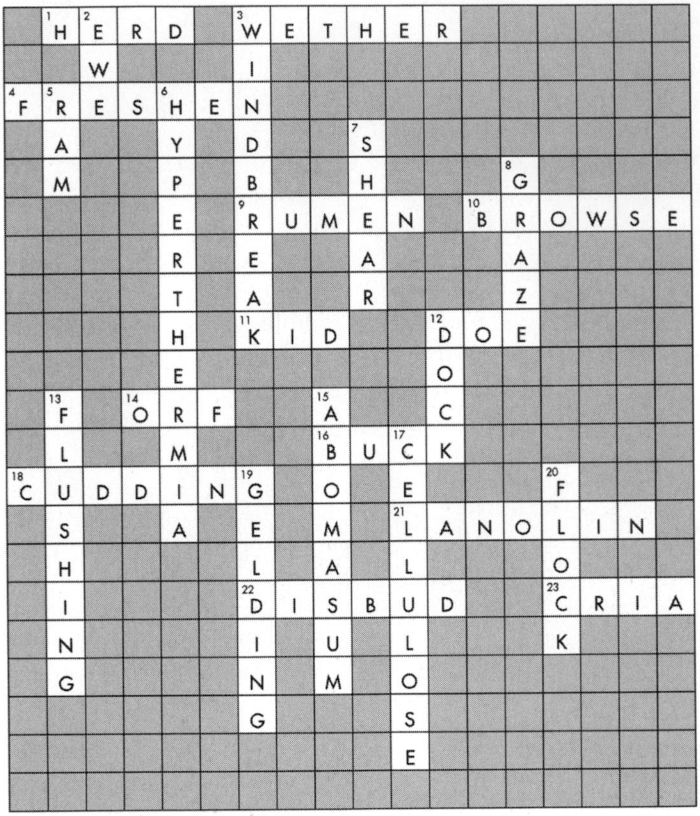

GLOSSARY

abomasum: the fourth compartment in the ruminant stomach; functions like the simple stomach in monogastric animals.

acute abdomen: a digestive disorder of llamas that is similar to colic in horses.

afterbirth: placental tissues that are expelled after the birth of a newborn.

artificial insemination: implanting of semen into the female reproductive tract by artificial means, as opposed to natural breeding.

aseptic technique: methods for creating and maintaining sterile conditions.

ballottement: a palpation method of pregnancy diagnosis in which the fetus is bounced gently away from the abdominal wall and felt as it rebounds.

berserk male syndrome: a condition seen in male bottle-fed llamas, who lose an instinctive fear of humans; the llamas perceive humans as a threat and attack accordingly.

bloat: distension in the rumen or abomasum caused by an accumulation of gas.

browser: animal that consumes bushes and shrubs rather than grasses.

buck effect: a natural method for synchronizing estrus in goats; does who have had no previous exposure to males begin to cycle soon after the introduction of a buck into the herd.

buckling: an immature male goat.

castration: removal of gonads, rendering animal incapable of reproduction.

cellulose: complex carbohydrate of the cell walls in plants.

chevon: goat meat.

cloning: the process of producing genetically identical progeny from a single organism, cell, or gene.

Clostridium perfringens: the bacteria that causes enterotoxemia.

Clostridium tetani: the bacteria that causes tetanus.

coccidiastat: a drug that controls coccidia.

coccidiosis: disease caused by the protozoan parasite coccidia.

colostrum: the thick yellow first milk at the time of parturition; it gives neonates passive immunity because it is rich in maternal antibodies.

communal dung pile: waste material deposited in one location.

conformation show: a competition in which animals are judged on their appearance, compared with desirable type and breed standards.

contagious ecthyma: a zoonotic, viral dermatitis affecting sheep, goats, and llamas; also known as *orf* or *sore mouth.*

creep-feed: a method of providing additional nutrients to young animals while denying access to mature animals.

cria: a young llama from birth to weaning age.

crotching out: clipping wool away from the udder and perianal areas of ewes before lambing.

cud: the regurgitated food bolus of ruminants.

culling: removing undesirable animals from the group.

cush: the sternally recumbent position a female llama assumes when she is receptive to the male for mating (cushing).

dehorn: to surgically amputate the horn.

dipping: briefly submerging the animal in a tank of insecticide to control external parasites.

disbud: to remove the horn bud in very young animals.

dock: to amputate the distal portion of the tail (verb); the part of the tail that remains on the body after docking (noun).

drug withdrawal time: the time needed for drug residues in food to fall to an acceptable level.

drylot: method of keeping livestock in a small area, as opposed to pasture; food and water are brought to the animals.

dry-off: the cessation of milk flow at the end of a dairy animal's lactation period.

dystocia: difficult parturition.

elastrator: an amputation device that applies an elastic band that restricts blood flow to the scrotum or tail.

emasculatome: bloodless castration device that crushes the spermatic cord without breaking the skin (also used for tail docking of lambs).

emasculator: surgical castration device that both cuts and crushes the spermatic cord (also used for tail docking of lambs).

embryo transfer: a reproductive process that harvests fertilized ova from donor females and transplants these ova into recipient females for the completion of gestation.

enterotoxemia: a disease that releases toxins from the intestinal tract into the blood.

epidermal growth factor (EGF): a potent growth factor for epithelial and fibroblast cells, used as a substitute for shearing wool from sheep.

extralabel drug use: a system that permits drugs to be used in species for which the Food and Drug Administration has not approved their use.

fleece: the coat of wool that is shorn off sheep in one piece.

flock: a group of sheep.

flushing: the practice of suddenly increasing nutrition to breeding animals to improve semen quality, ovulation, and conception rates.

fly strike: infestation of skin by fly larvae (also called cutaneous myiasis).

freshen: beginning of lactation cycle immediately after parturition.

grazers: animals that consume pasture or cereal crops (contrasted with browsers).

halter: a device made of rope or leather straps that fits around the head of an animal and is used to lead or restrain it.

hand mating: the practice of bringing a female in estrus to the male for the purpose of mating.

helminthiasis: a disease caused by parasitic worm infestation.

herd: a group of animals of the same species (e.g., a group of goats).

herd bound: tending to behave as a group rather than as individuals.

heterosis: see hybrid vigor.

hybrid vigor: the increased productivity and performance observed from the crossbreeding of animals of different breeds (same as heterosis).

hyperthermia: an abnormally high body temperature.

hypothermia: an abnormally low body temperature.

induced ovulation: a reproductive phenomenon in which ovulation occurs as a result of mating (as opposed to spontaneous ovulation).

ketosis: a metabolic disorder in which ketone bodies accumulate in the blood and tissues.

kid: a young goat from birth to weaning age (noun); the name for the act of parturition in goats (verb).

lanolin: wool grease that is processed for use in the cosmetics industry.

lamb: a young sheep from birth to weaning age (noun); the name given to the act of parturition in sheep (verb).

lingual torus: a swelling or pad on the tongue of ruminants.

mange: a skin disease caused by an infestation of mites.

mutton: meat obtained from adult sheep.

navel ill: an infection of the umbilicus (omphalitis).

omasum: the third chamber connecting the reticulum and the abomasum of the ruminant stomach.

open: a female animal of breeding age that is not pregnant.

orf: a zoonotic, viral dermatitis affecting sheep, goats, and llamas; also known as *contagious ecthyma* or *sore mouth.*

orgling: the guttural sound produced by male llamas during mating.

pasture or *pen bred:* males and females kept together so they can mate when ready (as opposed to hand mating).

pellet: a type of food in which concentrates are ground, mixed, and compressed into a small, uniform bullet.

pneumonia: an inflammation of the lungs.

polled: naturally hornless.

rabies: a zoonotic and fatal viral infection of the nervous system.

ram effect: a natural method for synchronizing estrus in sheep; ewes who have had no previous exposure to males begin to cycle soon after the introduction of a ram into the flock.

reticulum: the cranial portion of the ruminant stomach with a honeycomb appearance.

rumen: the largest chamber of the ruminant stomach, the one in which fermentation takes place.

ruminant: an animal having a multichambered stomach for digestion.

rumping: a restraint method in which a sheep is placed on its hindquarters.

run-in shed: a shed, usually three sided, that is placed in a pasture to provide shelter.

Sarcoptes scabiei: the mite that causes sarcoptic mange or scabies.

shearing: mechanical removal of the fleece from sheep.

spitting: regurgitating stomach contents; llamas do this as a means of defense when threatened.

spontaneous ovulation: a species characteristic in which ovulation occurs near the end of estrus whether mating occurs or not (as opposed to induced ovulation).

stanchion: a restraint device that secures an animal behind the head with two vertical bars.

standing heat: the stage of the estrous cycle when the female allows mounting by males or other females (synonymous with *estrus* in most species).

sweet feed: a mixture of whole, cracked, or rolled grains with molasses for increased palatability.

tetanus: a usually fatal disease caused by the neurotoxins of *Clostridium tetani.*

wattles: fleshy appendages that hang from the necks of goats.

white muscle disease: a disease caused by nutritional deficiency of selenium or vitamin E.

windbreak: shelter (usually three-sided) that an animal can stand behind to avoid the wind.

22 Rodents, Rabbits, and Laboratory Animal Science

CHAPTER OVERVIEW

This chapter describes rodents and rabbits commonly used as pets or laboratory animals. Mice, rats, hamsters, gerbils, and other small mammals kept in homes for companionship and enjoyment often are called pocket pets. As research animals, rodents and rabbits have made valuable contributions to human welfare.

RODENTS

Mice, rats, hamsters, gerbils, and guinea pigs are all rodents. *Rodents* characteristically have long front teeth or incisors. These teeth grow continuously and must be worn down by abrasion. *Malocclusion,* improper position of the teeth, causes overgrowth of the incisors. Malocclusion is common in the incisors of rodents and rabbits and in the cheek teeth of guinea pigs. Rodents are for the most part *nocturnal,* being more active at night than during the day. Most can be sexed by *anogenital distance.* Males have a longer distance between the anus and genitalia than do females. Rodents often are bred using either a *monogamous* mating system or a *polygamous* mating system. In the monogamous system, one female is paired with one male. In the polygamous (also known as the *harem*) mating system, two or more females are placed with one male. Most rodents give birth to *altricial,* blind, hairless, and helpless babies. The guinea pig, with its long gestation period, is the exception. Guinea pig babies are born *precocious,* which means they are fully furred, the eyes are open, and they are able to run around the cage and eat solid foods.

The term *murine* specifically refers to mice and rats. Young mice and rats are called *pups.* The mouse is the most commonly used laboratory animal. It is small and easily housed and handled and adapts readily to a laboratory environment. Its scientific name is *Mus musculus.* Varieties of mice are bred for specific characteristics or susceptibility to disease. *Inbred strains* are produced by brother-sister matings for at least 20 generations. Inbred mice of the same sex and strain are genetically identical. BALB/C and C57BL/6 are common inbred strains used in research. *Mutant* mice have naturally occurring genetic defects. *Nude* mice are mutant mice that are hairless and have deficiencies in their immune system. Nude mice often are used in *oncology,* cancer research, because they are capable of growing human tumors. Scientific technology has developed special mice called *transgenics* and *knockouts.* A transgenic carries genetic material *(DNA, deoxyribonucleic acid)* transplanted from the genes of another animal. The transplantation occurs at the fertilized egg stage of development. Transgenics are used to study the function of various genes. A knockout has a gene or portions of its genes removed or blocked. Knockouts are used to study diseases associated with defective genes. *Hybrid* mice are created by mating two inbred strains. *Random bred* or *outbred* mice are produced by mating mice as nonrelated as possible to maintain genetic diversity. Swiss Webster and ICR are common outbred stocks.

When handled gently, a rat is a quiet, clean, easily trained pet. The rat also has a long standing and important place in biomedical and behavior research. Its scientific name is *Rattus norvegicus. Albino* and *hooded* are the most common varieties used. Albino rats have white fur with pink skin and eyes. The Sprague-Dawley (SD) is a common albino outbred stock, and the Fischer 344 (F344) is an inbred albino strain. Hooded rats have pigmented eyes and are white with a black facial hood, shoulders, and dorsal stripe. The Long-Evans is an example of a hooded rat. Rats are communal animals and rarely fight when housed in groups. They are natural burrowers. Rats have no gallbladder. Behind the rat's eyeball is a pigmented lacrimal gland called the *harderian gland.* This red-brown gland secretes a red porphyrin-rich secretion that lubricates the eye. In times of stress or illness, red tears *(chromodacryorrhea)* overflow and stain the face.

The hamster has a stocky body, short tail, broad snout, and large cheek pouches in which food is transported or temporarily stored. The golden or Syrian hamster, *Mesocricetus auratus,* originated in the Middle East. As the name suggests, it is golden red in color. Color varieties and long-haired "teddy bears" often are kept as pets. With frequent handling, hamsters are readily tamed but often bite if startled. They are adept at escaping from enclosures and enjoy gnawing on caging and other items. They may *hibernate* and appear to be in a trancelike sleep if the room temperature drops to around 5° C. During hibernation, their body temperature drops and heart rate and metabolism slow. Females that are ready to be bred assume a *lordosis* posture. The female stands near the male with her back legs stretched outward in a fixed position, her hindquarters elevated, and her tail to one side. *Cannibalism,* killing and eating the young pups, is common during the first pregnancy or if the litter is disturbed.

The Mongolian gerbil, *Meriones unguiculatus,* is native to China and Mongolia. It is also known as the *jird.* Unlike most rodents, it has a hair-covered tail. It has strong claws for burrowing and stout hind limbs, which give it the ability to leap quickly. They love to dig and burrow in bedding material. Foot stomping is used as a means of communication with other gerbils. The *agouti* is the most common color variety seen in gerbils. Agouti is a naturally occurring coat color pattern that consists of brown hairs with bands of grayish yellow near the tips. Gerbils are nonaggressive, easy to handle, and simple to maintain as pets or in the laboratory. Gerbils are generally *monogamous,* which means they mate for life with one partner.

Guinea pigs are *hystricomorph,* or porcupinelike rodents. The guinea pig, or *cavy,* as it is commonly called, has short legs and a stocky body and is tailless. Its scientific name is *Cavia porcellus.* A variety of hair coats and colors exists. The most common pet and laboratory variety is the English or shorthaired. Abyssinians have short, rough hair arranged in whorls or rosettes, and the Peruvian variety has long hair resembling a rag mop. Male guinea pigs are called *boars;* females are called *sows.* Guinea pigs rarely bite or scratch and make good pets if handled gently. They live up to their name of "pig" by being messy eaters and scattering bedding material. They are more vocal than other rodents and often whistle to greet people entering their housing area. As a result of the long gestation period, newborns are fully furred and nearly self-sufficient. The act of giving birth is called *farrowing.*

RABBITS

The rabbit, *Oryctolagus cuniculus,* is a *lagomorph.* Lagomorphs are distinguished from rodents by having a second pair of incisors in the upper jaw. There are many breeds and varieties of rabbits. The New Zealand white, a medium-sized rabbit breed, is commonly used in research. The Dutch, a smaller breed that is white with a colored hooded head and belted hindquarters, is used both as a pet and in research. Male rabbits are called *bucks.* Female rabbits are called *does,* and their offspring are called *kits* or more commonly *bunnies.* The act of giving birth is called *kindling.* Rabbits are curious and spend a lot of time hopping around, exploring their environment. Wild rabbits are naturally nocturnal and are also *crepuscular,* being active in the twilight. Rabbits are *coprophagous,* ingesting large quantities of *night feces* directly from the anus. The night feces are rich in vitamins and proteins and are softer in consistency than the day feces.

REVIEW A

1. ________________________ characteristically have long chisel-shaped incisors that grow continuously.
2. An animal that is more active at night than in the day is described as ____________________ .
3. Mice and rats can be sexed by ________________________ distance.
4. A(n) ________________________ is an animal that results from the introduction of genetic material from one animal into the fertilized egg of a different animal and bred.
5. A(n) ________________________ mouse is created by breeding two inbred strains.
6. ________________________ animals have white fur and pink skin and eyes.
7. If the environmental temperature drops to around 5° C, a hamster may ____________________ and appear to be in a trancelike sleep.
8. The Mongolian gerbil is also known as a(n) ________________________ .
9. The guinea pig is commonly called a(n) ________________________ .
10. A male guinea pig is called a(n) ________________________ .
11. Young rabbits are called bunnies or ________________________ .
12. The act of giving birth in rabbits is called ________________________ .

HOUSING

Laboratory rodents often are housed in *shoebox* cages, which have solid flooring (Fig. 22-1, *A*) or in *suspended* cages, which hang and may have solid or wire flooring (Fig. 22-1, *B*). Shoebox cages have slotted, bar-type lids that hold food pellets and a water bottle. Individual shoebox cages or suspended cages are placed on a metal *rack* (Fig. 22-1, *C*). A rack generally accommodates 30 cages. *Microisolator* cages are a special type of shoebox cage covered by plastic filter tops that keep airborne disease agents out of the cages. They are used to house rodents such

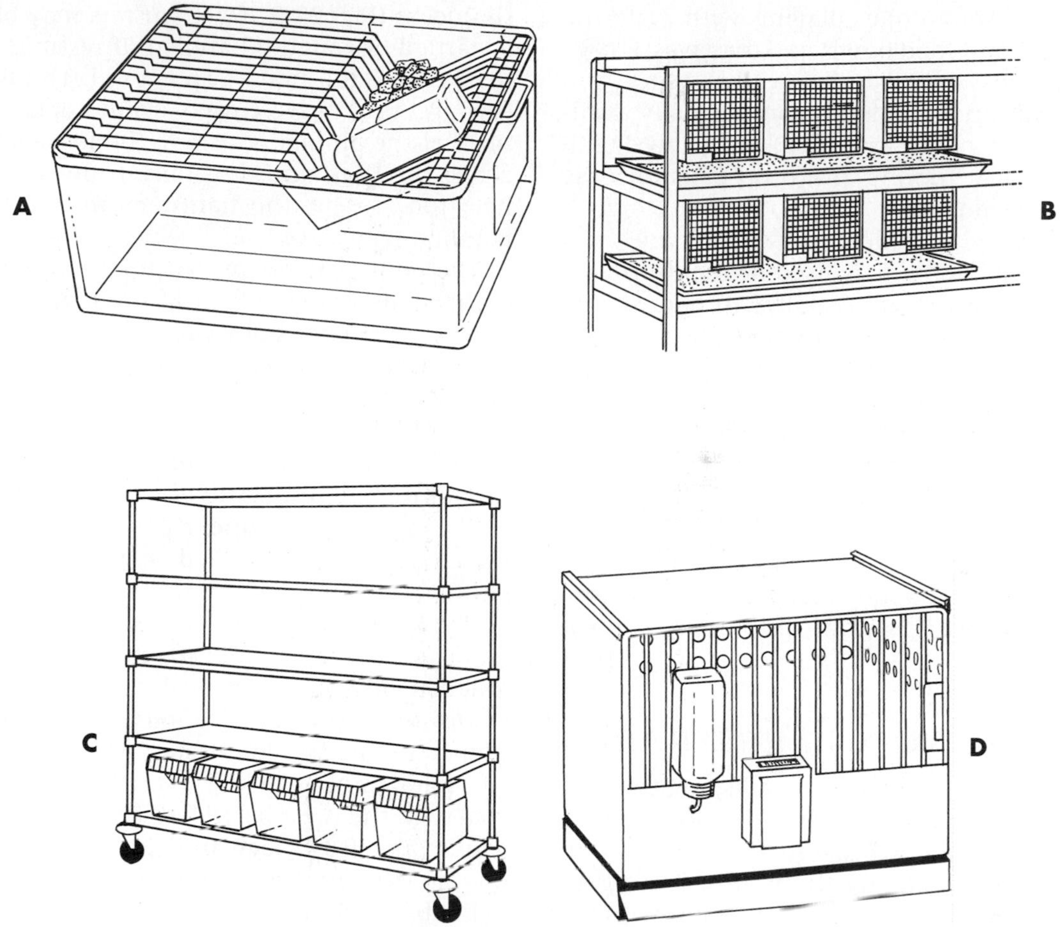

FIG. 22-1 Common types of caging. **A**, Shoebox cage; **B**, suspended cages; **C**, rack of cages; **D**, rabbit cage with J feeder and mesh floor.

as nude mice that are particularly susceptible to infection.

Pet rodents are housed in a variety of commercially available caging. Terraria with lids are a popular type of caging. Rodents can be housed singly, although they are more commonly housed in small groups. Exercise wheels can be placed in pet hamster or gerbil cages to allow activity. Plastic tubes that make up an exercise trail system can also be attached to hamster or gerbil cages. Rodents can drink water from water bottles with sipper tubes or from automatic watering devices.

To provide adequate space, guinea pigs are housed in tublike boxes with *direct* (also called *contact*) *bedding* material. When direct bedding is used, the animal comes into contact with the bedding material. Guinea pig cages normally do not need lids because guinea pigs are not climbers. Food can be placed in bowls or in a feeder attached to the cage. Guinea pigs can drink water from water bottles or from an automatic watering system. They enjoy playing with watering devices and food bowls and may waste large quantities of food and water.

A variety of caging is commercially available for rabbits. Assembled wire cages with suspended flooring and drop pans for easy waste removal are commonly used. *Indirect bedding,* with which the animal does not come into contact, is used in the drop pan. Laboratory rabbits usually are housed in *front-opening* cages with self-feeding J *feeders* (Fig. 22-1, *D*). Front-opening cages allow access to the animal from the front of the cage. They usually have slotted bar or wire mesh flooring, with trays under the flooring to catch the excreta. J feeders, shaped like the letter *J,* are attached to the front of the rabbit's cage to prevent the rabbit from soiling its food. Rabbits can drink water from water bottles or from an automatic watering system.

HANDLING AND RESTRAINT

Mice can be picked up by grasping the base of the tail with the fingers or with smooth-tipped forceps. Another method for examining or manipulating the mouse is to grasp the mouse by the scruff of the neck with the thumb and forefinger. The tail can be held by the opposite hand or between the fourth and fifth fingers of the same hand. If the skin is grasped too far from the head, the mouse can turn and bite the handler (Fig. 22-2, *A* and *B*).

Rats become tame when handled gently and rarely bite. They can be picked up by the base of the tail for short periods of time to transfer them from one cage to another. If manipulation is necessary, the rat is picked up by placing a hand firmly over the back and rib cage and restraining the head with thumb and forefingers immediately behind the jaws (Fig. 22-2, C).

Hamsters are easily moved by scooping them up or grasping the loose skin across the shoulders (Fig. 22-2, *D*). Hamsters may bite if startled or roughly handled. If restraint is needed, the full hand grip is used. The fingers and thumb are curled around opposite sides of the animal, grasping the loose skin across the back until it is taut. If the skin is held too loosely, the hamster can bite the handler.

The gerbil can be picked up by cupping both hands under it and lifting it from its cage. For injections or treatments, the gerbil is restrained like the mouse by scruffing the neck with one hand and firmly grasping the base of the tail with the other hand. Care should be taken not to pull on the tail. The skin of the tail, especially the tip, comes off easily, exposing the underlying muscle and vertebrae. This is called *degloving* (also known as *tail slip*).

The docile nature of guinea pigs makes them easier to restrain than most other rodents. One hand is placed under the thorax to support the body, and the other hand supports the hindquarters. Alternatively, one hand can be placed over the shoulder area with the thumb and forefingers directly behind the front legs and the other hand used to support the rump (Fig. 22-2, *E*).

Rabbits can be restrained by grasping the scruff of the neck with one hand and supporting the hindquarters and back with the other hand (Fig. 22-2, *F*). Occasionally, they resist handling and can endanger themselves or their handlers. If not restrained securely, rabbits can fracture their backs. They can also inflict painful scratches on the handler with their toenails. Rabbits are sensitive to noise and may react violently to sudden loud sounds. When frightened or stressed, they may attempt to bite or jump at a handler.

NUTRITION

Feed and water should be available *ad libitum.* Fresh, clean water should be provided

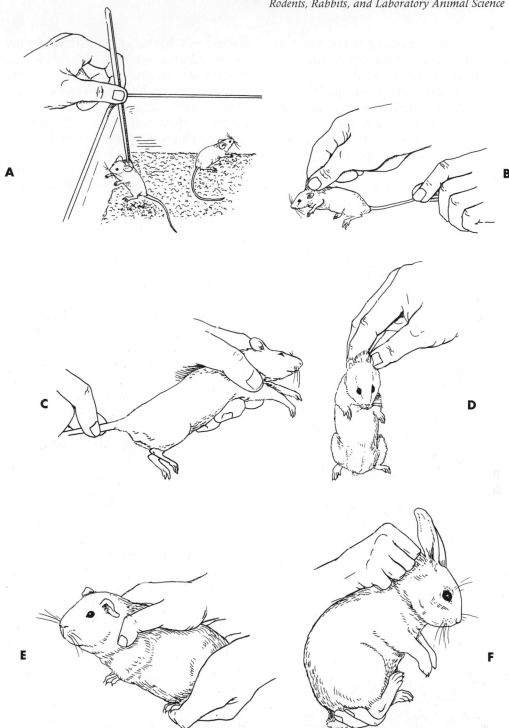

FIG. 22-2 Handling laboratory animals. **A,** Picking up a mouse with forceps; **B,** handling a mouse; **C,** restraining a rat; **D,** picking up a hamster; **E,** restraining a guinea pig; **F,** lifting a rabbit, using both hands.

to all rodents and rabbits by water bottle or automatic watering device. Rodents and rabbits should be fed a fresh, completely balanced, pelleted diet. A completely balanced diet provides all the nutrients the species needs. Supplementation of the diet is not recommended. Mice, rats, hamsters, and gerbils are fed block-type pellets, which are firm and must be gnawed by the animal. This type of food helps keep the incisor teeth worn down. Rabbits and guinea pigs are fed smaller pellets, which are more easily eaten by these species. Guinea pigs cannot synthesize vitamin C and must be fed a diet rich in this vitamin. Rabbits tend to overeat and become obese. Feeding rabbits measured amounts of feed and a diet that has a higher fiber content prevents obesity and promotes good health.

DISEASE

Most rodents and rabbits used in research studies are bred and raised in special environments to keep them healthy and disease free. In *specific pathogen free (SPF)* animals, a certain disease-causing agent has been eliminated. *Axenic* (also known as *germ-free*) animals are free of all detectable microorganisms and parasites. Axenic animals must be maintained under sterile conditions if they are to remain free of unwanted microorganisms.

Rodents and rabbits are susceptible to a number of bacterial, fungal, and viral diseases. *Murine mycoplasmosis* is a common respiratory disease in mice and rats. It is caused by the bacteria *Mycoplasma pulmonis. Snuffles* (also known as *pasteurellosis*) is a bacterial disease of rabbits that causes respiratory symptoms. Rodents and rabbits can also become infected with *parasites. Coccidiosis* is a protozoan parasitic disease that causes intestinal and liver lesions in rabbits. Mice can develop *alopecia,* hair loss, on their nose and face if infected with mites. *Acariasis* is an infestation of mites. Alopecia may also be caused by *barbering,* a common behavioral problem in many types of mice. A behaviorally dominant mouse will bite or chew the fur off a more subordinate mouse, usually in the facial region. Rabbits and guinea pigs can develop *sore hocks* when housed on wire flooring. Their foot pads and foot areas become ulcerated by the animal's weight pressing down on the foot. Hamsters are prone to *wet-tail,* a condition characterized by diarrhea and dehydration. Wet-tail is thought to be caused by a bacterial infection. Gerbils often *seizure* when handled or placed in a new environment. If not fed a diet high in vitamin C, guinea pigs can develop *scurvy.* Some bacterial, viral, and fungal organisms can be *zoonotic.* Zoonotic agents, such as *Microsporum,* which causes ringworm, are infectious agents that can be transmitted from animals to humans.

REVIEW B

1. Laboratory rodents often are housed in ______________ cages, which have a solid bottom flooring.
2. A(n) ______________ is a metal stand that supports a number of rodent cages.
3. The ______________ is a special type of shoebox cage that is used to house nude mice.
4. Bedding material with which the animal comes in contact is called ______________ bedding.
5. Laboratory rabbits often are housed in ______________ cages, which allow access to the animal from the front of the cage.
6. Care should be taken not to pull on the tip of the gerbil's tail because it comes off easily, exposing the underlying tissues. This condition is called ______________ .
7. If not restrained properly, the ______________ can fracture its back.
8. ______________ feeding means to free choice feeding. One species for which it is not recommended is the ______________ .
9. Acariasis is an infestation of ______________ .
10. Wet-tail causes diarrhea and dehydration in ______________ .
11. ______________ often seizure when placed in a novel environment.
12. Pasteurellosis or ______________ is a bacterial disease of rabbits that causes respiratory symptoms.

LABORATORY ANIMAL SCIENCE

Most of today's important medical and surgical advances were made possible through animal research. Research and testing are performed on animals that are similar to humans to attain comparable information. The majority of animals used in research are rodents and rabbits. Some research involves the use of other types of animals such as reptiles, amphibians, fish, chickens, pigs, goats, dogs, cats, and nonhuman primates (monkeys). Even though research benefits animals and humans, some people are against using animals for research. *Antivivisectionists,* for example, oppose using live animals for surgery for research purposes. *People for the Ethical Treatment of Animals (PETA)* is an organization that opposes the use of animals in research.

The use of animals in experimentation led to the development of *laboratory animal science.* Laboratory animal science is the scientific and technical information, knowledge, and techniques that apply to laboratory animal care. Organizations such as the *American Association for Laboratory Animal Science (AALAS)* promote improvement in the humane care and treatment of laboratory animals through educational programs and publications. *Laboratory animal medicine* is a specialty area of veterinary medicine that deals with the diagnosis, treatment, and prevention of diseases in laboratory animals.

Animals used in research are protected by federal regulations such as the *Animal Welfare Act (AWA)*. The Animal Welfare Act regulates the use of all warm-blooded vertebrates in research except purpose-bred rats and mice, birds, and farm animals used or intended for use as food or fiber. The AWA regulations deal with housing, handling, feeding, watering, sanitation, ventilation, transportation, separation of species, and veterinary care for these animals. Regulations require training for scientists and others using animals and consideration of *alternatives* that do not include the use of animals for experiments. Computer simulation and analytic chemical techniques are examples of alternatives. An *Institutional Animal Care and Use Committee (IACUC)* must also be established. The Institutional Animal Care and Use Committee inspects animal facilities, evaluates the animal care program, and reviews *protocols*.

In medical research, a protocol is a detailed description of the *principal investigator's (PI's)* proposed experimental plan. The *hypothesis* is an important component of the experimental plan and is the basis for the research. The hypothesis is a proposed explanation of the problem or question. Research can be done using *in vitro* or *in vivo* techniques. *In vitro* literally means within glass and refers to biologic work performed outside of the living organism, as in a cell culture. *In vivo* refers to biologic research work performed within living organisms. Scientists often use an animal that has the necessary biologic characteristics to answer the research question. An animal with such characteristics is called an *animal model*. Animal models can be categorized as natural or induced. *Natural animal models* possess the characteristic from birth and are said to have *congenital* conditions. Other models may have to be *induced* or created by surgical manipulation or injection of a chemical. In most experiments, there are *control* groups and *test* groups. The control groups are not subjected to the experimental manipulation. The control groups serve as standards against which the outcomes in the experimental groups can be compared.

Numerous research subjects are needed to provide statistically reliable conclusions. However, researchers try to use guidelines such as the *3R principle* of Russell and Burch. The 3R principle calls for *replacement* of animals by cell or tissue culture or mathematic models, *refinement* of procedures to minimize stress or pain to animals when possible, and *reduction* to the minimum number that will serve a useful purpose, yield statistically sound data, and produce scientific benefit.

At the end of the research study, the animals usually are *euthanized* and a *necropsy* is done. *Euthanasia* means to be put to death in a humane manner. A necropsy is an examination and dissection of a body after death, looking for signs of disease. *Pathology* is the study of changes in body tissues and organs as they relate to disease. Often, tissue samples are collected during the necropsy and analyzed at a later time.

REVIEW C

1. ______________________ is an organization that is against using animals in research.
2. ______________________ is a specialty area of veterinary medicine that deals with diagnosing, treating, and preventing disease in laboratory animals.
3. Animals used in research are protected by federal regulations such as the ______________ .
4. A special committee called the ______________________ inspects animals facilities, evaluates the animal care program, and reviews protocols.
5. A ______________________ is a detailed written description of the principal investigator's proposed experimental plan.
6. ______________________ refers to biologic work performed outside of the living organism.
7. ___________________________ refers to biologic research work performed within living organisms.
8. ______________________ groups are not subjected to the experimental manipulation.
9. The 3R principal involves ______________________ , ______________________ , and ______________________ .
10. ______________________ means to put to death in a humane manner.
11. ______________________ is an examination and dissection of a body after death.
12. ______________________ is the study of changes in body tissues and organs as they relate to disease.

Chapter 22 Answers

Review A

1. rodents
2. nocturnal
3. anogenital
4. transgenic
5. hybrid
6. albino
7. hibernate
8. jird
9. cavy
10. boar
11. kits
12. farrowing

Review B

1. shoebox
2. rack
3. microisolator
4. direct (contact)
5. front-opening
6. tail slip (degloving)
7. rabbit
8. *ad libitum,* rabbit
9. mites
10. hamsters
11. gerbils
12. snuffles

Review C

1. People for the Ethical Treatment of Animals (PETA)
2. laboratory animal medicine
3. Animal Welfare Act
4. Institutional Animal Care and Use Committee (IACUC)
5. protocol
6. *in vitro*
7. *in vivo*
8. control
9. replacement, refinement, reduction
10. euthanasia
11. necropsy
12. pathology

Chapter 22 — EXERCISES

RODENTS, RABBITS, AND LABORATORY ANIMAL SCIENCE

Exercise 1: Match the animals in the right column with the related terms in the left column by placing the appropriate letter in the space provided. Each letter will be used more than once.

_____ 1. *Oryctolagus cuniculus*
_____ 2. Susceptible to scurvy
_____ 3. Golden
_____ 4. Susceptible to snuffles
_____ 5. *Mus musculus*
_____ 6. Peruvian
_____ 7. Sprague-Dawley
_____ 8. Lagomorph
_____ 9. BALB/C
_____ 10. Sow
_____ 11. *Meriones unguiculatus*
_____ 12. Buck
_____ 13. Cavy
_____ 14. *Rattus norvegicus*
_____ 15. Boar
_____ 16. Parturition known as kindling
_____ 17. Susceptible to wet-tail
_____ 18. Parturition is known as farrowing
_____ 19. *Mesocricetus auratus*
_____ 20. Mongolian
_____ 21. Doe
_____ 22. Jird
_____ 23. Hystricomorph
_____ 24. Dutch

A. Mouse
B. Rat
C. Rabbit
D. Gerbil
E. Hamster
F. Guinea pig

Exercise 2: Select the correct answer.

1. ______________________ means hair loss.
   a. Crepuscular
   b. Altricial
   c. Malocclusion
   d. Alopecia
2. An animal that results from the removal of one or more genes from the fertilized egg is called a/an ______________________ .
   a. Hybrid
   b. Knockout
   c. Transgenic
   d. Inbred
3. All of the following are rodents *except* ______________________ .
   a. Rat
   b. Guinea pig
   c. Rabbit
   d. Hamster
4. ______________________ is a disease caused by a parasite.
   a. Lordosis
   b. Coccidiosis
   c. Scurvy
   d. Barbering
5. The breeding method in which one male is placed with two or more females is described as ______________________ .
   a. Polygamous
   b. Random
   c. Monogamous
   d. Outbred
6. All of the following terms are used to describe young *except* ______________________ .
   a. Kits
   b. Pups
   c. Bunnies
   d. Does
7. ______________________ are born precocious.
   a. Mice
   b. Guinea pig
   c. Gerbil
   d. Rabbit
8. Degloving can occur in ______________________ if it is not handled correctly.
   a. *Oryctolagus*
   b. *Mesocricetus*
   c. *Cavia*
   d. *Meriones*
9. Another word for germfree is ______________________ .
   a. Nude
   b. Specific pathogen free
   c. Axenic
   d. Hooded
10. ______________________ is an organization that promotes improvement in the humane care and treatment of laboratory animals through educational programs and publications.
    a. AALAS
    b. PETA
    c. AWA
    d. IACUC

CHAPTER 22 PUZZLE

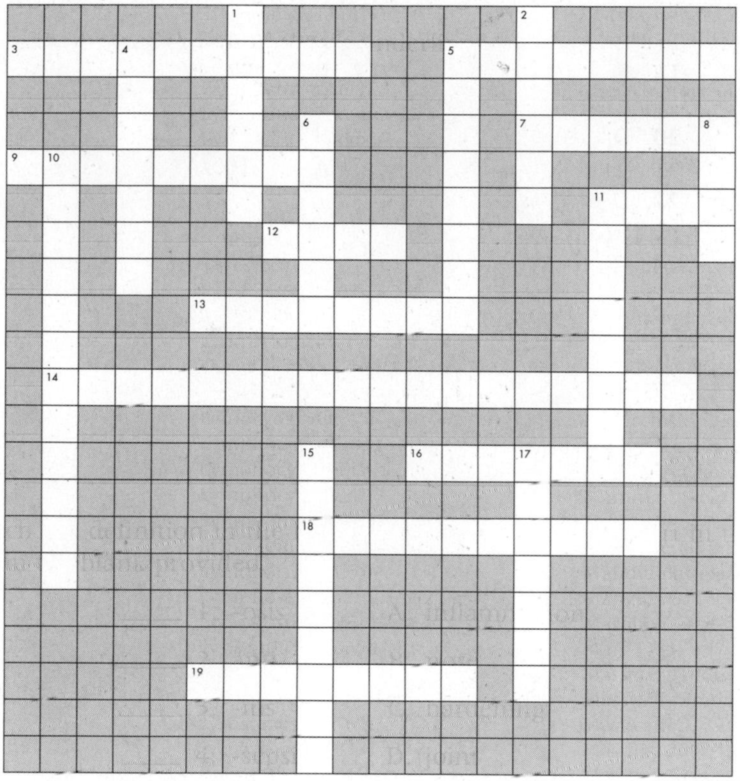
1
2
3
4
5
6
7
8
9
10
11
12
13
14
15
16
17
18
19

ACROSS CLUES

3. Proposed explanation for research question
5. Act of giving birth in rabbits
7. *Oryctolagus cuniculus*
9. Dominant animal chews fur off subordinate animal
11. Young mice
12. Male rabbit
13. Bedding with which the animal does not come in contact
14. One who opposes surgery on live animals for research purposes
16. Rodent with cheek pouches
18. Present at birth
19. Transmitted from animals to humans

DOWN CLUES

1. *Meriones unguiculatus*
2. Product of 20 or more brother/sister crosses
4. Synonym for *random bred*
5. Animal that results from the removal of one or more genes from the fertilized egg
6. Animal color pattern that consists of brown hair with bands of gray and yellow
8. Group that is subject to experimental manipulation
10. Experimental methods that do not involve the use of animals
11. Organism living on or in an animal and deriving nutrients from that animal
15. Active at night
17. Convulsion

Chapter 22 Answers

Exercise 1

1. C	9. A	17. E
2. F	10. F	18. F
3. E	11. D	19. E
4. C	12. C	20. D
5. A	13. F	21. C
6. F	14. B	22. D
7. B	15. F	23. F
8. C	16. C	24. C

Exercise 2

1. D	6. D
2. B	7. B
3. C	8. D
4. B	9. C
5. A	10. A

ANSWERS: CHAPTER 22 PUZZLE

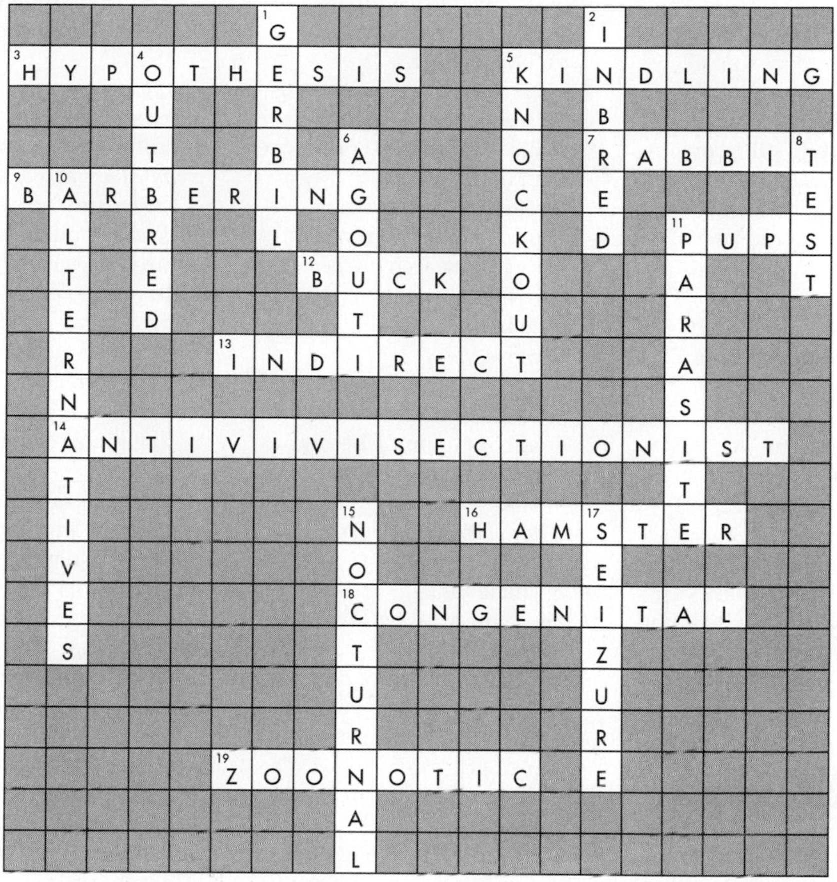
1 GERBIL
2 INBRED
3 HYPOTHESIS
4 OUTBRED
5 KINDLING
5 KNOCKOUT
6 AGOUTI
7 RABBIT
8 TEST
9 BARBERING
10 ALTERNATIVES
11 PUPS
11 PARASITE
12 BUCK
13 INDIRECT
14 ANTIVIVISECTIONIST
15 NOCTURNAL
16 HAMSTER
17 SEIZURE
18 CONGENITAL
19 ZOONOTIC

GLOSSARY

3R principle: a set of guidelines first enunciated by Russell and Burch that seek to reduce research animal use to a minimum while still providing scientifically valid results. The three R's are replacement, refinement, and reduction.

acariasis: an infestation with mites.

ad libitum: freely, as desired; refers to feeding or watering an animal.

agouti: naturally occurring coat color pattern of mammals, which consists of brown hairs with bands of gray and yellow near the tips.

albino: animal with a white hair coat and pink skin and eyes.

alopecia: condition in which hair is missing from a normally haired area.

alternative: method of experimentation that does not use animals, such as computer simulation or analytic chemical technique.

altricial: blind, hairless, helpless; most rodents are born in this developmental stage.

American Association for Laboratory Animal Science (AALAS): organization that promotes improvement in humane care and treatment of laboratory animals through educational programs and publications.

animal model: natural or induced disease or condition occurring in animals that is similar to a human disease or condition.

Animal Welfare Act (AWA): federal law that regulates use of all warm-blooded vertebrates in research except purpose-bred rats and mice, birds, and farm animals used or intended for use as food or fiber.

anogenital distance: distance between anus and genitalia; females have shorter distance than do males.

antivivisectionist: one who opposes surgery on live animals for research purposes.

axenic: free of foreign organisms, used interchangeably with *germfree*.

barbering: common behavioral problem in animals in which dominant animal bites or chews fur off subordinate animal; often seen in mice, where fur is chewed off face.

boar: male guinea pig.

buck: male rabbit.

bunny: young rabbit (also called *kit*).

cannibalism: the act of devouring one's own species.

Cavia porcellus: scientific name of guinea pig.

cavy: common name of guinea pig.

chromodacryorrhea: release of red tears; seen in rats that are stressed or ill.

coccidiosis: protozoan parasite infection affecting intestines and liver; commonly seen in rabbits.

congenital: present at birth; condition can be caused by genetic influence, disease transmission, or trauma during gestation.

contact bedding: bedding with which animal comes into contact (also called *direct bedding*).

control: the scientific standard against which all experimental results can be compared; procedure is identical to the experimental procedure except for the factor being studied.

coprophagous: animals that eat feces as a means of recycling protein, water, and vitamins.

crepuscular: active at twilight or before sunrise.

degloving: pulling skin of tail off through inappropriate handling (also called *tail slip*).

deoxyribonucleic acid (DNA): basic genetic material of life.

direct bedding: bedding with which animal comes into contact (also called *contact bedding*).

doe: female rabbit.

euthanasia: putting to death in a painless manner.

farrowing: act of giving birth in guinea pig.

front-opening: type of cage that allows access to animal from front, such as those commonly used to house rabbits.

germfree: free of foreign organisms (also called *axenic*).

harderian gland: red-brown lacrimal gland that secretes red porphyrin-rich tears to lubricate the eye.

harem: mating system in which one male is housed with two or more females (also called *polygamous*).

hibernation: dormant state characterized by reduced body temperature, heart rate, and metabolism.

hooded: having pigmented eyes and a white coat color with black facial hood, shoulders, and dorsal stripe.

hybrid: strain resulting from mating two inbred strains.

hypothesis: proposed explanation

for research problem or question.

hystricomorphs: porcupinelike rodents such as the guinea pig.

inbred: descended from progenitors who were siblings or close relatives to produce a narrow range of variations of genetic traits; refers to an animal descending from a line of 20 or more brother/sister crosses.

indirect bedding: bedding with which animal does not come into contact; usually used in catch or drop pan under caging unit.

induced animal model: an artificially caused disease in an animal that is used for research on human disease.

Institutional Animal Care and Use Committee (IACUC): special institutional committee that inspects animal facilities, evaluates animal care programs, and reviews research protocols.

in vitro: performed outside living organisms, such as tissue culture.

in vivo: performed within living organisms.

J feeder: feeder shaped like letter *J;* used for rabbits or guinea pigs.

jird: gerbil.

kindling: act of giving birth in rabbits.

kit: young rabbit (also called *bunny*).

knockout: animal that results from the removal of one or more genes from the fertilized egg.

laboratory animal medicine: specialty area of veterinary medicine that deals with diagnosis, treatment, and prevention of disease in laboratory animals.

laboratory animal science: scientific and technical information, knowledge, and techniques that apply to laboratory animal care.

lagomorph: animals, such as rabbits, distinguished from rodents by second pair of incisors in upper jaw.

lordosis: position of sexual receptivity in which animal lies down with rear legs extended and hips elevated.

malocclusion: improper occlusion of teeth.

Meriones unguiculatus: scientific name of Mongolian gerbil.

Mesocricetus auratus:

microisolator: shoebox caging system covered by a plastic filter top that limits air exchange between the room and the cage interior to protect the animals from pathogens.

monogamous: pairing with one mate, as do gerbils.

murine: pertaining to mice or rats.

murine mycoplasmosis: bacterial respiratory infection of mice and rats caused by *Mycoplasma pulmonis.*

Mus musculus: scientific name of mice.

mutant: an organism resulting from mutation.

mutation: a change of the DNA sequence within a gene of an organism resulting in the creation of a new trait not found in the parental type.

natural animal model: a naturally occurring animal disease that is sufficiently similar to a human disease to be used for research on that disease.

necropsy: dissection and examination of a body after death.

night feces: soft feces of rabbit produced at night that are high in protein and vitamins.

nocturnal: active primarily at night.

nude: having a naturally occurring genetic defect in mice in which the animal is hairless and has a deficiency in its immune system.

oncology: study of cancer.

Oryctolagus cuniculus: scientific name of rabbit.

outbred: descended from unrelated parents (also called *random bred*).

parasite: organism that lives on or in another organism from which it derives its nourishment.

pasteurellosis: bacterial disease of rabbits that causes respiratory symptoms; commonly called snuffles.

pathology: study of disease and its effects on organisms.

People for the Ethical Treatment of Animals (PETA): organization that opposes the use of animals in research.

polygamous: mating system in which one male is housed with two or more females (also called *harem*).

precocious: developmental stage of newborn babies in which they are fully furred, have their eyes open, and are able to move about and eat solid food.

principal investigator (PI): scientist who prepares the protocol and plans and coordinates all phases of the research work.

protocol: specified method or procedure for carrying out tasks or experiments.

pups: young mice and rats.

rack: metal structure that supports several caging units.

random bred: descended from unrelated parents (also called *outbred*).
Rattus norvegicus: scientific name of the rat.
reduction: one of the 3R principles of Russell and Burch, which states that the minimum number of animals in a study that will serve a useful purpose, yield statistically sound data, and produce scientific benefit should be used.
refinement: one of the 3R principles of Russell and Burch, which states that procedures used in animal research should focus on minimizing stress and pain to animals when possible.
replacement: one of the 3R principles of Russell and Burch, which states that animals used in research should be replaced when possible by cell or tissue culture or by mathematical models.
rodent: classification of mammals *(Rodentia)* characterized by chisel-shaped incisor teeth.
scurvy: disease caused by nutritional deficiency of vitamin C.
seizure: to undergo convulsions.
shoebox: type of caging used for rodents; has solid bottom flooring.
snuffles: bacterial disease of rabbits that causes respiratory symptoms (also called *pasteurellosis*).
sore hocks: ulceration of the foot pad or foot area caused by housing on wire flooring; occurs in rabbits and guinea pigs.
sow: female guinea pig.
specific pathogen free (SPF): free of specified disease-causing organisms.
suspended: type of caging used for rodents that is suspended from metal rack and has wire or solid flooring.
tail slip: external skin of tail is pulled off during inappropriate handling (also called *degloving*).
test group: group that is subject to experimental manipulation.
transgenic: animal that results from the introduction of genetic material (DNA) from one animal into the fertilized egg of a different animal.
wet-tail: disease of hamsters characterized by diarrhea and dehydration; thought to be caused by bacteria.
zoonotic: able to be transmitted between animals and humans.

23 Exotic Animals

CHAPTER OVERVIEW

This chapter introduces the wide variety of nondomestic animals that are customarily called exotics. Although small rodents and other pocket pets often are included in this designation, they have already been discussed in Chapter 22.

HERPETOLOGY

Scientists divide the animal kingdom into several major groups for classification purposes. By far the largest group is the *invertebrates.* This group contains about 95% of all known animals. It includes lobsters, oysters, sea sponges, jellyfish, and insects. Reptiles and amphibians are *vertebrates*. They belong to a group of animals that have a vertebral column, or backbone. Vertebrates include not only reptiles and amphibians but also fish, birds, and mammals. The differences between reptiles and amphibians generally are more obvious than their similarities. However, their joint study under the name *herpetology* (from the Greek word *herpes,* meaning a creeping thing) is a scientific tradition dating back 200 years. Many people are familiar with the major groups of amphibians and reptiles—salamanders, frogs, turtles, crocodiles, lizards, and snakes—from visits to the zoo or nature programs on television. This section describes some basic characteristics of these groups.

AMPHIBIANS

Amphibians have smooth, permeable, scaleless skin. The lack of a protective scaly covering determines their activities and habitat. Water evaporates quickly from the skin of amphibians. If an amphibian does not have access to water, it can dehydrate and die in a few hours. Consequently, most amphibians live in moist environments such as rain forests.

There are more than 4900 living (as opposed to extinct) species of amphibians. Herpetologists divide living amphibians into three groups. The best-known groups are the *caudates,* or salamanders and newts, and the *anurans,* or frogs and toads. The least known group is made up of wormlike, mostly secretive, burrowing animals called *caecilians.*

Anurans (Frogs and Toads)

There are nearly 4400 frog species (Fig. 23-1), and they form the largest group of amphibians. The names *frog, toad,* and *treefrog* are all common names (as opposed to scientific names) of anurans. In Europe, where there are few anuran species, the most obvious are the smooth-skinned, long-legged frogs of the genus *Rana* and the short-legged, warty toads of the genus *Bufo.* Consequently every European language has specific words for these two kinds. But

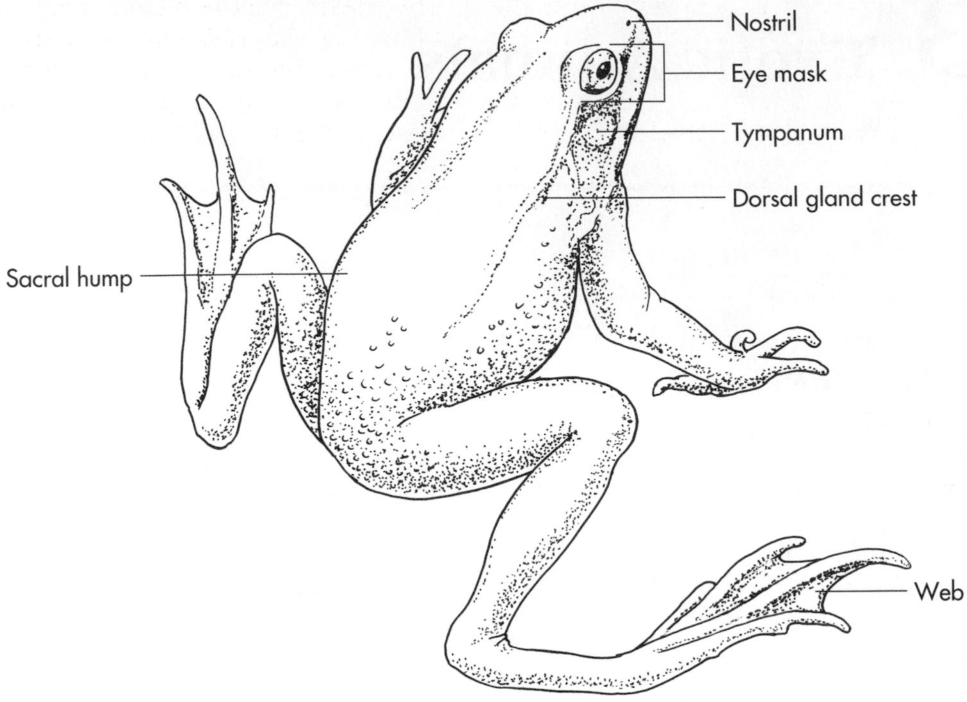
Nostril
Eye mask
Tympanum
Dorsal gland crest
Sacral hump
Web

FIG. 23-1 Adult frog.

where species are more diverse, this distinction breaks down, and it is not possible or necessary to force animals into either category. Generally species with short hind limbs that move by hopping or walking are loosely called toads. Species with long hind limbs are jumpers or swimmers and are called frogs.

Amphibians differ from reptiles in that most species (about 80% of all frogs) have a larval stage between the egg and adult. Most frogs develop from eggs into free-living aquatic larvae or *tadpoles* that *metamorphose* into adults. This transformation is more than simply growing limbs and resorbing the tail. Profound changes take place in anatomy and physiology. For example, the digestive tract shortens, becoming suited to a carnivorous diet instead of a vegetarian diet, the *gills* disappear, and respiration is taken over by the lungs.

Caudates (Salamanders and Newts)

As the scientific name *caudate* (from the Latin word *caudatus,* meaning "provided with a tail") suggests, *salamanders* and *newts* have long tails that are kept even after metamorphosis. Superficially they resemble lizards but are easy to distinguish because of their complete lack of scales. Species that are mostly aquatic are commonly called newts, and terrestrial species are known as salamanders. Caudates have tiny, saclike lungs or no lungs at all. As surprising as this may seem, they can breathe through their skin. Gas exchange of oxygen and carbon dioxide takes place on the moist skin as it does in the lungs of other animals.

Many salamanders achieve sexual maturity while still retaining many juvenile or larval characteristics. This absence or delay of metamorphosis is known as *neoteny.* The Mexican mole salamander, commonly known as the *axolotl,* is the best-known of the newts and salamanders exhibiting neoteny. It may retain gills and other larval features throughout life, even as a breeding adult.

REVIEW A

1. Species lacking a backbone are called ____________________ .
2. The study of reptiles and amphibians is called ____________________ .
3. The group of amphibians that includes frogs and toads is called ____________________ .
4. The change that a tadpole undergoes when it develops legs and loses its tail is called ____________________ ; the delay or absence of this process in some species is called ____________________ .
5. The word *caudate* indicates the presence of a(n) ____________________ .

REPTILES

The living reptiles are divided into four groups. The best-known orders are the *Testudinea,* or turtles; the *Crocodilia,* which include alligators and crocodiles; and the *Squamata,* which include lizards and snakes. The least-known group is the *tuatara.* These lizardlike animals are found only in New Zealand. However, they are different from lizards because their eggs take 11 to 16 months to hatch, and the young tuatara take 25 years to grow to the adult size of about 20 inches and 4 pounds.

Crocodilians are closely related to dinosaurs and birds, and a complete list of all living reptiles would have to include birds. However, birds are so different from the other groups of reptiles that scientists exclude them from herpetology. Consequently, the term *reptile* means all living reptiles except birds.

The common characteristic of all reptiles except crocodilians is a heart with one ventricle. Fishes and amphibians also have a heart with one ventricle, but crocodilians, birds, and mammals have a muscular wall known as the septum dividing the lower part of the heart into left and right ventricles. The single ventricle is advantageous for reptiles. Without a ventricular septum, a reptile can vary how much blood flows from the heart and goes to the body or the lungs. This ability is known as an *intracardiac blood shunt,* and it allows reptiles to increase their body heat and reduce heat loss by moving blood between the body and lungs.

Testudinea (Turtles and Tortoises)

Turtles are easy to recognize because of their shell (Figs. 23-2 and 23-3). It encloses the animal in a bony case with openings only at the front and rear. The dorsal part of the shell is called the *carapace;* the ventral part is the *plastron.* A turtle's habitat can be judged from its appearance. Terrestrial turtles, commonly known as *tortoises,* have high, domed

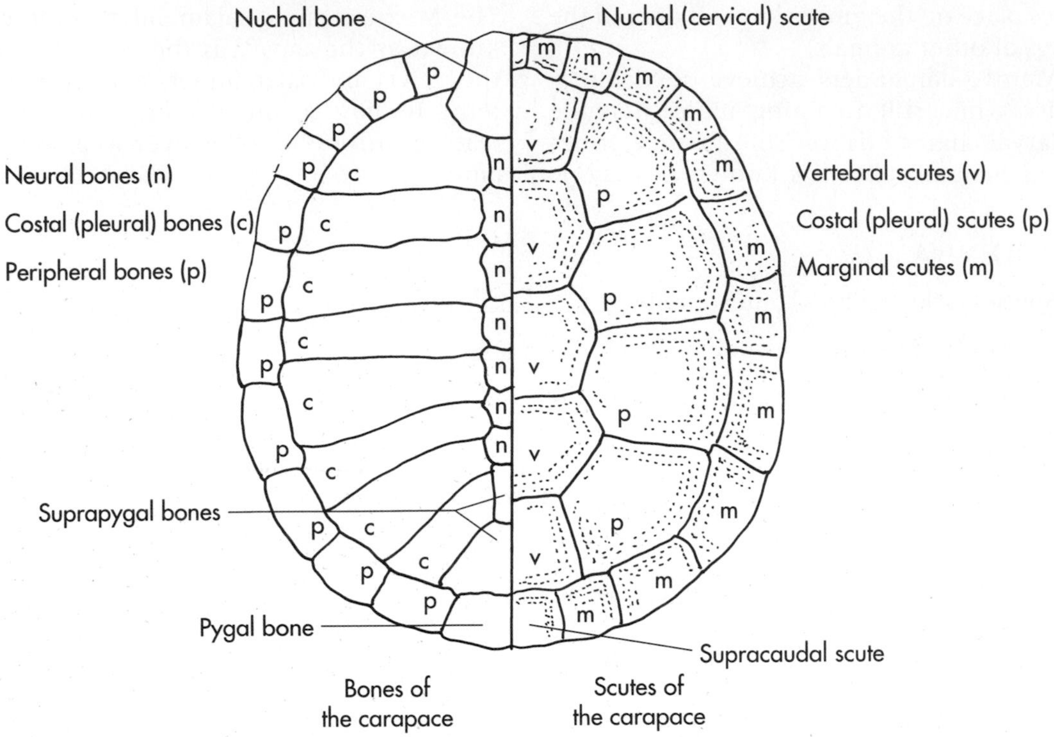
Nuchal bone
Nuchal (cervical) scute
Neural bones (n)
Costal (pleural) bones (c)
Peripheral bones (p)
Vertebral scutes (v)
Costal (pleural) scutes (p)
Marginal scutes (m)
Suprapygal bones
Pygal bone
Supracaudal scute
Bones of the carapace
Scutes of the carapace

FIG. 23-2 Dorsal view of the carapace with the scutes removed on the left side to show the underlying bones.

shells and sturdy legs. Aquatic turtles usually have webbed feet and flat shells that offer less resistance to movement in the water than do domed shells. All turtles lack teeth on the jaws. Instead they have horny ridges that cover the upper and lower jaws. In plant-eating species the outer edge of each horny ridge is serrated, making it easier to bite off sections of hard woody plants. In carnivorous turtles these horny ridges are knife-sharp and cut like shears.

Turtles lay eggs in a nest chamber, and the young develop in the eggs at a temperature corresponding to the surrounding sand or soil. The sex of most turtles, all crocodilians, and some lizards is determined by the temperature of the nest, not by genotype. This phenomenon is known as *temperature-dependent sex determination (TSD).* In most turtle species, males are produced at cooler temperatures and females in warmer ones. The opposite relationship occurs in many species of lizards exhibiting TSD: females are produced at cooler temperatures and males at higher temperatures. Crocodiles and alligators have a more complicated form of TSD: females are produced at the coolest temperatures, males at intermediate temperatures, and females again at the warmest ones.

Squamata (Lizards and Snakes)

Squamates, or scale reptiles, are the largest group of reptiles. In an evolutionary sense, snakes are specialized lizards. Furthermore, there is no scientific word describing the group that includes only lizards.

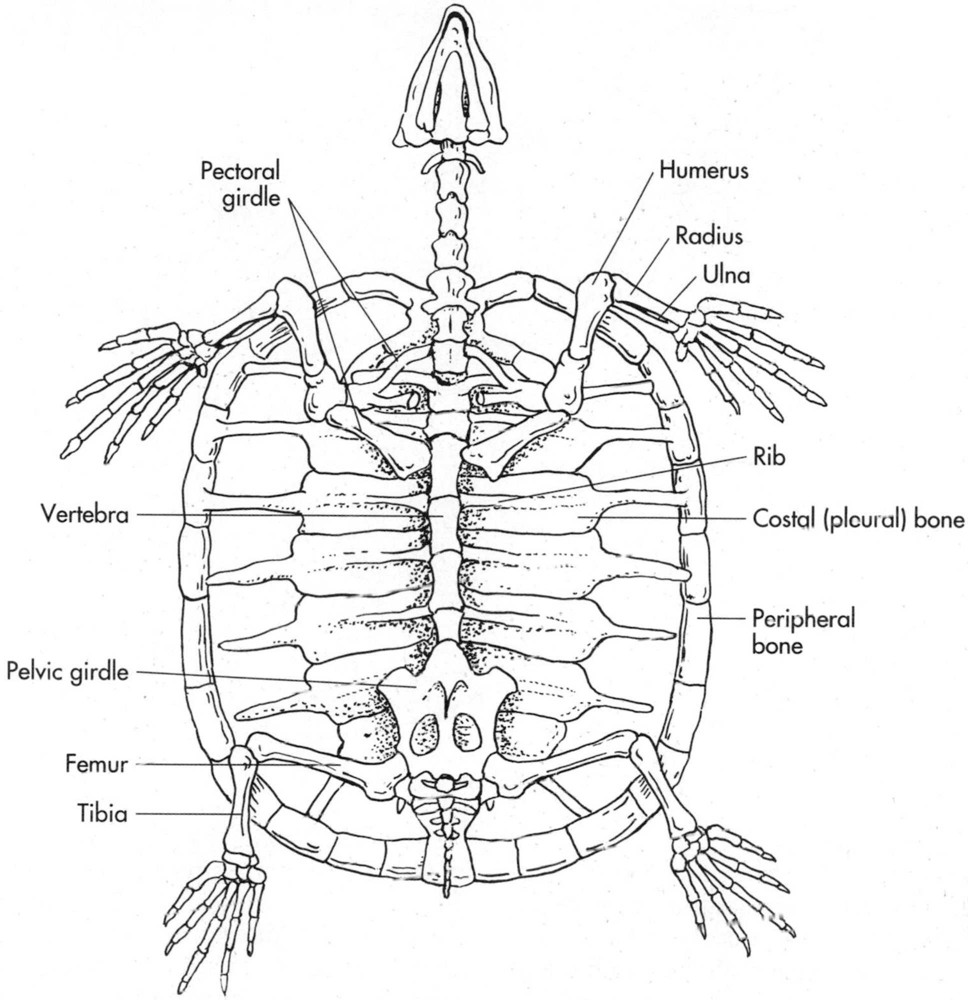
Pectoral girdle
Humerus
Radius
Ulna
Rib
Vertebra
Costal (pleural) bone
Peripheral bone
Pelvic girdle
Femur
Tibia

FIG. 23-3 Ventral view of turtle skeleton. All vertebrae except those of the neck and tail are fused into the carapace. The pectoral and pelvic girdles are enclosed within the rib cage (the pleural bones).

Lizards today are found on most continents except Antarctica and some Arctic regions (Fig. 23-4). There are almost 4300 species. During the mass extinction of dinosaurs that occurred 65 million years ago, lizards survived, but other large reptiles did not. The other surviving reptiles—turtles, crocodiles, and tuatara—have not evolved into as many different forms. Snakes evolved from lizards. Probably part of the reason for the great diversity of lizards is their small size: few living lizards are longer than 12 inches, and very few are longer than 3 feet.

Many lizards are *diurnal* and brightly colored. Snakes are more secretive and rely on scent rather than vision in their predatory and social behavior. Leglessness has evolved

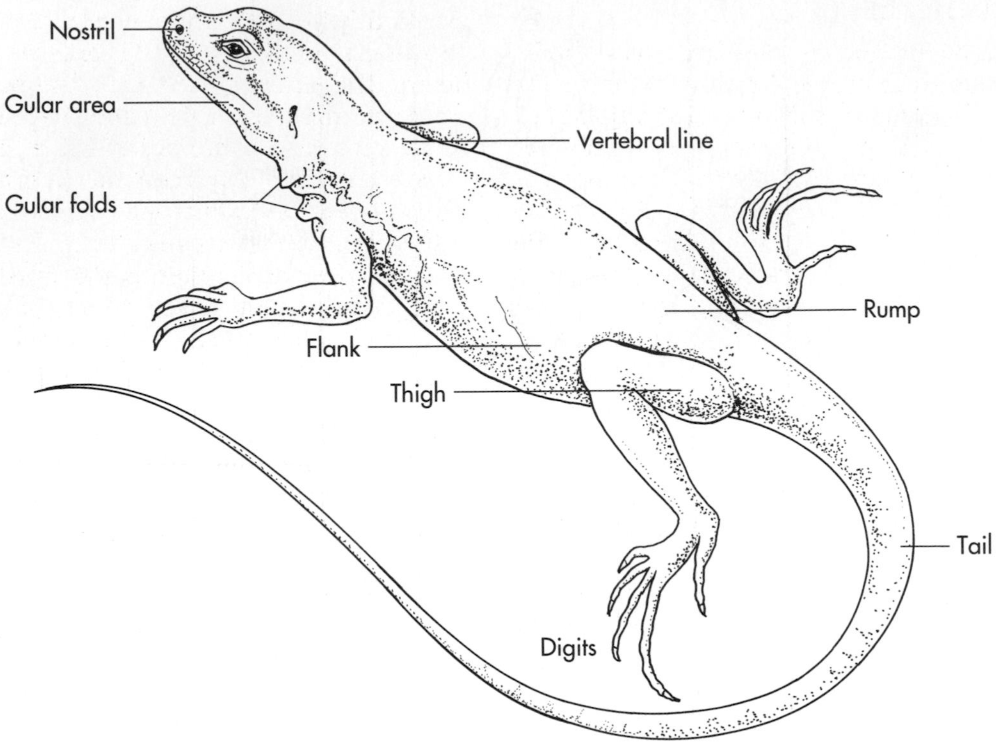
Nostril
Gular area
Vertebral line
Gular folds
Rump
Flank
Thigh
Tail
Digits

FIG. 23-4 External parts of a lizard.

often among squamates. All snakes are legless, and several lizard families are legless also. Legless squamates are generally long because they form curves along the length of their body to push against the ground during locomotion. Not all snakes are long and thin. Snakes swallow their prey whole, and the cartoon image of a snake with a lump representing a meal in its stomach is accurate. A short, thick body allows snakes to swallow large prey.

Crocodilia (Crocodiles)

Only 23 species of crocodiles, alligators, caimans, and gharials survive today, and scientists list most as endangered or threatened. The largest living crocodile is the Australian salt water crocodile, which can grow to 23 feet long and weigh 3300 pounds. The most obvious difference among crocodilians is the shape of their snout. Broad-snouted species such as the American alligator are generalized feeders and eat hard-bodied prey such as turtles, snails, and armored fish. Long-snouted species such as the Indian gharial are fish-eating experts that catch fast-moving prey with a quick sideways head movement.

Crocodiles are closely related to dinosaurs and birds. In contrast to other reptiles, crocodiles provide extensive parental care to their young. Some scientists believe that similar types of parental care were typical of dinosaurs.

Ectothermy

Amphibians and reptiles are cold-blooded animals, or *ectotherms*. In reality their blood is not cold. What is meant is that amphibians and reptiles get the energy to raise their body temperatures from outside sources, usually the sun. They do this either directly, by basking in sunlight, or indirectly, by lying on a warm surface that the sun previously heated. Until their body temperature is high enough, amphibians and reptiles cannot perform normal activities. In contrast, mammals and birds produce heat chemically by metabolizing carbohydrates, lipids, and protein from the food they eat. Mammals and birds are *endotherms*, or warm-blooded animals. Other words sometimes used to describe this difference are *poikilothermy* and *homeothermy*. As the word roots indicate, *poikilothermy* describes animals with variable temperature, and *homeothermy* refers to those that maintain a constant temperature.

Understanding ectothermy allows us to understand why the behavior, shape, physiology, and husbandry of amphibians and reptiles are different from those of birds and mammals. A lizard living in the desert has an advantage over a mammal such as a field mouse because it uses sunlight to maintain a high body temperature. In contrast, the field mouse uses metabolic heat production. Consequently, the amount of energy used by an ectotherm such as a lizard is only about one tenth the energy used by a similar-sized endotherm such as a field mouse. The difference means that the desert lizard uses far less energy per day than the field mouse. This is why amphibian and reptile owners often feed their pets only once or twice a week. Because endotherms generate heat by metabolic processes, about 98% of the energy a mammal obtains from its food is used to generate heat. Only 2% is left for producing and replacing cells and tissues. In contrast, ectotherms convert about 50% of the energy gained from eating into body tissue.

At night, when the temperature falls, the lizard's energy use also falls to about one third of its daytime rate. The field mouse also loses heat at night. However, instead of losing energy, the field mouse increases its energy use. It produces heat by metabolism to replace the heat lost to the cooling environment, and its energy consumption increases. This means that feeding an ectotherm does *not* help it deal with a cold environment. An external source of heat such as a heat lamp or electrical heating rock must always be used. Many health problems in reptiles and amphibians arise because the owners do not keep their pets warm enough.

REVIEW B

1. The name of the group of reptiles that includes living and extinct turtles is ______________ ; the group ______________________ includes lizards and snakes.
2. Terrestrial turtles are called ______________________ .
3. Two words to indicate the "cold-blooded" physiology of reptiles are ______________________ and ________________ ; the corresponding words for mammals are ________________ and ________________ .
4. The upper part of a turtle's shell is called the ______________________ ; the lower part is the ______________________ .

ORNITHOLOGY

In the first section of this chapter we looked at two types of vertebrates: reptiles and amphibians. The other vertebrates are fishes, birds, and mammals. As surprising as it may seem, birds are the closest living relatives of crocodilians among living animals. Fossil groups such as dinosaurs are more closely related to birds than are crocodilians. Some scientists claim that a complete list of living reptiles would have to include birds. However, birds are so different from other groups of reptiles that they are excluded from herpetology. The scientific study of birds is called *ornithology*. *Aviculture* refers to the hobby of raising and caring for birds.

Scientists have grouped birds for taxonomic classification into the class Aves. There are approximately 9000 bird species grouped into 24 orders. One order, the *Passeriformes* (known as *passerines* or songbirds) contains more than half the known bird species. Some examples of well-known passerines are larks, swallows, mockingbirds, finches, canaries, sparrows, starlings, and crows. The remaining 23 orders are collectively known as nonpasserines. In exotic veterinary practice the most common order of birds seen is the *Psittaciformes*. This order of birds is commonly known as *psittacines* or parrots.

External Appearance

Although birds vary in size from the tiny hummingbird to the ostrich and come in a rainbow variety of colors and fantastic array of patterns, they have a basic similarity in their body plan (Fig. 23-5). In fact birds vary far less in size and basic body structure than most other groups of animals.

The most common characteristic of a bird is the presence of feathers that make up the plumage. There are several types of feathers (Box 23-1), but the most important are *contour feathers* and *down feathers*. The contour or *flight feathers* streamline the body, reducing friction during flight or when moving on the ground or through water. Large flight feathers on the wings are known as *remiges* and are divided into *primaries* on the outer wing and *secondaries* on the inner wing (Fig. 23-5). Remiges are covered by feathers called *coverts*. When a bird flies, the wings provide lift and the tail steers. The tail feathers are known as *rectrices*. Many avian veterinarians recommend that all pet birds have their primary remiges clipped to decrease

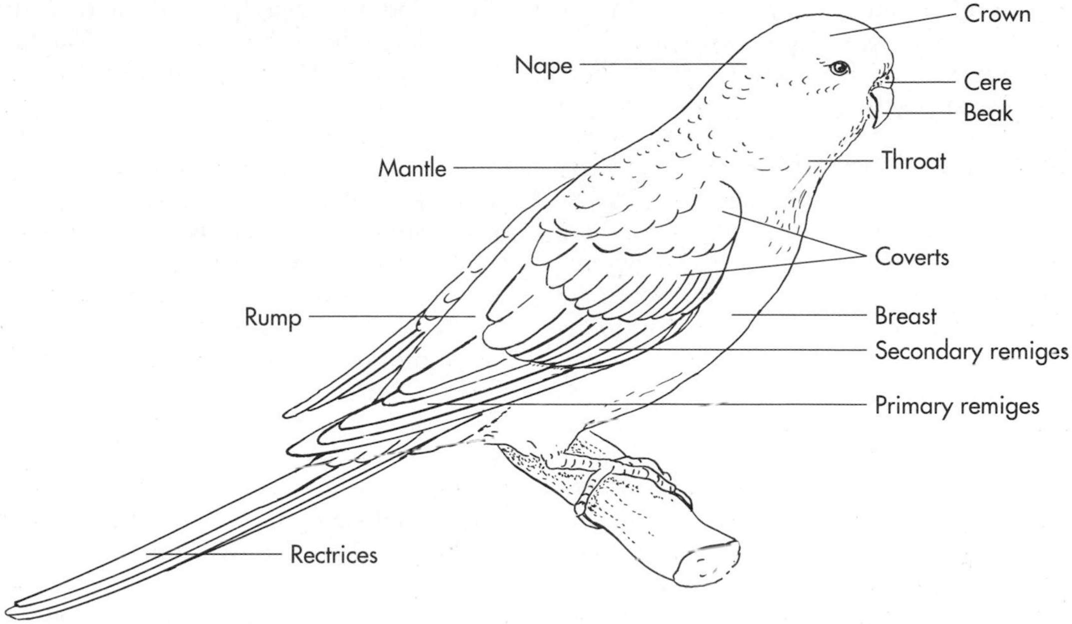
Crown
Nape
Cere
Beak
Mantle
Throat
Coverts
Rump
Breast
Secondary remiges
Primary remiges
Rectrices

FIG. 23-5 External features of a parakeet.

BOX 23-1 TYPES OF FEATHERS

contour feathers: the externally visible feathers that determine the bird's silhouette and the contours of the wings, body, and tail.

coverts: small feathers covering the bases of the longer feathers of a bird's wings or tail.

down feathers: fine, soft, fluffy feathers forming the first plumage of young birds and underlying the contour feathers in certain adult birds.

flight feathers: the strong feathers on the wings and tails of birds used in flight (also called *remiges*).

primary flight feathers: those inserting dorsally from the carpus along the carpometacarpus and phalanges.

rectrices (wreck'-trih-seez): the stiff main feathers of a bird's tail, used to control the direction of flight, singular, *rectrix* (wreck'-tricks).

remiges (rem'-ih-jeez): the large flight feathers (quills) of the wing; singular, *remex* (rem'-ex).

secondary flight feathers: those inserting dorsally along the ulna.

the potential for accidents and escape. Wing-clipping renders the bird unable to fly but still able to glide slowly to the ground without falling. It is a painless and temporary measure that must be repeated as the bird *molts*. Molting is the periodic (usually annual) shedding of feathers, which are then replaced by a new growth. Permanent surgical methods to prevent flight are called *pinioning*. The down feathers form a hidden underlayer in most adult birds and usually form the plumage of newly hatched chicks. Down feathers are important for providing warmth. In passerines the down feathers are absent, and in birds such as penguins or geese they cover the entire body surface.

Other distinctive features of a bird's external appearance are the beak and feet. The beak or bill is the horn-covered or keratinized projection of the face that forms the jaws or mouth parts. In the same way as our hands work for us, the beak functions for birds. It is used in nest building, for grooming or preening feathers, or as a weapon in combat, but its primary function is for food-gathering. Different bill shapes are adapted to eating different foods. Consider a woodpecker with a chisel-tipped bill that excavates holes in trees for nest sites and a pelican with its long bill and huge pouch, which it uses as a net to scoop fish from the water. Avian veterinarians may recommend regular beak-trimming or periodic filing (similar to fingernail filing in humans) to remove excessive flaking or correct a growth abnormality of the beak.

Variations are also present in the legs and feet. Birds that spend most of their time in trees have short, sturdy legs for climbing and perching, whereas ground-dwelling birds such as ostriches have long legs adapted to walking and running. Some birds, especially those living in cold climates, have feathered legs and even feathered toes. No bird has more than four toes; some have three, and the ostrich has only two. In most species, three toes point forward and the first toe is turned backward. However in parrots two toes point forward and two toes are turned backward. Other modifications of the feet are commonly seen in swimming species. Birds such as ducks and geese have webbed toes that function as paddles in the water. Overgrowth of the nails of the toes is very common in captive birds, and periodic nail trims are necessary in many pet birds.

The skeleton of a bird is highly modified to support powered flight (Fig. 23-6). The bones of the arm and hand support the wing, and the digits are fused to form a single large bone that supports the main flight feathers. Most birds have a large sternum or breastbone with a prominent *keel,* known as the *carina*. The keel provides an important surface area for attachment of the large pectoral or breast muscles, which supply power to the wings. Ostriches, emus, and similar ground-dwelling birds known as *ratites* do not have a keel because their wings are reduced in size and function. (The word *ratite* comes from the Latin word for raft, a boat without a keel.) The thoracic girdle in birds is formed from the coracoid bone, clavicle, and scapula. It has to be strong because it must support the bird's entire body weight when flying. The clavicles fuse to form the *furcula,* or wishbone. The furcula functions as a spacer bar to keep the wings apart. The bones of many birds are lightened by widespread *pneumatization,* a state in which the bones are hollow and contain *air sacs*. Although the bones of birds are hollow, they are strong structurally. Generally the bones are thin-walled and hollow but elaborately supported by fine internal bony cross-sections. This intricate bone pattern provides both lightness and strength that are essential for flight.

Internal Organs

All reptiles, except crocodilians, have a heart with a single ventricle, as do fishes and amphibians. Crocodilians, birds, and mammals have a solid septum or partition that divides the ventricle into left and right compartments. Consequently, the heart is four-chambered, although the arrangement is different anatomically from the four-chambered heart of mammals. Migratory birds that fly long distances have a larger heart than do birds that fly only short distances or do not fly at all.

Like mammals, birds are homeothermic.

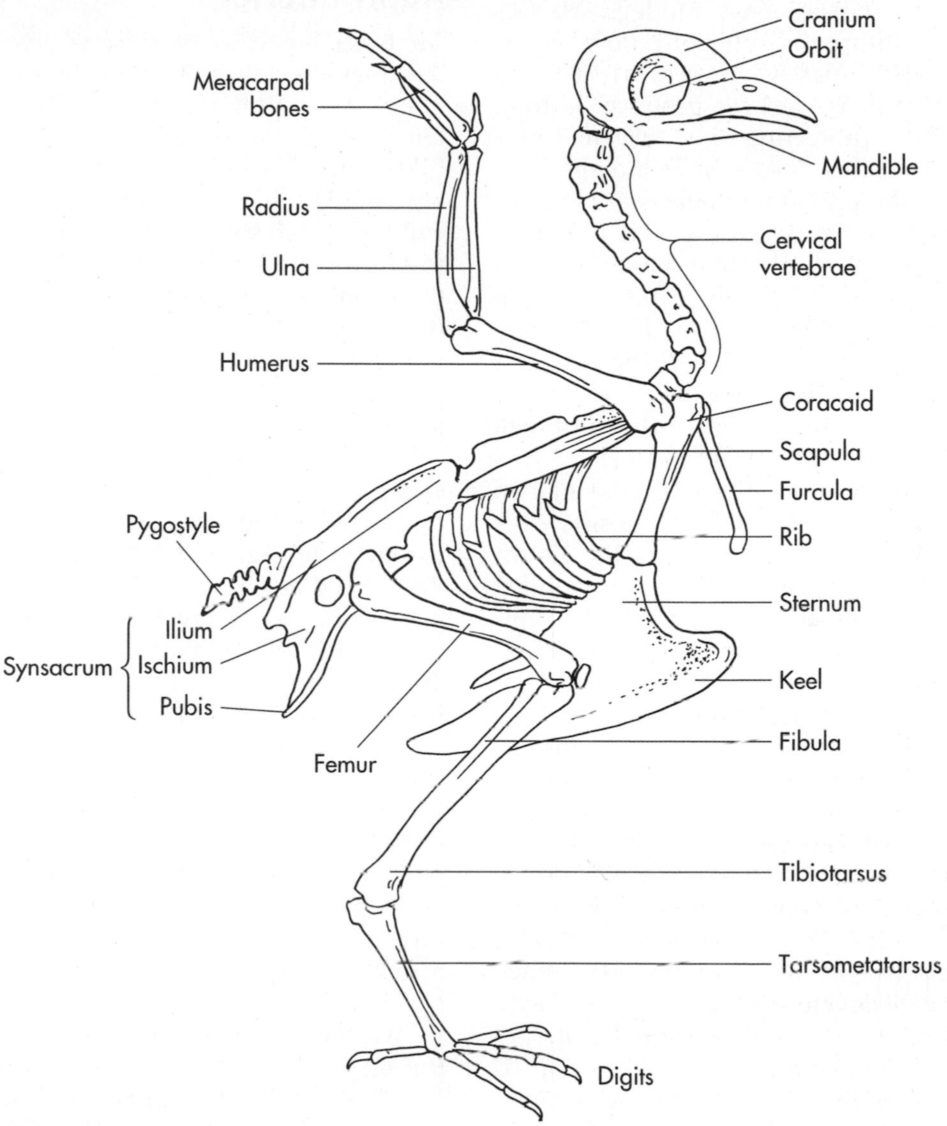
Cranium
Orbit
Metacarpal bones
Mandible
Radius
Ulna
Cervical vertebrae
Humerus
Coracaid
Scapula
Furcula
Pygostyle
Rib
Sternum
Ilium
Synsacrum
Ischium
Pubis
Keel
Fibula
Femur
Tibiotarsus
Tarsometatarsus
Digits

FIG. 23-6 Bird skeleton.

Although this ability to keep body temperature above the surroundings was achieved independently by the two groups during evolution, the physiology of thermoregulation in mammals and birds is similar.

Birds have a specialized respiratory system. They have small lungs that make up only 2% of the body. Connected to the lungs and found in various parts of the body are well-developed air sacs that may add up to 20% of the body volume. Most birds have 9 air sacs, but the number varies from 6 to 12 in different species. The abdominal and interclavicular air sacs are connected directly to the bones of the wings and legs. Air sacs allow a continuous, efficient flow of air through the lungs. They remove the potentially lethal body heat produced during flight while protecting the delicate internal organs. Birds do not have a diaphragm and rely on pressure changes in the air sacs (compared with atmospheric pressure) to move air through their nonexpansible lungs. Unlike in mammals, expiration is an active process in birds that requires contraction of the skeletal muscles of the ribs. It is important when holding a bird to allow the sternum to move freely, or the bird will suffocate.

The digestive tract of a bird is similar to that of other vertebrates. It consists of a coiled tube or gut extending from the mouth to the anus. Although the digestive tract organs are physiologically and anatomically similar to those of mammals, their names are different. Food passes from the mouth into the *gullet* (esophagus) and then to the *crop*. The crop is a thin-walled distensible pocket of the gullet in which food is stored for subsequent digestion or feeding of the young by regurgitation. In grain-eating and flesh-eating birds the crop is well developed, but it is absent in some insect-eating birds. Together the *proventriculus* and the *ventriculus* (or *gizzard*) make up the stomach and are well developed in grain-eating birds. From the gizzard, food passes to the duodenum and intestines, where digestion is completed before waste is excreted through the anus.

Birds have no urinary bladder, and like reptiles they do not produce urine. Nitrogenous wastes are excreted as *urea,* a semisolid, white, pastelike material, after water has been absorbed in the *cloaca*. The cloaca is a common opening through which the products of the digestive, excretory, and reproductive systems are passed.

Reproduction

All birds lay eggs, within which embryo development takes place. As in most vertebrates, the adult male has testes and the female has ovaries, although in nearly all birds, only the left ovary is functional. During copulation the cloaca of both sexes is everted so that sperm can transfer from male to female. However, in some birds such as ducks and ostriches, part of the male's cloaca is modified to form a penis. Fertilization of released ova takes place in the upper oviduct. As each egg passes along the oviduct, layers of albumin are deposited on it. Egg calcification, or the process of making the shell hard, occurs in the uterus. Pigment is also added in the uterus. The egg then passes through the vagina and cloaca and is deposited or laid into the nest.

For embryonic development to occur the egg must be kept at the correct temperature. This usually occurs through contact with the parent's body. The adults of many birds develop *brood patches,* areas without feathers supplied prolifically with blood vessels. *Brood* is an avian term meaning offspring or progeny. The parent bird settles on the nest so that its brood patch covers the eggs. King and emperor penguins lay only a single egg, incubated on top of their feet and covered by a muscular fold of abdominal skin. This is because these birds breed during the Antarctic winter; the males incubate the eggs for the 62 to 67 days of the harsh winter. The number of eggs a bird incubates is known as the *clutch*. With regular changeovers of the parents or short breaks away for feeding, the eggs are incubated until the chicks hatch. Incubation periods vary, from 80 days for an albatross to 10 days for some small passerines. Some birds such as cuckoos do not incubate their own eggs but parasitize other birds by laying their eggs in other birds' nests.

Parrots

The birds seen most often in exotic veterinary practice are parrots. Common pet parrots include parakeets, lovebirds, cockatiels, lorikeets, cockatoos, amazon parrots, conures, rosellas, and macaws. The small Australian parakeet, the *budgerigar* (the word is a mispronunciation of the word *gidjirrigaa,* from Gamilarraay, an Australian aboriginal language), is the most popular and ubiquitous member of the psittacines.

Parrots generally are easy to recognize because of the brilliant colors in their plumage. Other distinguishing features are the parrot's foot (two toes point forward and two toes turn backward) and the short, blunt beak with a downward-curved upper beak over a broad, straight lower beak. This design allows parrots to crush seeds and nuts that make up their diet. Parrots are famous for their ability to talk. This talent is actually the ability to mimic words or phrases. Parrots also mimic the sounds around them, and parrots kept in veterinary clinics often learn to meow, bark, or make guinea pig squeals. Despite their inclination for *mimicry,* the natural call-notes of parrots often are harsh squawks. Larger species are raucous and smaller species high-pitched.

In the wild, parrots are extremely social and spend their entire lives with a mate or in a flock. Many species are increasingly endangered in their natural habitat, and their importation is governed by strict laws. Most parrots sold as pets have been hand-raised as chicks and are very tame, having no fear of humans. Unfortunately, when pet parrots are confined and denied human or avian companionship and amusement, they develop behavior problems such as feather-plucking and self-mutilation. Behavioral disorders are one of the most common complaints for parrots seen in an exotic veterinary practice.

Diseases

Diseases of the crop are common in avian clinical practice. *Stasis,* or impairment of the normal motility and emptying of the crop, is common in juvenile psittacines. Baby bird formula that remains in the crop for prolonged periods becomes rancid from fungal and bacterial growth, a condition called *sour crop*. Bacterial and mycotic overgrowth in the crop result in an inflammation, called *ingluvitis*.

Chlamydiosis in birds is caused by the intracellular bacteria *Chlamydia psittaci.* The disease is also known as *parrot fever*. *C. psittaci* can infect many other animals, including mammals, reptiles, insects, and humans. The infection in people is called *psittacosis* or *ornithosis* and causes an influenzalike syndrome characterized by fever, headache, and myalgia.

Bacterial and fungal diseases in birds usually are secondary to stress, malnutrition, or other predisposing factors. The viral disease most frightening to aviculturists is *Pacheco's disease,* caused by an avian herpesvirus. Pacheco's disease has been known to kill as many as 7000 birds in one outbreak. Clinical signs may be nonspecific, with death occurring in less than 24 hours. Prevention of Pacheco's disease depends on vaccination and avoiding exposure.

REVIEW C

1. The scientific study of birds is ______________________.
2. Common songbirds are collectively called ______________________; parrots and similar birds are called ______________________.
3. The large flight feathers on the wings of birds are also called ______________________.
4. The periodic loss of a bird's feathers is called ______________________.
5. A surgical procedure that permanently prevents a bird from flying is called ______________.
6. The space in the hollow bones of birds contains ______________________.
7. *Gullet* is another name for ______________________.
8. The thin-walled pocket of the gullet used for food accumulation is the ________________.
9. The stomach of birds is divided into two parts, the ______________ and the ____________.
10. The digestive, excretory, and reproductive systems of birds terminate together in the ______________________.
11. Inflammation of the crop of birds is called ______________________.

WILDLIFE SCIENCE

There are many exotic animals that are inappropriate as pets. Animals like monkeys and big cats, for example, are better kept in zoos or wildlife centers. As humans expand their space, they encroach on the habitat of many wild species. Some of these animals may become endangered or extinct, and some end up in captivity. Still others become the focus of individuals intent on protecting their habitat. Managing wildlife has become a science of its own.

In the zoo world, the keepers have the most contact with the animals, but their relationship with the animals at the zoo is far different from the relationship they enjoy with their pets at home. Keepers work closely with these animals, even though they may have to avoid physical contact, to ensure that the animal is thriving in their exhibit.

Thriving is not just surviving. Animals that are not adapting well may show a range of signs. An obvious one is *stereotypic behavior,* in which boredom causes an animal to do repetitive actions such as pacing the perimeter of its enclosure for hours without interruption. Other symptoms are less obvious: the animal is not appropriately responsive, is failing to reproduce, or is not caring for its young. In the wild any animal showing weakness invites attention from predators. Animals instinctively know this, so they mask their symptoms when ill or injured. Environmental enrichment is used to reduce their stress and give them opportunities to do what they might do in the wild. This includes foraging or building their own shelters or nests from materials provided by the keeper. Other enrichment methods, such as hiding food items in an elaborate puzzle for primates, are used to challenge animals mentally.

Animals used in zoos and aquariums are

protected by the federal Animal Welfare Act (AWA), as described in Chapter 22. This act regulates the use of nonhuman primates and other mammals in zoos, circuses, and other exhibits. It mandates that attention be given to the psychological well-being of nonhuman primates. Each zoo must have its own Institutional Animal Care and Use Committee (IACUC) to oversee the care of animals and ensure that federal regulations are followed.

Organizations such as the *American Zoological Association (AZA)* have sought to bring uniformity to the standard of management and veterinary care at zoos by establishing a set of criteria and inspecting facilities before granting accreditation. Part of the cooperative standard for zoos and aquariums as overseen by the AZA is the need to share information. One of the ways in which information is shared between institutions is through the *International Species Inventory System (ISIS),* which gathers information such as blood count and chemistry values from participating facilities worldwide to build a database of "normal" traits for a given species. Although veterinarians and technicians have many references to what is normal for domestic animals, no such database exists for most wild species. The sharing of information via ISIS allows everyone to access the same information. *Species Survival Programs (SSPs)* exist to keep track of the management and breeding of many species, especially endangered animals who are losing their natural habitat and have become dependent on successful breeding in the captive environment. The SSP committees identify every representative of such species in captivity worldwide and painstakingly chart their lineage so that breeding decisions are based on creating or maintaining the best genetic diversity of each species.

Wildlife rehabilitators are people who work with wild animals that are ill, injured, or abandoned and are unable to fend for themselves. Rehabilitators face the daunting task of nursing and nurturing these animals through a recovery period and then returning them to the wild. Wildlife rehabilitation is a highly regulated activity, and rehabilitators must have the required permits and licenses to do their work. They must avoid the risk of *imprinting* on young animals. When this happens the animal considers the rehabilitator one of its own, and its chances of returning successfully to the wild are greatly reduced.

REVIEW D

1. A caged lion that paces back and forth constantly is demonstrating ____________________ behavior.
2. Providing food to a monkey in a way that mimics natural food gathering is a form of ____________________ .
3. The psychological well-being of wild animals in exhibits is mandated in the United States through the federal government by the ____________________ .
4. The national accrediting organization for zoos and aquariums in the United States is the ____________________ .
5. People who are licensed to care for injured wild animals are called ____________________ .

Chapter 23 Answers

Review A

1. invertebrates
2. herpetology
3. anurans
4. metamorphosis, neoteny
5. tail

Review B

1. Testudinea, Squamata
2. tortoises
3. ectothermy, poikilothermy, endothermy, homeothermy
4. carapace, plastron

Review C

1. ornithology
2. passerines, psittacines
3. remiges
4. molting
5. pinioning
6. air sacs
7. esophagus
8. crop
9. proventriculus, ventriculus (gizzard)
10. cloaca
11. ingluvitis

Review D

1. stereotypic
2. environmental (or psychological) enrichment
3. Animal Welfare Act
4. American Zoological Association (AZA)
5. wildlife rehabilitators

Chapter 23 EXERCISES

EXOTIC ANIMALS

Exercise 1: Match the description in the left column with its name in the right column by placing the appropriate letter in the blank space provided.

_____	1. Amphibians with tails	A. Anurans
_____	2. Frogs and toads	B. *Bufo*
_____	3. Rarely seen amphibian group	C. Caecilians
_____	4. Genus of frogs	D. Caudates
_____	5. Genus of toads	E. Invertebrates
_____	6. Turtles and tortoises	F. Passeriformes
_____	7. Lizards and snakes	G. Psittaciformes
_____	8. Songbird order	H. *Rana*
_____	9. Order containing parrots	I. Squamata
_____	10. Lacking a backbone	J. Testudinea

Exercise 2: Match the description in the left column with its name in the right column by placing the appropriate letter in the blank space provided.

_____	1. A change in form	A. Aviculture
_____	2. Avian progeny	B. Brood
_____	3. Body heat from outside source	C. Coverts
_____	4. Constant body temperature	D. Ectothermy
_____	5. Covering feathers	E. Endothermy
_____	6. Large flight feathers	F. Gills
_____	7. Metabolism provides body heat	G. Gizzard
_____	8. Nitrogenous waste	H. Homeothermy
_____	9. Respiratory organ of tadpoles	I. Metamorphosis
_____	10. Tail feathers	J. Poikilothermy
_____	11. The hobby of raising birds	K. Rectrices
_____	12. Variable body temperature	L. Remiges
_____	13. Ventriculus	M. Urea

Exercise 3: Fill in the blanks.

1. The three main groups of amphibians are ________________, ________________, and ________________.
2. The lizardlike reptile group found only in New Zealand is the ________________.
3. All reptiles have a heart with only one ventricle except the ________________, which have a septum dividing it into left and right sides. Reptiles lacking the septum can vary the proportion of blood pumped to the body or the lungs, an ability called ________________.
4. Terrestrial turtles are commonly called ________________.
5. In most turtles the sex of offspring is determined by a nongenetic process called ________________.
6. The externally visible feathers that determine a bird's silhouette are the ________________ feathers.
7. *Remiges* is another word for ________________ feathers, and rectrices are the ________________ feathers.
8. ________________ veterinarians are those who specialize in diseases of birds.
9. The maximum number of toes normally found on the foot of any bird species is ________________.
10. The incubation of bird eggs is facilitated by specialized featherless areas of skin called ________________.
11. The number of eggs that a bird incubates at a given time is called the ________________.
12. Information is shared between zoological institutions by means of the ________________; endangered species can be kept track of through the ________________.
13. When an injured wild animal learns to accept a wildlife rehabilitator as one of its own, the process is called ________________.
14. A disease of humans caused by *Chlamydia psittaci* is ________________.
15. Pacheco's disease is caused by an avian ________________.

CHAPTER 23 PUZZLE

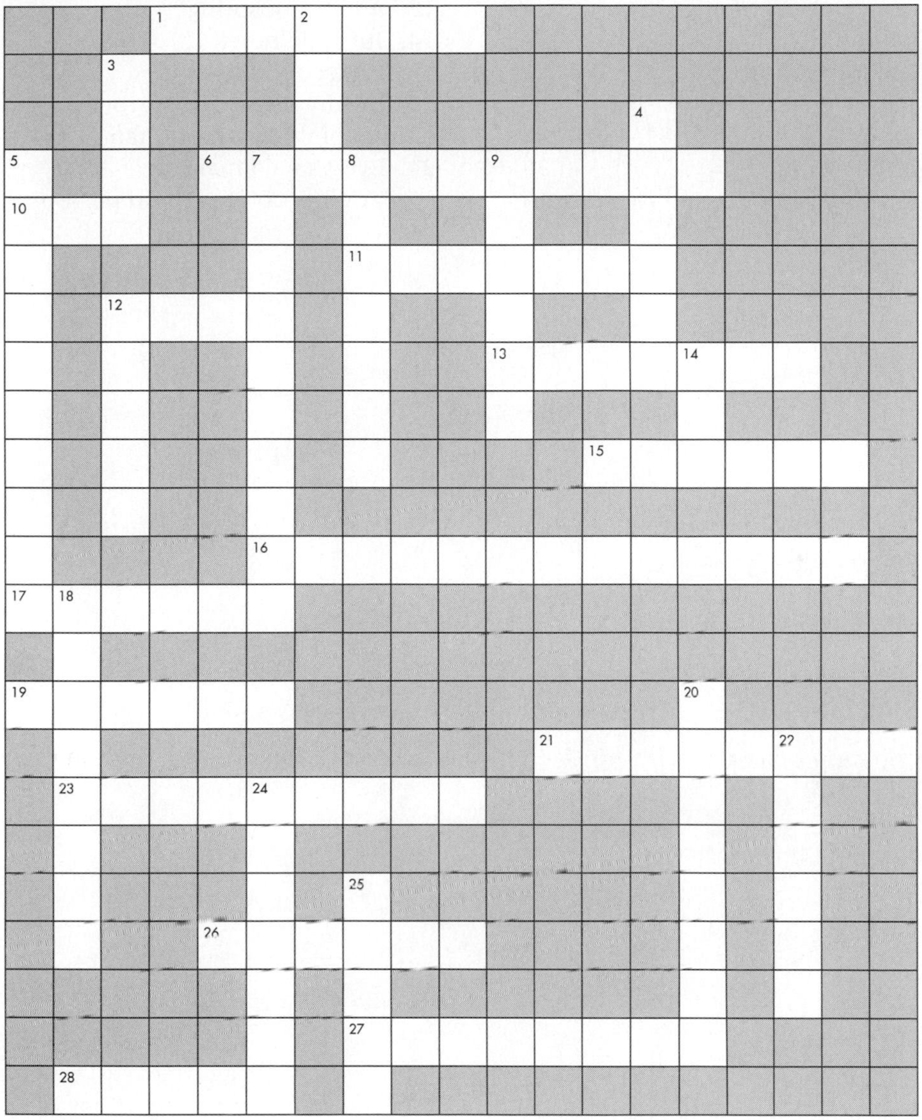
1
2
3
4
5
6
7
8
9
10
11
12
13
14
15
16
17
18
19
20
21
22
23
24
25
26
27
28

ACROSS CLUES

1. Amphibians with tails
6. Gizzard
10. Zoo group
11. Active during daytime
12. Toad
13. Retention of juvenile characteristics
15. Spasms and tremors
16. Change
17. On snakes but not on newts
19. Pregnant
21. Lizards and snakes
23. Procedure that prevents flying
26. Where egg meets the day

27. When frogs embrace
28. Useful under water

DOWN CLUES

2. Feathers for warmth
3. Frog
4. Esophagus
5. Songbirds
7. Animals that need the sun for warmth
8. Larval form
9. Keel
12. A bird's offspring
14. Juvenile newt
18. Protective shell
20. Deadly disease of parrots
22. Amphibian with no tail
24. Eye-shaped marking
25. Brightly colored, loud parrot

Chapter 23 Answers

Exercise 1

1. D
2. A
3. C
4. H
5. B
6. J
7. I
8. F
9. G
10. E

Exercise 2

1. I
2. B
3. D
4. H
5. C
6. L
7. E
8. M
9. F
10. K
11. A
12. J
13. G

Exercise 3

1. caudates, anurans, caecilians
2. tuatara
3. crocodilians, intracardiac blood shunt
4. tortoises
5. temperature-dependent sex determination
6. contour
7. flight, tail
8. Avian
9. four
10. brood patches
11. clutch
12. International Species Inventory System (ISIS), Species Survival Program (SSP)
13. imprinting
14. psittacosis (or ornithosis)
15. herpesvirus

ANSWERS: CHAPTER 23 PUZZLE

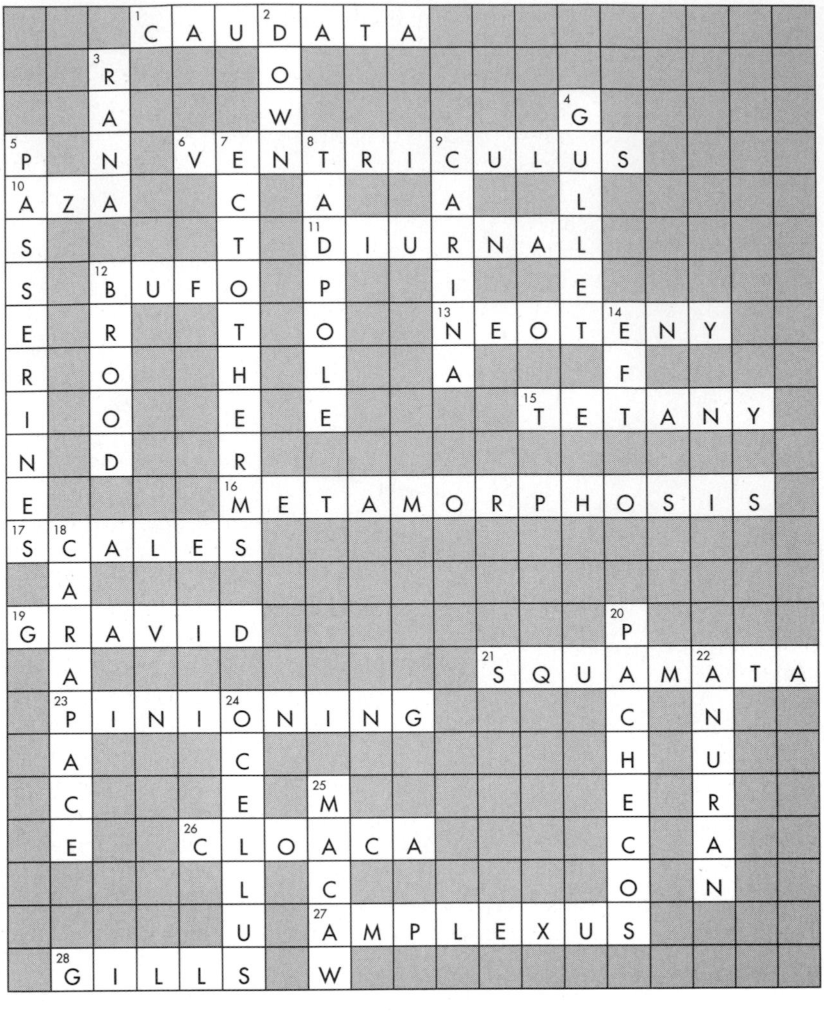
1 CAUDATA
2 DOW
3 RANA
4 GULLET
5 PASSERINE
6 VENTRICULUS
7 ECTOTHERMS
8 TADPOLE
9 CARINA
10 AZA
11 DIURNAL
12 BUFO
12 BROOD
13 NEOTENY
14 EFT
15 TETANY
16 METAMORPHOSIS
17 SCALES
18 CARAPACE
19 GRAVID
20 PACHECOS
21 SQUAMATA
22 ANURAN
23 PINIONING
23 PACE
24 OCELLUS
25 MACAW
26 CLOACA
27 AMPLEXUS
28 GILLS

GLOSSARY

air sacs: a part of the respiratory apparatus of birds consisting of a series of membrane-bound spaces located in the body cavity and bones and connecting with the lungs.

airsacculitis: inflammation of the air sacs.

American Zoological Association (AZA): international organization that promotes improvement and uniformity in the management of all species in zoological and aquarium settings.

amphibian: a cold-blooded, smooth-skinned vertebrate of the class Amphibia that characteristically hatches as an aquatic larva with gills and then transforms into an adult with air-breathing lungs. Includes frogs, toads, salamanders, and newts.

amplexus: the copulatory embrace of frogs and toads, during which the male fertilizes the eggs as they are released by the female.

anurans: living frogs and toads. With their extinct amphibian relatives they form a group of amphibians known as Salientia.

aspergillosis (ass-per-jill-oh'-sis): a disease caused by the fungus Aspergillus.

aviculture: the rearing of caged birds.

axolotl (ax'-oh-lott-ul): salamanders of the genus *Ambystoma,* which retain external gills and attain sexual maturity without undergoing metamorphosis.

brood: a group of young birds hatched at one time and cared for by the same mother.

brood patches: in birds, patches of featherless skin on the undersurface of the body that become highly vascular during brooding, facilitating the transfer of heat from the bird to the eggs.

budgerigar (budge'-uh-ree-gar): a parakeet *(Melopsittacus undulatus)* native to Australia and having green, yellow, or blue plumage (commonly called budgies).

Bufo: a genus of amphibians that includes toads.

bumblefoot: infection of the ball of the foot of birds, usually caused by *Staphylococcus* species.

Caecilia (see-sill'-ee-ah): the least known of the three orders of amphibians, consisting mostly of burrowing, wormlike forms.

carapace (kare'-uh-pace): the dorsal shell of turtles and tortoises.

carina: the large ventrally directed surface of a bird's sternum, the site of attachment of the major muscles of flight (also called *keel*).

Caudata (kow-dot'-uh): one of the three orders of amphibians, characterized primarily by having a tail; it includes salamanders and newts. *Caudata* is sometimes used interchangeably with *Urodela.* However, Urodela generally encompasses only living forms, whereas Caudata includes both living and fossil forms.

caudate (kow'-date): having a tail; used to refer collectively to salamanders and other tailed amphibians, as opposed to anurans, which lack tails.

cere: in budgerigars, the soft basal part of the beak above the nostril, blue in the male and brown in the female.

Chelonia: one of the four orders of reptiles; includes turtles and tortoises. Usually used to refer only to living forms (see Testudinea).

chelonian: belonging to the order Chelonia; turtles and tortoises.

Chlamydia psittaci (klam-id'-ee-uh sit'-uh-sigh): the causative agent of several diseases in many species, including psittacosis in birds and humans.

chlamydiosis (klam-id-ee-oh'-sis): any disease or infection caused by *Chlamydia psittaci,* including psittacosis, ornithosis, and parrot fever.

cloaca (klo-a'-ka): the compartment into which the products of the intestinal, genital, and urinary tracts pass before leaving the body. Present in birds, amphibians, and reptiles.

clutch: a setting of eggs.

cockatiel (kock'-uh-teel): a small crested Australian parrot *(Nymphicus hollandicus)* having gray and yellow plumage.

crest: a longitudinal ridge on the dorsal surface of the body formed by enlarged scales or a fold of skin.

Crocodilia: the order of reptiles that includes alligators, crocodiles, and others.

crop: a saccular diverticulum of the esophagus before it enters the thorax, present in birds.

diurnal (die-ur'-null): active during the daytime rather than at night.

dorsal gland crest: area of concentration of skin glands in certain amphibians.
ectotherm (eck'-toe-therm): an animal whose body temperature varies with that of its environment (same as *poikilotherm*).
eft: an immature newt, especially the juvenile red-spotted newt, which is called a red eft.
egg-bound: a disease of caged birds in which the female is unable to pass a mature egg.
endotherm: an organism that generates heat to maintain a constant body temperature, typically above the temperature of its surroundings (also called *homeotherm*).
eye mask: anatomical landmark produced by skin coloration; important in species identification.
femoral pores: in reptiles, pores occurring on the underside of the hind legs or preanal region; their size is an important sex difference in many lizards (*see pores*).
flank: the side of the body between the last rib and the ilium.
fledge: to grow the plumage necessary for flight.
fledgling: a young bird that is not fully feathered.
furcula: the united clavicles in birds (also called wishbone).
gills: the respiratory organ of aquatic animals, consisting of vascular membranes across which dissolved gases are exchanged.
gizzard: the muscular stomach of birds, often containing ingested grit and separated from the more cranial proventriculus by a constriction (also called *ventriculus*).
granular scales: convex scales formed like granules.
gravid: carrying developing young or eggs.
gular (goo'-lar): relating to the throat, as in *gular fold* or *gular area.*
gullet: esophagus.
hatchling: a newly hatched bird, amphibian, fish, or reptile.
herpetology: the study of reptiles and amphibians.
homeotherm (home'-ee-oh-therm): an organism that generates heat to maintain a constant body temperature, typically above the temperature of its surroundings (also called *endotherm*).
imprinting: a rapid learning process by which a newly hatched bird or other animal establishes a behavioral pattern of recognition and attraction to another animal, usually its parent.
ingluvitis (in-glue-vyte'-iss): inflammation of the crop.
International Species inventory System (ISIS): international inventory system on all species in captivity that enables zoos and wildlife centers worldwide to share information such as normal blood values.
intracardiac blood shunt: in reptiles, the ability to vary the proportion of blood flow from the ventricle that goes to either the lungs or the body.
invertebrate: an animal lacking a backbone or spinal column.
jowl: the flesh under the lower jaw or between the jaw and the ear.
keel: the large ventrally directed surface of a bird's sternum, the site of attachment of the major muscles of flight (also called *carina*).
macaws: large, brightly colored, long-tailed parrots of the genera *Ara* and *Anodorhynchus,* native to Central and South America.
metamorphosis: a change in the form of an animal during normal development after the embryonic stage, exemplified in amphibians by the changing of a tadpole into a frog.
mimicry: imitation by an animal of the sound, appearance, or behavior of another animal or structure.
molt: the physiological shedding of part or all of the integument, such as feathers, hair, cuticle, or skin, which is then replaced by a new growth. Includes the shedding of the skin by reptiles, of hair by many species, and of feathers by birds.
mucronate: ending abruptly in a sharp point, as mucronate feathers or mucronate scales.
nape: the back of the neck, immediately caudal to the head. Also called nucha.
neoteny (nee-ott'-en-nee): retention of juvenile characteristics in the adults of a species, as in certain amphibians.
Newcastle disease: an infectious, highly contagious disease of birds, and occasionally of humans, caused by a paramyxovirus.
newt: common name for several species of small, slender, brightly colored amphibians of the order Caudata.
nuchal (new'-kull): relating to the neck, as in *nuchal crest.*

ocellus (oh-sell'-us): a marking that resembles an eye, as on the tail feathers of a male peacock (plural *ocelli*).
ornithology: the branch of zoology that deals with the study of birds.
ornithosis: contagious, zoonotic disease of psittacine birds caused by *Chlamydia psittaci.*
oviparous (oh-vip'-ah-russ): producing eggs in which the embryo develops outside the maternal body, as in birds, amphibians, and most reptiles.
ovoviviparous (oh-vo-vie-vi'-pah-russ): producing eggs that develop and hatch within the female's body without obtaining nourishment from it, as in certain reptiles.
Pacheco's disease: a disease of parrots caused by a herpes virus and characterized by weakness, diarrhea, and focal necrosis of the liver and spleen.
parakeet: small parrots with long tails, in the family Psittacidae, and including the budgerigar.
parasitism: infestation with internal or external parasites.
parrot fever: infection with *Chlamydia psittaci.*
Passeriformes: the order of birds that includes perching birds and songbirds, including finches, sparrows, and canaries.
passerine: adjective referring to members of the order Passeriformes.
pinioning: a permanent alteration of a bird to prevent its flying. A common method is amputation of one distal wing at the carpus.
plastron: the ventral part of the shell of a turtle.
pneumatization (new-mat-tis-zay'-shun): the formation of air cavities in tissue.
poikilotherm (poy'-kill-oh-therm): an animal whose body temperature varies with that of its environment (same as *ectotherm*).
pores: in reptiles, small pits occupying part or all of a single scale, usually filled with a solid excrescence that may protrude as a small nodule *(see femoral pores).*
proventriculus (pro-ven-trick'-you-luss): the glandular stomach of birds, situated between the crop and the gizzard.
Psittaciformes: the order of birds that includes parrots and parakeets.
psittacine (sit'-uh-seen): adjective referring to members of the order Psittaciformes.
psittacosis: contagious, zoonotic disease of psittacine birds caused by *Chlamydia psittaci.*
pygostyle (pidge'-oh-style): in birds, the fused last four to eight spinal vertebrae to which the tail feathers are attached.
Rana: a genus of amphibians that includes frogs.
ratite: a running bird with a flat sternum and strong muscular legs, typified by ostriches and emus.
renal portal system: a system present in amphibians, reptiles, and birds in which part of the blood supply to the kidney comes from the hind limbs via veins that terminate in peritubular capillaries, where it is mixed with arteriolar blood coming from the glomeruli.
reptile: a cold-blooded, usually egg-laying vertebrate of the class Reptilia, having an external covering of scales or horny plates and breathing by means of lungs. Includes snakes, lizards, crocodiles, turtles, and dinosaurs.
sacral hump: external landmark produced by pelvic bones of frogs and toads.
salamander: common name for several species of lizardlike amphibians of the order Urodela.
Salientian: an amphibian of the order Salientia, which includes frogs, toads, and extinct forms *(see Anuran).*
salmonellosis: a highly contagious disease of all animal species caused by bacteria of the genus *Salmonella.* An important zoonosis, symptoms may include acute or chronic enteritis, septicemia, and abortion.
scales: small, platelike epidermal structures that form the external covering of fishes and reptiles.
scute: one of the thick epidermal plates on the head of snakes or the shell of tortoises and turtles (also called *scutum*).
snout-vent length (SVL): distance from the tip of the snout to the vent.
sour crop: stasis and distension of the crop with microbial overgrowth.
Species Survival Program (SSP): international organization that oversees endangered species in captivity and determines appropriate management and breeding of these species to preserve the highest level of genetic diversity.
spine: an acute projecting scale.
Squamata (skwa-mott'-tah): the order of reptiles that

includes lizards and snakes. (*Squama* is Latin for "scale.")

stasis: a stoppage or reduced flow, as with a body fluid or intestinal contents.

stereotypic behavior: excessive repetition or lack of variation of an animal's movements (also called *stereotypy*).

synsacrum (sin-sake'-rum): the fused lumbar and sacral vertebrae and pelvic girdle of birds.

tadpole: the limbless aquatic larva of a frog or toad, having gills and a long tail. As the tadpole approaches the adult stage, legs and lungs develop and the tail gradually disappears (also called *pollywog*).

tarsometatarsus: in birds, a compound bone between the tibia and the toes, formed by fusion of the tarsal and metatarsal bones.

temperature-dependent sex determination: a nongenetic means by which the sex of individuals of some species is set by their ambient temperature at an early stage in their development.

Testudinea: the order of reptiles that includes turtles and tortoises as well as extinct forms *(see Chelonia).*

tetany (tet'-uh-nee): an abnormal condition characterized by periodic painful muscular spasms and tremors, caused most often by faulty calcium metabolism.

tibiotarsus: in birds, a long bone in the leg between the femur and the tarsometatarsus, consisting of the tibia fused with the proximal bones of the tarsus.

tortoise: any of various terrestrial turtles, especially of the family Testudinidae, usually having a high, rounded carapace.

tuatara: lizard-like reptile found only in New Zealand.

turtle: any of various aquatic or terrestrial reptiles of the order Chelonia, having toothless jaws and a bony or leathery shell into which the head, limbs, and tail can be withdrawn.

tympanum: the membrane (ear drum) that transmits sound vibrations to the middle ear; it is readily visible in frogs and toads, which lack external ears.

urea: the major nitrogenous end product of protein metabolism in mammals.

Urodela: one of the three living orders of amphibians *(see Caudata).*

vent: the excretory opening of the digestive tract in birds, reptiles, amphibians, and fish.

ventriculus: the stomach or gizzard of birds.

vertebrate: an animal having a backbone or spinal column.

wildlife rehabilitator: a person with the education, training, and legal certification necessary to restore sick or injured wild animals to health with the goal of returning them to their wild state.

APPENDIX

A Abbreviations and Symbols

A

A angstrom unit; anode; anterior
a ampere; anterior; area
$\bar{\bar{a}}$ of each
AAHA American Animal Hospital Association
AALAS American Association for Laboratory Animal Science
ab antibody
ABO three basic human blood groups
a.c. before meals *(ante cibum)*
ACh acetylcholine
ACTH adrenocorticotropic hormone
ADH antidiuretic hormone
ad lib as much as desired *(ad libitum)*
A/G; A-G ratio albumin-globulin ratio
Ag silver
ag antigen
AHT animal health technician
AIDS acquired immune deficiency syndrome
AKC American Kennel Club
Al aluminum
ALAT assistant laboratory animal technician
Alb albumin
ALT alanine aminotransferase (formerly SGPT)
amp. ampere
ana so much of each, or $\bar{\bar{a}}$
A-P; AP; A/P anterior-posterior
APHIS Animal and Plant Health Inspection Service
Aq water *(aqua)*
As arsenic
ASD atrial septal defect
ASPCA American Society for the Prevention of Cruelty to Animals
AST aspartate aminotransferase (formerly SGOT)
Au gold
A-V; AV; A/V arteriovenous; atrioventricular
AVMA American Veterinary Medical Association

B

B boron; bacillus
Ba barium
Be beryllium
Bi bismuth
bid; b.i.d. twice a day *(bis in die)*
BMR basal metabolic rate
BP blood pressure
bp boiling point
BPH benign prostatic hypertrophy
BSA body surface area
BSP bromsulphalein
BUN blood urea nitrogen

C

C carbon; centigrade; Celsius
$\bar{c}$ with
Ca calcium, cancer
$CaCO_3$ calcium carbonate
Cal large calorie
cal small calorie
CBC; cbc complete blood count
cc cubic centimeter
CDC Centers for Disease Control
cf compare or bring together
CFT complement fixation test
Cg; Cgm centigram
$CHCl_3$ chloroform
ChE cholinesterase
CHF congestive heart failure
Cl chlorine
cm centimeter
CNS central nervous system
CO carbon monoxide
Co cobalt
CO_2 carbon dioxide
CPC clinicopathologic conference
CSF cerebrospinal fluid
CT; CAT computed (axial) tomography
Cu copper
$CuSO_4$ copper sulfate
CVA cerebrovascular accident
CVP central venous pressure
CVT certified veterinary technician

D

D dose; vitamin D; right *(dexter)*
DA displaced abomasum
DEA Drug Enforcement Administration
dg decigram
DIC disseminated intravascular coagulation

diff differential blood count
dim one half
dL deciliter
DNA deoxyribonucleic acid
DOA dead on arrival
DSH domestic short hair (cat)
DVM Doctor of Veterinary Medicine
Dx diagnosis

E

E eye
ECG electrocardiogram, electrocardiograph
ED effective dose
ED_{50} median effective dose
EEG electroencephalogram, electroencephalograph
EENT eye, ear, nose, and throat
EKG electrocardiogram, electrocardiograph
EMB eosin–methylene blue
EMG electromyogram
EMS emergency medical service
ENT ear, nose, and throat
ER emergency room (hospital); external resistance
ESR erythrocyte sedimentation rate
ext extract

F

F Fahrenheit; formula
FA fatty acid
FANA fluorescent antinuclear antibody test
F & R force and rhythm (pulse)
FBS fasting blood sugar
FD fatal dose; focal distance
FDA Food & Drug Administration
Fe iron
$FeCl_3$ ferric chloride
FeLV feline leukemia virus
FIP feline infectious peritonitis
FIV feline immunodeficiency virus
Fl fluid
fld fluid
fl oz; fl. oz. fluid ounce
FLUTD feline lower urinary tract disease
FR flocculation reaction
FSH follicle-stimulating hormone
ft foot
FUO fever of undetermined origin
FUS feline urological syndrome

G

g gram
Galv galvanic
GFR glomerular filtration rate
GH growth hormone
GI gastrointestinal
GLPs good laboratory practices
Gm; gm gram
GP general practitioner; general paresis
gr grain(s)
GSW gunshot wound
gt drop *(gutta)*
GTT glucose tolerance test
gtt drops *(guttae)*
GU genitourinary
Gyn gynecology

H

H hydrogen
H^+ hydrogen ion
H & E hematoxylin and eosin (stain)
Hb; Hgb hemoglobin
HBC hit by car
HCG human chorionic gonadotropin
HCT; Hct hematocrit
HDL high-density lipoprotein
He helium
Hg mercury
HIV human immunodeficiency virus
H_2O water
H_2O_2 hydrogen peroxide
H_2SO_4 sulfuric acid

I

I iodine
^{131}I radioactive isotope of iodine (atomic weight 131)
^{132}I radioactive isotope of iodine (atomic weight 132)
IB inclusion body
ICS; IS intercostal space
ICSH interstitial cell–stimulating hormone
ICU intensive care unit
ID intradermal
Id. the same *(idem)*
IH infectious hepatitis
IM intramuscular
in. inch
IP intraperitoneal
IOP intraocular pressure
IV intravenous

K

K potassium
k constant
Ka cathode or kathode
kc kilocycle
kev kilo electron volts
kg kilogram
km kilometer
kv kilovolt
kw kilowatt

L

L left; liter; length; lumbar; lethal; pound
LAT laboratory animal technician
LATG laboratory animal technologist
lb pound *(libra)*
LCM left costal margin
LD lethal dose
LDL low-density lipoprotein
LE lupus erythematosus
LFD least fatal dose of a toxin
LH luteinizing hormone
Li lithium
lig ligament
Liq liquor
LV left ventricle

M

M muscle; thousand
m meter
mcg; μg microgram
MCH mean corpuscular hemoglobin
MCHC mean corpuscular hemoglobin concentration
MCV mean corpuscular volume
MED minimal effective dose
mEq milliequivalent
mEq/L milliequivalent per liter
ME ratio myeloid-erythroid ratio
Mg magnesium
mg milligram
mmHg millimeters of mercury
MI myocardial infarction
MID minimum infective dose
ml milliliter
MLD median or minimum lethal dose
MLV modified live virus
MM mucous membrane
mm millimeter; muscles
Mn manganese
MRI magnetic resonance imaging
MT medical technologist
mu mouse unit

N

N nitrogen
n normal
Na sodium
NaCl sodium chloride
NAVTA North American Veterinary Technicians Association
Ne neon
NH_3 ammonia
Ni nickel
NPN nonprotein nitrogen
NPO; n.p.o. nothing by mouth *(non per os)*
NTP normal temperature and pressure

O

O oxygen; oculus; pint
O_2 oxygen
O_3 ozone
OB obstetrics
OD right eye *(oculus dexter);* optical density; overdose
OFA Orthopedic Foundation of America
Ol oil *(oleum)*
OR operating room
OS left eye *(oculus sinister)*
Os osmium
OSHA Occupational Safety and Health Administration
oz ounce; ℥

P

P phosphorus; pulse; pupil
P-A; P/A; PA posterior-anterior
P & A percussion and auscultation
PAB; PABA para-aminobenzoic acid
PAS; PASA para-aminosalicylic acid
Pb lead
PBI protein-bound iodine
p.c. after meals *(post cibum)*
PCV packed cell volume
PDA patent ductus arteriosus
PD/PU polyuria/polydipsia
PDR *Physician's Desk Reference*
PE physical examination
PET positron emission tomography
PFF protein-free filtrate
pH hydrogen ion concentration (alkalinity and acidity measure)
Pharm; Phar. pharmacy
PM postmortem; evening
PMN polymorphonuclear neutrophil leukocytes
PO; p.o. orally *(per os)*
POVMR problem-oriented veterinary medical records
PPB parts per billion
PPD purified protein derivative (TB test)
PPM parts per million
PRN, p.r.n. as needed *(pro re nata)*
pro time prothrombin time
PSP phenosulfonphthalein
Pt platinum; patient
pt pint
PTA plasma thromboplastin antecedent
PTC plasma thromboplastin component
Pu plutonium
PZI protamine zinc insulin

Q

q.d. every day *(quaque die)*
q.h. every hour *(quaque hora)*
Q4H every 4 hours (or other quantity)
qid, q.i.d. four times daily *(quater in die)*
q.l. as much as desired *(quantum libet)*
qns quantity not sufficient
q.p. as much as desired *(quantum placeat)*
q.s. sufficient quantity
qt quart
Quat four *(quattuor)*
q.v. as much as you please *(quantum vis)*

R

R respiration; right; *Rickettsia;* roentgen
℞ take
Ra radium
rad unit of measurement of the absorbed dose of ionizing radiation
RAI radioactive iodine
RAIU radioactive iodine uptake
RBC; rbc red blood cell; red blood count
RE right eye; reticuloendothelial tissue or cell
Re rhenium
Rect rectified
Rep. let it be repeated *(repetatur)*
RES reticuloendothelial system

Rh rhesus factor; rhodium
Rn radon
RNA ribonucleic acid
R/O rule out
RP retained placenta
RPM; rpm revolutions per minute
RT radiation therapy
RVT registered veterinary technician

S

S sulfur
S. sacral
s̄ without *(sine)*
S-A; S/A; SA sinoatrial
SC subcutaneous
SD skin dose
Se selenium
Sed rate; SR sedimentation rate
SGOT serum glutamic oxaloacetic transaminase (see *AST*)
SGPT serum glutamic pyruvic transaminase (see *ALT*)
Si silicon
Sn tin
SOAP subjective objective assessment plan
Sol solution
SP spirit
sp. gr. specific gravity
Sr strontium
s̄s̄ one half *(semis)*
Staph staphylococcus
Stat immediately *(statim)*
STD sexually transmitted disease
STH somatotropic hormone
Strep streptococcus
SubQ subcutaneous
Sym symmetrical

T

T temperature; thoracic
T_3 triiodothyronine
T_4 thyroxine
tab tablet
TB tuberculin; tuberculosis; tubercle bacillus
Th thorium
tid, t.i.d. three times daily *(ter in die)*
Tl thallium
TPR temperature, pulse, and respiration
tr tincture
TS test solution
TSH thyroid-stimulating hormone

U

U uranium; unit
UA urinalysis
ung ointment *(unguentum)*
URI upper respiratory infection
UTI urinary tract infection
US ultrasonic
USDA United States Department of Agriculture
USP *U.S. Pharmacopeia*
Ut. dict. as directed *(ut dictum)*

V

V vanadium; vision
v volt
VC vital capacity
VHD valvular heart disease
VLDL very low-density lipoprotein
VMD *Veterinariae Medicinae Doctor*
VS volumetric solution

W

w watt
WBC; wbc white blood cell; white blood count
Wt; wt weight

X

X-ray roentgen ray

Z

z atomic number
Zn zinc

Symbols

> Greater than
< Less than
♀ Female
♂ Male

APPENDIX

B Latin and Greek Combining Forms for English Numbers

Number	Latin term	Greek term
One	uni-	mon-, mono-
Two	duo-, du-	dy-, dyo-
Three	tri-	tri-
Four	quadri-, quadr-	tetr-, tetra-
Five	quinqu-	pent-, penta-
Six	sex-	hex-, hexa-
Seven	sept-, septi-	hept-, hepta-
Eight	octo-	oct-, octa-, octo-
Nine	novem-, noven-	ennea-
Ten	deca-, decem-	dek-, deka-
One half	semi-	hemi-
One and one half	sesqui-	
One hundred	centi-, cent-	hect-, hecto-, hecato-
One thousand	milli-, mill-	kilo-
One hundredth	centi-	
One thousandth	milli-	
First	primi-	prot-, proto-
Second	secundi-	deut-, deuto-, deutero
Third	tert-	
Fourth	quart-	
Fifth	quint-	
Ninth	non-, nona-	
Twice, duplication	di-, dis	di-

APPENDIX

C Metric Units and Equivalents

The International System of Units (SI) is the basis for most scientific measurement. However, the United States still uses its version of the English system (avoirdupois) for everyday purposes. Remnants of the apothecaries' system are still encountered as well. Therefore it may be necessary to convert from one system to another. The following tables provide abbreviations and equivalents for the most commonly used units.

SI Abbreviations

It is customary to use lowercase letters for abbreviations with one exception. The uppercase L is used for *liter* because the lowercase letter may be confused with the numeral 1.

Centimeter	cm
Cubic centimeter	cm^3 or cc
Cubic millimeter	mm^3
Deciliter	dL
Gram	g
Kilogram	kg
Kilometer	km
Liter	L
Meter	m
Microgram	mcg or µg
Milligram	mg
Milliliter	mL
Millimeter	mm

U.S. Avoirdupois and Apothecaries' Abbreviations

Fluid ounce	fl oz
Foot	ft
Grain	gr
Inch	in.
Mile	mi
Ounce	oz
Pint	pt
Pound	lb
Quart	qt

Length

SI Units and U.S. Equivalents

10 mm	= 1 cm	= 0.3937 in.
100 cm	= 1 m	= 39.37 in. (3.2808 ft)
1000 m	= 1 km	= 0.62137 mi
1 in	= 2.54 cm	= 25.4 mm
1 ft	= 30.48 cm	= 304.8 mm
1 mi	= 1.6093 km	

Weight

SI Units and U.S. Equivalents

1000 mcg	= 1 mg	= 0.015 gr
1000 mg	= 1 g	= 15.4324 gr
1000 g	= 1 kg	= 2.205 lb
1 gr	= 0.0648 g	= 64.8 mg
1 oz	= 28.349 g	
1 lb	= 0.453 kg	= 453.592 g

Volume

SI Units and U.S. Equivalents

1000 mm³	= 1 cc	= 1 mL
100 mL	= 1 dL	
1000 mL	= 1 L	= 1.056 qt
1 fl oz	= 29.57 mL	
1 pt	= 473.18 mL	
1 qt	= 946.36 mL	

Temperature Conversion Rules and Useful Equivalents

To convert Fahrenheit to Celsius, subtract 32 from the Fahrenheit temperature and multiply that figure by 5/9: °C = (°F − 32) × 5/9

To convert Celsius to Fahrenheit, multiply the Celsius temperature by 9/5 and add 32 to the total. °F = (°C × 9/5) + 32

USEFUL EQUIVALENTS

	Degrees Celsius	Degrees Fahrenheit
Freezing point of water	0	32
Refrigerator temperature	4.4	40
Room temperature	20	68
Human body temperature	37.0	98.6
Boiling point of water	100	212

APPENDIX

D Disease Terminology

These words are used to describe various aspects of disease. Their use is not confined to any one species or body system.

acute characterized by severe, rapid onset with short duration (cf *chronic*)
anorexia lack of appetite for food
asymptomatic without symptoms
benign not malignant
chronic of long duration (cf *acute*)
clinical visible, readily observed externally
enzootic affecting a nearly constant number of animals in a certain area (the equivalent of *endemic* in humans)
epizootic prevalent and spreading rapidly among large numbers of animals at the same time (the equivalent of *epidemic* in humans)
etiology study of the causes of disease; also used as a synonym for *cause*
febrile relating to fever
focus localizing region of disease (plural, *foci*)
idiopathic referring to a disease of spontaneous origin
incidence the number of new cases of a disease occurring during a certain period
lesion a wound or injury
lethal causing death
malignant harmful, threatening life
morbid pertaining to, or affected with, disease
morbidity the ratio of sick animals to well in a population
moribund near death
mortality rate death rate
necrosis death of a portion of the body
necrotic referring to dead tissue
palliative a treatment that gives relief, usually without removing the cause of the disease
pathogen a disease-producing microorganism
prevalence the total number of cases of a disease in a given population at a certain time
prognosis prediction of the course of a disease
prophylaxis treatment to prevent disease
purulent characterized by the presence of pus
sequela a consequence of a disease (plural, *sequelae*)
sign objective evidence of disease
symptom subjective evidence of disease (*sign* and *symptom* are used synonymously in veterinary medicine)
therapeutics the branch of medicine that deals with the treatment of diseases
therapy the treatment of disease
trauma a wound or injury
virulence ability of a microorganism to cause disease
zoonosis a disease that may be transmitted between animals and humans

APPENDIX

E Species Names

Common name	Scientific (generic)	Male/female terminology	Neutered male	Act of parturition	Young called
Cat	*Felis catus* (feline)	Tom/queen		Queening	Kitten
Cattle	*Bos taurus* *Bos indicus* (bovine)	Bull/cow	Steer	Calving	Calf
Chicken	*Gallus domesticus*	Rooster/hen	Capon	Laying/ hatching	Chick
Chinchilla	*Chinchilla laniger*				Kid
Dog	*Canis familiaris* (canine)	Dog/bitch		Whelping	Puppy
Ferret	*Mustela putoris furo*	Hob/jill	Gib female—sprite		Kit
Gerbil (jird)	*Meriones unguiculatus*				Pup
Goat	*Capra hircus* (caprine)	Buck/doe	Wether	Kidding	Kid (either sex) Buckling (male)
Guinea pig (cavy)	*Cavia porcellus*	Boar/sow		Farrowing	Pup
Hamster	*Mesocricetus auratus*				Pup
Horse	*Equus caballus* (equine)	Stallion/mare	Gelding	Foaling	Foal (either sex) Colt (male) Filly (female)
Llama	*Llama glama*		Gelding		Cria

Common name	Scientific (generic)	Male/female terminology	Neutered male	Act of parturition	Young called
Mouse	*Mus musculus*				Pup
Opossum	*Didelphis virginiana*				
Pig	*Sus scrofa* (porcine)	Boar/sow	Barrow	Farrowing	Piglet, pig (either sex) Gilt (female)
Rabbit	*Oryctolagus cuniculus*	Buck/doe		Kindling	Bunny
Rat	*Rattus norvegicus*				Pup
Sheep	*Ovis aries* (ovine)	Ram/ewe	Wether	Lambing	Lamb

APPENDIX

F Specialty Boards in Veterinary Medicine

The following groups are recognized by the American Veterinary Medical Association as areas of specialization for veterinarians. Each one has its own requirements for membership, which may include residency training, advanced degrees, publishing a scientific paper, and examinations.

American Board of Veterinary Practitioners
- Specialty, Avian Practice
- Specialty, Beef Cattle Practice
- Specialty, Canine and Feline Practice
- Specialty, Dairy Practice
- Specialty, Equine Practice
- Specialty, Feline Practice
- Specialty, Food Animal Practice
- Specialty, Swine Health Management

American Board of Veterinary Toxicology
American College of Laboratory Animal Medicine
American College of Poultry Veterinarians
American College of Theriogenologists
American College of Veterinary Anesthesiologists
American College of Veterinary Behaviorists
American College of Veterinary Clinical Pharmacology
American College of Veterinary Dermatology
American College of Veterinary Emergency and Critical Care
American College of Veterinary Internal Medicine
- Specialty of Cardiology
- Specialty of Internal Medicine
- Specialty of Neurology
- Specialty of Oncology

American College of Veterinary Microbiologists
American College of Veterinary Nutrition
American College of Veterinary Ophthalmologists
American College of Veterinary Pathologists
American College of Veterinary Preventive Medicine
American College of Veterinary Radiology
American College of Veterinary Surgeons
American College of Zoological Medicine
American Veterinary Dental College

BIBLIOGRAPHY

Aiello SE: *The Merck veterinary manual,* ed 8, Philadelphia, 1998, National Publishing.

Altman RB, ed: *Avian medicine and surgery,* Philadelphia, 1997, WB Saunders.

Anderson KN, ed: *Mosby's medical, nursing, and allied health dictionary,* ed 5, St. Louis, 1998, Mosby.

Battaglia RA, Mayrose VB: *Handbook of livestock management techniques,* Minneapolis, 1981, Burgess.

Belanger J: *Raising milk goats the modern way,* ed 10, 1994, Pownal, VT, Garden Way Publishing.

Blood DC, Studdert VP: *Saunders comprehensive veterinary dictionary,* ed 2, Philadelphia, 1999, WB Saunders.

Boyd JS: *A color atlas of clinical anatomy of the dog and cat,* London, 1994, Mosby-Wolfe.

Brooks ML: *Exploring medical language: a student-directed approach,* ed 4, Hanover, MD, 1998, Mosby Lifeline.

Budras KD, Fricke W: *Anatomy of the dog: an illustrated text,* Hanover, MD, 1994, Mosby-Wolfe.

Burt S: *Llamas: an introduction to care, training, and handling,* Loveland, CO, 1991, Alpine Publications.

Campbell JR, Lasley JF: *The science of animals that serve humanity,* ed 3, New York, 1985, McGraw-Hill.

Cochran PE: *Student's guide to veterinary medical terminology,* St. Louis, 1991, Mosby.

Committee on Pain and Distress in Laboratory Animals, ILAR, National Research Council: *Recognition and alleviation of pain and distress in laboratory animals,* Washington, DC, 1992, National Academy Press.

Cunningham M, Acker D: *Animal science and industry,* ed 5, Englewood Cliffs, NJ, 2000, Prentice Hall.

Dorland's pocket medical dictionary, ed 23, Philadelphia, 1982, Saunders.

Dyce KM, Sack WO, Wensing CJG: *Textbook of veterinary anatomy,* ed 2, Philadelphia, 1996, Saunders.

Ernst CH, Barbour RW: *Turtles of the world,* Washington, DC, 1989, Smithsonian Institution Press.

Fowler ME: *Zoo & wild animal medicine,* ed 2, Philadelphia, 1986, WB Saunders.

Fowler ME: *Restraint and handling of wild and domestic animals,* Ames, IA, 1987, Iowa State University Press.

Fowler ME: *Zoo & wild animal medicine: current therapy,* ed 3, Philadelphia, 1993, WB Saunders.

Frandson RD, Spurgeon TL: *Anatomy & physiology of farm animals,* ed 5, Philadelphia, 1992, Lea & Febiger.

Gill FB: *Ornithology,* ed 2, New York, 1995, WH Freeman.

Green T: *The Greek and Latin roots of English,* ed 2, New York, 1994, Ardsley House.

Guss SB: *Management and diseases of dairy goats,* Scottsdale, AZ, 1977, Dairy Goat Journal Publishing.

Haynes NB: *Keeping livestock healthy,* Charlotte, VT, 1978, Garden Way Associates.

Hoffman C, Amus I: *Caring for llamas: a health and management guide,* Fort Collins, CO, 1989, Pioneer Impressions.

Hofrichter R, ed: *Amphibians: the world of frogs, toads, salamanders and newts,* Buffalo, NY, 2000, Firefly Books.

Hudson LC, Hamilton WP: *Atlas of feline anatomy for veterinarians,* Philadelphia, 1993, Saunders.

Juniper T, Parr M: *Parrots: a guide to the parrots of the world,* New Haven, 1998, Yale University Press.

Low R: *Parrots: their care and breeding,* London, 1992, Blandford (Distributed in the United States by Sterling Publishing Company, New York).

Mader DR, ed: *Reptile medicine and surgery,* Philadelphia, 1996, WB Saunders.

Mattison C: *The encyclopedia of snakes,* New York, 1995, Facts on File.

Mattison C: *Frogs and toads of the world,* London, 1998, Blanford (Distributed in the United States by Sterling Publishing Company, New York).

McCurnin DM: *Clinical textbook for veterinary technicians,* ed 4, Philadelphia, 1998, Saunders.

Pasquini C, Spurgeon T: *Anatomy of domestic animals,* ed 4, LaPorte, CO, 1989, Sudz Publishing.

Pickett JP, ed: *The American heritage dictionary of the English language,* ed 4, Boston, 2000, Houghton Mifflin.

Pough FH, Andrews RM, Cadle JE, et al: *Herpetology,* ed 2, Upper Saddle River, NJ, 2000, Prentice-Hall.

Radostits OM, Leslie KE, Fetrow J: *Herd health, food animal production medicine,* ed 2, Philadelphia, 1994, Saunders.

Rogner M: *Lizards,* Malabar, Fla, 1997, Krieger Publishing Company.

Romich JA: *An illustrated guide to veterinary medical terminology,* Albany, NY, 2000, Delmar.

Ruckebusch Y, Phaneuf LP, Dunlop R: *Physiology of small and large animals,* Philadelphia, 1991, BC Decker.

Sims JA, Johnson LE: *Animals in the American economy,* Ames, 1972, Iowa State University Press.

Sisson S, Grossman D: *The anatomy of the domestic animals,* ed 3, Philadelphia, 1938, Saunders.

Welty JC, Baptista L: *The life of birds,* ed 4, New York, 1990, Saunders College Publishers.

Wildi T: *Metric units and conversion charts,* ed 2, 1995, IEEE Press.

Index

A

Page numbers followed by f indicate figures; t, tables; b, boxes.

C

D

E

F

G

H

I

M

P

Q

R

S

T

U

V

W

X

Y

Z